Cases and Concepts Step 1:
Basic Science Review

Cases and Concepts Step 1:
Basic Science Review

Aaron B. Caughey, MD, MPP, MPH, PhD
Associate Professor
Fellowship Program Director
Division of Maternal-Fetal Medicine
Department of Obstetrics, Gynecology, and Reproductive Services
University of California at San Francisco
San Francisco, California

Paul Baum, MD
Assistant Adjunct Professor of Medicine
Division of Experimental Medicine
UCSF School of Medicine
San Francisco, California

Christie del Castillo-Hegyi, MD
Attending Emergency Physician
Presbyterian Hospital
University of New Mexico
Albuquerque, New Mexico

Monica Ghandi, MD
Assistant Professor
Division of Infectious Diseases
Department of Medicine
University of California at San Francisco
San Francisco, California

Larissa R. Graff, PharmD
Assistant Clinical Professor
Department of Clinical Pharmacy
School of Pharmacy
University of California at San Francisco
Clinical Pharmacist—Hematology/Oncology
University of California at San Francisco Medical Center
San Francisco, California

C. Bradley Hare, MD
Assistant Professor
Division of Infectious Diseases
Department of Medicine
University of California at San Francisco
San Francisco, California

Jennifer Hoblyn, MB, MMSci, MRCPsych, MPH
VA Palo Alto Health Care System
Palo Alto, California
Department of Psychiatry and Behavioral Sciences
Stanford University School of Medicine
Stanford, California

Jonathan Z. Li, MD
Clinical and Research Fellow
Division of Infectious Disease
Brigham and Women's Hospital
Massachusetts General Hospital
Boston, Massachusetts

Jillian S. Main
Class of 2009
Chicago Medical School
Chicago, Illinois

Judith Neugroschl, MD
Assistant Professor of Psychiatry
Director of Medical Student Education in Psychiatry
Mount Sinai School of Medicine
New York, New York

Laetitia Poisson de Souzy, MD
Resident
Department of Obstetrics and Gynecology
University of California at San Francisco
San Francisco, California

Teresa Sparks
Class of 2009
UCSF School of Medicine
San Francisco, California

Annie Tan, MD
Clinical Fellow
Department of Obstetrics and Gynecology
University of Minnesota
Minneapolis, Minnesota

Susan H. Tran, MD
Fellow in Maternal-Fetal Medicine and Clinical Genetics
Department of Obstetrics, Gynecology,
   and Reproductive Sciences
University of California at San Francisco
San Francisco, California

Juan E. Vargas, MD
Assistant Clinical Professor
University of California at San Francisco School of Medicine
San Francisco, California

Jed T. Wolpaw, M.Ed
Class of 2010
UCSF School of Medicine
San Francisco, California

Katherine Y. Yang, PharmD, MPH
Assistant Clinical Professor
Department of Clinical Pharmacy
School of Pharmacy
University of California at San Francisco
Infectious Diseases Clinical Pharmacist
University of California at San Francisco Medical Center
San Francisco, California

Series Editor: Aaron B. Caughey, MD, MPP, MPH, PhD

Wolters Kluwer | Lippincott Williams & Wilkins
Health
Philadelphia · Baltimore · New York · London
Buenos Aires · Hong Kong · Sydney · Tokyo

Acquisitions Editor: Charles W. Mitchell
Senior Managing Editor: Stacey L. Sebring
Marketing Manager: Emilie J. Moyer
Production Editor: Beth Martz
Creative Director: Doug Smock
Compositor: International Typesetting and Composition

First Edition

Copyright © 2010 Lippincott Williams & Wilkins, a Wolters Kluwer business.

351 West Camden Street   530 Walnut Street
Baltimore, MD 21201   Philadelphia, PA 19106

Printed in the People's Republic of China

9 8 7 6 5 4 3 2 1

Library of Congress Cataloging-in-Publication Data

Cases and Concepts Step 1: Basic Science Review / Aaron B. Caughey . . . [et al.].
    p. ; cm.
  Includes index.
  ISBN-13: 978-0-7817-9391-9
  ISBN-10: 0-7817-9391-2
  1. Medicine—Case studies.   2. Medical sciences—Case studies.
I. Caughey, Aaron B.   II. Title: Basic science review.
  [DNLM: 1. Clinical Medicine—methods—Case Reports.   2. Clinical
Medicine—methods—Examination Questions.   WB 293 C338 2010]
  RC66.C365 2010
  610—dc22

                                        2008044380

DISCLAIMER

   Care has been taken to confirm the accuracy of the information present and to describe generally accepted practices. However, the authors, editors, and publisher are not responsible for errors or omissions or for any consequences from application of the information in this book and make no warranty, expressed or implied, with respect to the currency, completeness, or accuracy of the contents of the publication. Application of this information in a particular situation remains the professional responsibility of the practitioner; the clinical treatments described and recommended may not be considered absolute and universal recommendations.

   The authors, editors, and publisher have exerted every effort to ensure that drug selection and dosage set forth in this text are in accordance with the current recommendations and practice at the time of publication. However, in view of ongoing research, changes in government regulations, and the constant flow of information relating to drug therapy and drug reactions, the reader is urged to check the package insert for each drug for any change in indications and dosage and for added warnings and precautions. This is particularly important when the recommended agent is a new or infrequently employed drug.

   Some drugs and medical devices presented in this publication have Food and Drug Administration (FDA) clearance for limited use in restricted research settings. It is the responsibility of the healthcare provider to ascertain the FDA status of each drug or device planned for use in their clinical practice.

To purchase additional copies of this book, call our customer service department at **(800) 638-3030** or fax orders to **(301) 223-2320.** International customers should call **(301) 223-2300.**

Visit Lippincott Williams & Wilkins on the Internet: www.lww.com. Lippincott Williams & Wilkins customer service representatives are available from 8:30 am to 6:00 pm, EST.

PREFACE

The first 2 years of medical school are a demanding time for medical students. Whether the school follows a traditional curriculum or one that is case based, every student is expected to learn and be able to apply basic science information in a clinical situation.

Medical schools are increasingly using clinical presentations as the background to teach the basic sciences. Case-based learning has become more common at many medical schools, as it offers a way to catalogue the multitude of symptoms, syndromes, and diseases in medicine.

Cases and Concepts is a new series by Lippincott Williams & Wilkins designed to provide students with a textbook to study the basic science topics combined with clinical data. This method of learning is also the way to prepare for the clinical case format of USMLE questions. The books in this series will make the basic science topics not only more interesting but also more meaningful and memorable. Students will be learning not only the why of a principle but also how it might commonly be seen in practice.

The books in the *Cases and Concepts* series feature a comprehensive collection of cases that are designed to introduce one or more basic science topics. Through these cases, students gain an understanding of the coursework as they learn to:

- Think through the cases
- Look for classic presentations of most common diseases and syndromes
- Integrate the basic science content with clinical application
- Prepare for course exams and Step 1 USMLE
- Be prepared for clinical rotations

This series covers all the essential material needed in the basic science courses. Where possible, the books are organized in an organ-based system. Clinical cases lead off and are the basis for discussion of the basic science content. A list of thought questions follows the case presentation. These questions are designed to challenge the reader to begin to think about how basic science topics apply to real-life clinical situations. The **answers to these questions** are integrated within the **basic science review and discussion** that follows. This offers a clinical framework from which to understand the basic content.

The discussion section is followed by a high-yield **Thumbnail table and a Key Points box** that highlight and summarize the essential information presented in the discussion. The cases also include two to four multiple-choice questions that allow readers to check their knowledge of that topic. Many of the answer explanations provide an opportunity for further discussion by delving into more depth in related areas. Full answer explanations can be found at the end of the book.

This series was designed to provide comprehensive content in a concise and templated format for ease in learning. A dedicated attempt was made to include sufficient art, tables, and clinical treatment information, all while keeping the books from becoming too lengthy. We know you have much to read and that what you want is high-yield, vital facts.

Lippincott Williams & Wilkins and the authors wish you success in your studies and in your future medical career. Please feel free to offer us any comments or suggestions on these books at **www.lww.com**.

CONTENTS

Contents

PART IX: EPIDEMIOLOGY, BIOSTATISTICS, AND HEALTH POLICY

ABBREVIATIONS

5-FU	fluorouracil
5-HIAA	5-hydroxy indoleacetic acid
5-HT	5-hydroxy tryptamine, serotonin
7-DHC	7-dehydrocholesterol
A-aDO2	alveolar-arterial oxygen gradient
AA	Alcoholics Anonymous
AAC	antibiotic-associated colitis
Ab	antibody
ABG	arterial blood gas
ABPA	allergic bronchopulmonary aspergillosis
ABVD	Adriamycin (doxorubicin) + bleomycin + vinblastine + dacarbazine
AC	Adriamycin (doxorubicin) + cyclophosphamide
ACAT	acyl-CoA:cholesterol acyl transferase
ACE	angiotensin-converting enzyme
ACE-I	angiotensin-converting enzyme inhibitor
ACh	acetylcholine
AChEIs, ACE-I	acetylcholinesterase inhibitor
ACLS	advanced cardiac life support
ACP	acyl carrier protein
ACS	acute coronary syndrome
ACTH	adrenocorticotropic hormone
ACV	acyclovir
AD	Alzheimer disease
AD	autosomal dominant
ADA	adenosine deaminase
ADC	AIDS dementia complex
ADD	attention deficit disorder
ADH	alcohol dehydrogenase
ADH	antidiuretic hormone
ADHD	attention-deficit/hyperactivity disorder
ADLs	activities of daily living
ADP	adenosine diphosphate
AF	atrial fibrillation
AFB	acid-fast bacilli
AF	atrial flutter
AFP	alpha-fetoprotein
AH	auditory hallucination
AIDS	acquired immune deficiency syndrome
AIMS	Abnormal Involuntary Movement Scale
AIP	acute intermittent porphyria
ALA	aminolevulinic acid
Alb	albumin

Alkphos, AlkPhos	alkaline phosphatase
ALL	acute lymphocytic leukemia
ALT	alanine aminotransferase (SGPT)
AML	acute myelogenous leukemia
AMP	adenosine monophosphate
ampho B	amphotericin B
ANA	antinuclear antibody
ANC	absolute neutrophil count
ANS	autonomic nervous system
APC	antigen-presenting cell
APKD	adult polycystic kidney disease
ApoE	apolipoprotein E
APP	Alzheimer precursor protein
aPTT	activated partial thromboplastin time (may be PTT)
AR	autosomal recessive
AraC	cytarabine
ARB	angiotensin receptor blocker
ARV	antiretroviral
ASD	atrial septal defect
AST	aspartate aminotransferase (SGOT)
A-T	ataxia-telangiectasia
ATG	antithymocyte globulin
ATM	ataxia-telangiectasia mutated gene
ATP	adenosine triphosphate
ATPase	adenosine triphosphatase
AV node	atrioventricular node
BAL	blood alcohol level
BCG	Bacille Calmette-Guérin
BCR	B-cell receptor
BEA	bile esculin agar
Beta-HCG	beta-human chorionic gonadotropin
BID	twice daily
BMD	bone mineral density
BMI	body-mass index
BMR	basal metabolic rate
BMT	bone marrow transplant
BP	blood pressure
BPD	borderline personality disorder
BPG-2,3	bisphosphoglycerate
BPH	benign prostatic hypertrophy
BRA	bilateral renal agenesis
BTB	breakthrough bleeding
BUN	blood urea nitrogen
BV	bacterial vaginosis
BZD	benzodiazepine
c/o	complaints/complains of
C	Celsius
Ca	calcium
CA	cancer
CABG	coronary artery bypass graft

CAD	coronary artery disease
CAH	congenital adrenal hyperplasia
cAMP	adenosine 3c,5c-cyclic monophosphate (cyclic AMP)
CAT	computerized axial tomography
CBC	complete blood count
CBG	cortisol-binding globulin
CBS	cystathionine β-synthase
CBT	cognitive behavioral therapy
CBZ	carbamazepine
CC	chief complaint
CCK	cholecystokinin
CD	cluster differentiation
CD	conduct disorder
CD4	CD4+ cell count
CDC	Centers for Disease Control and Prevention
CDH	congenital diaphragmatic hernia
Cdk	cyclin-dependent kinase
CEE	conjugated equine estrogen
CF	cystic fibrosis
CFTR	cystic fibrosis transmembrane regulator
CGD	chronic granulomatous disease
cGMP	cyclic guanosine 3c, 5c-monophosphate
CHD	congenital heart disease
CHD	coronary heart disease
CHF	congestive heart failure
CI	confidence interval
CIA	Central Intelligence Agency
CIE	counter immune electrophoresis
CJD	Creutzfeldt-Jakob disease
CK	creatine kinase
CL	contralateral
Cl, Cl⁻	chloride
cm	centimeter
CML	chronic myelogenous leukemia
CMP	cytidylate
CMV	cytomegalovirus
CN	cranial nerve
CNS	central nervous system
CO	carbon monoxide
CO₂	carbon dioxide
CoA	coenzyme A
COC	combined oral contraceptive
COPD	chronic obstructive pulmonary disease
COX	cyclo-oxygenase
CP	chest pain
CPAP	continuous positive airway pressure
CPK	creatinine phosphokinase

CPR	cardiopulmonary resuscitation	EEG	electroencephalography	GE	gastroesophageal
CPS	carbamoylphosphate synthetase	EF	ejection fraction	GERD	gastroesophageal reflux disease
Cr	creatinine	EF	edema factor	GFR	glomerular filtration rate
CrAg	cryptococcal antigen (CrAg test)	EGD	esophagogastroduodenoscopy	GHB	gamma-hydroxybutyrate
CrCl	creatinine clearance	EHEC	enterohemorrhagic *E. coli*	GI	gastrointestinal
CRF	corticotropin-releasing factor	EIB	exercise-induced bronchospasm	Gi	inhibitory G protein
CRP	C-reactive protein	EIEC	enteroinvasive *E. coli*	GIST	gastrointestinal stromal tumor
CSA	cyclosporine	EKG	electrocardiogram	GMP	guanosine monophosphate
CSF	cerebrospinal fluid	ELISA	enzyme-linked immunosorbent	GpIIb/IIIa	glycoprotein IIb/IIIa
CT	computerized tomography		assay	Gs	stimulatory G protein
CTL	cytotoxic lymphocytes	EMG	electromyogram	GT	gastric tube
CVA	cerebrovascular accident	EMS	emergency medical services	GTD	gestational trophoblastic disease
CVS	chorionic villus sampling	ENT	ear, nose, throat (otolaryngology)	GTP	guanosine triphosphate
CXR	chest x-ray	EPEC	enteropathogenic *E. coli*	GU	genito-urinary
CYP450	cytochrome P450	EPS	extrapyramidal symptoms	GX	glycinexylidide
d	day	ER	emergency room	GXM	glucuronoxylomannan
D&C	dilation and curettage	ER	estrogen receptor	GxPy	gravida x para y
D2	dopamine	ESR	erythrocyte sedimentation rate	HA	headache
DDAVP	1-desamino-8-d-arginine	ETC	electron transport chain	HAARTS	highly active antiretroviral
	vasopressin	ETEC	enterotoxigenic *E. coli*		therapies
DES	diethylstilbestrol	EtOH	ethyl alcohol	HAV	hepatitis A virus
DFA	direct fluorescent antibody	F	female	HBeAg	hepatitis B envelope antigen
DHE	dihydroergotamine	FAC	fluorouracil + Adriamycin	HBsAg	hepatitis B surface antigen
DHF	dihydrofolate		(doxorubicin) +	hCG	human chorionic gonadotropin
DHFR	dihydrofolate reductase		cyclophosphamide	HCO3	hydrogen bicarbonate
DIC	disseminated intravascular	FADH$_2$	flavin adenine dinucleotide	Hct	hematocrit
	coagulation		(reduced)	HCTZ	hydrochlorothiazide
DID	dissociative identity disorder	FAE	fetal alcohol effect	HCV	hepatitis C virus
dL	deciliter	FAS	fetal alcohol syndrome	HDL	high-density lipoprotein
DLB	dementia with Lewy bodies	FASD	fetal alcohol spectrum disorder	HDV	hepatitis D virus
DM	diabetes mellitus	FBI	Federal Bureau of Investigation	HEENT	head, eyes, ears, nose, throat
DMARD	disease modifying antirheumatic	FCV	famciclovir	Hex A	hexosaminidase A
	drug	FDA	Food and Drug Administration	HgA1c	hemoglobin A1c
DMPA	depo-medroxyprogesterone	FEV$_1$	forced expiratory volume in the	Hgb	hemoglobin
	acetate		first second	HGE	human granulocytic ehrlichiosis
DNA	deoxyribonucleic acid	FFS	fee-for-service	HHV	human herpes virus
DNR	do not resuscitate	FGFR	fibroblast growth factor receptor	HI	homicidal ideation
DOT	directly observed therapy	FHx	family history	HIT	heparin-induced thrombocytopenia
DPH	diphenylhydantoin	FISH	fluorescent in situ hybridization	HIV	human immunodeficiency virus
DPT	diphtheria, pertussis, tetanus	FMN	flavin mononucleotide	HLA	human leukocyte antigen
DS	Down syndrome	FNA	fine needle aspirate	HME	human monocytic ehrlichiosis
dsDNA	double-stranded DNA	FSG	fasting blood glucose (not FBG)	HMG-CoA	hydroxymethylglutaryl-CoA
DSM-IV	*Diagnostic and Statistical*	FSH	follicle-stimulating hormone	HMO	health maintenance organization
	Manual, 4th edition	FTA-ABS	fluorescent treponemal antibody	HNPCC	hereditary nonpolyposis colon
DT	delirium tremens		absorption		cancer
dTMP	deoxythymidine monophosphate	FVC	forced vital capacity	HPA	hypothalamic-pituitary-adrenal
DTR	deep tendon reflex	G0	gap 0	HPI	history of present illness
DUI	driving under the influence	G1	gap 1	HR	heart rate
dUMP	deoxyuridine monophosphate	G2	gap 2	HRCT	high-resolution CT scan
DVT	deep vein thrombosis	G6P	glucose 6-phosphate	HRT	hormone replacement therapy
DWI	driving while intoxicated	G6PD	glucose-6-phosphate	HSV	herpes simplex virus
DZ	dizygotic		dehydrogenase	HTLV	human T-cell lymphotropic virus
EAggEC	enteroaggregative *E. coli*	GA	gestational age	HTN	hypertension
EBV	Epstein-Barr virus	GABA	gamma-aminobutyric acid	HVA	homovanillic acid
ECG	electrocardiogram	GAD	generalized anxiety disorder	I-FAB	intestinal fatty acid-binding
ECT	electroconvulsive therapy	GALT	galactose 1-uridyltransferase		protein
ED	emergency department	GALT	galactose-1-uridyltransferase	IADLs	instrumental activities of daily
EE	ethinyl estradiol	GCS	Glasgow Coma Scale		living

IBD	inflammatory bowel disease	LGV	lymphogranuloma venereum	MS	multiple sclerosis
ICD	implantable automatic cardioverter defibrillation	LH	luteinizing hormone	MSAFP	maternal serum alpha-fetoprotein
		LHON	Leber hereditary optic neuropathy	MSE	mental status examination
ICU	intensive care unit	LHRH	luteinizing hormone-releasing hormone	msec	millisecond
IDL	intermediate-density lipoprotein			MSLT	multiple sleep latency test
IE	infective endocarditis	LLE	left lower extremity	MSM	men who have sex with men
IEM	inborn error of metabolism	LMP	last menstrual period	MTB	mycobacterium tuberculosis
IF	intrinsic factor	LMWH	low molecular-weight heparin	mtDNA	mitochondrial DNA
IFG	impaired fasting glucose	LNG	levonorgestrel	MTHFR	methylenetetrahydrofolate reductase
IFN-γ	interferon-γ	LP	lumbar puncture		
Ig	immunoglobulin	LPN	licensed practicing nurse	MZ	monozygotic
IgA	immunoglobulin A	LPS	lipopolysaccharide	N/V	nausea/vomiting
IgE	immunoglobulin E	LR	likelihood ratio	Na	sodium
IgG	immunoglobulin G	LSD	lysergic acid diethylamide	nAchR	nicotinic acetylcholine receptor
IgM	immunoglobulin M	LT	leukotriene	NaCl	sodium chloride
IL-2	interleukin-2	Lytes	electrolytes	NAD	nicotinamide adenine dinucleotide
IL-6	interleukin-6	M	mitosis	NADH	nicotinamide adenine dinucleotide
IL-8	interleukin-8	MAC	membrane attack complex	NADPH	nicotinamide adenine dinucleotide phosphate, reduced
IM	intramuscular	MAO	monoamine oxidase		
IMI	inferior myocardial infarction	MAOI	monoamine oxidase inhibitor	NAPA	n-acetylprocainamide
IMP	inosine monophosphate	MBA	Masters of Business Administration	NBF	nucleotide-binding fold
IN	intranasal			NE	norepinephrine
INH	isoniazid	MCA	middle cerebral artery	NEJM	New England Journal of Medicine
iNOS	inducible nitric oxide synthase	MCAD	medium-chain acyl-CoA dehydrogenase	NF	neurofibromatosis
INR	international normalized ratio			NF1	neurofibromatosis type 1
IOP	intraocular pressure	MCV	mean corpuscular volume	NF2	neurofibromatosis type 2
IPA	Independent Practitioner Association	MD	myotonic dystrophy	NVS	nutritionally variant streptococci
		MDD	major depressive disorder	NGU	nongonococcal urethritis
IPT	interpersonal therapy	MDMA	3,4-methylenedioxymetham-phetamine (ecstasy)	NHL	non-Hodgkin lymphoma
IPV	inactive polio virus vaccine			NICU	neonatal ICU
IQ	intelligence quotient	MEGX	monoethylglycinexylidide	NIDDM	noninsulin-dependent diabetes mellitus
IRS	insulin receptor substrate	MELAS	**m**itochondrial **e**ncephalopathy, **l**actic **a**cidosis, and *stroke-like* syndrome		
IRS	Internal Revenue Service			NIMH	National Institute of Mental Health
ISA	intrinsic sympathomimetic activity				
		MFI	multifactorial inheritance	NK	natural killer
ISDN	isosorbide dinitrate	Mg	magnesium	NKDA	no known drug allergies
ISH	isolated systolic hypertension	mg	milligram	NMDA	N-methyl-D-aspartate
ISMO	isosorbide mononitrate	MHA-TP	microhemagglutination assay for *Treponema pallidum*	NMS	neuroleptic malignant syndrome
IV	intravenous			NNRTI	nonnucleoside reverse transcriptase inhibitor
IVDU	intravenous drug use	MHC	major histocompatibility complex		
IVF	in vitro fertilization	MHPG	3-methoxy-4-hydroxyphenylglycol	NPO	nothing by mouth, nil per os
IVIG	intravenous immune globulin	MI	myocardial infarction	NPV	negative predictive value
JVP	jugular venous pulsation	MIC	minimum inhibitory concentration	NRTI	nucleoside reverse transcriptase inhibitor
K	potassium	mL	milliliter		
kg	kilogram	MMPI	Minnesota Multiphasic Personality Inventory	NS	normal saline
KOH	potassium hydroxide			NSAID	nonsteroidal antiinflammatory drug
LAAM	levo-a-acetylmethadol or levomethadyl acetate	MOA	mechanism of action		
		MoAb	monoclonal antibody	NSR	normal sinus rhythm
lbs	pounds	MoM	multiples of the median	NSVD	normal spontaneous vaginal delivery
LC	locus ceruleus	MOTT	mycobacteria other than tubercle		
LCAT	lecithin-cholesterol acyltransferase	MPA	medroxyprogesterone acetate	NTD	neural tube defect
LCR	ligase chain reaction	MR	mental retardation	NtRTI	nucleotide reverse transcriptase inhibitor
LDH	lactate dehydrogenase	MRI	magnetic resonance imaging		
LDL	low-density lipoprotein	mRNA	messenger RNA	NVS	nutritionally variant streptococci
LDL-C	LDL cholesterol	MRSA	methicillin-resistant *Staphylococcus aureus*	O_2	oxygen
LES	lower esophageal sphincter			O_2sat	oxygen saturation
LF	lethal factor	MRSE	methicillin-resistant *Staphylococcus epidermidis*	OA	osteoarthritis
LFTs	liver function tests			OCD	obsessive-compulsive disorder

Abbreviations

OD	right eye	POAG	primary open angle glaucoma	SaO$_2$	oxygen saturation
ODD	oppositional defiant disorder	POS	point-of-service	SC, SQ	subcutaneous
OI	osteogenesis imperfecta	PPD	purified protein derivative	SCD	sequential compression device
OPV	oral polio virus vaccine	PPI	proton pump inhibitor	SCID	severe combined
OR	odds ratio	PPNG	penicillinase-producing		immunodeficiency
OR	operating room		*Neisseria gonorrhoeae*	SCLC	small cell lung cancer
OS	left eye	PPO	preferred provider organization	SE	status epilepticus
OTC	ornithine transcarbamoylase	PPV	positive predictive value	SERMs	selective estrogen receptor
	synthetase	PR	per rectum		modulators
OTC	over-the-counter	PR	progesterone receptor	SGOT	serum glutamic oxaloacetic
PA	protective antigen	PRPP	5-phosphoribosyl-		transferase
PABA	*P*-aminobenzoic acid		1-pyrophosphate	SH	somatic hallucination
PACU	postanesthesia care unit	PSGN	poststreptococcal	SHBG	sex hormone-binding globulin
PAH	phenylalanine hydroxylase		glomerulonephritis	Shh	Sonic hedgehog
PAS	para-aminosalicylic acid	PSHx	past surgical history	SHx	social history
PB	phenobarbital	PSVT	paroxysmal supraventricular	SI	suicidal ideation
PBG	porphobilinogen		tachycardia	SIADH	syndrome of inappropriate
PBP	penicillin-binding protein	PT	physical therapy		secretion of antidiuretic hormone
PCA	patient-controlled analgesia	PT	prothrombin time	SIDS	sudden infant death syndrome
PCI	percutaneous coronary intervention	PTH	parathyroid hormone	SL	sublingual
PCO$_2$	partial pressure of carbon dioxide	PTSD	posttraumatic stress disorder	SLE	systemic lupus erythematosus
PCP	phencyclidine	PTT	partial thromboplastin time	SLOS	Smith-Lemli-Opitz syndrome
PCP	primary care provider	PTU	propylthiouracil	SMA7	serum chemistries
PCP	*Pneumocystis carinii* pneumonia	PUD	peptic ulcer disease		(Na, K, Cl, HCO3, BUN, Cr, Glu)
PcP	*Pneumocystis jiroveci* pneumonia	PVD	peripheral vascular disease	SMBG	self-monitoring of blood glucose
PCR	polymerase chain reaction	PYR	pyrrolidonyl-beta-naphthylamide	SN	substantia nigra
PD	personality disorder	q12h	every 12 hours	SNRI	serotonin-norepinephrine
PDA	patent ductus arteriosus	qD	once daily		reuptake inhibitor
PDE	phosphodiesterase	QID	four times daily	snRNA	small nuclear RNA
PE	physical examination	r/o	rule out	snRNP	small ribonucleoprotein particle
PE	pulmonary embolism	R	regulatory	SNS	sympathetic nervous system
PEEP	positive end-expiratory pressure	RA	resident advisor	SOB	shortness of breath
PEP	phosphoenolpyruvate	RA	rheumatoid arthritis	SPECT	single photon emission
PERRLA	pupils equal, round, reactive to	RA	room air		computed tomography
	light and accommodation	RAI	radioactive iodine	SPS	sodium polystyrene sulfonate
PET	positron emission tomography	Rb	retinoblastoma	SSRI	selective serotonergic reuptake
PFK	phosphofructokinase	RBC	red blood cells		inhibitor
PFT	pulmonary function test	RCT	randomized controlled trial	STD	sexually transmitted disease
PG	prostaglandin	RDS	respiratory distress syndrome	STI	sexually transmitted infection
PGI2	prostaglandin I2; prostacyclin	REM	rapid eye movement	SuVT	sustained ventricular
PGT	per gastric tube	RF	rheumatoid factor		tachycardia
Ph+	Philadelphia chromosome	RFLP	restriction fragment length	T½	half-life
PI	paranoid ideation		polymorphism	T$_3$	triiodothyronine
PI	protease inhibitor	RNA	ribonucleic acid	T$_4$	tetra-iodo thyronine
PICC	peripherally inserted central	RNP	ribonucleoprotein	T$_4$	thyroxine (aka levothyroxine)
	catheter	ROC	receiver-operator curver	T, Temp	temperature
PID	pelvic inflammatory disease	ROS	review of systems	TB	tuberculosis
PK	pyruvate kinase	RPR	rapid plasma reagin test	TBG	thyroid-binding globulin
PKU	phenylketonuria		(for syphilis)	Tbili	total bilirubin
PLP	pyridoxal phosphate	RR	relative risk	TC	total cholesterol
Plt	platelets	RR	respiratory rate	TCA	tricarboxylic acid
PMDD	premenstrual dysphoric disorder	rRNA	ribosomal RNA	TCA	tricyclic antidepressant
PMH	past medical history	RSV	respiratory syncytial virus	TCR	T-cell receptor
PMN	polymorphonuclear	RT	reverse transcriptase	TD	tardive dyskinesia
PNS	parasympathetic nervous system	RUQ	right upper quadrant	Td	tetanus toxoid
PNS	peripheral nervous system	s/p	status post	TED	thromboembolic deterrent
PO	by mouth	S1, S2	heart sounds 1 and 2	TENS	transcutaneous electrical nerve
PO2	partial pressure of oxygen	S	synthesis		stimulation

TFT	thyroid function test	TXA2	thromboxane A2	VLDL	very low-density lipoprotein
TG	triglyceride	U.S.	United States	VP16	etoposide
THC	D-9-tetrahydrocannabinol	UA	urinalysis	VP	ventriculoperitoneal
THF	tetrahydrofolate	UC	ulcerative colitis	VPA	valproic acid
TIA	transient ischemic attack	UCD	urea cycle disorders	VRE	vancomycin-resistant enterococcus
TID	three times daily	UDP	uridine diphosphate glucose		
TIG	tetanus immune globulin	UFH	unfractionated heparin	VS	vital signs
TM	transmembrane	ULN	upper limit of normal	VSD	ventricular septal defect
TMP	trimethoprim	UMP	uridine monophosphate	VT	ventricular tachycardia
TMP-SMX	trimethoprim-sulfamethoxazole	URI	upper respiratory tract infection	VTA	ventral tegmental area
TNF	tumor necrosis factor	US	ultrasound	VZV	varicella zoster virus
TNF-a	tumor necrosis factor-alpha	UTI	urinary tract infection	WAIS	Wechsler Adult Intelligence Scale
TOF	tetralogy of Fallot	Utox	urine toxicology		
topo	topoisomerase	VACP	valacyclovir	WBC	white blood cell
ToRCHeS	toxoplasmosis, rubella, CMV, HSV, syphilis	VAD	vincristine + Adriamycin (doxorubicin) + dexamethasone	WHR	waist-to-hip ratio
				WISC	Wechsler Intelligence Scale for Children
TPN	total parenteral nutrition	VAPP	vaccine-associated paralytic polio (as in VAPP infection)		
TRH	thyrotropin-releasing hormone			WM	White male
tRNA	transfer RNA	VCFS	velocardiofacial syndrome	WNL	within normal limits
TS	Tourette syndrome	VDRL	Venereal Disease Research Laboratory [test (for syphilis)]	WNV	West Nile virus
TS	tuberous sclerosis			Wt	weight
TSH	thyroid-stimulating hormone	VF	ventricular fibrillation	XTC	ecstasy
TSST	toxic shock syndrome toxin	VH	visual hallucination	yo	year old

NORMAL RANGES OF LABORATORY VALUES

BLOOD, PLASMA, SERUM

Alanine aminotransferase (ALT, GPT at 30°C)	8–20 U/L
Amylase, serum	25–125 U/L
Aspartate aminotransferase (AST, GOT at 30°C)	8–20 U/L
Bilirubin, serum (adult) Total // Direct	0.1–1.0 mg/dL // 0.0–0.3 mg/dL
Calcium, serum (Ca2+)	8.4–10.2 mg/dL
Cholesterol, serum	Rec: <200 mg/dL
Cortisol, serum	0800 h: 5–23 g/dL // 1600 h: 3–15 g/dL
	2000 h: 50% of 0800 h
Creatine kinase, serum	Male: 25–90 U/L
	Female: 10–70 U/L
Creatinine, serum	0.6–1.2 mg/dL
Electrolytes, serum	
Sodium	(Na+) 136–145 mEq/L
Chloride	(Cl⁻) 95–105 mEq/L
Potassium	(K+) 3.5–5.0 mEq/L
Bicarbonate	(HCO3⁻) 22–28 mEq/L
Magnesium	(Mg2+) 1.5–2.0 mEq/L
Ferritin, serum	Male: 15–200 ng/mL
	Female: 12–150 ng/mL
Follicle-stimulating hormone, serum/plasma	Male: 4–25 mIU/mL
	Female: premenopause 4–30 mIU/mL
	midcycle peak 10–90 mIU/mL
	postmenopause 40–250 mIU/mL
Gases, arterial blood (room air)	
pH	7.35–7.45
PCO_2	33–45 mm Hg
PO_2	75–105 mm Hg
Glucose, serum	Fasting: 70–110 mg/dL
	2-h postprandial: <120 mg/dL
Growth hormone—arginine stimulation	Fasting: <5 ng/mL
	provocative stimuli: >7 ng/mL
Iron	50–70 g/dL
Lactate dehydrogenase, serum	45–90 U/L
Luteinizing hormone, serum/plasma	Male: 6–23 mIU/mL
	Female: follicular phase 5–30 mIU/mL
	midcycle 75–150 mIU/mL
	postmenopause 30–200 mIU/mL
Osmolality, serum	275–295 mOsmol/kg
Parathyroid hormone, serum, N-terminal	230–630 pg/mL
Phosphate (alkaline), serum (p-NPP at 30°C)	20–70 U/L
Phosphorus (inorganic), serum	3.0–4.5 mg/dL
Prolactin, serum (hPRL)	<20 ng/mL
Proteins, serum	
Total (recumbent)	6.0–7.8 g/dL
Albumin	3.5–5.5 g/dL
Globulin	2.3–3.5 g/dL
Thyroid-stimulating hormone, serum or plasma	0.5–5.0 U/mL
Thyroidal iodine (123I) uptake	8–30% of administered dose/24 h
Thyroxine (T_4), serum	5–12 g/dL
Transferrin	221–300 g/dL
Triglycerides, serum	35–160 mg/dL
Triiodothyronine (T_3), resin uptake	25–35%
Triiodothyronine (T_3), serum (RIA)	115–190 ng/dL
Urea nitrogen, serum (BUN)	7–18 mg/dL
Uric acid, serum	3.0–8.2 mg/dL

CEREBROSPINAL FLUID

Cell count	0–5 cells/mm^3
Chloride	118–132 mEq/L
Gamma globulin	3–12% total proteins
Glucose	40–70 mg/dL
Pressure	70–180 mm H$_2$O
Proteins, total	<40 mg/dL

HEMATOLOGIC

Bleeding time (template)	2–7 minutes
Erythrocyte count	Male: 4.3–5.9 million/mm^3
	Female: 3.5–5.5 million/mm^3
Erythrocyte sedimentation rate (Westergren)	Male: 0–15 mm/h
	Female: 0–20 mm/h
Hematocrit	Male: 41–53%
	Female: 36–46%
Hemoglobin A1C	6%
Hemoglobin, blood	Male: 13.5–17.5 g/dL
	Female: 12.0–16.0 g/dL
Leukocyte count and differential	
Leukocyte count	4500–11,000/mm^3
Segmented neutrophils	54–62%
Bands	3–5%
Eosinophils	1–3%
Basophils	0–0.75%
Lymphocytes	25–33%
Monocytes	3–7%
Mean corpuscular hemoglobin	25.4–34.6 pg/cell
Mean corpuscular hemoglobin concentration	31–36% Hgb/cell
Mean corpuscular volume	80–100 μm^3
Partial thromboplastin time (activated)	25–40 seconds
Platelet count	150,000–400,000/mm^3
Prothrombin time	11–15 seconds
Reticulocyte count	0.5–1.5% of red cells
Thrombin time	<2 seconds deviation from control
Volume	
Plasma	Male: 25–43 mL/kg
	Female: 28–45 mL/kg
Red cell	Male: 20–36 mL/kg
	Female: 19–31 mL/kg

SWEAT

Chloride	0–35 mmol/L

URINE

Calcium	100–300 mg/24 h
Chloride	Varies with intake
Creatine clearance	Male: 97–137 mL/min
	Female: 88–128 mL/min
Osmolality	50–1400 mOsmol/kg
Oxalate	8–40 g/mL
Potassium	Varies with diet
Proteins, total	<150 mg/24h
Sodium	Varies with diet
Uric acid	Varies with diet

PART I

Microbiology

HPI: SA is a 70-year-old man who presents to the office with right knee swelling and pain. SA complains of increasing pain and swelling in his right knee after accidentally falling 1 week ago. He also reports 3 days of fevers and chills, along with fatigue and generalized weakness. SA denies any cough, shortness of breath, nausea, vomiting, chest pain, bowel or urinary symptoms, rash, or other joint problems.

PMH: SA has taken carbidopa-levodopa (Sinemet) for Parkinson disease since 1992, lisinopril for hypertension, and glipizide for type II diabetes mellitus. No allergies to medications. Does not smoke; lives with wife.

PE: Temperature (T) 38.5°C; blood pressure (BP) 104/58; heart rate (HR) 75; respiratory rate (RR) 18; and oxygen saturation (SaO_2) on room air 96%

SA was somnolent, but arousable. Neurologic exam notable for marked tremor in hands and rigidity of his extremities with passive movement. Heart exam revealed no murmurs and lungs were clear. His right knee had a 1-cm healing laceration on the surface with noticeable swelling, warmth, and tenderness to palpation. Range of motion of SA's knee was limited secondary to pain and swelling. No rashes on skin exam.

Labs: White blood cell count (WBC) 18.1 with 90% neutrophils. Glucose 278. Aspiration of knee fluid showed 290,000 WBC with 96% neutrophils, 450,000 red blood cell count (RBC), and a Gram stain with 4+ WBC, 2+ gram-positive cocci in clusters. Blood and knee fluid cultures grew out gram-positive cocci in clusters on the day following admission. Chest X-ray was clear.

THOUGHT QUESTIONS

- How is *Staphylococcus* distinguished from the *Streptococcus* species?
- How are the different staphylococcal species distinguished?
- What are the key virulence factors of *Staphylococcus aureus*?
- What are the key clinical syndromes of the different staphylococci?
- What are treatment options for the staphylococci?

BASIC SCIENCE REVIEW AND DISCUSSION

Staphylococcus versus *Streptococcus*

There are two main distinguishing features between the two groups of gram-positive cocci:

- **The staphylococcal organisms are catalase positive, whereas the streptococcal bacteria are catalase negative.** The catalase enzyme helps bacteria convert hydrogen peroxide (H_2O_2) into oxygen and water. The catalase test involves adding H_2O_2 to a culture sample; if the bacteria in question produce catalase, they will cause conversion of the H_2O_2 to oxygen gas and bubbles will form.
- Staphylococcal species are usually found in **grape-like clusters**, whereas the streptococci tend to form **pairs and chains** (Fig. 1-1).

Staphylococcal Species The staphylococcal organisms of clinical interest include **S. aureus, S. epidermidis, S. saprophyticus,** and **S. lugdunensis.** *S. aureus* is distinguished from the other staphylococcal organisms mainly by its ability to produce **coagulase,** an enzyme that converts fibrinogen to fibrin in citrated plasma; **S. aureus is referred to as coagulase positive.** The other staphylococcal organisms usually do not produce this coagulase enzyme and are termed coagulase negative. The two main coagulase-negative staphylococcal species are distinguished by susceptibility to the antibiotic **novobiocin:** *S. epidermidis* is novobiocin susceptible and *S. saprophyticus* is novobiocin resistant (Fig. 1-2).

Staphylococcus Aureus *S. aureus* has some of the following distinguishing features:

- Forms a **golden yellow colony** on agar
- Ferments **mannitol**
- Causes complete hemolysis (**β-hemolysis**) on blood agar
- Contains an **IgG-binding protein called protein A** in the cell wall
- Produces a **clumping factor** (different from coagulase) that binds fibrinogen

Microbiology labs either use the coagulase test (slide or tube) or watch for agglutination of latex beads coated with IgG against protein A, fibrinogen, and capsule-specific antibodies to distinguish *S. aureus* from the other staphylococcal species.

The clinical syndromes of *S. aureus* are multifarious and include **skin infections, abscesses, endocarditis, septic arthritis, osteomyelitis, sepsis, meningitis, pneumonia, food poisoning,** and **toxic shock syndrome.** *S. aureus* forms part of the normal flora in humans and is usually found in **nasal passages and on the skin.** Skin infections include impetigo, furuncles, carbuncles, cellulitis, paronychia, surgical wound infections, blepharitis, and breast mastitis. Endocarditis from *S. aureus* can occur on normal or prosthetic heart valves and can be quite destructive; **right-sided S. aureus endocarditis** (tricuspid or aortic valve involvement) is commonly seen in intravenous drug users. Septic arthritis or osteomyelitis can occur from hematogenous spread from another source or secondary to local trauma, as in the case of our patient. *S. aureus* pneumonia is seen in postoperative patients or following viral respiratory infections, especially influenza. Staphylococcal abscesses can be seen in any organ and often follow bacteremia. The syndromes of **food poisoning, toxic shock syndrome,** and **scalded skin syndrome from S. aureus are all**

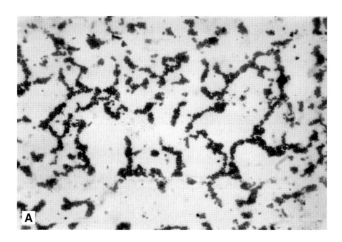
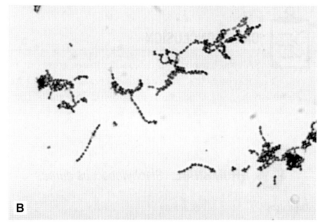

• **Figure 1-1.** Panel **(a)** shows the clustered gram-positive cocci typical of *Staphylococcus;* panel **(b)** shows the gram-positive cocci in pairs and chains typical of streptococcal species. (Image in public domain from Centers for Disease Control and Prevention Public Health Image Library, http://phil.cdc.gov/phil/home.asp)

"nonsuppurative" infections in that they are toxin mediated instead of a direct effect of bacterial replication.

Virulence factors of *S. aureus* include:

- **Enterotoxins** (six types, A–F), which cause the vomiting and watery diarrhea that characterize the food poisoning syndrome of *S. aureus*. The enterotoxin is preformed in foods and has a short incubation period (1–8 hrs).
- **Toxic shock syndrome toxin** (TSST), which causes toxic shock, seen in individuals with wound infections or, formerly, menstruating women using tampons. TSST is indistinguishable from enterotoxin F and causes the release of large amounts of interleukin-1 (IL-1), IL-2, and tumor necrosis factor-alpha (TNF-α). Toxic shock syndrome is characterized by fever, hypotension, a desquamating rash, and multiorgan failure.
- **Exfoliatin,** which causes scalded skin syndrome, in which the superficial layers of the epidermis are sloughed off.
- **Invasins** that promote bacterial spread through tissues (leukocidin, hyaluronidase, and fibrinolysin).
- **Surface factors** that inhibit phagocytic engulfment (capsule and protein A).

Coagulase-negative Staphylococci Multiple coagulase-negative staphylococcal species exist in nature. The main species that are pathogenic in humans are *S. epidermidis*, *S. saprophyticus*, and *S. lugdunensis*. *S. schleiferi* and *S. haemolyticus* can also rarely cause disease in humans.

S. epidermidis is part of the normal flora on the skin and mucous membranes and forms a **glycocalyx** ("slime") layer that coats foreign surfaces. Hence, *S. epidermidis* is a frequent cause of **endocarditis on prosthetic heart valves** and of foreign body infections, including intravenous catheter and prosthetic implant infections. *S. epidermidis* can cause peritonitis in patients with renal failure undergoing peritoneal dialysis through an indwelling peritoneal catheter.

S. saprophyticus causes **urinary tract infections (UTIs)**, mainly in young, sexually active women and elderly men. It is distinguished from the other coagulase-negative staphylococcal species by its resistance to novobiocin.

S. lugdunensis is increasingly reported as a cause of **infective endocarditis** (IE). *S. lugdunensis* causes a more virulent form of IE than the other coagulase-negative staphylococci, with high morbidity rates despite its in vitro susceptibility to penicillins and multiple other antibiotics. *S. lugdunensis* is frequently misidentified as *S. aureus*, as the former is also yellow pigmented, causes β-hemolysis on blood agar, and agglutinates with protein A and the clumping factor. The two organisms are distinguished by the coagulase test. Of note, *S. lugdunensis* may be weakly coagulase positive on a slide test because it has a clumping factor that binds fibrinogen, but the organism will be clearly coagulase negative on the tube test.

Treatment

Ninety percent of *S. aureus* strains are resistant to penicillin G because of production of plasmid-derived **β-lactamases.** Such organisms can be treated with β-lactamase–resistant penicillins, such as **nafcillin, dicloxacillin, oxacillin, cephalosporins,** or **vancomycin.** Adding a **β-lactamase inhibitor** (such as clavulanic acid) to a β-lactamase–sensitive penicillin (such as amoxicillin) will also treat β-lactamase–producing staphylococci. Some staphylococcal species are **"methicillin resistant"** (e.g., "nafcillin resistant") secondary to alteration in penicillin-binding proteins; such species are treated with **vancomycin, linezolid,** or **daptomycin,** depending on the nature of the infection. *S. epidermidis* infections are often highly antibiotic resistant and most likely will require vancomycin or another agent. *S. saprophyticus* UTIs can be treated with trimethoprim-sulfamethoxazole (TMP-SMX) or a fluoroquinolone.

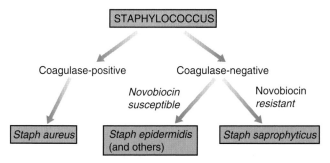

• **Figure 1-2.** Classification scheme of staphylococci.

CASE CONCLUSION

SA's knee aspirate and blood cultures grew out methicillin-susceptible *S. aureus*. He was treated with appropriate antibiotics (nafcillin and then cefazolin) for a total of 4 weeks with clearance of his joint infection and bacteremia. A transesophageal echocardiogram showed no signs of IE.

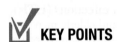

THUMBNAIL: *Staphylococcus aureus*

Organism	*S. aureus*
Type of organism	Gram-positive cocci in clusters; coagulase positive
Diseases caused	Skin infections, abscesses, endocarditis, septic arthritis, osteomyelitis, sepsis, meningitis, pneumonia, food poisoning, and toxic shock syndrome
Epidemiology	Normal flora found mainly in nasal passages and on skin; right-sided endocarditis found mostly in intravenous drug users; compromised immune systems favor infection
Diagnosis	Culture of appropriate specimen
Treatment	Nafcillin, cephalosporins, amoxicillin-clavulanate for methicillin-susceptible species; vancomycin, linezolid, or daptomycin for methicillin-resistant species

KEY POINTS

- Staphylococcal species are distinguished from streptococcal organisms by the presence of catalase and the formation of clusters instead of pairs and chains
- *S. aureus* is the only coagulase-producing staphylococcal species and is generally more virulent than the others, with multiple suppurative and toxin-mediated presentations

- The two main coagulase-negative staphylococcal species that cause human disease are *S. epidermidis* (foreign body infections) and *S. saprophyticus* (UTIs in sexually active women and elderly men)
- Methicillin-resistant *S. epidermidis* species are common, and methicillin-resistant *S. aureus* (MRSA) species are on the rise

QUESTIONS

1. Which of the listed antibiotics is the drug of choice for methicillin-sensitive staphylococci?

   A. Vancomycin
   B. Cefazolin
   C. Linezolid
   D. Ampicillin
   E. Penicillin

2. What is the general carriage rate of MRSA in the general population?

   A. 1%
   B. 10%
   C. 25%
   D. 80%
   E. 100%

3. Which of the following is not a risk factor for the development of MRSA?

   A. Injection drug use
   B. Dermatologic conditions
   C. Frequent use of antibiotics
   D. Diabetes mellitus
   E. Nasal herpes

4. What is the rate of methicillin resistance in *S. epidermidis*?

   A. 1%
   B. 10%
   C. 25%
   D. 80%
   E. 100%

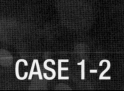

CASE 1-2
Streptococcus Pyogenes and the Other β-hemolytic Streptococci

HPI: SP is a 21-year-old woman who presents with a 3-day history of a painful sore throat. She has pain with swallowing and even with talking. She also has felt feverish for the past 2 days and somewhat listless. She does not have a cough, runny nose, or shortness of breath. She just started a new job as a nanny and notes that the 18-month-old baby has been fussy, feverish, and not eating well.

PMH: Had eczema as a child. Takes no medications and has no drug allergies. Not sexually active.

PE: T 38.4°C; HR 88; BP 100/70; RR 12

On oropharyngeal exam, her posterior pharynx is erythematous, swollen, and coated with a whitish exudate. Bilateral tonsils are also edematous, red, and covered with a similar exudate. The lymph nodes in her neck are swollen and tender just beneath the angles of the mandibles. Lung exam is clear.

Labs: WBC 10.0 with 80% neutrophils. Throat culture pending.

THOUGHT QUESTIONS

- What are the leading organisms that cause acute pharyngitis?
- How would you distinguish between the major bacterial etiologies in the lab?
- What are some of the virulence factors of the relevant bacteria?
- What are some long-term complications of these infections?
- What are the best options for treating these organisms?

BASIC SCIENCE REVIEW AND DISCUSSION

Pharyngitis

Acute pharyngitis is an inflammatory disease of the pharynx, and infectious causes include a multitude of viruses and bacteria. The most important viral etiology is **rhinovirus,** which is the most common agent of the common cold. The pharyngitis of a viral upper respiratory infection is often accompanied by a runny nose (called **coryza**), sneezing, and itchy eyes. Other viral etiologies of pharyngitis associated with the common cold are **coronavirus, parainfluenza virus, and adenovirus. Herpes simplex virus** can cause pharyngitis, often with distinct vesicular ulcerations on the posterior pharynx. **Coxsackie virus** can cause herpangina, characterized by fever, sore throat, and tender vesicles in the oropharynx, as well as hand-foot-and-mouth disease, manifesting as a vesicular rash on the hands and feet and mouth ulcerations. **Epstein-Barr virus and cytomegalovirus** can lead to pharyngitis in the setting of the infectious mononucleosis syndrome, and the "flu" syndrome of influenza virus can include an inflamed pharynx. Finally, **primary human immunodeficiency virus (HIV)** infection can manifest with a host of nonspecific symptoms, including fever, rash, lymphadenopathy, pharyngitis, fatigue, myalgias/arthralgias, nausea, vomiting, diarrhea, night sweats, and oral and genital ulcers.

Bacterial Causes Bacterial etiologies of pharyngitis may include mixed anaerobic infections (called **Vincent angina**). Sexually transmitted etiologies of pharyngitis include *Neisseria gonorrhoeae* and *Chlamydia trachomatis,* usually in the setting of orogenital contact. *Mycoplasma pneumoniae* and *Chlamydia pneumoniae* both cause atypical pneumonia syndromes, which can include a pharyngitis component. ***Corynebacterium diphtheriae*** was a frequent cause of bacterial pharyngitis prior to mass immunization of the populations of most industrialized nations with diphtheria toxoid. **The hallmark of diphtheria pharyngitis is a thick, grayish exudate called a pseudomembrane.** Finally, ***Arcanobacterium haemolyticum*** (formerly called *Corynebacterium haemolyticum*) has been increasingly recognized as an agent of pharyngitis in young people, **almost always accompanied by a scarlatiniform rash.**

The most important bacterial etiology of acute pharyngitis, however, is the **group A β-hemolytic streptococcus, called** *Streptococcus pyogenes.* Strains of other serogroups of β-hemolytic streptococcus, especially **group C and group G,** are increasingly implicated in bacterial pharyngitis as well.

Streptococci The **streptococci** species have been classified since 1919 into three different groups based on their hemolytic patterns on blood agar. **α-Hemolytic streptococci** create a greenish zone around their colonies on blood agar secondary to incomplete lysis of the red blood cells in the agar. **β-Hemolytic streptococci** form a clear zone around their colonies representing complete lysis of the red blood cells. **γ-Hemolytic** streptococci are generally nonhemolytic or variably hemolytic. A general classification scheme for the α-, β-, and γ-hemolytic streptococci is shown in Figure 1-3, along with the appropriate laboratory tests to distinguish each organism from another within a hemolytic class. Of note, Optochin and bacitracin are antibiotics to which different streptococcal species have varying susceptibility patterns, and a bile esculin-positive species hydrolyzes the esculin in bile esculin agar (BEA), resulting in a characteristic black discoloration.

The grouping of the **β-hemolytic streptococci** is based on antigenic differences in the **C carbohydrate** (located in the cell wall) from **Lancefield's** 1933 classification scheme; the distinct Lancefield groups A through U of the β-hemolytic streptococci are distinguished in the clinical laboratory by precipitin tests with specific antisera or by immunofluorescence. Additional methods of distinguishing the β-hemolytic streptococci include the diagnostic biochemical/antibiotic susceptibility tests in the

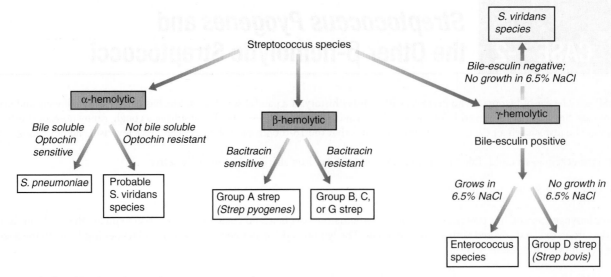

• **Figure 1-3.** Classification scheme of streptococcus species.

figure above. For instance, group A streptococcus (*S. pyogenes*) is distinguished from the other β-hemolytic streptococcus by its susceptibility to **bacitracin.** The species name for group B streptococcus is **S. agalactiae,** which can colonize the female genital tract and cause neonatal meningitis and sepsis. **Group C streptococcus** species cause some of the same syndromes as group A streptococcus (e.g., pharyngitis and skin infections) and include *S. dysgalactiae* (rare in humans), *S. equisimilis* (most common group C streptococcus species in humans), and *S. zooepidemicus* (causes epidemic infections in domestic animals).

S. pyogenes Group A streptococcus (**S. pyogenes**) is the most common bacterial cause of **pharyngitis,** and can resolve spontaneously or extend to otitis, sinusitis, mastoiditis, and meningitis if untreated. *S. pyogenes* can also produce **skin infections,** such as cellulitis, impetigo, erysipelas, necrotizing fasciitis, scarlet fever, or lymphangitis. The **M protein** protrudes from the outer surface of the cell in *S. pyogenes* and is the most important **virulence factor** of group A streptococci; the factor impedes phagocytosis by host macrophages and polymorphonuclear leukocytes, and strains that do not express this protein are avirulent. Group A streptococci elaborate a number of extracellular products important in the pathogenesis of the organism. For instance, **erythrogenic toxin** causes the rash of **scarlet fever** and can lead to a toxic shock-like syndrome. Streptolysin O (oxygen-labile) and streptolysin S (oxygen-stable) are hemolysins that contribute to β-hemolysis when group A strains are grown on blood agar plates; antibody to the streptolysin O (called **ASO**) develops soon after group A infections, and its titer is important in the diagnosis of nonsuppurative complications (see below). Hyaluronidase degrades hyaluronic acid, which is the ground substance of subcutaneous tissue, facilitating spread of *S. pyogenes* in skin infections. **Streptokinase** activates plasminogen to form plasmin, dissolving the fibrin structure of clots.

Nonsuppurative disorders can follow acute infections with the group A streptococcus and are usually caused by an immunologic response to streptococcal M proteins that cross-react with human antigens. Nonsuppurative diseases include **poststreptococcal glomerulonephritis (PSGN)** and **acute rheumatic fever;** the group A strains that cause pharyngitis are more typically associated with rheumatic fever and the strains that cause scarlet fever are more likely to give PSGN. Most cases of PSGN resolve completely, but **rheumatic fever can lead to permanent aortic or mitral valve defects.** If streptococcal infections are treated within 8 days after onset, the complication of rheumatic fever is usually prevented, making early diagnosis and treatment of streptococcal pharyngitis important. **ASO titers and the antihyaluronidase Ab titers are usually elevated in the presence of poststreptococcal nonsuppurative complications** and aid in diagnosis.

Diagnosis and Treatment

Diagnosis of group A pharyngitis is usually made by **throat culture,** and there has never been a reported case of penicillin-resistant *S. pyogenes*. Hence, **penicillin is the drug of choice** in the treatment of streptococcal infections, given its safety, narrow spectrum, low cost, and efficacy in the prevention of acute rheumatic fever. Penicillin can be administered either as a single dose of **benzathine penicillin G intramuscularly** (1.2 million units IM given once) or as a 10-day course of **oral penicillin** (penicillin V 500 mg PO two to three times a day for 10 days). **Amoxicillin is usually easier to administer in children** for group A streptococcus, as its liquid formulation tastes better than the oral suspension of penicillin. Other antibiotics (such as second- or third-generation cephalosporins) may be administered in short courses with equal efficacy. **Erythromycin is the drug of choice in penicillin-allergic patients.**

CASE CONCLUSION

SP's throat culture was positive for β-hemolytic streptococcus that was bacitracin susceptible. She was given a 10-day course of oral penicillin, with resolution of her symptoms within 2 days of starting antibiotics. The baby under her care was also positive for group A streptococcal pharyngitis and received a 10-day course of oral amoxicillin.

THUMBNAIL: Streptococcal Pharyngitis

Organism	*S. pyogenes* (group A streptococcus)
Type of organism	Gram-positive cocci in pairs and chains; catalase negative; β-hemolytic; bacitracin susceptible
Diseases caused	Pharyngitis, skin infections (including scarlet fever), nonsuppurative complications (PSGN and rheumatic fever)
Epidemiology	Most common cause of bacterial pharyngitis; disease primarily occurs among children ages 5 to 15; spread by direct person-to-person contact, usually through saliva or nasal secretions
Diagnosis	Throat culture
Treatment	Intramuscular benzathine penicillin or 10-day course of oral penicillin or amoxicillin; erythromycin for penicillin-allergic patients; can use azithromycin, cefuroxime, cefixime, and cefpodoxime for 5-day courses

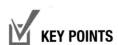 **KEY POINTS**

- Group A streptococcus is the most frequent etiology of acute bacterial pharyngitis
- Group A streptococcus is a β-hemolytic streptococcus and can usually be distinguished from the other β-hemolytics by its bacitracin susceptibility or by precipitation with specific antisera (against its Lancefield antigen)

- Group A streptococcal infections can lead to nonsuppurative complications following acute *S. pyogenes* infection, including PSGN and rheumatic fever
- The treatment of choice for *S. pyogenes* is penicillin

QUESTIONS

1. Which of the following substances contributes to the complete lysis of red blood cells on blood agar plates by the β-hemolytic streptococcus?

   A. Streptokinase
   B. M protein
   C. Erythrogenic toxin
   D. Streptolysin O
   E. Hyaluronidase

2. Which of the following features does not help distinguish group A streptococcus from other streptococcal species?

   A. Bacitracin susceptibility
   B. Most likely infection to trigger immunologic disorders, such as rheumatic fever and acute glomerulonephritis
   C. Catalase negativity
   D. M protein is a virulence factor
   E. Species name of *S. pyogenes*

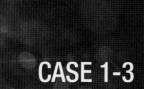

CASE 1-3 α-Hemolytic Streptococci

HPI: SV is a 48 year-old man with a history of mitral valve regurgitation who presents to your office with a 10-day history of fatigue, fever, and generalized malaise. He also notes some reddish lesions on his palms, which he has never noticed before. He denies any cough, but has mild new shortness of breath with exertion and with lying down flat at night in bed. SV is generally in good health except for a root canal approximately 3 weeks previously.

PMH: History of mitral valve regurgitation thought secondary to rheumatic fever as a child; SV takes no medications and has no drug allergies.

PE: T 38.6°C; HR 115; BP 110/78; RR 12

Heart exam is notable for a loud systolic murmur best heard at the left sternal border with radiation over to the left axilla. Lungs are clear and abdominal exam is normal. Skin exam is significant for several scattered reddish lesions over his palms and soles that are not painful when palpated.

Labs: WBC 14.8 with 86% neutrophils; blood cultures grew out gram-positive cocci in chains that are α-hemolytic on blood agar.

THOUGHT QUESTIONS

- Which species of gram-positive cocci are α-hemolytic?
- What syndromes does *Streptococcus pneumoniae* cause?
- What are the treatment options for *S. pneumoniae*?
- How are the *Streptococcus viridans* species classified?
- How is *S. viridans* endocarditis treated?

BASIC SCIENCE REVIEW AND DISCUSSION

α-Hemolytic Streptococci

The classification of streptococcal species has been reviewed elsewhere in this text (see Case 1-2: *Streptococcus pyogenes*) and the **α-hemolytic streptococci** flowchart (Fig. 1-4) is replicated here. α-Hemolytic streptococci create a greenish zone around their colonies on blood agar secondary to incomplete lysis of the red blood cells in the agar. The two main species of α-hemolytic streptococci are **S. pneumoniae** and the **S. viridans group.**

Streptococcus pneumoniae

Properties Gram-positive **lancet-shaped cocci** are arranged in pairs or short chains. As indicated above, *S. pneumoniae* is lysed by bile, and growth is inhibited by Optochin. Pneumococci possess a prominent polysaccharide capsule, and more than 80 antigenically distinct types of pneumococci exist.

Transmission and Epidemiology There is no animal reservoir for the pneumococcus. Immunocompromised patients, HIV-infected patients, and alcoholics are predisposed to disseminated pneumococcal illness. Splenectomized patients lack the ability to develop specific antibody to opsonize the organism's polysaccharide capsule and these patients are susceptible to overwhelming pneumococcal sepsis.

Clinical *S. pneumoniae* causes a variety of clinical syndromes, including pneumonia (usually lobar), bacteremia, meningitis, otitis media, sinusitis, and bronchitis. Immunocompromised patients are more prone to the overwhelming pneumococcal sepsis syndrome.

Diagnosis Typical pneumococcal species (lancet-shaped gram-positive cocci in pairs and short chains) should be seen on Gram stains of sputum, cerebrospinal fluid (CSF), or blood. Culture can confirm the diagnosis (see Fig. 1-5).

Treatment Although penicillin was formerly the drug of choice for the pneumococcus, there is emerging **penicillin resistance** within this species. The minimal inhibitory concentration (MIC) is a measure of antibiotic sensitivity and is defined as the lowest concentration of drug that inhibits the growth of the organism. A pneumococcal species is considered highly penicillin susceptible if the MIC to penicillin is less than 0.1 µg/mL. Intermediate resistance of a pneumococcal strain to penicillin is defined as having an MIC of between 0.1 and 1 µg/mL. A strain is highly resistant to penicillin if the MIC is greater than or equal to 2 µg/mL. The rate of intermediate- and high-level penicillin resistance varies by institution, with cumulative rates of up to 20 to 30% in some parts of the United States.

Table 1-1 summarizes the MIC cutoffs for determination of penicillin resistance in the pneumococcus. The rates of penicillin resistance given in the table are rates reported from a major public institution in San Francisco in 1999.

Penicillin-resistant strains of the pneumococcus tend to also have high rates of resistance to other antibiotics. Ceftriaxone can be used for strains of pneumococcus with intermediate resistance to penicillin for most infections, but vancomycin is usually required for high-level resistance to penicillin, especially in the setting of meningitis.

Classification of *S. viridans* Species

Viridans streptococci are part of the normal flora of the upper respiratory tract, oral cavity, gastrointestinal tract, and female genital tract. These organisms are generally of low virulence, but the most common syndrome of *S. viridans* is **infective endocarditis** or **subacute bacterial endocarditis** in patients with underlying valvular heart disease. Subacute bacterial endocarditis often follows a history of dental work, as the latter causes

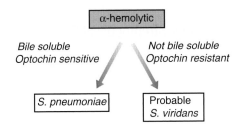

● **Figure 1-4.** Classification of α-hemolytic streptococci.

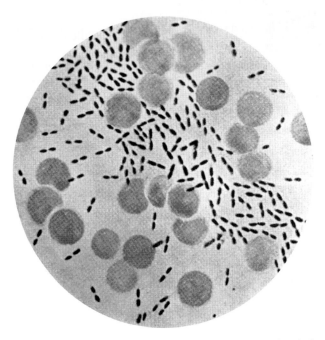

● **Figure 1-5.** Gram stain showing lancet-shaped diplococci typical of *S. pneumoniae*. (Image in public domain from Centers for Disease Control and Prevention Public Health Image Library, http://phil.cdc.gov/phil/home.asp.)

transient viridans streptococcal bacteremia that may seed abnormal valvular tissue. Viridans streptococci have rarely also been associated with meningitis, pneumonia, and abscess formation. Organisms in the *S. milleri* group have a proclivity for forming localized purulent collections.

The classification of viridans streptococci species has undergone multiple revisions, given that the viridans group is composed of a number of disparate α-hemolytic and sometimes nonhemolytic species of streptococcal organisms. The evolution of *S. viridans* taxonomy is shown in Table 1-2.

Treatment

Most viridans streptococci are **highly penicillin susceptible,** with a MIC to penicillin of less than 0.1 μg/mL. Some species of streptococci are nutritionally variant, defined by their requirement for pyridoxal or thiol group supplementation for growth. These streptococcal species are less susceptible to penicillin than other species of streptococcus, with MICs ranging from 0.2 to 1 μg/mL. Although these nutritionally variant streptococci were formerly classified under the viridans streptococci group of organisms, they have recently been reclassified into their own genus called **Abiotrophia** (main species are *Abiotrophia adiacens* and *A. defectiva*).

The treatment for *S. viridans* endocarditis is as follows:

- For penicillin-susceptible streptococcal species (MIC <0.1 μg/mL):
  - Penicillin, 12–18 million units intravenously (IV) total per day for 4 weeks

- or penicillin plus gentamicin, 1 mg/kg IV every 8 hours for 2 weeks
- or ceftriaxone, 2 g IV every day for 4 weeks
- or vancomycin, 30 mg/kg IV total per day for 4 weeks (in penicillin-allergic patients)
- For penicillin intermediate-resistance streptococcal species (e.g., *Abiotrophia* species; MIC >0.1 and ≤1 μg/mL):
  - Penicillin, 18 million units IV total per day plus gentamicin for 4 weeks
  - or vancomycin, IV for 4 weeks

TABLE 1-1 MIC Ranges of Penicillin Susceptibility in Pneumococcus and Prevalence in a City Hospital

MIC to Penicillin	Level of Resistance	Rate at SFGH
0.1 μg/mL	Penicillin susceptible	84.5%
0.1–1 μg/mL	Intermediate resistance	11.6%
≥2 μg/mL	Highly resistant	3.9%

Modified from Winston LG, Perlman JL, Rose DA, et al. Penicillin-nonsusceptible Streptococcus pneumoniae at San Francisco General Hospital [SFGH]. Clin Infect Dis 1999;29:580–585.

TABLE 1-2 Evolving Classification Schemes for the Viridans Streptococcal Species

1st Classification Scheme	2nd Classification Scheme	Current Taxonomic Name
S. mitior	{ *S. mitis* *S. sanguis II*	{ *S. mitis* *S. oralis*
S. sanguis	*S. sanguis I*	*S. sanguis* *S. gordonii* **S. crista**
S. salivarius *S. mutans* *S. milleri*	*S. salivarius* *S. mutans* *S. MG-intermedius* *S. anginosus-constellatus*	*S. salivarius* *S. mutans* group[a] *S. intermedius* } *S. intermedius* *S. constellatus.* } group *S. anginosus*
		S. vestibularis *S. parasanguis*
	S. morbillorum	*Gemella morbillorum*

[a]*S. mutans group strongly associated with dental caries*

CASE CONCLUSION

SV's blood cultures were confirmed as positive for viridans streptococci (*S. salivarius* species) and his cardiac echocardiogram showed a vegetation on the mitral valve. He was given the diagnosis of *S. viridans*-infective endocarditis. As the MIC of the *S. viridans* species to penicillin was less than 0.1 μg/mL, SV was treated with penicillin and gentamicin for a 2-week course, with complete resolution.

THUMBNAIL: Subacute Bacterial Endocarditis

Organism	Species of viridans streptococci group
Type of organism	Catalase-negative gram-positive cocci in pairs and chains
Diseases caused	Infective endocarditis on heart valves with underlying defects; rarely, pneumonia, meningitis, and abscess (the latter more with the *S. milleri* group)
Epidemiology	Part of normal flora in oral cavity, gastrointestinal tract, respiratory tract, and female genital tract; pathogens are of low virulence and usually require damaged heart valve prior to causing endocarditis
Diagnosis	Gram stain to look for gram-positive cocci in pairs and chains; α-hemolytic; insoluble in bile and resistant to Optochin
Treatment	Penicillin

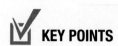

KEY POINTS

- α-Hemolytic streptococci include *S. pneumoniae* and species in the viridans streptococci group
- *S. pneumoniae* species are developing increasing penicillin resistance
- Viridans streptococci species cause infective endocarditis on structurally damaged valves
- Viridans streptococci are highly penicillin susceptible; nutritionally variant streptococci (*Abiotrophia* genus) often have intermediate resistance to penicillin

QUESTIONS

1. Nutritionally variant streptococci will grow under the following conditions:

   A. On sheep blood agar
   B. Around a *Staphylococcus aureus* streak on a blood agar plate
   C. In tryptic soy broth
   D. Around a *Streptococcus pneumoniae* streak on a blood agar plate
   E. On a charcoal yeast extract agar plate

2. The erythematous painless lesions on SV's palms in the setting of infective endocarditis are called:

   A. Osler nodes
   B. Roth spots
   C. Splinter hemorrhages
   D. Janeway lesions
   E. Palpable purpura

Enterococci

HPI: A 63-year-old male is admitted to the hospital overnight for pacemaker placement. He is discharged the following day with no problems. At his follow-up appointment a week later, he complains of pain at the pacemaker insertion site.

PE: T 38.4°C; BP 116/76; HR 80 paced; RR 18

The pacemaker pocket is warm, erythematous, and tender. There is a 2/6 systolic murmur.

Labs: Labs and blood cultures are drawn in the office. WBC 12.2 with a left shift. He is admitted to the hospital and put on vancomycin and gentamicin. The following day, his blood cultures grow gram-positive cocci in chains.

THOUGHT QUESTIONS

- What laboratory tests help distinguish *Enterococcus* from related species?
- What are the mechanisms of drug resistance in *Enterococcus*?
- What parameters for the use of antibiotics can reduce the incidence of vancomycin-resistant enterococci (VRE)?

BASIC SCIENCE REVIEW AND DISCUSSION

Originally classified in the 1930s as group D streptococci, enterococci possess a group D-specific cell wall carbohydrate (glycerol teichoic acid linked to the cytoplasmic membrane). In 1984, hybridization studies showed a more distant relationship to streptococci, and enterococci were officially given their own genus. **Enterococci are facultatively anaerobic, nonmotile, gram-positive, spherical bacteria that grow in pairs or in short chains.** Enterococci are catalase negative and have complex nutritional requirements. **They are able to grow in high concentrations of salt** (termed **halotolerant**) **and bile acids,** both adaptive to their ecological niche in the intestinal environment.

In the laboratory, colonies of *Enterococcus* are white in color and are typically nonhemolytic, but may be α- or β-hemolytic. They can be distinguished from other species of streptococci by their growth on **BEA** slants with blackening of the medium due to hydrolysis of esculin; production of acid from several sugars, including glucose, maltose, and lactose; growth in **SF broth** (*Streptococcus faecalis* broth) with production of acid; resistance to **Optochin** (differentiates from *S. pneumoniae*); and hydrolysis of **pyrrolidonyl-β-naphthylamide** (PYR; differentiates from *S. pneumoniae*). See Figure 1-3 (Case 1-2) for a general classification of streptococcal species.

Although they are not considered to be highly virulent, their **intrinsic resistance and ability to develop resistance** to several types of broad-spectrum anti-infectives allow them to cause superinfections in patients already receiving antimicrobial therapy. Infections containing enterococcal species are often **polymicrobial** and may contain anaerobes, such as *Bacteroides* species.

Currently, enterococcal infections account for 12% of all nosocomial infections, second only to *Escherichia coli* infections. *Enterococcus* can cause complicated abdominal infections, skin and skin structure infections, urinary tract infections, infections of the bloodstream, and subacute bacterial endocarditis. **Risk factors for enterococcal infections include urinary or intravascular catheterization, long-term hospitalization, and use of broad-spectrum antibiotics.**

Two species of enterococci cause the majority of human infections: ***E. faecalis* (which accounts for 80% of enterococcal infections) and *E. faecium* (which accounts for 10% of enterococcal infections).** Clinical isolates of *E. faecium* are becoming increasingly common, which is a particular concern because of its high resistance to antibiotics, especially in nosocomial settings (e.g., intensive care units). In a study conducted between 1995 and 1997, data were collected from more than 15,000 *Enterococcus* isolates. Of those, less than 2% of *E. faecalis* were found to be resistant to ampicillin and vancomycin, whereas 83% of the *E. faecium* isolates were resistant to ampicillin and 52% were resistant to vancomycin.

VRE emerged first in Europe in 1988 and became one of the most important nosocomial pathogens of the 1990s. Broad-range multidrug antibiotic resistance is **mediated by R plasmids** that are promiscuously spread between bacteria—both within species and across species.

There are five described **phenotypes of vancomycin resistance.** VanA and VanB are the most common phenotypes associated with clinical isolates of *E. faecium*. VanC is the intrinsic phenotype of *E. gallinarum* and *E. casseliflavus/E. flavescens*. Less common are the acquired VanD and VanE phenotypes. **The mechanism of resistance is alteration of the terminal dipeptide of the precursors of the peptidoglycan cell wall from D-Ala-D-Ala to D-Ala-D-lactate (in VanA, VanB, and VanD) or to D-Ala-D-serine (in VanB and VanE).** With the incorporation of these new dipeptides, the binding affinity of vancomycin is greatly reduced.

E. faecium is the most frequently isolated species of VRE in hospitals and typically produces high vancomycin MICs (>128 µg/mL). These isolates typically contain *vanA* genes. A *vanB*-containing isolate typically produces lower-level resistance to vancomycin (MICs 16–64 µg/mL). Newer agents, such as quinupristin-dalfopristin, linezolid, and daptomycin, have been developed with activity against VRE.

Enterococci are also **intrinsically resistant to aminoglycosides,** but the addition of a β-lactam antibiotic (e.g., ampicillin) allows entry of the aminoglycoside into the bacterial cell, producing a synergistic combination that results in cell death. Enterococci that are highly resistant to aminoglycosides pose an important clinical problem, as these organisms are resistant to synergistic killing by β-lactam/aminoglycoside combinations. The resistance is due to the production of plasmid-mediated aminoglycoside-modifying enzymes.

CASE CONCLUSION

Our patient's pacemaker is removed, and the wires are culture positive for *Enterococcus*. His blood cultures from admission are speciated as *E. faecalis*, with an MIC to ampicillin of 64 μg/mL and to vancomycin of 4 μg/mL. A transthoracic echocardiogram demonstrates a small vegetation on his mitral valve. After his pacemaker is removed, he is treated for 6 weeks with vancomycin and gentamicin for endocarditis and a new pacemaker is placed without complication.

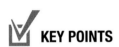

THUMBNAIL: *Enterococcus*

Organism	*E. faecalis, E. faecium*
Type of organism	Gram-positive cocci in chains; group D streptococci
Diseases caused	Urinary and biliary tract infections, septicemia, endocarditis, wound infection, intra-abdominal abscesses complicating diverticulitis or appendicitis
Epidemiology	Normal flora of the gastrointestinal tract
Diagnosis	Isolation of organism from sterile site; distinguished from other streptococci in the laboratory by ability to grow in 6.5% NaCl and in bile esculin
Treatment	β-lactam (e.g., ampicillin) plus aminoglycoside (e.g., gentamicin), vancomycin, quinupristin-dalfopristin, daptomycin, linezolid

KEY POINTS

■ Enterococci have high levels of resistance to salt and bile acids, making them particularly well suited to their environment in the human gastrointestinal and biliary tracts

■ Increasing rates of vancomycin resistance are common in hospital settings, and treatment is difficult

QUESTIONS

1. According to the CDC guidelines for the appropriate use of vancomycin, which of the following cases would be considered appropriate use?

   A. Primary treatment of antibiotic-associated colitis
   B. Continued use in a patient with methicillin-sensitive *S. epidermidis*
   C. Once-weekly treatment in a hemodialysis patient with a streptococcal infection
   D. Methicillin-sensitive *S. aureus* endocarditis in a patient with a history of anaphylaxis to penicillin
   E. Attempt to eradicate MRSA colonization in a patient on chronic hemodialysis

2. The *Enterococcus* phenotype that expresses high-level vancomycin resistance is:

   A. VanA
   B. VanB
   C. VanC
   D. VanD
   E. VanE

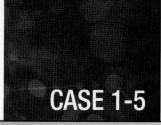

HPI: NA is a 65-year-old woman who presents to your clinic with a 2-week complaint of cough and shortness of breath. The cough is described as occasionally productive of greenish sputum, although it is mostly dry. NA also complains of low-grade fevers, worse at night, and accompanied by night sweats. Her recent history is significant for a diagnosis of temporal arteritis—a medium and large vessel vasculitic syndrome that can lead to blindness—5 weeks ago, for which she has been treated with corticosteroids. She denies any abdominal pain, nausea, vomiting, diarrhea, constipation, or urinary symptoms.

PMH: Temporal arteritis diagnosed 5 weeks ago as above; NA also has a history of adult-onset diabetes mellitus and hypertension. Medications include prednisone at a dose of 40 mg orally per day currently, two antihypertensive medications, and an oral hypo-glycemic medication. NA has no known drug allergies and does not smoke.

PE: T 38.3°C; BP 150/95; HR 90; RR 18; SaO$_2$ on room air 92%

NA is generally a chronically ill-appearing woman who looks older than her stated age. The main findings on her physical exam are crackles in the right upper lobe with egophony changes in that area. Moderate soft tissue swelling is noted over her right scapular area. No rashes. Heart, lung, and neurologic exam are all normal.

Labs: WBC 8.5 with a normal differential; chest roentgenogram shows a large, cavitating nodule in the right upper lobe with surrounding pneumonitis; Gram stain of the sputum sample shows branching, slender, gram-positive rods.

THOUGHT QUESTIONS

- What is a classification scheme for the gram-positive rods?
- Which gram-positive rods are filamentous and how are they distinguished?
- What are the clinical syndromes caused by the filamentous gram-positive rods?
- How should these infections be treated?

BASIC SCIENCE REVIEW AND DISCUSSION

Classification of Gram-Positive Rods

The diagram (Fig. 1-6) below shows a classification scheme for gram-positive rods.

Filamentous Gram-positive Rods The filamentous gram-positive rods are in the *Nocardia* and *Actinomyces* genera.

Nocardia

Nocardia is a genus of **aerobic** actinomycetes and its main species include *N. asteroides, N. brasiliensis, N. farcinica, N. oti-tidiscaviarum,* and *N. transvalensis.*

Properties *Nocardia* species are filamentous, branching, beaded, gram-positive rods. These organisms also stain weakly positive with a modified **acid-fast** bacteria (AFB) stain, which is a distin-guishing characteristic of *Nocardia* from *Actinomyces* species.

Transmission and Epidemiology *Nocardia* species are ubiquitous **envi-ronmental** saprophytes, living in soil, organic matter, and water. Human infection usually arises from direct inoculation of the skin or soft tissues or by inhalation of the organism.

Clinical *Nocardia* infections tend to occur in immunocompro-mised hosts (e.g., patients on steroids, organ transplant recipi-ents, or patients with advanced HIV infection). The three main clinical syndromes of *Nocardia* infection are:

1. **Skin/soft tissue infections and mycetoma:** *N. aster-oides* tends to cause self-limited skin infections; *N. brasiliensis* is the most common cause of progressive cuta-neous and lymphocutaneous (*sporotrichoid*) disease.

    Mycetoma (**Madura foot**) is a local, chronic, slowly progressive, often painless destructive infection that begins in the subcutaneous tissue and spreads to contiguous struc-tures. Causative organisms from plant debris or soil are inoculated into the subcutaneous tissue by minor trauma. A defining characteristic of mycetoma is the presence of tiny grains seen in the drainage from **sinus tracts** (repre-senting clumps of organisms). Mycetoma can be caused by two groups of organisms: (1) **actinomycetoma** is caused by filamentous, aerobic branching bacteria (such as *N. brasiliensis, N. asteroids, Streptomyces somaliensis, Actino-madura madurae,* and *Actinomadura pelletieri*); (2) **eumyce-toma** is caused by soil fungi (such as *Pseudoallescheria boydii, Madurella mycetomatis, Madurella grisea, Fusarium, Acremonium,* and *Corynespora*).

2. **Respiratory infections:** pulmonary disease is the promi-nent clinical finding of nocardiosis, with more than 90% of such cases caused by *N. asteroides*. Pulmonary nocardiosis has manifold manifestations, including suppurative pneu-monia, lung abscess, and **cavitary disease** with contigu-ous extension to surrounding areas, causing pleural effusion, empyema, and overlying soft tissue swelling.

3. **Neurologic infections:** central nervous system (CNS) manifestations of nocardiosis often accompany respiratory disease and include distinct granulomas or abscesses in the brain. Neurologic manifestations can progress very slowly and result in a chronic, debilitating neurologic syndrome. Diagnosis of nocardial infection in the brain lesion is usu-ally made by biopsy or aspiration.

Diagnosis *Nocardia* can be isolated from respiratory secretions, skin biopsies, or brain lesion aspirations. Direct smears should show gram-positive, beaded, branching filaments that are usually acid fast.

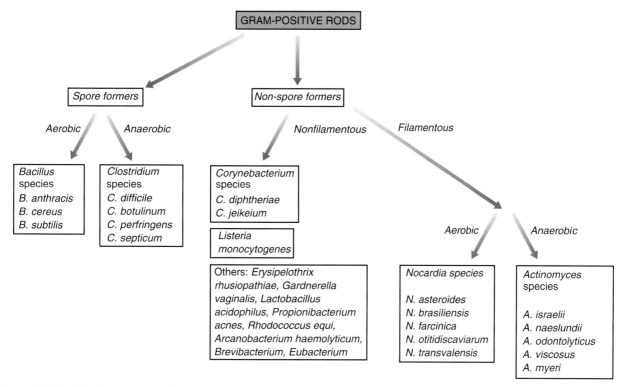

• **Figure 1-6.** Classification of gram-positive rods.

Treatment The mainstay of treatment for nocardial infections is **sulfonamides. TMP-SMX** is the formulation most often used for these agents, although sulfadiazine and sulfisoxazole demonstrate equal efficacy in the treatment of nocardiosis. Alternative agents in the face of sulfa allergies include amikacin and imipenem.

Actinomyces

Actinomycosis is an indolent infection caused by the following **anaerobic** or microaerophilic bacterial species: *Actinomyces israelii, A. naeslundii, A. odontolyticus, A. viscosus,* and *A. meyeri.*

Properties When *Actinomyces* organisms invade tissue, they form tiny but visible grains called **"sulfur granules"** because of their yellow color. Classic features of actinomycosis infections include extension to contiguous structures by crossing anatomic boundaries with the formation of fistulae and sinus tracts.

Transmission and Epidemiology *Actinomyces* species are part of the **endogenous human flora** that normally colonize the mouth, colon, and vagina. The peak incidence of actinomycosis is reported to be in the mid-decade with a male-to-female predominance, thought to be secondary to poorer oral hygiene in this age group. No person-to-person transmission has been documented, and immunocompromise is not a precondition for actinomycosis infections.

Clinical The major clinical syndromes of *Actinomyces* include the following:

1. **Orocervicofacial disease:** soft tissue swelling, abscesses, or mass lesions in the head and neck area, especially the **angle of the jaw,** are the most common manifestations of actinomycosis. Chronic, recurring abscesses and spread to adjacent structures are common. Extension of orofacial actinomycosis can lead to brain abscesses.
2. **Thoracic involvement:** indolent infection usually involving a combination of the pulmonary parenchyma and pleural space, with spontaneous drainage of an empyema through the chest wall serving as a diagnostic clue.
3. **Abdominal and pelvic disease:** actinomycosis in these regions most often manifests as an abscess or hard mass lesion with fistula and sinus tract formation to contiguous structures and through the overlying skin.
4. **Musculoskeletal disease:** actinomycotic infection of the bone is usually a result of adjacent soft tissue infection and can involve prosthetic joints.

Diagnosis As *Actinomyces* infections are exquisitely sensitive to antibiotics, aspiration of the involved tissue for Gram stain and culture should be performed prior to the administration of antibiotics. Branching, gram-positive, filamentous rods should be cultured out under anaerobic conditions. A diagnostic clue to actinomycosis is the presence of visible sulfur granules in the pus or tissue from a biopsy.

Treatment **Penicillin** is the mainstay of treatment. Use tetracycline or erythromycin for penicillin-allergic patients.

 CASE CONCLUSION

Modified acid-fast staining and culture of the organism from NA's sputum confirmed *N. asteroides* and she was treated with a 4-week-long course of TMP-SMX with complete resolution. Her steroid therapy was also tapered off.

THUMBNAIL: Pulmonary Nocardiosis

Organism	*N. asteroides*
Type of organism	Branching, beaded, filamentous gram-positive rod that is acid-fast positive
Diseases caused	Skin and soft tissue infections, including mycetoma, respiratory infections such as cavitary nodules, and brain abscesses
Epidemiology	Respiratory, neurologic, and disseminated infections usually occur in immunocompromised hosts; actinomycetoma occurs from inoculation of *Nocardia* (usually *N. brasiliensis*) from soil into skin of foot through minor trauma
Diagnosis	Gram stain to look for typical morphology and modified acid-fast stain; culture
Treatment	Sulfonamides (usually TMP-SMX)

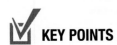

KEY POINTS

■ Gram-positive rods can be divided initially into spore-forming rods and non–spore-forming rods, with the latter being divided into filamentous and nonfilamentous rods

■ The filamentous gram-positive rods include *Nocardia* species (aerobic; soil organisms) and *Actinomyces* species (anaerobic; endogenous flora)

■ The main clinical findings of nocardiosis are skin and soft tissue infections, including mycetoma, and respiratory and neurologic infections in immunocompromised hosts

■ The treatment of choice for nocardial infections is sulfonamides

QUESTIONS

1. The most common site of *Actinomyces* abscesses is the:

   A. Brain
   B. Perimandibular region
   C. Tongue
   D. Maxillary sinus
   E. Pleural cavity

2. *Listeria* is a common etiology of meningitis in:

   A. Neonates
   B. Adults
   C. Patients with complement deficiencies
   D. Patients after a neurosurgical procedure
   E. Splenectomized patients

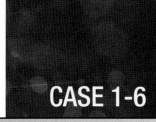

CASE 1-6 *Clostridium Difficile*

HPI: A 49-year-old man recently fell while hiking. He scraped his leg and was unable to clean the wound properly at the time. Several days later, he developed a low-grade fever and erythema and swelling around the wound. He was diagnosed with cellulitis, and as he is allergic to penicillin, he was prescribed a 10-day course of clindamycin. His cellulitis promptly resolved, but he returns to his primary care doctor 1 week later with low-grade fever, abdominal pain, and nonbloody diarrhea. He denies any recent travel or suspicious meals. No one else at home has diarrhea.

PE: T 38.0°C; BP 130/70; HR 85; RR 12

The patient appears well. There is no rash. Mucous membranes are moist. Heart and lung exam are normal. Abdominal exam shows diffuse mild tenderness, but no peritoneal signs. There are no masses or hepatosplenomegaly. Rectal exam shows trace guaiac-positive brown stool. The patient's cellulitis has completely resolved, with no erythema, exudate, or edema.

Stool cultures show no pathogens.

A test for C. *difficile* toxin in the stool is positive.

Labs: WBC 12, normal differential. Hematocrit is 47. Platelets are 350.

THOUGHT QUESTIONS

- What bacteria can cause infectious diarrhea?
- What predisposed this patient to get C. *difficile* colitis?
- Why should this patient not receive antimotility agents to relieve his symptoms?

BASIC SCIENCE REVIEW AND DISCUSSION

Clostridium species are anaerobic, spore-forming gram-positive rods that can be found in soil and, in certain cases, as intestinal colonizers. They can cause a wide variety of **toxin**-mediated illnesses, including gas gangrene (C. *perfringens*), tetanus (C. *tetani*), botulism (C. *botulinum*), food poisoning (C. *perfringens*), and pseudomembranous colitis (C. *difficile*).

Antibiotic use is frequently associated with diarrhea, because of alterations in the bowel flora. Most of these cases will resolve once the antibiotics are withdrawn, but approximately 10 to 30% of antibiotic-associated diarrhea is caused by C. *difficile* colitis, one of the serious **complications of antibiotic use.** (Other complications of antibiotic use include allergic reactions, renal or hepatic toxicity, systemic fungal infections, and creation of antibiotic-resistant pathogens.) For an expanded discussion of bacterial causes of infectious diarrhea, see Case 1-8.

Pseudomembranous colitis is caused by overgrowth of C. *difficile* after antibiotics have disrupted the normal ecology of the gut. Even a single dose of virtually any antibiotic can lead to C. *difficile*, although clindamycin and the third-generation cephalosporins are the classic offenders. Once the gut ecology has been altered, C. *difficile* colonization occurs through fecal-oral transmission of the organism. Toxigenic strains of C. *difficile* elaborate two toxins, A and B, which inactivate Rho small GTP (guanosine triphosphate) signaling proteins and lead to intestinal epithelial cell death. The symptoms of C. *difficile* colitis are fever, abdominal pain, and diarrhea. On endoscopic exam, the colon mucosa is covered with a yellow coating, known as a **pseudomembrane.** If untreated, C. *difficile* colitis can lead to **toxic megacolon,** which can be life threatening if bowel necrosis or perforation occurs. To avoid precipitating toxic megacolon, antimotility agents are relatively contraindicated.

C. *difficile* is rarely diagnosed via endoscopy. More commonly, stool is sent for an assay that detects C. *difficile* toxin either through a cytotoxicity assay or with an enzyme-linked immunosorbent assay (ELISA). Culture for C. *difficile* is more sensitive, but many strains of C. *difficile* do not produce toxins and are subsequently not virulent, so the test is less specific.

To underscore that C. *difficile* colitis is due to ecological disruption in the colon, the infection can actually be treated by enemas containing stool from a healthy person. A more palatable and commonly used treatment consists of a course of antibiotics that kill C. *difficile* in the intestinal lumen. **Oral metronidazole** is the treatment of choice. Oral vancomycin will also work, but it is expensive and runs the risk of selecting for vancomycin-resistant enterococci in the patient's gut. If the patient is unable to take oral medication, IV metronidazole can be secreted into the gut, and has some efficacy. Oral supplements of *Lactobacillus* or *Saccharomyces* have been used to try to restore ecological order in the gut, but these treatments remain unproven. If at all possible, the broad-spectrum antibiotics that precipitated the C. *difficile* infection should be withdrawn.

 CASE CONCLUSION

The patient is treated with a 10-day course of metronidazole and his diarrhea resolves.

THUMBNAIL: Clostridial Infections

Organism	C. Difficile	C. Perfringens	C. Tetani	C. Botulinum
Type of organism	Anaerobic, spore-forming, motile, gram-positive rod	Anaerobic, spore-forming, nonmotile, gram-positive rod	Anaerobic, spore-forming, motile, gram-positive rod	Anaerobic, spore-forming, gram-positive rod
Diseases caused	Pseudomembranous colitis	Gas gangrene (also can cause enterotoxin-mediated food poisoning)	Tetanus (lockjaw)	Botulism
Epidemiology	Illness follows antibacterial antibiotic treatment	Organism is ubiquitous in soil and common in stool; infection usually follows traumatic injury	Sporadic cases worldwide among unimmunized or partially immunized persons after exposure to organism or spores in contaminated wound	Infection via contaminated food (particularly infants fed honey) or via wounds
Diagnosis	Stool assay for *C. difficile* toxin; pseudomembranes visualized on endoscopy	Clinical diagnosis; presence of gas or crepitus in wounds; gram-positive rods on Gram stain of exudate	Clinical; may culture organism from wound	Clinical; may culture organism or detect toxin from samples of serum, stool, or implicated food or wound
Treatment	PO metronidazole; PO vancomycin; IV metronidazole	Emergent surgical debridement; penicillin; hyperbaric oxygen	Penicillin; tetanus immune globulin (TIG); tetanus toxoid (Td); supportive care	Antitoxin immune globulin; penicillin; wound debridement

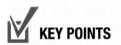 **KEY POINTS**

■ *C. difficile* colitis is a potentially lethal complication of antibiotic use

■ The treatment of choice is oral metronidazole; oral vancomycin or IV metronidazole are alternatives

QUESTIONS

1. Which antibiotic is least likely to cause *C. difficile* colitis?

   A. Clindamycin
   B. Ceftriaxone
   C. Metronidazole
   D. Cefoxitin
   E. Cefotaxime

2. What is the life-threatening complication of *C. difficile* infection?

   A. Gas gangrene
   B. Toxic megacolon
   C. Sepsis
   D. Pneumonia
   E. Appendicitis

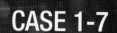

CASE 1-7 *Neisseria Meningitidis*

HPI: NM is a 19-year-old female college student who presents to the emergency department with a 1-day history of high fever, headache, stiff neck, rash, and fatigue. She was observed to have a characteristic rash upon presentation to the ER and was quickly moved to an isolation room. Blood cultures were drawn, NM was started on antibiotics, and a lumbar puncture to obtain CSF was performed.

PMH: NM has no significant past medical history and takes no medications. She has no allergies. She is not sexually active and lives in the sophomore dormitory at her college with two roommates.

HPI: T 39.5°C; HR 135; BP 85/58; RR 20

NM is acutely ill in appearance. Notable physical findings include photophobia, stiff neck, and a diffuse rash composed of multiple large purpura and petechiae, which looked like she was bleeding underneath her skin.

Labs: WBC 24.0 with 95% neutrophils.

THOUGHT QUESTIONS

- What is the most likely diagnosis of this patient?
- Why was she moved into an isolation room?
- What are some risk factors for this condition?
- Should her roommates be contacted?
- What is the treatment for this condition?

BASIC SCIENCE REVIEW AND DISCUSSION

The most likely diagnosis in this patient is meningococcemia with *Neisseria meningitides* meningitis.

Characteristics

Neisseria meningitides is a **gram-negative coccus** with a prominent polysaccharide capsule and at least 13 different serologic types. The most important serologic groups of *N. meningitides* (based on their capsular polysaccharides) are the A, B, C, Y, and W-135 groups. The **endotoxin** in the cell wall of the gram-negative *N. meningitides* is a **lipopolysaccharide** similar to that found in gram-negative rods, with a corresponding ability to cause a **sepsis-like syndrome.** Both *N. meningitides* and *N. gonorrhoeae* species require culture on heated sheep blood agar (called "**chocolate agar**"), and they are both **oxidase positive.**

Transmission and Epidemiology

N. meningitides organisms are transmitted from person to person by **airborne respiratory droplets,** after which time they can temporarily colonize the **nasopharynx** in the exposed individual (although carriers are usually asymptomatic). The organism then enters the bloodstream from the nasopharynx and is disseminated either widely or just to the meninges. Approximately **5% of the population are chronic carriers** of *N. meningitides* and serve as a source of infection to others.

Epidemics of meningococcal disease still occur around the world, especially in **sub-Saharan Africa.** Infection in the United States is associated with individuals living in close contact, such as among **military recruits and college students living in dormitories.** The spleen is important for opsonization of the polysaccharide-enclosed organism as an initial defense mechanism. Hence, **splenectomized patients** have an increased susceptibility to *N. meningitides* infection. Individuals with complement deficiencies, particularly in the **late-acting complement components (C5–C9),** also have an increased incidence of severe meningococcal disease.

Clinical

The two most important clinical manifestations of *N. meningitides* infection are **meningitis and meningococcemia.** *N. meningitides* and *Streptococcus pneumoniae* are the most common etiologies of bacterial meningitis in adults. *N. meningitides* causes the typical symptoms of a bacterial meningitis, including fever, headache, stiff neck, photophobia, and **polymorphonuclear pleocytosis** in the CSF. Meningitis can occur alone or with the syndrome of meningococcemia.

Meningococcemia can be quite severe in its presentation, including high fever, shock-like symptoms, **widespread purpura and petechiae, disseminated intravascular coagulation** (DIC), and **adrenal insufficiency** caused by hemorrhagic necrosis of the adrenal glands **(Waterhouse-Friderichsen syndrome)** usually in the setting of DIC and septic emboli. The massive DIC and septic emboli can lead to the worse-case scenario of digit and extremity gangrene (Fig. 1-7). Meningococcemia can occur either alone or with the syndrome of meningitis. *N. meningitides* bacteremia without the syndrome of sepsis can also occur and is usually manifested by a low-grade fever and an upper respiratory illness. The serum level of bacteremia is low in this condition (e.g., 22–325 organisms/mL of blood in one small series in children).

Therapy

Penicillin or ampicillin were the former mainstays of treatment for *N. meningitides,* but there has been increasing **penicillin resistance** with the meningococcus, mainly secondary to the alteration of penicillin-binding proteins or high-level β-lactamase production. Hence, **high-dose ceftriaxone** is the initial therapy of choice for serious meningococcal infections until the susceptibility of the organism to penicillin can be determined.

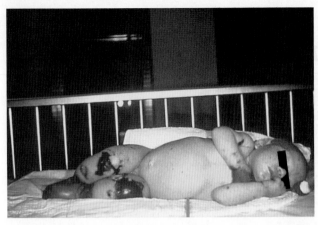

● **Figure 1-7.** Four-month-old infant with petechiae and gangrene of lower extremities of meningococcemia. (Image in public domain from Centers for Disease Control and Prevention Public Health Image Library, http://phil.cdc.gov/phil/home.asp)

THUMBNAIL: Meningococcemia

Organism	*N. meningitides*
Type of organism	Gram-negative cocci, oxidase positive
Diseases caused	Meningitis; meningococcemia with sepsis-like syndrome, widespread purpura and petechiae, DIC, adrenal insufficiency; bacteremia without sepsis
Epidemiology	Common cause of meningitis in adults; can occur in epidemic form, especially in sub-Saharan Africa; outbreaks in military recruits and college students in dormitories; splenectomy and late complement deficiencies are risk factors
Diagnosis	Blood and CSF culture; gram-negative cocci, oxidase positive, only grows on chocolate agar; capsular polysaccharide (five important serotypes)
Treatment	High-dose ceftriaxone until susceptibilities available (then high-dose penicillin if susceptible)

Chemoprophylaxis for close contacts of the index patient is indicated to eliminate the nasal carriage of the *N. meningitides* organism and prevent further infection and transmission. Individuals qualifying for chemoprophylaxis include household and close contacts, fellow children and adults in a daycare facility, individuals in a closed population such as a boarding school, dormitory, or military unit, and any hospital personnel who had close contact with the patient's respiratory secretions (e.g., respiratory technologist or physician who intubated the patient). In addition, the index patient will require chemoprophylaxis before he or she leaves the hospital to clear the nasal carriage of *N. meningitides* if solely treated with penicillin (or chloramphenicol, which is mainly used in nonindustrialized settings), which does not reliably eliminate nasal carriage. Adequate chemoprophylaxis regimens include **rifampin** 600 mg twice a day for 3 days, a single 500-mg dose of **ciprofloxacin,** or 250 mg of **intramuscular ceftriaxone** administered once.

The **meningococcal vaccine** contains the capsular polysaccharides of **groups A, C, Y, and W-135 strains, but not group B,** which is a major cause of disease but poorly immunogenic. Groups qualifying for the vaccine are military personnel, individuals who travel to endemic regions, splenectomized patients, and individuals with C5–C9 or properdin deficiency. College freshmen are often offered the vaccination upon entry to college depending on the institution.

CASE CONCLUSION

NA quickly entered a full septic shock syndrome and was intubated and continued on high-dose ceftriaxone. She died 18 hours after admission despite vigorous attempts to reverse the syndrome of septic shock. All close contacts and fellow dormitory dwellers underwent chemoprophylaxis with single doses of ciprofloxacin administered within several days of NA's presentation.

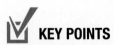 **KEY POINTS**

■ *N. meningitides* causes meningitis and meningococcemia, often accompanied by septic shock with widespread purpura and petechiae

■ Risk factors for *N. meningitides* infection include close, crowded conditions, splenectomy, and late complement and properdin deficiencies

■ Increasing rate of penicillin resistance in the meningococcus, necessitating initial treatment with ceftriaxone

■ Chemoprophylaxis indicated for close contacts of the index patient to eliminate nasal carriage of *N. meningitides* and further transmission and infection. Meningococcal vaccination is indicated for patients with the risk factors listed above.

QUESTIONS

1. Which of the following side effects occurs commonly with the administration of rifampin for *N. meningitides* chemoprophylaxis?

   A. Liver failure
   B. Renal failure
   C. Orange discoloration of secretions
   D. Anemia
   E. Leukopenia

2. Which of the following organisms is also a gram-negative coccus?

   A. *Pseudomonas aeruginosa*
   B. *Listeria monocytogenes*
   C. *Streptococcus pneumoniae*
   D. *Chlamydia trachomatis*
   E. *Moraxella catarrhalis*

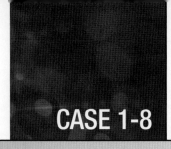

CASE 1-8

Gram-Negative Rods that Cause Gastrointestinal Infections

HPI: SS is a 34–year-old woman normally in good health who presents to your office with a 3-day history of diarrhea. She first started having small amounts of brown, watery stools 3 days ago, and noted blood and mucus in her stool over the past 2 days. SS also reports 2 days of fever and severe abdominal cramping, which is often relieved by defecation. She does not have any cough, shortness of breath, nausea, vomiting, pain with urination, or rash. She has been trying to keep fluids down but has not eaten much over the past 3 days. One of her children had a 2- to 3-day history of watery diarrhea last week without accompanying blood in the stool or fever.

PMH: Had appendectomy at age 14; SS does not take any regular medications and has no drug allergies. Married with two children (ages 4 and 6).

PE: T 38.6°C; HR 116; BP 98/68; RR 12

SS's abdomen is diffusely tender to palpation and no masses are appreciated. Bowel sounds are present. Rectal exam significant for brownish-green stool with streaks of blood and mucus. No rashes. Lung and heart exam within normal limits.

Labs: WBC 13.5 with 90% neutrophils; all other lab tests within normal limits.

THOUGHT QUESTIONS

- How would you distinguish between an upper gastrointestinal (GI) syndrome and a lower GI syndrome?
- What are the types of organisms that cause either upper or lower GI syndromes?
- What are the bacterial etiologies of diarrhea?
- Which of these bacterial organisms tend to cause bloody diarrhea?

BASIC SCIENCE REVIEW AND DISCUSSION

The major clinical manifestations of **upper GI infections (gastroenteritis)** are usually nausea, vomiting, and watery diarrhea. A number of pathogens and preformed toxins can lead to such syndromes. The most common viral pathogens that cause upper GI infections are Norwalk virus, calicivirus, astrovirus, and rotavirus: **Norwalk virus** infection is characterized mainly by nausea and vomiting, and **rotavirus** is the most common cause of pediatric diarrhea worldwide.

The **toxin-mediated** upper GI infections are usually caused by enterotoxin-producing strains of ***Staphylococcus aureus, Bacillus cereus,*** or ***Clostridium perfringens.*** The mean time to illness from ingestion of preformed *S. aureus* toxin is 2 to 7 hours, and the staphylococcal food poisoning syndrome is characterized mainly by vomiting with occasional mild diarrhea. *B. cereus* strains can produce two different toxins: a heat-stable toxin that can result in diarrhea after 2 to 7 hours and a heat-labile toxin that can result in disease manifestations 8 to 14 hours after ingestion. The classic food associated with *B. cereus* poisoning is reheated fried rice. Finally, the enterotoxin of *C. perfringens* is heat labile and usually results in clinical manifestations 8 to 14 hours after food consumption. The syndrome of enterotoxigenic *C. perfringens* is usually dominated by mild to moderate diarrhea with abdominal cramping; vomiting is less common with *B. cereus* and *C. perfringens* infections.

Lower GI syndromes (enterocolitis) are manifested mainly by the symptom of diarrhea, and the responsible pathogens can be bacterial, viral, or parasitic. The most common viral agent of diarrhea

in the immunocompetent patient is **rotavirus,** although this infection is rarely seen in adults. Rotavirus infections are major causes of dehydration and mortality in children in the developing world. **Adenoviruses** are increasingly recognized as agents of pediatric diarrhea as well, especially in industrialized regions.

In terms of **protozoal** causes of diarrhea, ***Cryptosporidium*** has been associated with waterborne outbreaks of diarrhea in both immunocompetent and immunocompromised hosts. ***Cyclospora*** is increasingly reported in foodborne diarrhea outbreaks, especially associated with imported berries. ***Giardia lamblia*** infection can manifest as both an acute and chronic syndrome: acute giardiasis presents with loose, foul-smelling stools accompanied by flatulence, abdominal cramping, bloating, nausea, anorexia, and malaise. Chronic giardiasis can present with just malaise and diffuse epigastric abdominal discomfort without diarrhea. ***Entamoeba histolytica*** infection usually presents as **dysentery** (bloody diarrhea mixed with mucus) accompanied by lower abdominal cramping, tenesmus, fever, and flatulence. The differential for acute diarrhea in the immunocompromised host broadens to include a wide variety of other viral and parasitic pathogens.

In terms of **bacterial** etiologies of diarrhea, the most common agents are enteric gram-negative rods. These syndromes are typically divided into **invasive** infections and **noninvasive** infections, with the former more likely to cause bloody diarrhea. Noninvasive enteric bacterial infections are typically caused by enterotoxigenic *Escherichia coli* (ETEC), enteropathogenic *E. coli* (EPEC), and enteroaggregative *E. coli* (EAggEC) strains, all acquired from ingestion of contaminated water or food. Other bacterial etiologies of noninvasive enterocolitis include *Vibrio cholerae* (cholera), *Clostridium difficile* toxin (antibiotic-associated diarrhea that can also lead to an invasive syndrome), *Salmonella enteritides* (a fast-growing organism with a fairly short time period of 14 to 21 hours from ingestion to symptoms), and *Vibrio parahaemolyticus* (usually acquired from ingestion of contaminated undercooked or raw seafood). The cholera toxin is an enterotoxin that is found in many other bacterial species and causes watery diarrhea, either alone or in combination with mucosal invasion.

TABLE 1-3 Bacterial Organisms

Organism	Source of Infection	Pathogenesis	Syndrome	Comments
Shigella dysenteriae, S. flexneri, S. boydii (mostly in travelers); *S. sonnei* (most common in U.S.—more mild disease)	Transmitted by the "4 F's:" food, finger, feces, and flies	Organism invades mucosa of distal ileum and colon; also has a cholera toxin-like enterotoxin	Fever, crampy abdominal pain, diarrhea—watery at first, but then with blood and mucus	Low infectious dose (ingestion of as few as 100 organisms causes disease)
Salmonella typhi, Salmonella paratyphi A, B, and C; *Salmonella choleraesuis*	Ingestion of fecally contaminated food or water	Enterocolitis characterized by invasion of small and large intestinal tissue	Variety of syndromes: typhoid fever has few GI symptoms, with constipation predominating; enterocolitis causes abdominal pain and diarrhea, with or without blood (mostly *Salmonella typhimurium*)	Infectious dose is 10^4 to 10^5 organisms
Campylobacter jejuni	Contaminated water and raw food (especially poultry); domestic animals (cattle, chickens, and dogs) serve as a source of human transmission	Organism often invades intestinal mucosa, but also has cholera toxin-like enterotoxin	Enterocolitis begins as a watery, foul-smelling diarrhea followed by bloody stools, severe abdominal pain, and fever	*C. jejuni* GI infection is associated with Guillain-Barré syndrome; organism is a comma- or S-shaped gram-negative rod
Enteroinvasive *E. coli*	Ingestion of contaminated food and water	Plasmid-mediated invasion of epithelial cells	Fever, cramping, watery diarrhea as initial syndrome, followed by scant bloody stools	Common in travelers returning from Europe and Latin America
Enterohemorrhagic *E. coli*, including the 0157:H7 serotype	Ingestion of contaminated food (e.g., undercooked hamburger) and water	Verotoxin (called this because it's toxic to Vero [monkey] cells in culture), which blocks protein synthesis	Diarrhea is bloody, but often without leukocytes; fever is uncommon; severe cases can lead to hemolytic-uremic syndrome, hallmarked by microangiopathic hemolytic anemia, thrombocytopenia, and acute renal failure	Antibiotic treatment of children with *E. coli* 0157:H7 infection seems to increase the risk of the hemolytic uremic syndrome

Wong CS, Jelacic S, Habeeb RL, et al. The risk of the hemolytic-uremic syndrome after antibiotic treatment of Escherichia coli *0157:H7 infections. N Engl J Med 2000;342:1930–1936.*

This enterotoxin ribosylates GTP-binding protein and causes a sustained increase in adenylate cyclase activity and intracellular accumulation of cyclic AMP, triggering a molecular cascade that ultimately manifests in the symptom of diarrhea.

Table 1-3 presents some of the distinguishing characteristics of bacterial organisms in the United States that can lead to mucosal invasion and dysentery.

CASE CONCLUSION

Stool culture from SS revealed **Shigella sonnei,** a non–lactose-fermenting gram-negative rod. She was treated with fluids and given a 5-day course of ciprofloxacin for treatment. Her child's diarrhea had resolved completely, so he was not given any treatment. SS's diarrhea, fever, and abdominal pain resolved 2 days after starting the antibiotics.

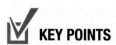 **THUMBNAIL:** Bloody Diarrhea

Organism	Shigella (S. dysenteriae, S. flexneri, S. boydii, S. sonnei)
Type of organism	Non–lactose-fermenting gram-negative rods
Diseases caused	All cause an acute lower GI syndrome; after an incubation period of 1 to 4 days, symptoms begin with abdominal cramps followed initially by watery diarrhea and then diarrhea mixed with blood and mucus; fever is common
Epidemiology	S. dysenteriae, S. boydii, and S. flexneri are usually only seen in recently returned travelers from abroad; S. sonnei, which causes a more mild disease than the others, is isolated from approximately 75% of all individuals with shigellosis in the United States; Shigella has a very low infectious dose, with only about 100 organisms required to produce illness in 25% of exposed patients
Diagnosis	Stool culture
Treatment	The main treatment for shigellosis is fluid and electrolyte replacement; antibiotics are not needed in mild cases but may reduce the duration of symptoms in more severe cases; ciprofloxacin is now the drug of choice given increasing TMP-SMX resistance in the organism; antiperistaltic agents may prolong the excretion of the organism and prolong the symptoms of fever and diarrhea

KEY POINTS

- Upper GI syndromes are accompanied by nausea and vomiting with or without watery diarrhea and usually are caused by viral infections or bacteria-derived enterotoxins, such as S. aureus toxin, B. cereus toxin, and C. perfringens toxin

- Lower GI syndromes can be caused by adenoviral or rotaviral infections, intestinal protozoa, or bacteria; latter infections can be either noninvasive or invasive, leading to bloody diarrhea in the latter

- Main bacterial etiologies of bloody diarrhea in the United States include Shigella, Salmonella, Campylobacter, enteroinvasive E. coli (EIEC), and enterohemorrhagic E. coli (EHEC)

- Shigella species are non–lactose-fermenting gram-negative rods that cause dysentery with a very low infectious dose of 100 organisms; accompanying symptoms include fever and abdominal cramping

QUESTIONS

1. Which of the following pathogens are associated with watery diarrhea after an incubation period of 8 to 14 hours?

    A. Rotavirus and Norwalk virus
    B. Shigella and Salmonella
    C. EIEC and EHEC
    D. S. aureus and B. cereus
    E. B. cereus and C. perfringens

2. If SS's stool culture showed comma- or S-shaped gram-negative rods, which of the listed agents is the most likely etiology of her diarrhea?

    A. Giardia lamblia
    B. Salmonella typhi
    C. Bacillus cereus
    D. Campylobacter jejuni
    E. Shigella dysenteriae

HPI: PA is an 18-year-old female with cystic fibrosis who presents to the emergency department with 2 days of worsening shortness of breath and cough. Her cough is productive of greenish sputum and she also complains of a low-grade fever. PA denies any abdominal pain, nausea, or vomiting. She has chronic diarrhea controlled by pancreatic enzymes, which has not changed in any way. PA is usually admitted to the hospital two or three times a year for pneumonia and worsening pulmonary function in the setting of her chronic lung disease.

PMH: As stated above, PA has cystic fibrosis with a history of multiple pneumonias and hospital admissions. Chronic medications include Pancrease enzymes and various bronchodilators. No allergies to medications.

PE: T 38.4°C; HR 118; BP 95/60; RR 20; SaO$_2$ on room air 89%

PA is generally thin and chronically ill in appearance. Her lung exam is significant for diffuse crackles and wheezing throughout both lung fields.

Labs: WBC 11.5 with 80% neutrophils. Sputum shows slender Gram-negative rods on Gram stain and the chest X-ray shows patchy pneumonia in both lower lobes on top of PA's chronic lung disease.

THOUGHT QUESTIONS

- What is the most likely etiology of PA's pneumonia?
- What are the characteristics of this organism?
- What kind of infections does this organism cause?
- How would you diagnose this infection?
- How would you treat this infection?

BASIC SCIENCE REVIEW AND DISCUSSION

The most likely etiology of PA's pneumonia is a *Pseudomonas* species given the fact that cystic fibrosis patients are susceptible to pseudomonal infections and given the characteristic Gram stain.

Characteristics

Pseudomonas species are **aerobic** Gram-negative rods that do not ferment glucose for energy. These organisms are called **nonfermenters** as compared with the *Enterobacteriaceae*, which ferment glucose for energy. *Pseudomonas* species derive their energy by oxidation of sugars rather than by fermentation, so they are **oxidase positive**. *Pseudomonas aeruginosa* is one of the major species in the *Pseudomonas* genus and derives its name from the production of various pigments, including **pyoverdin**, a yellow-green pigment, and **pyocyanin**, a blue or green pigment. *P. aeruginosa* is motile, nutritionally versatile, and can grow at a variety of temperatures (optimally at 37°C, but can also grow at 42°C).

Transmission and Epidemiology

P. aeruginosa is found in soil, water, plants, and animals and can be found in various **water supplies,** including disinfectants, in the hospital setting. Given its minimal nutritional requirements, *P. aeruginosa* can exist in a number of different environmental settings and is a major etiology of **nosocomial infections.** *P. aeruginosa* can also compose part of the normal microbial flora of humans, with rates of colonization enhanced in hospitalized patients.

Although *P. aeruginosa* is ubiquitous in the environment, pseudomonal infections are mainly **opportunistic and affect compromised hosts.** For instance, **patients with extensive burns** have impaired skin host defense mechanisms, predisposing them to *P. aeruginosa* invasion. **Cystic fibrosis patients** or other patients with chronic lung disease have impaired respiratory clearance mechanisms, predisposing them to *P. aeruginosa* colonization and subsequent disease.

Clinical Syndromes

P. aeruginosa can cause a variety of clinical syndromes, including:

1. **Respiratory infections:** *P. aeruginosa* pneumonia occurs almost exclusively in patients with compromised lung function or systemic immunocompromise. Exposure to the hospital environment, especially in ICUs, **endotracheal intubation, and prior use of antibiotics** increase the likelihood of *P. aeruginosa* pneumonia. Other risk factors for this condition include cystic fibrosis, chronic bronchiectasis or other chronic lung diseases, **neutropenia,** administration of cancer chemotherapy, and **AIDS.** Cystic fibrosis patients tend to develop lower respiratory tract infections with **mucoid strains** of *P. aeruginosa*.

2. **Urinary tract infections:** *P. aeruginosa* infections of the urinary tract are often nosocomial, iatrogenic, and related to prolonged **urinary tract catheterization.** *Pseudomonas* UTIs occur frequently in chronic care facilities and frequently plague spinal cord injury victims. *P. aeruginosa* UTIs are often recurrent, and clearance may require removal of urinary tract catheters.

3. **Skin and soft tissue infections:** *Pseudomonas* bacteremia can produce distinctive skin lesions called **ecthyma gangrenosum,** which involve local hemorrhage, necrosis, surrounding erythema, and vascular invasion by the *Pseudomonas* bacteria. Bacteremia can also be associated with subcutaneous nodules, deep abscesses, cellulitis, bullae, necrotizing fasciitis, and vesicular or pustular lesions. Primary *P. aeruginosa* skin and soft tissue infections can be localized

or diffuse, and predisposing factors include burns, trauma, decubitus ulcers, dermatitis, and **frequent swimming or exposure to water.**

4. **Ear infections:** *P. aeruginosa* is the predominant bacterial pathogen of **external auditory canal otitis** and is usually associated with injury, meatal maceration, inflammation, chronic humid conditions in the ear, and swimming (**"swimmer's ear"**). This infection is manifested by an itchy or painful ear with discharge and edema and is treated with **topical application of antibiotic-** and steroid-containing otic solutions. **"Malignant" external otitis** is defined by locally invasive *P. aeruginosa* infections of the external auditory canal, with destruction of underlying soft tissues. This condition occurs mainly in **elderly diabetic patients** and requires **systemic therapy.**

5. **Other:** Other *P. aeruginosa*-associated conditions include endocarditis, meningitis, brain abscess, eye infections, **bone and joint infections,** and **necrotizing enterocolitis,** especially in young infants and **neutropenic cancer patients.**

Diagnosis

Diagnosis of *P. aeruginosa* infection is made by Gram stain and culture. *P. aeruginosa* grows as **non–lactose-fermenting, oxidase-positive colonies,** and these Gram-negative rods have a **typical slender morphology** (Fig. 1-8).

Treatment

P. aeruginosa is resistant to a number of antibiotics. The four classes of antibiotics that are most commonly used against *Pseudomonas* species are listed below (Table 1-4). Serious infections often require combination therapy among these classes of antibiotics.

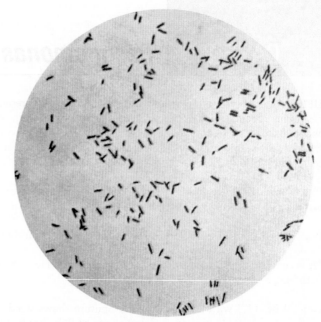

● **Figure 1-8.** Slender Gram-negative rods typical of *Pseudomonas aeruginosa*. (Image in public domain from Centers for Disease Control and Prevention Public Health Image Library, http://phil.cdc.gov/phil/home.asp)

TABLE 1-4 Antibiotic Classes Effective for *Pseudomonas*

Drug Class	Examples
1. Aminoglycosides	Gentamicin, tobramycin
2. Fluoroquinolones	Ciprofloxacin
3. Antipseudomonal penicillins	Ticarcillin, piperacillin,
4. Third- and fourth-generation cephalosporins	Ceftazidime and cefepime, respectively
Other active agents include:	
5. Aztreonam (monobactam)	
6. Imipenem-cilastatin	

THUMBNAIL: *P. aeruginosa* Pneumonia

Organism	*P. aeruginosa*
Type of organism	Oxidase-positive, aerobic Gram-negative rod
Diseases caused	Respiratory tract infections, especially in patients with cystic fibrosis and chronic lung disease, UTIs, external otitis and malignant external otitis, bacteremia, ecthyma gangrenosum, skin and soft tissue infections, bone and joint infections, eye infections, and necrotizing enterocolitis in young infants and neutropenic patients
Epidemiology	*P. aeruginosa* mainly causes disease in hosts with impaired immune function, impaired respiratory tracts, and impaired skin defenses; major cause of nosocomial infections; found ubiquitously in soil and water, including water supplies in hospital environment
Diagnosis	Oxidase-positive, non–lactose-fermenting slender Gram-negative rod seen on Gram stain of affected tissue
Treatment	Fluoroquinolones; aminoglycosides; antipseudomonal penicillins; third- and fourth-generation cephalosporins and imipenem; serious infections may require combination therapy with an aminoglycoside and an appropriate β-lactam antibiotic

CASE CONCLUSION

Culture of PA's sputum grew out a mucoid strain of *P. aeruginosa*. She was treated with a combination of piperacillin and tobramycin in-house and discharged on a course of oral ciprofloxacin with gradual improvement.

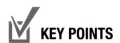 **KEY POINTS**

- *P. aeruginosa* is an oxidase-positive, aerobic, non–lactose-fermenting Gram-negative rod with minimal nutritional requirements and the ability to live in hospital water supplies
- Major cause of infection in nosocomial setting and in compromised hosts
- Major clinical syndromes are respiratory, skin, and soft tissue infections; UTIs; bone and joint infections; and eye and ear infections
- Resistant to multiple antibiotics, and mainstays of treatment are fluoroquinolones, aminoglycosides, antipseudomonal penicillins, and third- and fourth-generation cephalosporins

QUESTIONS

1. Which of the following combination would be most appropriate for a serious *P. aeruginosa* pneumonia with bacteremia in a bone marrow transplant recipient?

   A. Penicillin and gentamicin
   B. Cefepime and tobramycin
   C. Cefepime and piperacillin
   D. Ciprofloxacin and cefuroxime
   E. Imipenem and ticarcillin

2. Which of the following is a risk factor for *P. aeruginosa*-associated necrotizing enterocolitis?

   A. Use of prior antibiotics
   B. Mesenteric ischemia
   C. Neutropenia
   D. Ulcerative colitis
   E. Pseudomembranous colitis

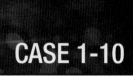

CASE 1-10 *Salmonella Typhi*

HPI: A 27-year-old man returns from a 2-week trip to India with a fever and abdominal pain. He also complains of constipation.

The patient had full immunizations, including typhoid and hepatitis A, before leaving on his trip. He took mefloquine for malaria prophylaxis during the trip, and used insect repellent. His friend did not become ill on the trip. He has no past medical history. He works as a prep cook in a salad bar restaurant.

PE: T 40.0°C; BP 120/70; HR 85; RR 16

A toxic-looking man in no acute distress. The skin of his trunk shows some faint salmon-colored macules. His oropharynx is benign. He has some mild cervical and axillary lymphadenopathy. Lungs are clear. Heart is regular in rhythm, but the relatively slow heart rate for his fever is noted. His belly is diffusely tender, but there are no peritoneal signs. There is mild hepatosplenomegaly but no masses. No peripheral edema; no embolic stigmata on the extremities.

Labs: His complete blood count shows a leukopenic white count of 2.1, anemia with a hematocrit of 38, and thrombocytopenia with platelets of 95.

Thick blood smears are negative for malaria.

Dengue serologies are negative. An HIV test is negative.

One of two blood cultures, a stool culture, and a skin biopsy of his rash grow out *Salmonella typhi*.

THOUGHT QUESTIONS

- What are common causes of fever to consider in a returning traveler?
- What clinical syndromes can *Salmonella* cause?
- Why is the patient's occupation important in this case?

BASIC SCIENCE REVIEW AND DISCUSSION

See Table 1-14 (in Case 1-26) for a differential of fever in a traveler. **Typhoid fever** is a febrile illness caused by *S. typhi*, a gram-negative rod. It is spread through fecal-oral transmission. It should not be confused with unrelated but similarly named febrile illnesses collectively known as **typhus,** caused by the rickettsial species. Murine typhus (*Rickettsia typhi*), scrub typhus (*Orientia tsutsugamushi*), and epidemic typhus (*Rickettsia prowazekii*) are all spread by arthropod vectors.

Salmonella strains can be distinguished on the basis of serologic and biochemical tests. They can cause two clinical presentations. **Gastroenteritis** is caused by strains such as *S. enteritidis* and *S. typhimurium*, along with others collectively known as the nontyphoidal salmonellae. This self-limited illness is characterized by nausea, vomiting, and nonbloody diarrhea, along with fevers and abdominal cramping. The other presentation, **typhoid fever,** is caused by *S. typhi* and *S. paratyphi*. Typhoid fever is more serious than *Salmonella* gastroenteritis; about 10% of untreated patients die. Patients commonly suffer high fevers and abdominal pain. Although diarrhea can occur, constipation is actually more common. Patients often manifest **relative bradycardia**—their heart rate does not increase in proportion to their body temperature. One third of patients have **rose spots,** a faint salmon-pink maculopapular rash, usually over the trunk. Blood counts often show leukopenia, anemia, and thrombocytopenia. Typhoid fever causes swelling of gut-associated lymphoid tissue, which can result in intestinal perforation or necrosis.

Typhoid fever is diagnosed by culture of *Salmonella* from blood, stool, urine, or skin biopsy of a rose spot. Bone marrow and duodenal cultures are more invasive but higher yield sites . Unfortunately, serology is not reliable in making the diagnosis.

Whereas the nontyphoidal salmonellae can grow in animals and may be transmitted by poultry, eggs, or reptilian pets, *S. typhi* and *S. paratyphi* only grow in humans. Typhoid fever is spread through fecal-oral transmission, but this is usually indirect, through contaminated food or water. Typhoid vaccines are available and are recommended by the Centers for Disease Control and Prevention before travel to endemic countries, although they are not highly protective as seen in our patient. Three forms, a heat-killed whole-organism vaccine, a live-attenuated oral vaccine, and a capsular polysaccharide vaccine, are available. Typhoid fever is generally treated with fluoroquinolone antibiotics. **Carriage** of the organism can persist for weeks, particularly in patients with gallstones or other anatomic derangements of the gallbladder; carriers can subsequently potentially infect many other people.

CASE CONCLUSION

The patient is given a course of fluoroquinolone treatment and his fever resolves after 2 days. His case is reported to the Department of Public Health. To minimize the risk of spreading his illness, he is switched to a non-food handling position until follow-up stool cultures are negative for *S. typhi*.

THUMBNAIL: *Salmonella typhi* and *Salmonella paratyphi*

Organism	*S. typhi* and *S. paratyphi*
Type of organism	Aerobic, gram-negative rods
Disease caused	Typhoid fever
Epidemiology	Fecal-oral spread, usually via food or water; a major role is played by asymptomatic carriers; there is no animal reservoir; most typhoid fever in the United States is contracted through developing-world travel
Diagnosis	Blood culture; stool culture to show carriage; serology is not reliable
Treatment	Fluoroquinolone
Prevention	Typhoid vaccine

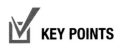

KEY POINTS

- Most serotypes of *Salmonella* cause gastroenteritis, but *S. typhi* and *S. paratyphi* cause typhoid fever, a more serious, systemic illness
- Typhoid fever is spread through fecal-oral transmission

QUESTIONS

1. What biochemical feature of *Salmonella* distinguishes it from most of the enteric flora (other enterobacteraciae)?

    A. Lactose nonfermenter
    B. Glucose fermenter
    C. Oxidase negative
    D. Nitrate reducer
    E. Failure to produce hydrogen sulfide

2. Which of the following is caused by *S. typhimurium*?

    A. Murine typhus
    B. Epidemic typhus
    C. Scrub typhus
    D. Typhoid fever
    E. Gastroenteritis

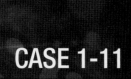

CASE 1-11 *Mycobacterium Tuberculosis*

HPI: A 36-year-old woman, born in the Philippines, is admitted to the hospital for a work-up of bloody stools. Although this is her first episode of frank blood, she has had episodes of melena over the past 6 months. She notes a 30-pound weight loss over the last 6 months, with occasional fevers and night sweats. She denies cough, hemoptysis, abdominal pain, or orthostasis. She has no family history of cancer.

PE: T 37.9°C; BP 120/70; HR 80; RR 14

The patient is a thin woman in no distress. Lungs are clear. There is no abdominal tenderness or palpable masses. A rectal exam shows a small amount of bloody stool, with no palpable masses.

Labs: WBC 12, normal differential. She has a microcytic anemia, with a hematocrit of 29 and a mean corpuscular volume (MCV) of 75. Electrolytes are normal. Amebic serologies are negative.

A chest X-ray shows small, calcified upper lobe nodules interpreted as evidence of old granulomatous disease.

The patient undergoes colonoscopy. A large 8-cm fungating lesion is seen in her right colon, with an appearance classic for colon cancer. Biopsies are taken and sent to pathology. After the endoscopy, the gastroenterologist tells the patient she likely has cancer. To the gastroenterologist's surprise, the pathologist calls the biopsies inconclusive. Because of her chest X-ray, a purified protein derivative (PPD) tuberculosis is placed, and is positive. The pathologist stains the colon specimens for AFB (acid-fast bacilli), but no organisms are seen. Unfortunately, the colonic lesion was not sent for culture. Nonetheless, the patient is started on empiric four-drug TB therapy, with isoniazid, rifampin, pyrazinamide, and ethambutol.

THOUGHT QUESTIONS

- Which parts of the body are most commonly affected by tuberculosis (TB)?
- Is this patient contagious?
- If four drugs are necessary to treat a case of active TB, why is only one drug necessary to treat latent TB infection?

BASIC SCIENCE REVIEW AND DISCUSSION

Mycobacteria are rod-shaped bacteria with a thick, waxy coat. The chemical properties of this coat allow them to be detected with an **acid-fast stain**—hence the name acid-fast bacilli (of note, the acid-fast stain can also stain *Nocardia.*) The traditional acid-fast technique is being replaced by a more sensitive fluorescent stain.

Mycobacteria are divided into two groups. The first group is the ***Mycobacterium tuberculosis* complex** (made up of *M. tuberculosis* and the difficult-to-distinguish *M. bovis*), which causes TB, the leading cause of infectious mortality in the world. One third of the world's population is infected with TB. *M. tuberculosis* is only found in humans and is acquired by person-to-person contact. A positive culture for *M. tuberculosis* indicates infection that must be treated. The second group is the **nontuberculous mycobacteria,** which by contrast are free-living and acquired from the environment. The nontuberculous mycobacteria usually affect immunocompromised hosts. Their presence in a culture may reflect disease but can also be caused by colonization or contamination.

M. tuberculosis may be distinguished on culture by its slow rate of growth (taking up to 6 weeks to detect), lack of pigment, and "cording" morphology (the long edges of the bacilli are aligned parallel to each other). *M. tuberculosis* is usually sensitive to the drug isoniazid, whereas many species of nontuberculous mycobacteria are resistant.

Almost all transmission of TB is due to inhalation of infectious respiratory droplets from an infected patient. The droplets are small, requiring specialized masks to filter them from the air. The droplets may also persist for hours after an infected person has left the room. However, TB is not easily caught, and transmission usually requires exposure for many hours. Primary infection occurs at the site of inhalation in the lungs and usually resolves, with the body walling off the bacteria. At a later time, however, the infection can **reactivate,** causing disease. The most frequent site of reactivation is in the lungs, particularly in the apices where the oxygen tension is highest. TB can also spread from the lung parenchyma to the pleural space. TB can affect almost any part of the body, however. After the lungs, other common sites include the genitourinary system, GI tract, meningeal space, lymph nodes, or bone. In some cases, TB is spread through the bloodstream, creating many tiny foci of infection, referred to as **miliary** TB. The pathologic hallmark of TB infection is **caseating granuloma** formation at the site of infection.

The **PPD** test can be used to identify people who have ever had primary TB infection. This test measures cellular immunity against a purified protein derivative of *M. tuberculosis*. The test measures the size of the cell-mediated hypersensitivity response several days after intradermal injection of the PPD. Cutoffs in millimeters for a positive test differ depending on the patient population; in general, patients who are immunocompromised or who have a higher likelihood of reactivation are screened with a lower cutoff, resulting in a more sensitive test. Patients who are anergic as a result of immunocompromise or overwhelming mycobacterial infection may have false-negative tests. Patients who are identified as PPD positive but have no signs of active infection are considered to have latent **TB infection,** and are usually given a course of treatment to kill the remaining tubercle bacilli at the site of primary infection to prevent later reactivation disease. The treatment is usually isoniazid for 6 to 9 months. The long course is necessary because of the slow growth rate of the mycobacteria.

Patients who have active disease are usually diagnosed by AFB smears or cultures from the suspected site of infection. Rarely, patients are treated empirically, and the diagnosis is made by clinical improvement after TB therapy is started. In contrast to latent TB infection, patients with active TB have a much larger number of mycobacteria in their bodies and must be treated with a combination of drugs to avoid the selection of antibiotic-resistant organisms. Usually, a patient is treated with four drugs (isoniazid, rifampin, pyrazinamide, and ethambutol) until the susceptibilities of the infecting strain are known. Other drugs exist to treat TB but are second line because of lower efficacy and difficulties of administration, side effects, or cost. In particular, patients with **multidrug-resistant TB** (defined as TB resistant to both isoniazid and rifampin) are difficult to treat. Because of the long courses of treatment required for active TB and the risk of creating resistant strains if partial treatment is given, patients are often given **directly observed therapy** (DOT) if there is any doubt about their ability to adhere to the treatment regimen. Patients with active TB who are in institutional settings (hospitals, nursing homes, or prisons) must be isolated. Epidemiologic investigation of all new TB cases and evaluation of close contacts for disease are crucial measures in preventing the spread of TB in the community.

The major recent issues in TB control have been a rise in urban TB rates coinciding with the HIV epidemic and a rise in multidrug-resistant TB. These problems have been addressed by increased surveillance and treatment of latent TB in HIV-positive patients and by an increase in spending on DOT to improve adherence and prevent the emergence of resistant strains. Recently, most new cases of TB in the United States have been in immigrants who acquired their disease in countries with higher prevalence rates of TB.

A TB vaccine, **Bacille Calmette-Guérin (BCG),** exists but is not used in this country. It decreases the incidence of extrapulmonary TB, especially TB meningitis, but has not been shown to reduce the incidence of pulmonary disease. The vaccination may cause false-positive PPDs but will usually not cause a PPD of greater than 10 mm unless the vaccine has been recently administered. In a patient from a country of high TB prevalence, a positive PPD is more likely to reflect latent TB infection than represent a false-positive test due to the BCG immunization.

CASE CONCLUSION

The patient continues on four-drug TB therapy for 1 month, with an improvement in her weight loss and fevers. On repeat endoscopy after 1 month of TB therapy, the colonic lesion has almost completely resolved. The patient finishes a 6-month course of TB therapy.

THUMBNAIL: *Mycobacterium tuberculosis*

Type of organism	*Mycobacterium*; acid-fast bacillus
Disease caused	Tuberculosis
Epidemiology	Spreads person to person through aerosol droplets
Diagnosis	Latent infection is diagnosed through PPD skin testing; active infection is diagnosed via acid-fast smears and mycobacterial cultures from the affected site, usually sputum
Treatment	Latent infection is treated with 6 to 9 months of isoniazid; active infection is usually treated with combination therapy; initially, isoniazid, rifampin, pyrazinamide, and ethambutol are given; pyrazinamide and ethambutol usually can be discontinued once antibiotic susceptibilities return

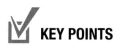

KEY POINTS

■ *M. tuberculosis* is a slow-growing mycobacterium that is transmitted from person to person via respiratory aerosols

■ Most active TB disease results from reactivation of a previous primary infection; the most common site for active TB is the lungs, but infection can be seen at many other sites

■ Patients who have been exposed to TB but have no active disease are said to have latent TB infection and are treated to reduce their chances of active TB in the future

■ Active TB must be treated with multiple drugs to avoid selection for drug-resistant organisms

QUESTIONS

1. Which of the following patients is most infectious?

   A. An 18 year old with tuberculous lymphadenitis of the neck (scrofula)
   B. A 36 year old with HIV, a negative PPD, lung cavities on chest X-ray, and sputum with a positive AFB smear
   C. A 46 year old with a positive PPD and no cough
   D. A 71 year old with a positive PPD, a right upper lobe infiltrate, and sputum that is AFB smear negative but culture positive
   E. A 24 year old with TB meningitis

2. Which of the following drugs is a first-line agent against TB?

   A. Streptomycin
   B. Pyrazinamide
   C. Para-aminosalicylic acid (PAS)
   D. Levofloxacin
   E. Cycloserine

3. Which toxicity do all of the first-line TB drugs have in common?

   A. Neuropathy
   B. Optic neuritis
   C. Hepatotoxicity
   D. Serious drug-drug interactions
   E. Hyperuricemia

4. Which of the following patients needs to be started on multidrug therapy for TB?

   A. An asymptomatic 9-year-old Philippine immigrant with a positive PPD and a normal chest X-ray
   B. A 43 year old with a history of TB treated with three drugs for 6 months, who has calcified granulomas on his chest X-ray
   C. A 17 year old with a lymph node biopsy growing *M. tuberculosis*
   D. A 51-year-old nurse who was inadvertently exposed to a patient with active pulmonary TB in an emergency room for 30 minutes
   E. A 34-year-old man who sat on a bus for 2 hours next to a man with a hacking cough

Nontuberculous Mycobacteria

HPI: MF is a 28-year-old woman who presents to your office with complaints of recurrent boils on her lower extremities. You have seen this patient four times in the past 6 months for recurrent furuncles on both lower extremities. Cultures of these lesions have been negative for bacterial growth. The skin boils seem to have no response to the antibiotics that are commonly used for bacteria that cause skin infections. The lesions seem to resolve spontaneously but have led to scarring on MF's lower legs. She presents again today with recurrence of the skin boils on both legs. MF does not have any fevers or chills. She has never had any problems with skin infections or any other skin conditions prior to 6 months ago. MF receives manicures and pedicures every month and has not changed salons. She has not changed her skin lotion, soap, or detergent. MF shaves her legs with a disposable razor that she changes frequently and she does not use depilatories.

PMH: Intrauterine device infection 3 years ago, requiring removal. MF only takes oral contraceptive pills and has no allergies. Lives with boyfriend and is monogamous. Works at cosmetics counter.

PE: T 37.1°C; BP 115/78; HR 70; RR 16

MF has multiple scattered violaceous boils on both her lower extremities. Her lesions are only found below the knee in both legs, and several boils have areas of ulceration and bleeding. Multiple scars are visible around the boils on both legs.

Labs: WBC 9.0 with normal neutrophil count. You take cultures of the boil and the lab calls you in 3 days saying that an acid-fast organism is growing on routine bacterial media. The lab subsequently identifies this organism as a mycobacterial species and asks you if MF needs respiratory isolation.

THOUGHT QUESTIONS

- How do nontuberculous mycobacteria differ from *Mycobacterium tuberculosis*?
- How are the nontuberculous mycobacteria classified?
- What are the clinical syndromes caused by nontuberculous mycobacteria?
- What are the main species of rapidly growing mycobacteria that cause human disease?
- What are the clinical syndromes caused by rapidly growing mycobacteria?

BASIC SCIENCE REVIEW AND DISCUSSION

Nontuberculous Mycobacteria versus *M. Tuberculosis*

Nontuberculous mycobacteria (NTM) are defined as mycobacteria species other than the *M. tuberculosis* complex (comprised of the species *M. tuberculosis* and *M. bovis*); these species have also been called mycobacteria other than tubercle (MOTT) bacilli. Most of the NTM organisms have been isolated from water and soil and are **ubiquitous in the environment.** Hence, even potentially pathogenic isolates of NTM may be found as contaminants or colonizers as well as etiologic agents of infection. Most infections with NTM appear to be acquired by aspiration or inoculation of the organisms from a natural reservoir, and there is little evidence of person-to-person transmission of disease.

As a group, NTM differ in several respects from the classic tubercle bacilli:

1. NTM present with **varying degrees of acid fastness.**
2. NTM have a wider temperature range for growth and often grow comfortably at temperatures not found in the human body.
3. **Growth rates tend to be variable:** some species grow in less than 7 days; others have generation times similar to or longer than *M. tuberculosis*.
4. Many of the NTM have colonies that are pigmented yellow to orange.
5. NTM fail to produce progressive disease in guinea pigs, which is the traditional animal model for *M. tuberculosis*.
6. The majority of NTM will produce lesions in mice, however, depending on the route of inoculation.
7. **NTM show a general pattern of resistance to many of the first-line antituberculous agents,** such as rifampin, isoniazid, streptomycin, and ethambutol.
8. Human infections with NTM are frequently associated with preexisting disease or trauma.
9. Infected persons may or may not show skin hypersensitivity to protein derivatives of these mycobacterial species (analogous to the PPD delayed-type hypersensitivity reaction seen with *M. tuberculosis*).
10. NTM generally produce smooth colonies (some rough variants exist) and emulsify readily.

Clinical Syndromes of NTM

Dr. Ernst Runyon devised a scheme in the mid-1950s to classify NTM into four groups based on essentially two criteria: **pigment production and speed of growth.** "Rapid growers" are characterized by the ability to grow rapidly (2 to 7 days) at temperatures ranging from 25°C to 42°C. Colonies of the organisms in this group are generally smooth but rough variants may occur. The colonies may be pigmented or nonpigmented.

The typical clinical syndromes of NTM, along with their geographic distribution, are presented in Table 1-5.

TABLE 1-5 Classification of Nontuberculous Mycobacteria

Common Etiologic Species	Geography	Unusual Etiologic Species
Pulmonary disease		
M. avium-intracellulare	Worldwide	M. simiae, M. chelonae
M. kansasii	U.S., coal mining regions, Europe	M. szulgai, M. fortuitum
		M. celatum, M. asiaticum
M. abscessus	Worldwide, but mostly U.S.	M. shimodii
M. xenopi	Europe, Canada	M. haemophilum
M. malmoense	UK, northern Europe	M. smegmatis
Lymphadenitis		
M. avium intracellulare	Worldwide	M. fortuitum
M. scrofulaceum	Worldwide	M. chelonae, M. kansasii
M. malmoense	UK, northern Europe (especially Scandinavia)	M. abscessus
		M. haemophilum
Skin and soft tissue infection		
M. fortuitum, M. chelonae	Worldwide, mostly U.S.	M. smegmatis
M. abscessus		M. haemophilum
Abscesses, ulcers, sinus tracts		M. nonchromogenicum
M. marinum	Worldwide	
Swimming pool granuloma or sporotrichoid presentation		
M. ulcerans	Australia, tropics, Africa, S.E. Asia	
Chronic ulcer		
Mycobacterium Avium-Intracellularae (MAC), M. kansasii	Worldwide or U.S.	
Hyperimmune reactions		
Skeletal (bone, joint, and tendon infections)		
MAC	Worldwide	M. marinum
M. kansasii	Worldwide	M. scrofulaceum
M. fortuitum, M. chelonae	Worldwide, mostly U.S.	
Disseminated infection		
MAC	Worldwide	M. fortuitum
M. kansasii	U.S.	M. xenopi, M. simiae
M. chelonae	U.S.	M. malmoense
M. haemophilum	U.S., Australia	M. genavense
		M. conspicuum
		M. marinum

Syndromes of Rapidly Growing Mycobacteria

Rapidly growing mycobacteria are acid-fast rods that resemble diphtheroids on Gram stain. They usually grow as fast as in 1 to 7 days and thrive on most routine laboratory media, as well as on special media for isolation of mycobacteria. The ubiquitous rapid growers survive nutritional deprivation and extremes of temperature. They are recovered readily from soil, dust, and water and have also been isolated from tap water, municipal water supplies, moist areas in hospitals, contaminated biological solutions, aquariums, domestic animals, marine life, and even **contaminated whirlpool foot baths in nail salons.**

Most of the disease caused by rapid growers is sporadic and community acquired, although nosocomial outbreaks or clustered cases have been reported. For instance, there is a recognized association between rapidly growing mycobacterial wound infections

and the procedures of breast augmentation or coronary artery bypass grafting. A recent report[1] described a cluster of cases of lower extremity M. fortuitum furunculosis in women who received **pedicures** at a certain nail salon in northern California; the whirlpool foot bath in this facility was found to be contaminated with M. fortuitum. More than 90% of disease caused by rapid growers originates from three species: **M. fortuitum, M. chelonae, and M. abscessus.**

Rapid growers are the most common NTM species to cause **skin and subcutaneous tissue infections.** M. fortuitum, M. chelonae, and M. abscessus are, again, the three most frequently implicated species. The organisms often form abscesses at the site of puncture wounds (e.g., after stepping on a nail) or after open traumatic injuries or fractures. They can also cause nosocomial skin and soft tissue disease, including infections of long-term intravenous or peritoneal catheters, postinjection abscesses, or surgical wound infections. Incubation periods from the time of injury to clinical infection vary from 1 week to 2 years, but most infections occur within the first month. Infections may resemble pyogenic abscesses with an acute inflammatory reaction and suppuration, or they may progress slowly, with chronic granulomatous inflammation, ulceration, sinus tract formation, and exudates that resemble sporotrichosis. Patients may require **both antibiotic therapy and surgical management** to achieve cure.

Bronchopulmonary infections caused by the rapid growers usually occur following aspiration events. The largest epidemiologic group of patients with lung disease are **elderly (>60 years), Caucasian, female nonsmokers with no predisposing conditions or known lung disease.** Another epidemiologic group of patients susceptible to lung infection with the rapid growers are those with some underlying lung conditions. These patients tend to develop disease at a younger age (<50 years). Predisposing underlying disorders associated with these infections include lung damage produced by prior mycobacterial infection (usually TB or MAC), gastroesophageal (GE) disorders with chronic vomiting, lipoid pneumonia, cystic fibrosis, and bronchiectasis. Of note, these rapid growers may just colonize respiratory secretions without playing a clinical role in disease.

M. abscessus accounts for approximately 80% of rapidly growing mycobacterial respiratory disease isolates, whereas *M. fortuitum* accounts for approximately 15% of these syndromes. In the small group of patients with GE disorders and chronic vomiting, however, *M. abscessus* and *M. fortuitum* infection occur with equal frequency. The usuall presenting symptoms of these pulmonary infections are cough and fatigue, fevers, night sweats, and weight loss (similar to TB). Chest roentgenograms in these syndromes usually show multilobar, patchy, reticulonodular or mixed interstitial-alveolar infiltrates with an upper lobe predominance; cavitation occurs in approximately 15% of cases. High-resolution CT (HRCT) of the lung frequently shows associated cylindrical bronchiectasis and multiple small (<5 mm) nodules. The clinical course is highly variable—in most patients, the course is chronic and inexorably progressive; in others, more fulminant, rapidly progressive disease can occur, especially in association with GE disorders. Spontaneous recovery may rarely occur.

Other clinical syndromes of the rapid growers include lymphadenitis, keratitis, endophthalmitis, suppurative arthritis, osteomyelitis, endocarditis (on natural, prosthetic, or porcine valves), aortitis, meningitis, peritonitis, chronic urinary infections, solid pulmonary nodules, bacteremia related to in-dwelling IV catheters, or ventriculoperitoneal (VP) shunts.

CASE CONCLUSION

You tell the lab that respiratory isolation is not necessary for MF and ask for further identification of the mycobacterial organism. The species is identified as *M. fortuitum*. You start MF on ciprofloxacin and doxycycline and notify the local health department to initiate an investigation of the cleanliness of the nail salon frequented by MF.

THUMBNAIL: Rapidly Growing Mycobacteria

Organism	*M. fortuitum, M. chelonae, M. abscessus*
Type of organism	NTM (Runyon group IV)
Diseases caused	Skin and soft tissue infections, pulmonary infections
Epidemiology	Found in soil, dust, and water and can contaminate hospital water supplies; skin and soft tissue infections usually occur secondary to trauma or surgery; pulmonary infections occur in elderly, Caucasian females without underlying risk factors and in younger patients with underlying lung disease
Diagnosis	Culture drainage material, tissue biopsy, or sputum; will grow out in 1 to 7 days even on routine bacterial media
Treatment	Take out foreign bodies and débride extensive soft tissue infections; rapid growers are resistant to typical TB therapy and usually are susceptible to newer macrolides, quinolones, doxycycline, and minocycline, and sulfonamides; IV options for serious infections include amikacin, cefoxitin, and imipenem

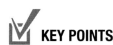 KEY POINTS

- NTM are ubiquitous in the environment and are classified by their speed of growth and pigment production
- The clinically significant rapidly growing mycobacteria are *M. fortuitum*, *M. chelonae*, and *M. abscessus*; growth occurs in 1 to 7 days and can occur on routine lab media for bacterial cultures
- The main clinical syndromes of the rapid growers are skin and soft tissue infections, usually preceded by some sort of trauma or surgery, and pulmonary infections
- Rapid growers are usually resistant to typical agents used for TB and may respond to macrolides, fluoroquinolones, tetracyclines, and sulfonamides

QUESTIONS

1. The duration of treatment for infections caused by rapidly growing mycobacteria is usually:

   A. 7 to 10 days
   B. 10 to 14 days
   C. 14 to 28 days
   D. 1 to 3 months
   E. 4 to 6 months

2. Which drug is currently approved for administration once a week as prophylaxis for MAC in HIV infection?

   A. Rifabutin
   B. Azithromycin
   C. Clarithromycin
   D. Ethambutol
   E. Rifampin

REFERENCES

1. Winthrop KL, Abrams M, Yakrus M, et al. An outbreak of mycobacterial furunculosis associated with footbaths at a nail salon. N Engl J Med 2002;346:1366–1371.

CASE 1-13 *Mycoplasma*

HPI: A 24-year-old man presents to a medical school teaching clinic with complaints of a cough that has lasted 2 weeks, accompanied by fatigue and malaise. The cough is incessant and productive of small amounts of yellow sputum. These symptoms were preceded by several days of rhinitis and a sore throat. He has taken his temperature at home, and it reached a maximum of 100°F.

The patient has no past medical history and has been taking an over-the-counter decongestant and expectorant.

PE: T 37.3°C; BP 120/60; HR 65; RR 14; SaO$_2$ 98% on room air

Physical exam shows a young man in no respiratory distress. There is no conjunctival injection. The oropharynx shows slight erythema. Ear exam shows bullous myringitis of the right tympanic membrane. Lungs are clear to auscultation and percussion. Abdomen is benign, with no hepatosplenomegaly. There is no rash.

The physician initially suspects viral bronchitis but decides to check a chest X-ray.

The chest X-ray shows a diffuse interstitial infiltrate, which looks "much worse than the patient."

Although diagnostic testing usually would not be performed in this case, the physician demonstrates some diagnostic tests for the edification of his students. He checks a sputum Gram stain, which shows normal flora and no predominant species. Next, he draws blood into an anticoagulated tube and places the tube on ice. Within minutes, the red blood cells have clumped together. The clumping reverses with warming.

THOUGHT QUESTIONS

- Which infections could cause these symptoms and the findings on chest X-ray?
- What did the blood clumping test show?
- Which antibiotics would be reasonable to prescribe?
- Why was this patient not admitted to the hospital?

BASIC SCIENCE REVIEW AND DISCUSSION

Pneumonia pathogens are often divided into typical and atypical etiologies. **Typical** causes of pneumonia are bacterial: *Streptococcus pneumoniae* (pneumococcus), *Haemophilus influenzae*, and *Moraxella*. **Atypical pneumonia** can be caused by viruses, such as influenza, parainfluenza, adenovirus, and respiratory syncytial viruses, *Mycoplasma*, or *Chlamydia*. *Legionella*, often grouped with the atypical agents, is a gram-negative bacterium that usually causes more severe disease than the other atypical agents. *Legionella* is grouped with the other atypical agents, however, because it is an intracellular bacterium that is difficult to diagnose and is treated with similar antibiotics. The clinical distinction between the typical and atypical pneumonias is difficult to make in practice, but classically atypical pneumonia presents as a milder, more subacute illness, sometimes described as "walking pneumonia." Fever is less pronounced and patients are less likely to die of the illness. Chest X-rays show patchy or interstitial infiltrates (unlike the classic lobar infiltrates of pneumococcal pneumonia) and are often described as "looking worse than the patient." Sputum Gram stains do not reveal the etiologic organism. Because of the milder severity of illness and the difficulty of culturing mycoplasma and chlamydia, most diagnoses of atypical pneumonia are made clinically and without cultures. Such patients are usually well enough to be treated as outpatients.

Regardless of whether a patient appears to have a "typical" or "atypical" presentation of pneumonia, most patients will be treated with an antibiotic regimen that covers both types of agents. Because the atypical pneumonia agents such as *Chlamydia* and *Legionella* live within mammalian cells, antibiotics with good intracellular penetration, such as the macrolides, tetracyclines, and fluoroquinolones, are the most effective. β-Lactams, although excellent drugs against most typical causes of bacterial pneumonia, do not penetrate mammalian cells. In addition, β-lactams have no activity against mycoplasma, which do not have a cell wall.

Mycoplasma pneumoniae is the most frequent cause of atypical pneumonia. The other pathogenic *Mycoplasma* species (*M. hominis*, *M. genitalium*, and *Ureaplasma urealyticum*) all infect the genitourinary tract. Mycoplasma are the smallest known free-living organisms. They have no cell wall, which renders them resistant to β-lactam antibiotics, and are invisible on Gram stain. They have no DNA homology with typical bacteria. Unlike viruses, mycoplasma are able to grow in defined, noncellular media; they are extracellular parasites and contain both DNA and RNA.

M. pneumoniae infection can also lead to serious skin rashes, such as **erythema multiforme** and **Stevens-Johnson syndrome.** Mycoplasma is also associated with an infection of the tympanic membrane known as **bullous myringitis, and** with immunologic phenomena, most strikingly **cold agglutinins,** as described in this case. Cold agglutinins are IgM antibodies directed against the modified I antigen found on the red blood cells of infected patients. If severe, the cold agglutinins may be associated with Raynaud phenomenon (spontaneous vasoconstriction of the extremities, associated with cold). The pneumonia of mycoplasma is self-limited without treatment, but treatment shortens the illness and probably reduces spread.

Chlamydia pneumoniae is another major cause of atypical pneumonia. Chlamydia are obligate intracellular parasites distantly related to eubacteria. They have very small genomes for prokaryotes; only mycoplasma genomes are smaller. They cannot synthesize their own energy and must rely on the host cell to supply ATP and GTP. The organisms have a biphasic life cycle. The inert, hardy, extracellular state, known as an elementary body, is stabilized by disulfide cross-linking between membrane proteins. Once taken up into a cell by receptor-mediated endocytosis, the elementary bodies transform into larger reticulate bodies, which are metabolically active and reproduce by binary fission, ultimately giving rise to more elementary bodies. Unlike *C. psittaci*, the agent of psittacosis associated with birds, *C. pneumoniae* has no animal reservoir and is spread from human to human through respiratory secretions. The organism may be present with or without causing disease. Most initial infections occur during school age. Clinical presentations tend to be mild and similar to mycoplasma pneumonia. Some preliminary research suggests that chlamydia pneumonia infection may be associated with the development of atherosclerosis.

Legionella pneumophila is a gram-negative aerobic rod bacterium, often lumped with the other causes of atypical pneumonia because, like chlamydia and mycoplasma, it is difficult to culture and is resistant to β-lactam antibiotics. *Legionella* can survive for years in water and is tolerant of chlorine, so it may colonize plumbing or air conditioning systems. *Legionella* may require symbiotic microorganisms for survival in these habitats. Aerosols from these colonized sources, or aspiration of contaminated water, lead to pneumonia. Unlike the other atypical pneumonias, *Legionella* pneumonia tends to be very severe, with almost all patients requiring hospital admission. As with other intracellular pathogens, cell-mediated immunity is the major defense against *Legionella*, and the illness is more severe in patients lacking cell-mediated immunity. *Legionella* may also cause a self-limited febrile illness without pneumonia, known as Pontiac fever.

Unexplained hyponatremia may be a clue to Legionella infection. *Legionella* tends to be underdiagnosed because it will not grow with standard blood or sputum culturing techniques. *Legionella* can be cultured but requires a special medium made from a charcoal yeast extract at pH 6.9. The organism may be detected with direct fluorescent antibodies, but the test requires a large number of organisms. A urine test for the presence of *Legionella* antigen is a convenient new way to diagnose the illness, although the available test only detects *L. pneumophila* serogroup 1 species.

CASE CONCLUSION

The patient is sent home with a 5-day course of azithromycin and instructions to return if he gets worse. His cough resolves several days after finishing the azithromycin course. (Because of its long half-life, azithromycin is still present in the blood days after the patient stops taking the pills.)

THUMBNAIL: Nonviral Agents of Atypical Pneumonia

Organism	*Legionella pneumophila*	*Mycoplasma pneumoniae*	*Chlamydia pneumoniae*	*Chlamydia psittaci*
Diseases caused	Atypical pneumonia or lobar pneumonia, often severe	Atypical pneumonia	Atypical pneumonia; possibly linked to atherosclerosis	Psittacosis (usually resembles atypical pneumonia)
Epidemiology	Lives in water and may be spread through plumbing or air conditioning	Endemic	Endemic	Exposure to birds
Diagnosis	*Legionella* urinary antigen; *Legionella* culture (special media)	Cold agglutinins; may be detected through serology, culture, or polymerase chain reaction (PCR), but usually empirically treated	May be detected through serology, culture, or PCR, but usually empirically treated	Serology
Treatment	Macrolides, tetracyclines, fluoroquinolones	Macrolides, tetracyclines, fluoroquinolones	Macrolides, tetracyclines, fluoroquinolones	Tetracyclines

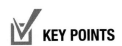

KEY POINTS

- The major causes of atypical pneumonia include viral infections, such as influenza, parainfluenza, respiratory syncytial virus (RSV), and adenovirus, and *Mycoplasma*, *Chlamydia*, and *Legionella*

- A typical pneumonia classically presents with prolonged cough and malaise; fevers are less common than in typical pneumonia; although chest X-rays are supposed to show patchy or interstitial infiltrates rather than the lobar infiltrates caused by pneumococcus, the distinction is not reliable

- Although it can be difficult to distinguish typical and atypical pneumonia agents by their clinical presentation, the distinction is useful because antibiotic therapies differ for the two classes

QUESTIONS

1. Which of these antibiotic classes, often used to treat pneumonia, misses atypical agents?

   A. Macrolides
   B. Ketolides
   C. Fluoroquinolones
   D. Tetracyclines
   E. β-lactams

2. Which of the following organisms, if found on a sputum culture, definitely indicates infection?

   A. *Chlamydia pneumoniae*
   B. *Pneumococcus*
   C. *Haemophilus influenzae*
   D. *Legionella pneumophila*
   E. *Moraxella*

3. Which of the following organisms lacks a cell wall?

   A. *Klebsiella pneumoniae*
   B. *Mycoplasma pneumoniae*
   C. *Pneumococcus*
   D. *Moraxella*
   E. *Candida albicans*

4. Which of the following agents of pneumonia is extracellular?

   A. *Chlamydia pneumoniae*
   B. *Mycoplasma pneumoniae*
   C. *Chlamydia psittaci*
   D. *Legionella pneumophila*
   E. Influenza A

CASE 1-14 | *Treponema Pallidum*

HPI: FS is a 29-year-old man who presents with a red, mildly itchy widespread rash. He denies any new laundry detergents or other causes of contact dermatitis. He has not had any fevers, night sweats, sore throat, or abdominal pain.

PE: On exam, he has a papular erythematous rash over his torso and extremities involving his palms and soles. His mouth shows some white painless mucous patches on his buccal mucosa. Exam of his genitalia shows some new, fleshy wart-like lesions, which appear to be condyloma lata.

Further history reveals that 6 weeks ago he had a painless ulcer on his penis, along with some nontender swelling in his groin, presumably lymphadenopathy. The ulcer went away and so the patient did not relate it to the present rash until asked. Upon further questioning, he admits to multiple female sex partners, including prostitutes. He often does not use a condom during vaginal sex.

THOUGHT QUESTIONS

- What are the major treponemal diseases?
- What is the differential diagnosis of genital ulcerations?
- What are the stages of syphilis, and what are their manifestations?
- How is the diagnosis of syphilis made?
- How is syphilis treated?
- How is he going to explain this to his wife?

BASIC SCIENCE REVIEW AND DISCUSSION

Syphilis is caused by a **spirochete**, *Treponema pallidum* (Table 1-6). Unique among the spirochetal diseases, it is sexually transmitted. Other spirochetal diseases are **zoonoses** transmitted by insect bites (Lyme disease and relapsing fever) or by exposure to rodent urine (leptospirosis). The other diseases caused by the *Treponema* family are spread through nonsexual contact and consequently are diseases of childhood (Table 1-7).

Syphilis has several well-defined stages. Although the symptoms of early syphilis (**primary** and **secondary** stages) will resolve without treatment, the infection is still present. Up to one third of patients with untreated **latent** infection will develop the feared complications of **tertiary** syphilis, years after their initial infection. Staging of syphilis is important because it determines proper patient management (Fig. 1-9).

The diagnosis of syphilis can be made by identifying **treponemes** from a patient's lesions. These are usually found by scraping the base of a **chancre** of primary syphilis but can also be

found by scraping the **condyloma lata** lesions of secondary syphilis. In practice, this is rarely done, as treponemes are too narrow to be seen by standard light microscopy and a special **dark-field microscope** is required. *T. pallidum* cannot be cultured. Most cases of syphilis are diagnosed by means of serologic tests. The **RPR** (rapid plasma reagin test) and venereal disease research laboratory **(VDRL)** tests are examples of "**nontreponemal**" tests, which are used for initial screening. These tests are easily performed but are frequently falsely positive. A second set of confirmatory "**treponemal**" tests, such as the **MHA-TP** (microhemagglutination assay for *T. pallidum*) or **FTA-ABS** (fluorescent treponemal antibody absorption), are used to rule out false-positives.

Although other drugs are effective, the mainstay of syphilis treatment is parenteral penicillin. For patients with early syphilis (primary, secondary, or less than 1 year of latent syphilis), a one-time dose of **benzathine penicillin** is given intramuscularly. The benzathine formation ensures that the patient receives the entire dose while providing sustained antibiotic levels that are necessary to kill this slow-growing organism. Patients who have tertiary syphilis or have had latent syphilis for more than 1 year require longer courses of penicillin therapy.

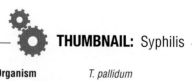

THUMBNAIL: Syphilis

Organism	*T. pallidum*
Type of organism	Spirochete
Diseases caused	Syphilis; closely related organisms cause bejel, yaws, and pinta
Epidemiology	Sexually transmitted; may also be transmitted transplacentally, causing congenital syphilis
Diagnosis	Characteristic chancre of primary syphilis or rash of secondary syphilis; demonstration of treponemes in lesion by dark-field microscopy; serologies; organism is not culturable
Treatment	Penicillin; no resistance reported; route and duration of therapy depend on stage of disease; doxycycline is used for penicillin-allergic patients.

CASE CONCLUSION

His doctor happens to have a dark-field microscope in the office, and scrapings of the condyloma lata are positive for treponemes. A stat RPR is also performed and is positive. Tests are also sent for gonorrhea, chlamydia, and HIV. The patient is diagnosed with secondary syphilis and is treated with a single dose of benzathine penicillin IM. He is asked to report the names of his recent sexual contacts, and public health workers call these women in for evaluation and treatment.

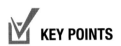

TABLE 1-6 The Spirochetes

Genus	Morphology	Diseases
Borrelia	Thick, loose coils	Lyme disease (ticks); relapsing fever (lice)
Leptospira	Tight coils, hooked ends	Leptospirosis
Treponema	Slender, tight coils	Syphilis; bejel (endemic syphilis); pinta; yaws

✓ KEY POINTS

- Syphilis is caused by a spirochete, *T. pallidum*; other spirochetal diseases include Lyme disease and leptospirosis

- Diagnosis is made on the basis of clinical symptoms suggesting a stage of syphilis, serology, and dark-field microscopy, if available; the organism cannot be cultured

- The treatment of choice is penicillin; resistance has not been reported

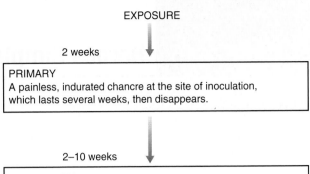

EXPOSURE

↓ 2 weeks

PRIMARY
A painless, indurated chancre at the site of inoculation, which lasts several weeks, then disappears.

↓ 2–10 weeks

SECONDARY
A maculopapular rash, which may involve palms and soles and which lasts several weeks.
Flat, wart-like lesions at the groin or axilla called condyloma lata.

LATENT

↓ Years

TERTIARY
30% of untreated patients may eventually develop complications:
a) proximal aortic aneurysm
b) tabes dorsalis (dorsal column injury)
c) general paresis (insanity)
d) gummas (destructive lesions of bone and soft tissue)

• **Figure 1-9.** Staging of syphilis.

TABLE 1-7 The Treponemal Diseases

	Venereal Syphilis	Bejel (Endemic Syphilis)	Yaws	Pinta
Organism	*T. pallidum pallidum*	*T. pallidum endemicum*	*T. pallidum pertenue*	*T. carateum*
Transmission	Sexual; congenital	Skin contact	Skin contact	Skin contact
Organ involvement	Skin; bone; heart; CNS	Skin; bone	Skin; bone	Skin

QUESTIONS

1. A patient presents with bony lesions consistent with a treponemal infection. Which of the following lists would be a reasonable differential diagnosis in descending order of probability?

   A. Pinta, syphilis, bejel (endemic syphilis)
   B. Syphilis, yaws, pinta
   C. Bejel (endemic syphilis), yaws, syphilis
   D. Yaws, pinta, syphilis, bejel (endemic syphilis)
   E. Pinta, yaws, bejel (endemic syphilis)

2. A patient is diagnosed with syphilis based on a positive RPR, confirmed by FTA-ABS. His treatment depends on his stage of disease, which is determined by his symptoms. Which of the following is characteristic of secondary syphilis?

   A. Aortic aneurysm
   B. Gummas
   C. Tabes dorsalis
   D. Condyloma lata
   E. Painless chancre

3. When should a patient with syphilis be treated with a drug other than penicillin?

   A. Pregnancy
   B. Penicillin-resistant syphilis is suspected
   C. Neurosyphilis
   D. Patient has a penicillin allergy
   E. Topical treatment of syphilitic chancre in primary syphilis

HPI: HS is a 21-year-old female who presents to your office with complaints of "blisters" in her vulvar area. These lesions appeared in this area with some extension to her inner thighs on the day prior to presentation. She also has had 2 days of low-grade fevers and feels that she has swelling of the lymph nodes in her groin. She denies any abnormal vaginal discharge or bleeding. HS has never experienced these symptoms before. She just became sexually active for the first time approximately 2 months ago with a male partner who told her that he had never had sexual relations before they met. She stopped using condoms with this partner 1 month ago.

PMH: HS has no significant medical history. Just started taking oral contraceptive pills a month ago and has no allergies.

PE: T 38.0°C; HR 86; BP 118/75; RR 14

Generally anxious, tearful young woman in no acute distress. Genital exam reveals crops of vesicles bilaterally around the inner vulva with scattered vesicles on both upper inner thighs. Lymph nodes are swollen bilaterally in the inguinal region.

Labs: No blood laboratory tests performed on this visit. A smear of the fluid from the base of one of the vesicles was sent for culture and fluorescent antibody staining.

THOUGHT QUESTIONS

- What are the infectious etiologies of genital ulceration?
- How would you make the diagnosis of herpes simplex virus (HSV) infection?
- What are the characteristics of the HSV-1 and HSV-2 viruses?
- What are some of the clinical syndromes associated with HSV and are there differences between the manifestations of HSV-1 and HSV-2?
- What is the mechanism of antivirals used in the treatment of HSV infections?

BASIC SCIENCE REVIEW AND DISCUSSION

Differential of Genital Ulcers

In the United States, the two major infections on the differential of genital ulceration are **herpes** lesions (60–70%) and primary **syphilis** (10–20%). The differential is more expansive in nonindustrialized settings and in travelers returning to the United States. Other agents that cause genital ulceration include the following:

1. **Granuloma inguinale (Donovanosis):** this infection is a major cause of genital ulceration in the tropics and is caused by *Calymmatobacterium granulomatis,* an encapsulated pleomorphic gram-negative rod. The primary lesion begins as a small **painless** papule or indurated nodule and then ulcerates to form an exuberant, beefy-red, granulomatous ulcer with rolled edges and with a characteristic satin-like surface that bleeds easily on contact. Interestingly, even large ulcerative lesions are painless. However, spontaneous healing is accompanied by scar formation, which can produce gross genital deformities. This infection can cause lymphedema; subcutaneous spread of granulomas into the inguinal region can cause groin swellings called **pseudobuboes,** The diagnosis is made by demonstrating typical intracellular **Donovan bodies** in Giemsa-stained smears obtained from lesions, and the treatment is doxycycline for 21 days.
2. **Lymphogranuloma venereum (LGV):** this sexually transmitted disease is caused by **invasive serovars** of *Chlamydia trachomatis* and is found mainly in the tropical and subtropical nations of Africa and Asia. The initial manifestation of LGV is a short-lived papular genital lesions followed by massive **painful inguinal lymphadenopathy,** often with systemic symptoms. Diagnosis is made serologically and treatment is doxycycline or erythromycin for 21 days.
3. **Chancroid:** this sexually transmitted infection is caused by *Haemophilus ducreyi,* a small gram-negative rod that is more common in tropical countries. Chancroid infection has been found in the United States in association with the use of crack cocaine and selling sex for drugs. This infection is initially manifested by **painful,** nonindurated **(soft) genital ulcers** and local lymphadenitis. The diagnosis is made by culturing the organism from the genital ulcer or a lymph node and treatment is with a single dose of high-dose azithromycin. See Figure 1-10 for an example of a typical chancroid ulcer.

Herpes Simplex Virus 1 and 2 Infections

Properties There are two serotypes of herpes simplex virus: **types 1 and 2.** All herpes viruses are structurally similar, with an **icosahedral** core surrounded by a **lipoprotein envelope** and a genome composed of **linear double-stranded DNA.** These viruses are large (120–200 nm in diameter) and HSV-1 and -2 are structurally and morphologically indistinguishable. However, the two HSV serotypes can be differentiated by restriction endonuclease patterns of their genomes and type-specific monoclonal antisera.

After entry into the cell, the HSV virions are uncoated and the genome DNA enters the nucleus, where virus mRNA is transcribed by host cell RNA polymerase. Two of the early viral proteins translated are **thymidine kinase** and viral DNA polymerase, which helps replicate the viral genome DNA. Virion assembly occurs in the nucleus, leading to the formation of **intranuclear inclusions.** During **latent** herpes infection, HSV virions are transported to the **dorsal root ganglion** (HSV-1 goes to **trigeminal ganglia** and HSV-2 goes to **lumbar and sacral ganglia**) along peripheral sensory nerves, and multiple copies of HSV DNA are found in the cytoplasm of infected neurons in episomal form.

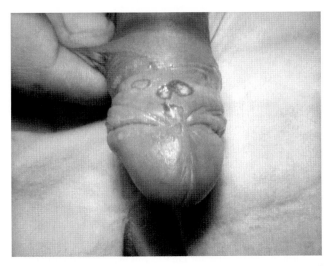

• **Figure 1-10.** Chancroid ulcers of *Haemophilus ducreyi* on the penis. (Image in public domain from Centers for Disease Control and Prevention Public Health Image Library, http://phil.cdc.gov/phil/home.asp)

Transmission and Epidemiology HSV-1 infections are transmitted primarily in **saliva,** and HSV-2 infections are transmitted mainly by **sexual contact.** Oral-genital contact can lead to HSV-1 infection in the genital area and HSV-2 lesions in the oral cavity in 10 to 20% of cases. **Asymptomatic shedding** of both HSV-1 and HSV-2 can occur and plays an important role in transmission, although these agents are more easily transmitted in the presence of active herpetic lesions. Approximately 80% of the U.S. population is infected with HSV-1, with most of these infections occurring during childhood; half of these infections are manifested by recurrent **herpes labialis (cold sores).** Approximately 20 to 25% of the U.S. population is infected with HSV-2, with 20% of these infections being asymptomatic.

Clinical HSV-1 causes the following conditions:

1. **Gingivostomatitis:** this syndrome is often the manifestation of primary HSV-1 infection and occurs primarily in children. Gingivostomatitis is characterized by fever, irritability, and multiple vesicular lesions in the mouth.
2. **Herpes labialis:** the term describes **fever blisters** or cold sores, which primarily represents recurrent HSV-1 disease.
3. **Keratoconjunctivitis:** a syndrome characterized by corneal ulcers and lesions of the conjunctival epithelium, with recurrences leading to scarring and blindness.
4. **Encephalitis:** HSV-1 is the most common cause of sporadic focal encephalitis in the United States, with a proclivity for the **temporal lobes.** Symptoms include altered mentation, anosmia, bizarre behavior, and fever; the syndrome has a high mortality rate, with neurologic sequelae in those who survive.
5. **Herpetic whitlow:** this condition is a painful infection of the hand involving one or more fingers initiated by viral inoculation of the host through exposure to infected body fluids via a break in the skin. Whitlow is typically seen in **healthcare workers** after touching a patient's active herpetic lesion.
6. **Disseminated infection:** HSV-1 can cause disseminated conditions in immunocompromised patients, such as esophagitis, hepatitis, and pneumonia.

HSV-2 causes the following conditions:

1. **Genital herpes:** this condition is manifested by painful vesicular lesions of the male and female genitalia and the anal area. Lesions are more severe, extensively distributed, and protracted in primary HSV-2 infection than in recurrent disease. Primary HSV-2 infection can also cause fever, inguinal lymphadenopathy, dysuria, urethral discharge, cervicitis, and vaginal discharge. The genital ulcers manifest initially as vesicles, which eventually crust over. Recurrent genital herpes infections are often heralded with a prodrome of localized tingling and are more localized than primary infections, with fewer systemic symptoms.
2. **Neonatal herpes:** the risk of transmission of HSV-2 to the fetus is 33% in the setting of primary HSV-2 infection in the mother, compared with 3 to 5% in the setting of recurrent HSV-2 infection. Hence, cesarean sections are recommended for pregnant women with active HSV-2 lesions to decrease the risk of transmission to the fetus in either situation. Manifestations of neonatal herpes include localized skin, eye, and/or mouth lesions, encephalitis, and disseminated disease.
3. **Aseptic meningitis:** the syndrome of herpes meningitis is usually caused by HSV-2 rather than HSV-1. The syndrome is usually mild and self-limited without subsequent development of neurologic sequelae.

Diagnosis The most important diagnostic procedure is isolation of the virus from the lesion by growth in cell culture; the typical **cytopathic effect** occurs in 1 to 3 days, after which the virus is identified by **fluorescent antibody staining** of the infected cells. **Tzanck smear** on cells from the base of the vesicle show **multinucleated giant cells** when stained with Giemsa stain. Immunity to HSV-1 and HSV-2 is type specific, and current serologic tests can detect acute infection with either virus by measuring type-specific IgM levels. Diagnosis of encephalitis is best made by PCR analysis of the CSF for HSV-1; the sensitivity of PCR for HSV is 98% and the specificity is 94%.

Treatment The following agents are used to treat HSV-1 and HSV-2 infections: (*a*) oral agents: acyclovir (ACV; Zovirax); valacyclovir (VACV; Valtrex; prodrug of ACV); famciclovir (FCV; Famvir) and (*b*) IV agents: acyclovir; foscarnet (Foscavir; for resistant viruses); cidofovir (Vistide; restricted because of renal toxicity); penciclovir (Denavir; investigational; no oral bioavailability). In addition to reducing the frequency of recurrences of herpetic outbreaks in the treated individual, use of these oral agents also reduces the incidence of viral shedding in genital secretions and reduces transmission of herpes to sexual partners.

The following diagram (Fig. 1-11) schematizes the mechanism of action of these antivirals.

ACV is phosphorylated by viral thymidine kinase to ACV-monophosphate, which is then phosphorylated to ACV-triphosphate (ACV-TP) by host cell enzymes. ACV-TP inhibits viral DNA polymerase and blocks replicating viral DNA. Most **ACV-resistant** strains have lost the viral thymidine kinase, although drug resistance in HSV can also occur at the level of the viral DNA polymerase. VACV and FCV have better oral availability than ACV, but all reduce shedding and hasten time to lesion healing. **Cidofovir** is a nucleotide analog that already exists in the monophosphate form, so that its activation only occurs through cellular enzymes. **Foscarnet** is a DNA polymerase phosphorylation binder and is the only drug that can be used against ACV-resistant virus.

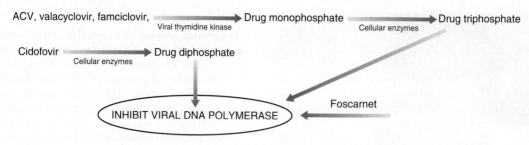

• **Figure 1-11.** Schematization of the mechanisms of action of these antivirals.

CASE CONCLUSION

Direct fluorescent antibody (DFA) staining of HS's vesicular lesion was positive for HSV-2. She was treated with acyclovir and she promptly broke up with her boyfriend.

THUMBNAIL: Herpes Simplex Virus Infections

Organisms	HSV-1 and HSV-2
Type of organism	Large double-stranded DNA virus
Diseases caused	Acute gingivostomatitis, recurrent herpes labialis, keratoconjunctivitis, encephalitis, genital herpes, neonatal herpes, aseptic meningitis, disseminated infection
Epidemiology	80% of the U.S. population is infected with HSV-1, with primary infections occurring in childhood predominantly; 20 to 25% of the U.S. population is HSV-2 infected, with primary infections occurring predominantly in young, sexually active adults
Diagnosis	DFA staining in cell culture of fluid scraped from the base of the vesicle
Treatment	Acyclovir, famciclovir, valacyclovir; foscarnet for acyclovir-resistant virus

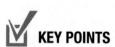

KEY POINTS

■ The major causes of genital ulceration in the United States are herpes simplex virus infections and primary syphilis (although genital ulcers in the rest of the world can also be caused by *Chlamydia trachomatis*, *Haemophilus ducreyi*, and *Calymmatobacterium granulomatis*)

■ HSV-1 is typically spread by saliva and causes oral ulcerations, and HSV-2 is typically spread by sexual contact and causes

genital ulcerations, although each virus can cause the converse syndrome

■ Asymptomatic shedding of virus can occur and is a major source of transmission when active lesions are not visible

■ Effective antivirals exist for HSV, although drug resistance is emerging

QUESTIONS

1. What degree of HSV resistance to acyclovir is seen in the U.S. population?

   A. 0%
   B. 5%
   C. 15%
   D. 50%
   E. Depends on the host

2. Asymptomatic shedding of HSV-2 occurs in what percentage of days out of a year?

   A. 1.2%
   B. 4.3%
   C. 6.7%
   D. 10.2%
   E. 18.5%

CASE 1-16 Cytomegalovirus

HPI: A 41-year-old woman with AIDS and a CD4 count of 20 presents with new onset of diarrhea, up to 10 small stools a day. She also has crampy abdominal pain and low-grade fevers. She has been prescribed antiretroviral therapy but has not been taking it.

PE: T 38°C; BP 120/75; HR 95; RR 14

The patient is cachectic and in no acute distress. Her funduscopic exam is normal. Her oral mucosa is dry with some thrush in the oropharynx. She has a few shotty inguinal nodes but otherwise no lymphadenopathy. Heart and lung exam are normal. Her abdomen has mild left lower quadrant tenderness, but no peritoneal signs. There are no masses or hepatosplenomegaly. Rectal exam shows no masses; stool is brown and guaiac positive.

Labs: White count is 3. Hematocrit is 32. Platelets are 340. She has an elevated BUN (blood urea nitrogen) of 25, consistent with dehydration. Stool samples are sent for bacterial culture, which is negative for pathogens. A test for *Clostridium difficile* toxin is negative. Stool is also examined for ova and parasites, including cryptosporidium and microsporidium (parasites that can cause diarrhea in advanced AIDS), but none are found. A Giardia stool antigen is negative.

A chest X-ray shows no signs of tuberculosis.

The patient is sent for endoscopy, which shows signs of inflammation. Several biopsies are taken. On pathology, characteristic large nuclear inclusion bodies are seen, consistent with cytomegalovirus (CMV) infection. The biopsies ultimately grow out CMV virus.

THOUGHT QUESTIONS

- What opportunistic organisms can cause diarrhea in advanced AIDS?
- How will this patient be treated?
- What would be the best strategy for preventing this infection from recurring?

BASIC SCIENCE REVIEW AND DISCUSSION

CMV is a member of the **herpes virus family.** The other known herpes viruses are the herpes simplex viruses (HSV-1 and -2), varicella-zoster virus (VZV), Epstein-Barr virus (EBV), and human herpes viruses (HHV-6, -7, and -8). These are all large DNA viruses, and CMV is the largest human pathogenic virus. CMV uses its many proteins to down-regulate the host immune response. For example, one CMV protein prevents cellular major histocompatability (MHC) complexes from being exported to the cell membrane. This prevents T lymphocytes from detecting evidence of viral infection. At the same time, CMV manufactures a "decoy" MHC complex to prevent host natural killer cells (which kill cells *lacking* MHC) from neutralizing the infected cell. CMV is named for the large nuclear inclusion bodies it makes when replicating in infected cells.

CMV infection is common; most people have serologic evidence of prior infection. Lower socioeconomic status is associated with infection; infection prevalence can approach 80 to 90% in urban areas and up to 100% in regions of Africa. Although primary infection is usually asymptomatic, acute CMV can cause a mononucleosis-type syndrome in immunocompetent hosts. Whereas EBV is the cause of four out of five cases of mononucleosis, CMV is responsible for the remainder. Compared with EBV, CMV mononucleosis tends to produce more fever, with less adenopathy and splenomegaly. The monospot test for EBV antibodies is negative in CMV mononucleosis. After the acute infection is cleared, the virus is still present in a latent form and secondary infection can occur when the host's defenses are weakened.

CMV is much more serious in immunosuppressed hosts. If a pregnant woman sustains primary CMV infection, the virus can cause systemic and CNS infection in her fetus, with devastating results. The virus can also be transmitted to neonates at birth. CMV pneumonitis is a major scourge of bone marrow and organ transplant recipients. The more immunosuppressed the patient, the worse the infection can be. Prophylaxis with ganciclovir has been shown to reduce the risk of CMV disease in this population. Blood is screened for CMV antibodies to avoid infecting previously unexposed patients who may undergo bone marrow transplantation in the future. In HIV patients with CD4 counts below 50, CMV can cause retinitis or colitis. Pneumonitis is more rare in this population. HIV patients at risk for retinitis should receive regular eye exams.

All drugs active against CMV are inhibitors of the viral DNA polymerase. CMV lacks a viral thymidine kinase to activate acyclovir, valacyclovir, and famciclovir, so these herpes drugs are not active against CMV. **Ganciclovir** (and its new oral formulation valganciclovir) are the drugs of choice against CMV. In cases of ganciclovir-resistant CMV, other agents, such as foscarnet and cidofovir, can be used. However, these drugs have serious toxicities, including nephrotoxicity.

CASE CONCLUSION

The patient is started on IV ganciclovir and the diarrhea improves after several weeks of therapy. She is referred to an ophthalmologist for a dilated retinal exam, which is negative for CMV retinitis. Her thrush is treated, and because of her low CD4 count, she is put on prophylaxis for PCP and mycobacterium avium-intracellularae (MAC). After this unpleasant experience, she agrees to take HIV antiretroviral therapy. A year later, her CD4 count is over 300 and her prophylactic medications are discontinued.

THUMBNAIL: Cytomegalovirus

Organism	Cytomegalovirus
Type of organism	Herpes DNA virus
Diseases caused	Mononucleosis; opportunistic infections in transplant recipients (pneumonitis) and AIDS patients (retinitis and colitis); congenital infection (TORCH)
Epidemiology	Transmission through intimate contact; infected blood transfusions or organ transplants
Diagnosis	CMV culture; CMV antigenemia; CMV PCR
Treatment	Ganciclovir, valganciclovir, cidofovir, foscarnet

KEY POINTS

- CMV is a member of the herpes virus family
- CMV infection is common and symptoms are usually mild, except in immunocompromised patients (transplant recipients, AIDS patients, and neonates)
- All anti-CMV drugs are active against HSV, but many HSV drugs are not active against CMV because CMV lacks a viral thymidine kinase to activate them
- Ganciclovir (or its new oral formulation, valganciclovir) is the drug of choice for CMV because it has fewer toxicities than the alternatives

QUESTIONS

1. Which of the following antiviral drugs is active against CMV?

   A. Acyclovir
   B. Foscarnet
   C. Famciclovir
   D. Lamivudine
   E. Valacyclovir

2. How are asymptomatic HIV patients screened for CMV disease?

   A. Digital rectal exams every month while the absolute neutrophil count is less than 500
   B. Monthly chest X-rays while the HIV viral load is detectable
   C. Quarterly blood cultures for CMV while the CD4 count is less than 100
   D. Eye exams every 6 months while the CD4 count is less than 50
   E. A one-time lumbar puncture when the CD4 count drops below 200

46

HPI: HV is a 22-year-old man presenting to the ER with 4 days of fever, rash, sore throat, fatigue, muscle pain, joint pain, and swollen lymph nodes. He denies any night sweats, headache, cough, shortness of breath, abdominal pain, nausea, vomiting, diarrhea, or urinary symptoms. No one around him is sick and he has not started any new medications, or had any recent animal exposures or recent travel. HV has sex with men only and recently entered a relationship with a new boyfriend.

PMH: HV had syphilis 4 years ago, which was treated. He does not take any regular medications or have any drug allergies. Condom use is inconsistent.

PE: T 39.2°C; BP 120/85; HR 115; RR 12

HV appears acutely ill with a diffuse, erythematous rash over his trunk, back, and upper and lower extremities. His oropharyngeal exam is significant for severe redness in the posterior pharynx and a small ulcer on the inside of his right cheek. Swollen lymph nodes are noted diffusely.

Labs: WBC 3.5 with normal differential.

THOUGHT QUESTIONS

- What are the infectious agents that can lead to HV's constellation of symptoms and how would you test for them?
- What are the symptoms of acute HIV infection?
- Why is acute HIV syndrome symptomatic?
- How is acute HIV infection diagnosed?

BASIC SCIENCE REVIEW AND DISCUSSION

Differential Diagnosis

Possible infectious etiologies of HV's syndrome include viral syndromes, such as primary EBV or CMV infection, primary HSV infection, acute hepatitis A or B infection, human herpes virus-6 (roseola) infection, acute HIV infection, or rubella. Possible bacterial infections include secondary syphilis, severe (streptococcal) pharyngitis, leptospirosis, meningococcemia, disseminated gonococcal infection, or brucellosis. Protozoal etiologies include acute toxoplasmosis or malaria, although HV has no risk factors for the latter. HV could also be suffering from a severe acute drug reaction (although he reports taking no new medications) or an acute presentation of an autoimmune illness.

Tests to exclude the above-listed infectious causes are cited in Table 1-8.

Symptoms of Acute HIV Infection

Acute HIV infection can have a number of clinical manifestations but usually causes a **mononucleosis-like illness** of rapid onset and varying severity. Approximately **80%** of patients manifest some symptoms during HIV seroconversion. Table 1-9 lists the frequency of the most common signs, symptoms, and laboratory values associated with primary HIV infection.

Among the most prominent signs and symptoms of acute HIV seroconversion are fever, skin and mucosal lesions, generalized lymphadenopathy, and headache associated with retro-orbital pain. A **maculopapular rash** with primary HIV infection occurs in 30 to 50% or more of patients and is most often non-pruritic, with macular or maculopapular lesions predominantly on the trunk, neck, and face. The acute seroconversion rash is frequently associated with mucocutaneous oral, genital, and anal ulcers and should resolve spontaneously within 15 days. In most cases, the **acute retroviral syndrome** is self-limited, with a mean duration of 2 to 3 weeks.

Process of HIV Seroconversion

HIV seroconversion is marked by the appearance of anti–HIV-specific antibodies in the plasma, which usually occurs 5 to 10 days after the acute retroviral syndrome and 3 to 8 weeks after initial infection. Following exposure to the HIV virus, the sequence of markers to identify HIV infection, in chronologic order of appearance in the serum, is as follows: (*a*) HIV viral RNA; (*b*) **p24 antigen** (a viral core protein encoded by the HIV *gag* gene); and (*c*) anti-HIV antibody.

Approximately 2 weeks after the initial infection, **HIV viremia** increases exponentially and then declines to a steady-state level as the host's humoral and cell-mediated immune response controls HIV replication (Fig. 1-12). This time interval, the serologic **"window period,"** is characterized by seronegativity for HIV antibody, detectable p24 antigenemia, detectable HIV RNA levels, and variable CD4 lymphocyte concentrations. The detection of specific antibody to the HIV virus signals the end of the window period and identifies the individual as seropositive. The symptoms of the acute HIV seroconversion syndrome manifest during the stage of massive viremia that follows the initial HIV exposure.

Diagnosis of Acute HIV Infection

As can be extrapolated from Figure 1-12, the diagnosis of primary HIV infection is made by the detection of a high HIV RNA level with a negative HIV antibody titer.

TABLE 1-8 Tests to Exclude Infectious Causes

Infectious Agent	Diagnostic Test
Bacterial causes	Blood cultures (serology for *Brucella* and throat culture for streptococcal pharyngitis)
Acute EBV infection	Monospot and acute EBV titers
Acute CMV infection	Acute CMV titers
Primary HSV infection	HSV-1 and HSV-2 IgM titers
Acute hepatitis A infection	Hepatitis A IgM and IgG titers
Acute hepatitis B infection	Hepatitis B surface antigen (HepBsAg); Hepatitis B "e" antigen (HepBeAg); Hepatitis B core antibody (HepBcAb); Hepatitis B surface antibody (HepBsAb)
Acute HIV infection	HIV antibody and HIV RNA levels
Syphilis	RPR or VDRL serologic test for syphilis as well as the FTA-ABS
Toxoplasmosis	Toxoplasma IgM and IgG titers
Malaria (*Plasmodium* infection)	Thick and thin Giemsa-stained blood smears
Autoimmune disease	ANA titer or other specific serologies

TABLE 1-9 Signs, Symptoms, and Laboratory Abnormalities Associated with Acute HIV Syndrome

Signs, Symptoms, and Laboratory Values	Frequency (%)
Fevers	>90%
Fatigue	>90%
Rash	>70%
Headache	32–70%
Lymphadenopathy	40–70%
Pharyngitis	50–70%
Myalgias, arthralgias	50–70%
Nausea, vomiting, or diarrhea	30–60%
Night sweats	50%
Oral ulcers	10–20%
Genital ulcers	5–15%
Thrombocytopenia	45%
Leukopenia	40%
Elevated hepatic enzymes	21%

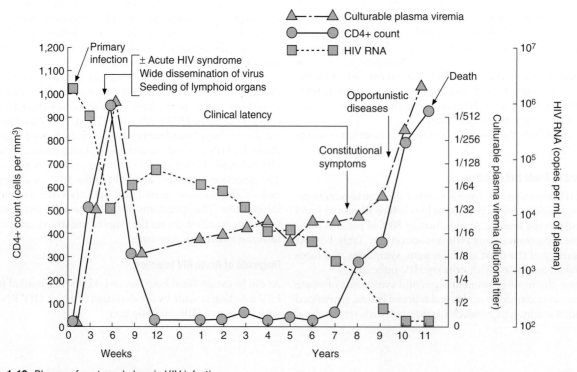

• **Figure 1-12.** Phases of acute and chronic HIV infection.

CASE CONCLUSION

The results of HV's laboratory work-up were as follows: blood cultures × 3 negative; monospot and acute EBV titers negative, hepatitis A IgM negative, hepatitis A IgG positive; HepBsAg negative, HepBeAg negative, HepBsAb and HepBcAb both positive, HIV antibody negative, HIV RNA by PCR greater than 100,000 copies/mL; RPR negative, specific FTA-ABS positive; toxoplasma IgM negative, toxoplasma IgG positive; ANA (antinuclear antibody) 1:40 with a speckled pattern. These results indicate that HV is undergoing the acute retroviral syndrome of primary HIV infection.

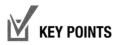

THUMBNAIL: Acute HIV Seroconversion Syndrome

Organism	Human immunodeficiency virus
Type of organism	Retrovirus (single-stranded RNA virus)
Diseases caused	Primary HIV infection; AIDS
Epidemiology	High-risk groups for acquisition of HIV infection include men who have sex with men (MSM), IV drug users (IVDU), heterosexuals with high-risk sex behaviors (e.g., selling sex for money), individuals who received a blood transfusion prior to 1985 (e.g., hemophiliacs)
Diagnosis	HIV antibody test for chronic HIV infection; high HIV RNA level and negative HIV antibody test for acute HIV infection
Treatment	Therapy for acute HIV infection symptomatic; treatment for acute infection with antiretroviral therapy is controversial; chronic infection should be treated with combination antiretroviral therapy

KEY POINTS

- Primary HIV infection manifests with a variety of symptoms in 80% of patients, including fever, rash, fatigue, headaches, lymphadenopathy, pharyngitis, myalgias, gastrointestinal symptoms, and oral or genital ulcers
- Syndrome of acute HIV seroconversion corresponds to the phase of massive viremia that occurs approximately 2 weeks after initial infection with HIV

- Diagnosis of acute HIV infection is made by detecting high HIV plasma viral load in the face of a negative anti-HIV antibody
- Treatment of acute HIV syndrome with antiretroviral therapy is controversial and under study

QUESTIONS

1. What is the appropriate *initial* clinical management for this syndrome?

   A. Starting combination antiretroviral therapy immediately
   B. Symptomatic therapy
   C. Prednisone
   D. Cidofovir
   E. High-dose acyclovir

2. The term "retrovirus" refers specifically to the presence of:

   A. Reverse transcriptase
   B. *gag* gene complex
   C. Viral envelope
   D. Incorporation of the viral genome into the host genome
   E. Plasmids

CASE 1-18 West Nile Virus

HPI: WN is a 58-year-old man who was brought to the ER by his wife because of a 4-day history of fevers, chills, night sweats, and myalgias. WN has also developed significant asymmetric weakness in the right lower leg and left arm. WN does not have a cough but feels short of breath and is having difficulty swallowing. No changes in speech, no visual changes, abdominal pain, diarrhea, rash, joint pains, or urinary symptoms. Wife notes that WN has seemed confused over the past 2 days. WN has had no recent gastrointestinal or upper respiratory tract infections.

PMH: WN has a history of hypertension and smoking. Takes an antihypertensive medication and has an allergy to sulfa-containing medications, to which he develops a severe rash. Lives with his wife and works as a civil engineer.

PE: T 38.6°C; HR 112; BP 142/90; RR 18

WN appears in mild respiratory distress with obvious difficulties swallowing. His main physical findings are flaccid paralysis in his left arm and the distal portion of his right leg with loss of reflexes throughout. Sensation is intact throughout. He is alert, but oriented only to self and year. His heart, lung, and abdominal exam are all normal.

Labs: Studies: MRI of the brain was normal, and blood and CSF samples were sent for serology.

THOUGHT QUESTIONS

- What is the differential of acute flaccid paralysis?
- What is the definition of an arbovirus?
- What are some medically important arboviral infections?
- When was West Nile virus detected in the United States and how has it spread since then?

BASIC SCIENCE REVIEW AND DISCUSSION

Differential of Acute Flaccid Paralysis

The differential for **acute flaccid paralysis** is limited and includes **paralytic polio virus** infection, enterovirus 71 infection, vaccine-associated paralytic polio (VAPP) infection, **Guillain-Barré syndrome,** transverse myelitis, botulism (although *Clostridium botulinum* infection is associated with descending **symmetric** paralysis), and some other causes of encephalitis. **West Nile virus encephalitis** has recently been identified as an infection associated with acute flaccid paralysis.

Arboviruses

Arboviruses are arthropod-borne viruses (i.e., spread by mosquitoes and ticks) that include members of the following viral families: **Alphaviridae, Flaviviridae, Bunyaviridae, and Reoviridae.** Table 1-10 lists the important known arboviruses.

The life cycle of the arbovirus is based on the ability of these viruses to multiply in both the vertebrate host and the blood-sucking vector. Only the female of the species serves as the vector of viral transmission to humans, because only females require a blood meal for progeny production. Humans are often dead-end hosts for the arbovirus because viremia is so low in humans that a mosquito or tick cannot ingest enough virus for transmission. In the syndromes of yellow fever and dengue, however, humans have a high-level viremia and the transmitting arthropods are able to acquire the virus through biting humans.

The diseases of arboviruses range in severity from mild to rapidly fatal. The clinical picture of arboviral infections usually fits into one of three categories: (*a*) **encephalitis;** (*b*) **hemorrhagic fever;** and (*c*) fever with myalgia, arthralgias, and nonhemorrhagic rash. Arboviruses have a tendency to cause sudden outbreaks of disease, generally at the interface between human communities and jungle or forest areas where arthropods are found in abundance (Table 1-11).

West Nile Virus

Properties West Nile virus (WNV) is a member of the **flavivirus** family (single-stranded RNA virus).

Transmission and Epidemiology WNV was first identified as a cause of an encephalitis outbreak on the U.S. eastern seaboard in 1999. The flavivirus had first been identified in a patient in Uganda in 1937 but was not previously recognized in the western hemisphere prior to this outbreak. The virus has spread throughout most of the United States and Canada as of the winter of 2002. WNV is primarily an infection of **birds and *Culex* mosquitoes,** with humans and horses serving as incidental hosts. The incidence of human disease peaks in the late summer and early fall after the emergence of mosquitoes and birds provides an efficient means of geographic distribution of the virus. As of October 2002, there have been 2703 laboratory-positive confirmed human cases of WNV infection and 146 deaths since the beginning of 2001. Besides transmission of infection to humans from mosquito bites, case reports have linked transmission to the **transplantation** of four organs from a single donor during the 2002 outbreak.

Clinical Twenty percent of WNV infections are manifested by a mild, febrile illness, which can include malaise, anorexia, nausea, vomiting, headache, lymphadenopathy, eye pain, and rash. The rash is generally an erythematous macular, papular, or morbilliform eruption involving the neck, trunk, arms, or legs. The incubation period of the infection is thought to range from 3 to 14 days and symptoms of the mild illness usually last 3 to 6 days.

More severe infection manifests as meningitis or encephalitis and develops in approximately 1 out of 150 infections. The neurologic illness develops only rarely in young persons; incidence is higher among persons older than 50 years of age and in immuno-suppressed individuals. Encephalitis is more commonly reported

TABLE 1-10 Arboviruses

Viral Family	Examples
Alphaviridae	Eastern equine encephalitis, Western equine encephalitis, Venezuelan equine encephalitis
Flaviviridae	Yellow fever virus, dengue virus, Japanese encephalitis virus, St. Louis encephalitis virus, WNV, tick-borne encephalitis
Bunyaviridae	California encephalitis virus (La Crosse encephalitis)[a]
Reovirus	Colorado tick-borne virus

[a]Hantaviruses are in the bunyavirus family, but they are not considered arboviruses; Hantaviruses are roboviruses (rodent-borne viruses).

than meningitis and is often accompanied by fever, GI symptoms, rash, and mental status changes. Other notable features of the syndrome of WNV encephalitis include severe muscle weakness and **flaccid paralysis,** which may serve to distinguish the syndrome of WNV encephalitis from other etiologies. Other neurologic presentations include ataxia and extrapyramidal signs, cranial nerve abnormalities, myelitis, optic neuritis, areflexia, polyradiculitis, and seizures. Case reports from former outbreaks (not in the United States) have observed myocarditis, pancreatitis, and fulminant hepatitis with WNV infection.

Case fatality rates range from 4 to 14%, with advanced age being the most important risk factor for death (especially age greater than 70 years). In the New York outbreak of 1999–2000, persons 75 years of age and older were nearly nine times more likely to die than younger persons. Clinical risk factors for death are encephalitis with severe muscle weakness and change in the level of consciousness. Diabetes mellitus and immunosuppression may also be independent risk factors for death. Furthermore, recovery from WNV encephalitis is marked by significant long-term neurologic sequelae.

TABLE 1-11 Characteristics of Important Arboviral Diseases

Organism	Vector	Animal Reservoir	Region
Alphaviridae			
Eastern equine encephalitis	Swamp mosquito (*Culiseta*)	Wild birds	Atlantic and Gulf states
Western equine encephalitis	*Culex* mosquito	Wild birds	West of Mississippi river
Venezuelan equine encephalitis	Various mosquitoes	Wild birds	South America
Flaviviridae			
St. Louis encephalitis	*Culex* mosquito	Wild birds	Widespread in southern, central, and western states
Japanese encephalitis	*Culex* mosquito	Birds and pigs	Asia, especially southeast Asia
Dengue virus	*Aedes aegypti*	Monkeys/humans	Tropics
Yellow fever	*Aedes aegypti*	Monkeys/humans	Africa/South America
Tick-borne encephalitis; CEE: Central Europe encephalitis; and RSSE: Russian spring summer encephalitis	*Ixodes* tick	Vertebrates	Central Europe
West Nile virus	*Culex* mosquito	Crows and domestic birds; variety of animals	Most eastern and midwestern states
Bunyaviridae			
California encephalitis virus (La Crosse encephalitis)	*Aedes* mosquito	Small mammals	North-central states
Reoviridae			
Colorado tick fever: *Coltivirus* subfamily	*Dermatocentor* tick	Small mammals	Rocky Mountain states

Diagnosis The most efficient diagnostic method for WNV infection is **detection of IgM antibody** to WNV in the serum or CSF, using the IgM antibody capture enzyme-linked immunosorbent assay (MAC-ELISA). Approximately 75% of patients with WNV encephalitis have detectable IgM in serum or CSF during the first 4 days of illness, and nearly all test positive by 7 to 8 days after the onset of illness. IgM antibodies may persist for a year or more after infection. WNV-specific IgM in the CSF is confirmatory for diagnosis of a current WNV infection, but identification of virus-specific IgM in serum indicates only a probable infection and requires confirmation with acute and convalescent phase antibodies (to identify a change by a factor of four or more in the antibody titer). Patients with recent vaccination against related Flaviviruses (e.g., yellow fever, Japanese encephalitis, dengue) may have positive WNV MAC-ELISA results.

Treatment Treatment is supportive, often involving hospitalization, IV fluids, and respiratory support. Ribavirin in high doses and interferon α-2b were found to have some activity against WNV in vitro, but no controlled clinical trials have been performed.

CASE CONCLUSION

Our patient developed respiratory paralysis on the second day of admission, requiring intubation for mechanical ventilation. WNV-specific IgM antibodies were positive in WN's CSF on the 13th day of hospitalization, confirming the diagnosis of WNV encephalitis. One month after the onset of WN's weakness, he remains in a long-term rehabilitation facility on continued respiratory support.

THUMBNAIL: West Nile Virus Encephalitis

Organism	West Nile virus
Type of organism	Flavivirus (single-stranded RNA virus)
Diseases caused	Mild febrile illness, meningitis, encephalitis notable for severe muscle weakness, and flaccid paralysis
Epidemiology	The virus was first detected in the United States in 1999; since then, WNV has been identified in almost every state; associated with birds and transmitted to humans by the bite of the *Culex* mosquito; transmission has also been linked to the transplantation of four organs from a single donor
Diagnosis	Detection of WNV-specific IgM antibodies in the CSF or a four-fold rise in antibody titer of IgM in serum acute to convalescent phase samples
Treatment	Supportive

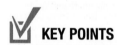

KEY POINTS

- The differential for acute flaccid paralysis is limited, including paralytic polio virus infection, transverse myelitis, Guillain-Barré syndrome, and WNV encephalitis
- Arboviruses are arthropod-borne viruses (spread by mosquitoes or ticks) and include members of the Alphaviridae, Flaviviridae, Bunyaviridae, and Reoviridae families
- WNV was first detected in the United States in 1999 and is associated with an encephalitic syndrome hallmarked by severe muscle weakness and flaccid paralysis
- Definitive diagnosis of WNV encephalitis is made by detection of virus-specific IgM in the CSF

QUESTIONS

1. Which of the following measures can be protective against the acquisition of WNV infection?

    A. Mosquito repellant
    B. Not handling dead birds
    C. Testing pets for latent infection
    D. Avoiding zoos
    E. Never keeping pet birds

2. Which of the following host factors is most strongly linked to increased morbidity and mortality of WNV encephalitis?

    A. HIV
    B. Diabetes mellitus
    C. Iatrogenic immunosuppression
    D. Older age
    E. Young age

CASE 1-19 Hepatitis A Virus

HPI: A 34-year-old-woman comes to the ER because of nausea and jaundice. She has had 4 days of anorexia and malaise. Nausea developed 2 days ago, and this morning she noticed that her eyes were yellow. On questioning, she also notes dark urine and generalized pruritus. She works at a daycare center but does not recall any of the children being ill with similar symptoms. She takes only oral contraceptive pills.

PE: T 36.6°C; BP 108/62; HR 88; RR 16

She is notably jaundiced with icteric sclerae and nail beds. She has mild right upper quadrant tenderness. The remainder of her exam is normal.

Labs: Notable labs include: aspartate aminotransferase (AST) 890; alanine aminotransferase (ALT) 1202; total bilirubin 5.4; alkaline phosphatase 216. Serologies are sent.

THOUGHT QUESTIONS

- What are potential sources for this infection?
- What are potential long-term sequelae of this infection?
- What can be done to prevent infection in people at risk?

BASIC SCIENCE REVIEW AND DISCUSSION

Hepatitis A virus (HAV) is a **nonenveloped, 27- to 30-nm, heat-resistant RNA virus of the Picornavirus (picorna = pico + rna = small RNA) family.** There is only one serotype. **Replication of the virus is limited to the liver,** although virus can be detected in the liver, bile, stool, and blood during active infection. Unlike other hepatitis viruses, HAV will replicate in tissue culture, albeit poorly.

Transmission of HAV occurs almost exclusively from the **fecal-oral route. Person-to-person spread easily occurs** under conditions of poor hygiene and overcrowding. Both large outbreaks and sporadic cases can be traced to contaminated food, water, milk, and shellfish. **Filter-feeding shellfish are an important reservoir for HAV** because they may concentrate large amounts of virus from contaminated water sources during feeding.

Clinically, HAV presents similarly to other types of acute hepatitis with anorexia, nausea, vomiting, and jaundice. The incubation period for HAV ranges from 15 to 45 days, with a mean of 30 days.

Specific diagnosis of HAV is made on the basis of serology. **IgM antibodies to HAV can be detected during the acute illness and are diagnostic of acute infection.** These IgM antibodies persist for several months. During convalescence, IgG titers rise and become the predominant class. Detectable IgG persists indefinitely and indicates immunity to reinfection.

Unlike hepatitis B and C, **there is no carrier state for HAV and no chronic infection occurs,** eliminating the risk of hepatocellular carcinoma that is seen in other chronic viral hepatitides. In general, the prognosis is excellent, with fulminant hepatitis occurring in only 0.1% of cases, more commonly in patients with preexisting hepatitis C or other forms of liver disease. HAV is most often diagnosed in children and young adults, and many infections are clinically mild or silent.

The disease is **self-limited,** and therapy for acute HAV is supportive, consisting of symptom management and ensuring adequate hydration. Because of its potential importance to public health, any case of acute HAV should be reported to local health officials and consideration should be given to preventive therapy in exposed, nonimmune contacts.

All preparations of pooled serum immune globulin contain antibodies to HAV. **Postexposure immunoprophylaxis with immune globulin** should be offered within 2 weeks of exposure to household or childcare center contacts or those exposed to a common source. Casual contacts and medical personnel do not routinely require immune globulin.

Vaccination against HAV is recommended for at-risk populations (healthcare workers, childcare workers, sexually active gay men, and travelers to endemic areas) and populations in whom disease may be more severe (chronic liver disease, hepatitis C infected).

CASE CONCLUSION

The patient was hydrated in the ER and sent home. At follow-up with her primary physician 2 days later, labs from the emergency room demonstrated IgM to hepatitis A virus. She was negative for hepatitis C and showed hepatitis B surface antibody from prior vaccination. Her symptoms continued for 1 week, after which her jaundice slowly resolved. She remained profoundly fatigued for several weeks and was unable to return to work for 5 weeks. Other workers at her daycare center, as well as the children and family members of the children, were offered immunoprophylaxis.

THUMBNAIL: Hepatitis A

Organism	Hepatitis A
Type of organism	Picornavirus: single-stranded RNA virus
Disease caused	Acute hepatitis
Epidemiology	Transmission via fecal-oral route; foodborne outbreaks (shellfish, water, milk) and sexual transmission (oral-anal contact) are common
Diagnosis	HAV IgM antibodies; HAV IgG indicates prior infection or vaccination with subsequent immunity
Treatment	Supportive care; no specific therapy

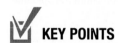

KEY POINTS

■ Hepatitis A is the most common cause of acute infectious hepatitis in adults

■ At-risk populations should be vaccinated

QUESTIONS

1. A 41-year-old man presents to the ER with sudden onset of anorexia, abdominal pain, nausea, and dark urine. He lives with his wife and 2-year-old son who is in daycare, neither of whom are ill. He works as a phlebotomist at your hospital and has been successfully immunized for hepatitis B. He drinks one glass of wine daily with dinner and denies IVDU. He takes no medications. On exam he is afebrile with obvious scleral icterus, mild jaundice, and right upper quadrant tenderness. Labs show normal CBC (complete blood count) and creatinine, AST 1420, ALT 1824, total bilirubin 4.8, alkaline phosphatase 312. What is the most likely source of his infection?

    A. Tick
    B. Sexual partner
    C. Mother
    D. Occupational exposure
    E. Food

2. A healthy 35-year-old woman is going to a remote village in Mexico for hiking in 2 weeks. She has no history of hepatitis A disease or vaccination. Which of the following strategies for prevention of hepatitis A is appropriate?

    A. Hepatitis A vaccine only
    B. Serum immune globulin only
    C. Both hepatitis A vaccine and serum immune globulin
    D. Give her rimantadine to begin taking immediately if she feels ill
    E. No prevention strategy is necessary, as she is not at risk

CASE 1-20 Hepatitis B Virus

HPI: A 35-year-old Taiwanese man presents with fatigue, nausea, and right upper quadrant abdominal pain and bloating over a 2-week period. He has been unable to eat much and has lost 10 pounds. He does not drink alcohol and denies recent ingestions such as Tylenol, wild mushrooms, or herbal medications.

PE: T 37.0°C; BP 120/75; HR 90; RR 14

The patient has scleral icterus but no jaundice. There are no signs of hepatic failure such as gynecomastia, palmar erythema, testicular atrophy, or asterixis. Abdominal exam shows hepatomegaly with a tender smooth liver edge 8 cm below the costal margin.

Labs: White count is 8.0. Hematocrit is 45. Platelets are 200. Electrolytes and renal function are normal. Liver function tests show albumin 3.8, AST 540, ALT 930, alkaline phosphatase 110, and bilirubin of 3.2. International normalized ratio (INR) is 1.0.

Hepatitis serologies are: **HBsAg** (hepatitis B surface antigen) positive; **HBeAg** (hepatitis B e antigen) positive; **anti-HBs** (anti-hepatitis B surface antibody) negative; **anti-HBc** (anti-hepatitis B core antibody) negative. He is HAV IgG positive. Tests for HCV (hepatitis C virus) and HDV (hepatitis D virus) are negative.

Ultrasound is negative for hepatic masses or blood clots affecting perfusion of the liver.

He is offered a liver biopsy to help stage his hepatitis, but he declines and says he would want treatment "no matter what."

THOUGHT QUESTIONS

- What does each test in the hepatitis serology panel tell you about this patient?
- When was this patient likely infected?
- Why do HIV drugs work against hepatitis B virus?

BASIC SCIENCE REVIEW AND DISCUSSION

Hepatitis B is a partially double-stranded DNA virus that infects hepatocytes. Although it is a DNA virus, it replicates through an RNA intermediate, and its polymerase must reverse transcribe the RNA to make new DNA. Therefore, some of the HIV reverse transcriptase inhibitors are also active against HBV.

Hepatitis B can be transmitted through blood or sexual contact. The virus is highly infectious because it reproduces at a very high titer. Its titer and infectivity are approximately 10-fold higher than HCV and 100-fold higher than HIV.

Hepatitis B can cause acute or chronic hepatitis. A useful mnemonic is: H<u>A</u>V causes <u>A</u>cute hepatitis, H<u>C</u>V causes <u>C</u>hronic, and H<u>B</u>V causes <u>B</u>oth.

Rare patients, particularly those with underlying liver disease, may die of fulminant hepatic failure from primary infection with HBV. Most adults make a full recovery; however, neonates or immunocompromised patients infected with HBV are less likely to clear the infection. These patients risk becoming chronically infected, with HBV integrated into hepatocyte genomes. Neonatal infection leading to chronic infection is most common in Asia. Patients with chronic HBV infection have a greatly increased risk of **cirrhosis.** Interestingly, liver damage in hepatitis B is thought to be due solely to the **host's immune response** to the virus; the virus itself is not harmful to liver cells. Another long-term complication of chronic HBV infection is **hepatocellular carcinoma.**

The incidence of this cancer is directly correlated with the duration of chronic HBV infection. Hepatocellular carcinoma can occur independently of cirrhosis, and the virus may increase cancer risk through genetic means—either through disruption of tumor suppressor genes during integration or possibly through the activity of one of its own genes. See Figure 1-13 and Table 1-12 for a diagram and an explanation of hepatitis B serologic tests.

A recombinant HBV vaccine has been very effective in reducing new cases of hepatitis B. Because it contains only the surface antigen and not other parts of the virus, people who have been immunized will exhibit anti-HBs but will not demonstrate anti-HBc, unless they were exposed to the virus in the past.

Treatment for hepatitis B used to be limited to **interferon alfa-2b,** a very toxic therapy with low rates of success. More recently, new antiviral drugs, particularly **lamivudine, adefovir, and tenofovir,** which inhibit the HBV reverse transcriptase, have shown efficacy in reducing viral replication. It is not yet clear whether these drugs should be used sequentially or whether combination therapy modeled after HIV would be better. Compared with HIV, HBV is slower to develop resistance to these drugs. For patients with life-threatening complications of HBV, such as cirrhosis or hepatocellular carcinoma, liver transplantation is an option; recurrence of the HBV infection post-transplant can be prevented by administration of hepatitis B immune globulin.

Patients with multiple hepatitis viral infections have a worse prognosis. All patients with chronic hepatitis should be immunized against hepatitis A. **Hepatitis D** is a defective single-stranded RNA virus that cannot replicate on its own. However, in patients with concomitant HBV infection, HDV is able to replicate and can lead to hepatic decompensation. Hepatitis D is most common in the Mediterranean and is transmitted by blood.

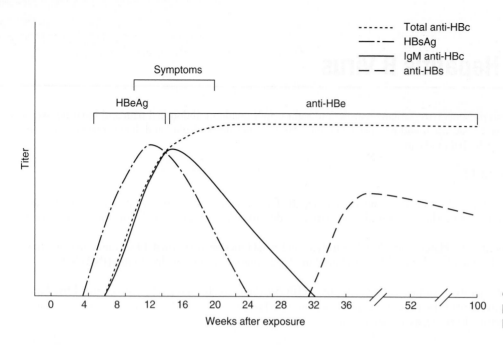

Figure 1-13. Immune response to hepatitis B. (Courtesy of Centers for Disease Control and Prevention.)

Legend:
- Total anti-HBc
- HBsAg
- IgM anti-HBc
- anti-HBs

CASE CONCLUSION

The patient is started on lamivudine. Within a week, the patient is feeling much better. A repeat HBV viral load shows that the viral DNA has become undetectable. Eighteen months later, the patient develops fatigue, nausea, and right upper quadrant tenderness. An HBV viral load is again detectable. His doctor suspects lamivudine resistance has taken root. Lamivudine is continued to select for "less fit" mutant virus, and tenofovir is added in an attempt to suppress the viral load again.

TABLE 1-12 Interpretation of Hepatitis Serologies

Results	Interpretation
Anti-HBs +; anti-HBc +	Past infection; now immune
Anti-HBs +; anti-HBc −	Immunization with recombinant HBV vaccine
Anti-HBs −; anti-HBc +	1. "Window period" after acute infection where anti-HBc has appeared before anti-HBs 2. Distant infection with waning anti-HBs titer 3. Chronic HBV infection, often seen in HBV patients co-infected with HIV or HCV
HBsAg +	Acute or chronic HBV infection
Anti-HBs −; anti-HBc −; HBsAg −	Never exposed or immunized to HBV
HBeAg +	Active HBV infection at high titer; therefore, more infectious

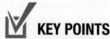

THUMBNAIL: Hepatitis B

Organism	Hepatitis B virus
Type of organism	Hepadna virus (DNA)
Diseases caused	Acute or chronic hepatitis; hepatocellular carcinoma
Epidemiology	In the United States, primarily transmitted through blood exposure or sexual contact; primarily transmitted vertically in many Asian countries
Diagnosis	Serology
Treatment	Lamivudine, adefovir, tenofovir, interferon
Prevention	Vaccination

KEY POINTS

- HBV is a DNA virus that requires a reverse transcriptase for replication; hence, some HIV drugs are active against HBV
- HBV can cause acute or chronic hepatitis; mortality stems from acute fulminant liver failure, cirrhosis, or hepatocellular carcinoma
- HBV is transmitted through blood exposure or through sex, similar to HIV
- An effective recombinant HBV vaccine is available, although not always accessible in developing nations

QUESTIONS

1. Which serologic marker shows immunity to HBV?

   A. Anti-HBe
   B. Anti-HBs
   C. Anti-HBc
   D. HBeAg
   E. HBsAg

2. Which HIV drug is also active against HBV?

   A. ddI
   B. Indinavir
   C. AZT
   D. 3TC (lamivudine)
   E. Nevirapine

HPI: A 16-year-old boy is brought in to the doctor's office one December morning by his mother. For the past 3 days he has been feeling "terrible," staying in bed all day with fever, headache, fatigue, and severe myalgias. "This is the worst cold I've ever had." He has also had a runny nose and mild nonproductive cough.

The mother's parents live with the family. The grandfather has emphysema and the grandmother has had a recent myocardial infarction. Their health is tenuous, and the mother is concerned they could catch his illness.

PE: T 38.5°C; BP 120/60; HR 65; RR 14; SaO_2 sat 99% on room air

Physical exam shows a young man in no respiratory distress, but looking quite fatigued and uncomfortable. The patient is flushed, but there is no rash. His conjunctivae are injected, and his nose has clear discharge. The oropharynx is red but there is no exudate. The neck is supple, with mild enlargement of anterior cervical lymph nodes. Lungs are clear, and heart exam is regular. Abdomen is benign. There is no edema.

A nasal wash is sent for a viral DFA panel, which tests for influenza A and B, parainfluenza 1, 2, and 3, adenovirus, and RSV. The test is positive for influenza A.

THOUGHT QUESTIONS

- Which viruses can cause respiratory symptoms?
- How can a patient with influenza be clinically distinguished from a patient with a cold?
- What measures can be taken to prevent or treat influenza?
- Why is the influenza vaccine required yearly? Who should receive it?
- What are the complications of influenza?

BASIC SCIENCE REVIEW AND DISCUSSION

Influenza is an **orthomyxovirus,** with a segmented negative-sense single-stranded RNA genome. The virus has a membrane envelope embedded with multiple protein spikes called **hemagglutinin** and **neuraminidase.** These are the major viral antigens and are used by researchers to distinguish viral strains. The body uses them to drive its immune response, but viral strains with changes in these proteins are able to re-infect people with an immune response to previous strains of virus. The hemagglutinin functions as a viral adhesion molecule, used to bind sialic acid on the host cell surface as a prelude to infection; the neuraminidase is necessary to cleave off sialic acid from already infected cells to allow the virus to spread to new, uninfected cells.

Influenza is an acute illness that is usually much more severe than a cold, presenting with fevers, malaise, myalgias, and fatigue. Usually the illness is self-limited and resolves in about a week. The major complication of influenza is **pneumonia,** which is the primary cause of mortality. Pneumonia is most common in patients with chronic heart or lung disease. The virus itself may cause pneumonia. Viral infection may also predispose patients to secondary bacterial pneumonia, which usually follows 1 to 2 weeks after the viral infection. Whereas any of the usual bacterial pathogens can cause postviral pneumonia, there is an increased incidence of *Staphylococcus aureus* pneumonia, which is an unusual lung pathogen in other settings.

Influenza has a pattern of **epidemic** spread, every 1 to 3 years. These epidemics are caused by **antigenic drift** in the virus, moderate changes in the viral coat proteins that allow the virus to infect people who have previously had influenza. Every few decades, an influenza **pandemic** occurs, thought to be due to an **antigenic shift,** wherein a brand new subtype of viral coat proteins occurs. The pandemic viruses are always influenza A, and they are thought to be due to recombination of avian and human influenza viruses in swine in Southeast Asia. The new virus usually receives a new designation for its coat proteins. For example, the Spanish pandemic of 1918 was caused by an H1N1 (hemagglutinin type 1, neuraminidase type 1) virus, and was succeeded by the 1968 Hong Kong flu, which was an H2N2 virus. After an antigenic shift, the new virus is able to spread widely because the population has no effective immunity. Such pandemics can be devastating. The 1918 pandemic killed 21 million people, many of them younger individuals.

Influenza may be prevented by vaccinations. Experts survey viruses in human and animal populations to guess in advance which viruses will be circulating the following winter. A vaccine is then manufactured according to these predictions; most years these predictions turn out to be correct and the vaccine is protective. Because of yearly changes in the circulating virus, the vaccine must be administered on a yearly basis as well.

Two sets of antiviral medications are available for influenza. All must be prescribed within 48 hours of symptom onset to have any effect on the course of the illness. The medications may also be used for prophylaxis during influenza outbreaks to prevent illness in those who were not vaccinated. Two drugs, amantadine and rimantadine, act by preventing viral **uncoating.** They are only effective against influenza A. Two newer drugs, the neuraminidase inhibitors oseltamivir and zanamivir, are active against both types of influenza. They inhibit **neuraminidase,** which the virus requires to cleave off sialic acid molecules on the host cell membrane. Without the ability to cleave these receptor molecules off, the virus is trapped on the cell, unable to move to another cell and spread the infection.

THUMBNAIL: Respiratory Viruses

Organism	Influenza A and B	Parainfluenza 1, 2, and 3	Respiratory syncytial virus	Adenovirus	Rhinovirus	Coronavirus
Type of organism	Orthomyxovirus (negative-sense, ssRNA virus)	Paramyxovirus (negative-sense, ssRNA virus)	Paramyxovirus (negative-sense, ssRNA virus)	Adenovirus (dsDNA virus)	Picornavirus (positive-sense, ssRNA virus)	Coronavirus (positive-sense, ssRNA virus)
Diseases caused	Influenza	URI (upper respiratory tract infection), croup, bronchiolitis	Pneumonia, bronchiolitis, tracheobronchitis	Tracheitis, bronchiolitis, pneumonia; subclinical infection common	URI	URI
Epidemiology	Spread by person-to-person contact; pigs serve as a reservoir in which new strains can be generated; annual winter epidemics; regular pandemics every few decades	Person-to-person contact; subtype of outbreaks changes in a yearly pattern	Person-to-person contact; newborns almost universally infected; yearly predictable pattern of outbreaks	Person-to-person contact	Person-to-person contact	Person-to-person contact
Diagnosis	DFA; ELISA; culture	DFA; ELISA; culture; serologies	DFA; ELISA; culture; serologies	DFA; ELISA; culture; serologies	Culture (rarely performed); serology only possible if infecting serotype is known	All rarely performed: culture, antigen detection, RT-PCR
Treatment	Amantadine (A only); rimantadine (A only); oseltamivir; zanamivir		Ribavirin			
Prevention	Immunization; prophylaxis with antiviral agents		Hyperimmune globulin or monoclonal antibody in high-risk infants	Oral vaccine used in the military		

CASE CONCLUSION

Because the boy has had symptoms for more than 48 hours, it is too late for him to benefit from antiviral medication. He is also at low risk of complications. However, the physician is concerned about the grandparents, in whom influenza could be life-threatening. When he hears they did not receive influenza vaccinations this year, he prescribes them prophylactic rimantadine to decrease their chances of contracting the virus. (He chooses rimantadine over amantadine because it is less likely to have CNS side effects in the elderly.)

The grandparents are admonished to have influenza vaccinations every year from now on.

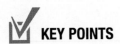

KEY POINTS

■ Viruses that cause respiratory symptoms include influenza, parainfluenza, RSV, adenovirus, coronavirus, and rhinovirus; influenza tends to cause more systemic symptoms than other causes of viral URIs

■ Influenza can be prevented with immunization or with prophylactic antiviral medication

■ The course of illness can be ameliorated if antivirals are administered within 48 hours of onset: Amantadine and rimantadine inhibit viral uncoating but are only active against influenza A; the neuraminidase inhibitors oseltamivir and zanamivir are active against both influenza A and B

QUESTIONS

1. Which of the following patients is likely to have influenza?

   A. A 34 year old with 3 days of vomiting and diarrhea
   B. A 12 year old who has trouble paying attention in class because of his nasal congestion and cough
   C. A 25 year old with anorexia, nausea, right upper quadrant abdominal pain, and jaundice
   D. A 21-year-old recent Mexican immigrant with cough, conjunctivitis, runny nose, and a macular erythematous rash
   E. A 29 year old confined to bed with headache, myalgias, fatigue, and high fever

2. Which enzyme is inhibited by zanamivir?

   A. Reverse transcriptase
   B. Hemagglutinin
   C. Protease
   D. Neuraminidase
   E. Dihydrofolate reductase

3. Which of the following is a contraindication to influenza vaccination?

   A. AIDS
   B. Receipt of the vaccine within the previous 5 years
   C. Pregnancy
   D. Allergy to eggs
   E. Severe pulmonary or cardiac disease

4. Which of the following drugs is active against influenza B?

   A. Amantadine
   B. Stavudine
   C. Oseltamivir
   D. Nelfinavir
   E. Rimantadine

CASE 1-22 *Aspergillus Fumigatus*

HPI: AF is a 55-year-old man who had a cadaveric renal transplant a year ago for kidney disease related to his long-standing diabetes mellitus. He is on multiple immunosuppressive medications and has recently needed several courses of steroids to treat rejection of his transplanted organ. AF presents to the office today complaining of 5 days of severe shortness of breath with a cough productive of blood-tinged sputum with black streaks, fevers and chills, severe fatigue, and sharp chest pain with deep breathing or coughing.

PMH: Type II diabetes mellitus and hypertension; medications include insulin injections, atenolol, hydrochlorothiazide, cyclosporine, tacrolimus, and prednisone at a current dose of 6 mg orally every day. No allergies to medications.

HPI: T 38.9°C; HR 114; BP 98/62; RR 24; SaO$_2$ 86% on room air

AF is a very ill-appearing, cachectic man, breathing rapidly and having problems speaking secondary to shortness of breath. His lung exam is significant for crackles in the right lung field. Skin is dry without any rashes.

Labs: WBC 14.2 with 82% neutrophils. Sputum Gram stain shows septate hyphae branching at acute angles. Chest X-ray has a cavitary lung lesion in the right upper lobe and peripheral consolidations.

THOUGHT QUESTIONS

- What are the possible etiologies of pneumonia in patients on immunosuppressives?
- What is the most likely etiology in this patient?
- What is the microbiology of this organism?
- What is the epidemiology of disease with this organism and what are its syndromes?
- What are its possible treatments?

BASIC SCIENCE REVIEW AND DISCUSSION

Differential

The differential for lower respiratory infections in immunocompromised patients is vast. Although neutropenia is an additional risk factor for many of the fungal or viral pathogens, the use of prednisone or potent immunosuppressive therapy can predispose patients to a number of respiratory infections even without neutropenia. Besides the bacterial agents associated with typical community-acquired and atypical pneumonias, immunocompromised patients are also susceptible to a number of additional pathogens, including **gram-negative bacilli,** *Pneumocystis carinii, Staphylococcus* **species, fungal infections, including the dimorphic fungi and molds, viruses (especially cytomegalovirus),** *Nocardia* **species,** *Rhodococcus equi,* **and** *Legionella.* The septate acute-angle branching hyphae in the sputum of this immunosuppressed patient on steroids probably indicates a respiratory tract infection with the dreaded *Aspergillus.*

Microbiology

Aspergillus **is an ubiquitous mold** and serves as a saprophytic fungus in soil, its natural ecological niche. *Aspergillus fumigatus* is the usual cause of aspergillosis, although there are several disease-causing species of *Aspergillus* in humans. *A. fumigatus* is characterized by green conidia, approximately 2.5 to 3 μm in diameter, produced in chains from greenish stalks. A rare isolate of this organism is pigmentless and produces white conidia. The chains of conidia are borne on broad vesicles of approximately 20 to 30 μm in diameter. **Replication is achieved by a process**

of budding, and there is no sexual stage. *A. fumigatus* grows relatively rapidly and can reach a colony size of approximately 4 cm within 1 week when grown on special media at 25°C. In nature, *A. fumigatus* is a thermophilic species, with growth occurring at temperatures as high as 55°C and survival maintained at temperatures up to 70°C. *Aspergillus* **forms septate, true hyphae with acute-angle branching at 45°** with clusters of conidia topping the fungal stalks (Figure 1-14). *Aspergillus* cell walls are more or less parallel, in contrast to *Mucor* and *Rhizopus* walls, which are more irregular.

Epidemiology

Environmental surveys indicate that all humans will inhale at least several hundred *A. fumigatus* conidia per day. As the airborne conidia have a small enough diameter to reach the lung alveoli, **most susceptible patients manifest disease with *A. fumigatus* in the respiratory tract.** However, *Aspergillus* can also **invade the nose and paranasal sinuses, external ear, or traumatized skin,** leading to subsequent infection in these organs. *Aspergillus* can also disseminate to virtually any organ in the severely compromised patient.

The most important determinant in *Aspergillus* infection is the immune status of the host. A fourfold increase in invasive aspergillosis has been observed in developed countries over the past two decades secondary to increased iatrogenic immunosuppression. The incidence of aspergillosis in certain transplant populations is shown in Table 1-13.

Neutropenia in acute leukemics and bone marrow transplant (BMT) patients is the most important risk factor for aspergillosis, just as the return of bone marrow function is vital to the therapeutic response to antifungals. In solid organ transplant patients, immunosuppression predisposes to infection; **high-dose corticosteroids alone** may predispose to aspergillosis in some patients. Previously normal children with invasive aspergillosis should be evaluated for **chronic granulomatous disease.** Patients in the **late stages of HIV infection** (usually with CD4 counts of less than 50 cells/μL) have an increased susceptibility to invasive aspergillosis, although half of them usually have a secondary predisposing factor, such as leukopenia or corticosteroid

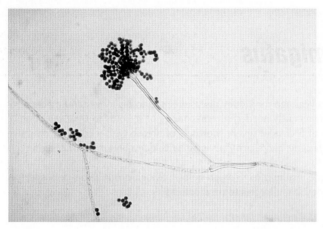

• **Figure 1-14.** Conidia of *Aspergillus fumigatus*. (Image in public domain from Centers for Disease Control and Prevention Public Health Image Library, http://phil.cdc.gov/phil/home.asp)

therapy. In addition to immunosuppression, **prolonged use of broad-spectrum antibiotics and parenteral nutrition** predispose to this fungal infection. Patient-to-patient spread of *Aspergillus* has not been documented.

Clinical Syndromes

Aspergillus **can invade tissue planes** or spread hematogenously, leading to a myriad of clinical syndromes. One prominent feature of these infections is **growth of hyphae into and along blood vessels,** leading to hemorrhagic infarction and necrosis of affected tissue. The following organ systems are predominantly infected.

Ear and Sinus Mucosal invasion by *A. fumigatus* in the nose and sinus can spread rapidly to contiguous structures, causing vascular invasion and necrosis. Infection can ultimately lead to proptosis and monocular blindness.

Eye Minor trauma to the cornea can lead to deep stromal invasion with *Aspergillus* in susceptible patients. Endophthalmitis due to *Aspergillus* can occur hematogenously in immunosuppressed patients or can be a late complication of cataract extraction.

Lungs Four main clinical syndromes:

1. ***Allergic bronchopulmonary aspergillosis*** (ABPA): this disease is defined more as an **allergic response to *Aspergillus*** antigens rather than direct invasion by the organism and usually occurs in immunocompetent asthmatics. The clinical syndrome of ABPA is manifested by **peripheral eosinophilia,** fleeting pulmonary infiltrates from bronchial plugging, an immediate-type skin test response to *Aspergillus* antigens, and **elevation in total serum IgE and anti-*Aspergillus* IgG levels.** Septate hyphae can be seen microscopically in expectorated sputum plugs, with *Aspergillus* growth on culture. **Treatment is usually a combination of high-dose steroids and antifungals.**

2. *Aspergilloma:* this syndrome is described as a **"fungus ball"** in the lungs and is usually caused by growth of *Aspergillus* in a preexisting lung cavity (e.g., from TB, sarcoidosis, histoplasmosis, bronchiectasis). Aspergillomas can also occur de novo and are marked by severe hemoptysis, intermittent *Aspergillus* in the sputum, and elevated peripheral titers of anti-*Aspergillus* IgG.

3. *Aspergillus pneumonia:* patients with prolonged neutropenia are the highest risk group for acute, rapidly progressing *Aspergillus* pneumonia. This process results in **dense consolidations and cavitations,** with clues to the diagnosis being pleuritic chest pain secondary to extension of the infection to the visceral pleura and hemoptysis from blood vessel invasion.

4. *Pseudomembranous tracheobronchitis:* this condition can be seen in HIV infection or in less severely immunocompromised patients, and is manifested by fever, dyspnea, cough, expectorated sputum plugs, and hemoptysis. Bronchoscopy reveals yellowish plaques or membranes (**"cotton balls"**) on hyperemic tracheobronchial mucosa.

CNS The most common manifestation of CNS aspergillosis is the formation of **brain abscesses** from hematogenous spread of the fungus. **Cerebral infarction** can also occur by occlusion of the cerebral blood vessels by the organism.

Cardiac Cardiac manifestations of *Aspergillus* include endocarditis, myocarditis, and coronary artery embolization by the hyphae.

Other *Aspergillus* can also lead to esophageal or GI ulcerations, necrotizing skin ulcers, osteomyelitis, or infection of the kidneys, bone marrow, thyroid gland, adrenal glands, and pancreas.

Diagnosis and Treatment

Diagnosis of *Aspergillus* infection usually is made by culturing the organism from the appropriate sample and by viewing septate hyphae with dichotomous 45°-angle branching invading tissue under histologic examination. **Blood vessel or tissue invasion by the organism is highly suggestive of true *Aspergillus* infection, rather than colonization.** However, the presence of any *Aspergillus* organisms in the sputum of a highly immunosuppressed patient should be investigated carefully. Serology is helpful in the diagnosis of ABPA or aspergilloma if an increase in anti-*Aspergillus* IgG antibodies is observed.

The mainstay of treatment for invasive *Aspergillus* infections has been intravenous amphotericin B (ampho B), although a recent study suggests that the new triazole, **voriconazole,** is more effective than ampho B for the initial treatment of this infection.[1] As voriconazole is much better tolerated than ampho B and can be given both intravenously and orally, the development of this antifungal may be a major breakthrough in the treatment of invasive aspergillosis. In fact, treatment with voriconazole, caspofungin, or both together is often the treatment

TABLE 1-13 Incidence of Aspergillosis	
Iatrogenic Procedure	Incidence of Invasive Aspergillosis
Allogeneic BMT	4–6%
Autologous BMT	0.7%
Renal transplantation	3.9%
Heart or lung transplant	1.7%
Liver transplant	1.5%

of choice in this setting. As ABPA was thought to be primarily an allergic response to *Aspergillus* antigen, this condition was initially treated with only high-dose corticosteroids. However, recent data indicates that adding **itraconazole to steroid therapy for ABPA improves treatment response.**[2] Oral itraconazole

can be administered for more indolent *Aspergillus* infections, although *Aspergillus* resistance to this agent is emerging. Finally, **surgical resection** of an aspergilloma, an isolated *Aspergillus* pulmonary lesion, or invasive aspergillosis of the brain or sinuses may improve the prognoses of these grim conditions.

CASE CONCLUSION

AF had a bronchoscopy for diagnostic purposes and was found to have acute-angle branching septate hyphae with blood vessel invasion on bronchial biopsies. He was started on intravenous voriconazole therapy for invasive pulmonary aspergillosis. AF's respiratory function grew increasingly compromised, requiring intubation upon admission. He suffered respiratory arrest on his third day of hospitalization and expired.

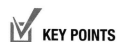

THUMBNAIL: Aspergillosis

Organism	*A. fumigatus*
Type of organism	Thermophilic mold; forms septate hyphae that branch at 45° dichotomous angles
Diseases caused	Sinus infections; eye infections; pulmonary infections, including allergic bronchopulmonary aspergillosis, aspergillomas, cavitations, tracheobronchitis, and invasive pneumonias; CNS infections, myocarditis, and endocarditis
Epidemiology	Invasive infection occurs primarily in severely immunocompromised hosts on corticosteroids, immunosuppressive therapy, or with neutropenia
Diagnosis	Culture and demonstrating tissue invasion on biopsy
Treatment	Intravenous or oral voriconazole or intravenous ampho B for serious infections; oral itraconazole for indolent infections; steroids and itraconazole for ABPA

KEY POINTS

- *A. fumigatus* is a thermophilic mold identified by its septate hyphae that branch at acute angles
- Invasive aspergillosis occurs in the severely immunocompromised host and carries a poor prognosis
- Intravenous or oral voriconazole will probably replace intravenous ampho B as the mainstay of therapy for severe *Aspergillus* infections

QUESTIONS

1. Amphotericin B is notable for the following toxicity:
   A. Hepatotoxicity
   B. Renal tubular acidosis
   C. Hyperkalemia
   D. Pulmonary fibrosis
   E. Lupus-like syndrome

2. Mucormycosis can be distinguished from aspergillosis in that *Mucor* branches at angles of:
   A. 15°
   B. 30°
   C. 60°
   D. 90°
   E. 150°

REFERENCES

1. Herbrecht R, Denning DW, Patterson TF, et al. Voriconazole versus amphotericin B for primary therapy of invasive aspergillosis. N Engl J Med 2002;347:408–415.

2. Stevens DA, Schwartz HJ, Lee JY, et al. A randomized trial of itraconazole in allergic bronchopulmonary aspergillosis. N Engl J Med 2000;342:756–762.

HPI: A 37-year-old gay man with long-standing AIDS presents with 10 days of gradually worsening headache, fever, and weakness. He called your office today for an appointment because he began vomiting last night. Despite the fact that he has been compliant with his antiretroviral regimen of didanosine, abacavir, indinavir, and ritonavir, his CD4 count was 74 cells/μL at last check. He also takes TMP-SMX and weekly azithromycin as well as pravastatin (Pravachol) for hyperlipidemia and atenolol for hypertension.

PE: T 38.6°C; BP 148/96; HR 86; RR 12

The patient is groggy, but oriented. Mild meningismus is present. Fundi exam is normal. There are three papular, ulcerated skin lesions, less than 1 cm long, on his upper extremities. Otherwise the exam is normal.

Labs: Opening pressure 280 cm H_2O, WBC 12 (100% lymphocytes), RBC 22, glucose 30, protein 84. Cultures and serology sent.

THOUGHT QUESTIONS

- Where did this patient's infection originate?
- How is the causative organism identified?
- What features of this organism add to its virulence?

BASIC SCIENCE REVIEW AND DISCUSSION

Cryptococcus neoformans is a round, yeast-like **fungus,** 4 to 6 μm in diameter with a large **polysaccharide capsule. Smooth, creamy white, mucoid colonies** appear within 36 to 72 hours on most simple culture media, including **Sabouraud's agar,** at 37°C.

Microscopically, *Cryptococcus* appears as **spherical, budding, encapsulated yeast cells.** The capsule varies in size among different strains but may be up to twice the width of the individual cell. There are four capsular serotypes (A, B, C, and D), with **serotype A being the most commonly isolated in human disease.** The capsule is composed primarily of glucuronoxylomannan (GXM), and the degree of mannosyl substitution of the GXM determines the serotype. Capsular GXM has been shown to inhibit both phagocytosis of the yeast cells and production of antibody.

All *Cryptococcus* species are **nonfermentative, hydrolyze starch, assimilate inositol, and produce urease.** These are the characteristics that distinguish *Cryptococcus* from other medically important yeasts. Additionally, *C. neoformans* produces a **phenoloxidase** that converts catecholamines into dark pigments. This may be important in the virulence of the organism, as mutants lacking phenoloxidase activity may be killed by the epinephrine oxidase system.

Cases of cryptococcal infection occur sporadically worldwide, and the yeast is ubiquitous in soil and **avian fecal material.** Disease may occur in normal hosts but is more commonly seen in patients with some degree of **immunosuppression** such as AIDS (usually with CD4 counts of less than 200 cell/μL), hematologic malignancies, autoimmune disease, or corticosteroid therapy. Among persons with AIDS, the annual incidence is 2 to 4 cases per 1000.

Infection is acquired by **inhalation** of cells into the lung. Pulmonary infection may be clinically silent and resolve spontaneously, but hematogenous spread to the CNS may lead to a **meningoencephalitis** with scant inflammatory response by the host.

Clinically, patients with cryptococcal meningitis present **subacutely** with headache, fever, nausea, blurred vision, irritability, and gait changes. Because of a mild inflammatory response, nuchal rigidity is often mild. Papilledema is present in only one third of cases. Cerebral edema and/or hydrocephalus may occur in untreated cases, which are invariably fatal.

Lumbar puncture (LP) often reveals a **minimally inflammatory CSF with few lymphocytes.** CSF glucose is low in over half of cases, and protein may be normal to slightly high. **Opening pressure must be carefully measured, as values greater than 250 mm H_2O correlate to poor neurologic outcome and death.** In cases with increased pressure, repeated LPs or continuous CSF drainage must be considered.

Culture of the organism from CSF is the most common means of diagnosis. Blood cultures are often positive, as up to 40% of cases of meningitis involve concurrent fungemia and up to 60% show disseminated infection. The **cryptococcal antigen** (CrAg) test is better than 95% sensitive on either serum or CSF. High titers are often seen, but serum titers are not correlated to clinical or microbiologic response to therapy. **India ink** preparation and mucicarmine staining of the CSF often demonstrates the encapsulated yeast cells (Fig. 1-15) but is not frequently used currently because of the widely available CrAg, which has superior sensitivity and specificity.

Isolated pulmonary cryptococcal infection mimics malignancy. Serum CrAg and culture are less reliable, and biopsy is often required to make the diagnosis. *Cryptococcus* may also cause ulcerated papular skin lesions or bone lesions similar to tuberculosis. In these forms of disease, biopsy is the diagnostic tool of choice.

Initial therapy for cryptococcal meningitis in AIDS patients consists of an induction phase with **amphotericin B** with **flucytosine.** The major side effects of amphotericin are renal toxicity with acidosis and elevated creatinine, infusion-associated rigors, hypokalemia, and hypomagnesemia. The major toxicity of flucytosine is bone marrow suppression. After an induction period of 2 weeks or until clinical improvement occurs, suppressive therapy with **fluconazole** is initiated at high doses, and then set at lower doses. Suppressive therapy should continue indefinitely or until a patient is asymptomatic and has a sustained (>6 month) increase in CD4 cells to greater than 100–200 cells/μL while on antiretroviral therapy. Some experts suggest repeating an LP prior to discontinuation of suppressive therapy to ensure clearance of the organism from the CSF.

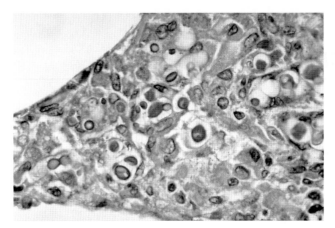

• **Figure 1-15.** Mucicarmine stain of *Cryptococcus neoformans* on histopathology of lung from an AIDS patient. (Image in public domain from Centers for Disease Control and Prevention Public Health Image Library, http://phil.cdc.gov/phil/home.asp, courtesy of Dr. Edwin P. Ewing, Jr.)

In patients without AIDS, treatment is with amphotericin alone or in combination with flucytosine. Therapy continues until four weekly CSF cultures (or India ink stains) are negative and CSF glucose is normal. Up to 70% of non-AIDS patients achieve cure. The mortality rate is approximately 12%.

CASE CONCLUSION

Our patient was admitted to the hospital and started on amphotericin B and flucytosine. Serum and CSF CrAg tests were both positive. Cultures of both CSF and blood grew *C. neoformans*. LP was repeated three more times over the next week with 10 mL of CSF removed each time, in order to control the elevated intracranial pressure. The patient made a gradual recovery and was transferred to a rehabilitation facility 2 weeks later on high-dose fluconazole.

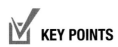

THUMBNAIL: *Cryptococcus neoformans*

Organism	*C. neoformans*
Type of organism	Encapsulated yeast
Diseases caused	Meningoencephalitis; pneumonia; skin and bone lesions
Epidemiology	Common environmental organism in soil worldwide; associated with pigeon droppings; infection via inhalational route; most disease among immunosuppressed patients: AIDS (CD4 counts <200 cell/μL), hematologic malignancies, autoimmune disease, or corticosteroid therapy
Diagnosis	Culture of CSF or blood; India ink examination of CSF; cryptococcal antigen in serum or CSF; biopsy may be necessary in pulmonary or skin infection
Treatment	Induction therapy with amphotericin B and flucytosine, then high-dose fluconazole, followed by maintenance therapy with lower-dose fluconazole

KEY POINTS

■ In addition to specific antifungal therapy, control of elevated intracranial pressure is an important determinant of clinical outcome with cryptococcal meningitis

■ In patients with AIDS and cryptococcal meningitis, long-term suppressive therapy is required until sustained increases in CD4 count on antiretroviral therapy are achieved

QUESTIONS

1. A patient with AIDS and cryptococcal meningitis is started on amphotericin B and flucytosine. Which of the following is the major toxicity of flucytosine?

   A. Renal tubular acidosis
   B. Infusion-related fevers and rigors
   C. Hypokalemia
   D. Hypomagnesemia
   E. Pancytopenia

2. Which of the following properties of *Cryptococcus* does not contribute to its virulence?

   A. The capsular polysaccharide inhibits phagocytosis of the yeast
   B. The capsular polysaccharide inhibits antibody production to the yeast
   C. The yeast secretes a toxin that directly kills macrophages
   D. The yeast phenoloxidase enzyme breaks down host catecholamine, which are toxic to the yeast

HPI: A 52-year-old diabetic woman undergoes emergency surgery for a perforated gallbladder, secondary to cholelithiasis. During the surgery, her peritoneum is irrigated with antibiotic solution. She is treated with broad-spectrum antimicrobial therapy with IV piperacillin-tazobactam. Because she cannot be fed, total parenteral nutrition is started through a central intravenous catheter in her right internal jugular vein. She has a persistent fever, and a follow-up CT scan shows the development of several abdominal abscesses. She is brought back to the OR for a repeat laparotomy during which the abscesses are drained. Cultures of the abscesses grow *Escherichia coli* and *Enterococcus* sensitive to piperacillin-tazobactam. Three days after the second operation, she develops new fevers and becomes hypotensive, requiring both epinephrine and phenylephrine to maintain a blood pressure of 110/50. Her diabetes is being managed with an insulin drip.

She has had normal respiratory secretions. She has started to have loose bowel movements over the past 2 days.

PE: T 39°C; BP 110/50 on multiple pressors; HR 110

Intubated and sedated patient. On a ventilator, requiring increasing support, with a delivered FiO_2 of 70% and a positive end-expiratory pressure (PEEP) of 10. The patient has no rashes. Her central line site shows no erythema. Her lung sounds are coarse due to the ventilator. Her heart has a regular rhythm with no murmur. Her abdomen is soft. The abdominal incision shows pink tissue with no exudate or erythema; she is not forming granulation tissue, however. Wound drains are showing minimal output of serosanguinous fluid.

Labs: WBC 18, Hct (hematocrit) 31, platelets 140. Electrolytes are within normal limits.

A chest X-ray shows some bibasilar atelectasis, but no effusions or infiltrates.

A sputum Gram stain shows mixed flora. A stool test for *Clostridium difficile* toxin is negative.

Two of two blood cultures grow yeast.

THOUGHT QUESTIONS

- What is the difference between yeast and mold?
- What is the range of infections caused by yeast?
- Where could this patient's yeast have come from?
- What options do the doctors have for treating her infection?
- What are common causes of fever in the intensive care unit (ICU)?

BASIC SCIENCE REVIEW AND DISCUSSION

Fungi can be divided into **yeast** (e.g., *Candida*, *Cryptococcus*), which have an oval or round cellular shape, and **molds** (*Aspergillus*), which form long filamentous structures. Some fungi, the **dimorphic fungi** (e.g., *Coccidioides*, *Blastomyces*, *Histoplasma*) are able to grow in both forms. Mycologists make many identifications by morphology rather than by biochemical testing. *Candida* is an oval budding yeast with pseudohyphae, whereas *Cryptococcus* are round in shape. A **germ tube** test looks for the development of tube-like projections from the *Candida* yeast cells when they are put in a special medium. A positive germ tube test confirms that the yeast is *Candida albicans*. If the test is negative, then the yeast species is determined by chemical tests. The speciation is important because certain yeast species, such as *C. glabrata* and *C. krusei*, are resistant to fluconazole, a drug frequently used to treat yeast infections. Yeast speciation is often used to choose therapy because the determination of antifungal susceptibilities is time consuming and often not standardized.

Most yeast infections are superficial minor infections, affecting the skin or mucous membranes of the mouth (thrush) or vagina. These infections are more common in patients with impaired cellular immunity, such as diabetics, patients on steroids or other immunosuppressive agents, and AIDS patients. These infections can often be treated with topical azoles or with nystatin.

Systemic yeast infections are uncommon. They tend to occur in seriously compromised hosts, like the patient described in this case. **Risk factors** for infection include recent abdominal surgery (as the gut can be a source of infecting yeast) or in-dwelling central lines (another potential portal of entry). Impaired cell-mediated immunity (from AIDS, diabetes, steroids, and immunosuppression) or neutropenia can also predispose a host to fungal infection. Finally, high blood lipid levels from total parenteral nutrition (TPN), high blood sugar levels from diabetes, and alteration of normal bacterial flora due to administration of broad-spectrum antibiotics can also create favorable circumstances for yeast.

There are several classes of antifungal drugs. The **azoles** (both topical drugs such as miconazole and econazole and systemic drugs such as fluconazole and voriconazole) act by inhibiting synthesis of **ergosterol,** an analog of cholesterol that is a required component of fungal membranes but is not found in mammalian cell membranes. The **polyenes** (amphotericin and nystatin) act by binding to ergosterol in the fungal cell membrane and creating holes in the membrane, thereby killing the cell. Amphotericin causes both infusion-related toxicity (fever and chills) and renal toxicity (decreased glomerular filtration rate [GFR], along with magnesium and potassium wasting). Newer lipid-based forms of amphotericin have been developed in an attempt to reduce the toxicity of this drug. Finally, a new class of drugs, the **echinocandins** (caspofungin), block b-glycan synthesis in the fungal cell wall.

CASE CONCLUSION

The patient's central intravenous line is removed and a temporary line is placed. Another set of blood cultures is drawn before amphotericin B is started. The original cultures are speciated as *C. albicans*, using the germ tube test; the follow-up blood cultures are negative. The patient tolerates the amphotericin poorly, with her creatinine rising above 2.0 after 3 days of therapy. She is switched to IV fluconazole. A dilated funduscopic exam is done to rule out the complication of *Candida* endophthalmitis, which would necessitate additional local treatment in the eye. Despite treatment of her infections, the patient develops an increasing requirement for vasopressors and for ventilatory support. Several days later, her family decides to withdraw aggressive care, and the patient dies.

THUMBNAIL: *Candida*

Organism	*C. albicans*
Type of organism	Yeast (fungus)
Diseases caused	Local infections of perineum, vagina, or oropharynx; line-related bacteremia; hepatosplenic infections
Epidemiology	More prevalent in patients with defects in cellular immunity (AIDS, transplant immunosuppression, steroids)
Diagnosis	Culture
Treatment	Topical treatment with azoles or nystatin; fluconazole or voriconazole; amphotericin B; caspofungin

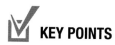

KEY POINTS

- Fungi can be divided into yeast (e.g., *Candida*, *Cryptococcus*) and molds (*Aspergillus*); some fungi, the dimorphic fungi (e.g., *Coccidioides*, *Blastomyces*, and *Histoplasma*) are able to grow in both forms
- Most yeast infections are superficial, affecting the skin or mucous membranes of the mouth or vagina
- Systemic yeast infections are usually only seen in patients with breaches in their defenses (e.g., in-dwelling lines that provide a route of entry through the skin) or with deficiencies in cell-mediated immunity
- Minor *Candida* infections are treated topically; serious infections may be treated with azoles, amphotericin, or caspofungin

QUESTIONS

1. A physician is obligated to treat yeast grown from which culture site?

   A. Stool
   B. Sputum
   C. Skin
   D. Urine
   E. Blood

2. Which yeast antibiotic has the most toxicity?

   A. Amphotericin B
   B. Miconazole
   C. Nystatin
   D. Econazole
   E. Caspofungin

3. Which of the following drugs acts by blocking yeast cell wall synthesis?

   A. Amphotericin B
   B. Penicillin
   C. Fluconazole
   D. Nystatin
   E. Caspofungin

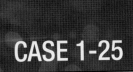

CASE 1-25

Coccidioidomycosis and the Endemic Mycoses

HPI: A 35-year old-woman who lives in Arizona had a cadaveric renal transplant 8 months ago for end-stage renal disease from rapidly progressive glomerulonephritis. She has been on immunosuppression with FK506 and prednisone. She presents to the hospital with a 3-day history of progressive shortness of breath, productive cough, and fevers.

PE: T 39.0°C; HR 125; BP 95/50; RR 25; SaO$_2$ 89% on room air

On exam, she is tired, anxious, and in moderate respiratory distress. She can speak in 2- to 3-word sentences and is using accessory muscles to breathe.

Labs: WBC 18 with a left shift; ABG (arterial blood gas) pH 7.30; pCO$_2$ 45; pO$_2$ 65 on room air

Chest X-ray shows bilateral fluffy infiltrates.

The patient is intubated. Bronchoscopy is done and sputum is sent for culture. Several days later, a mold grows from the culture and is identified as *Coccidioides*.

THOUGHT QUESTIONS

- Which infectious agents cause diffuse, bilateral pneumonia?
- Which unique types of organisms cause pneumonia in immunocompromised patients?
- What are the endemic fungi and where in the United Sates are they found?
- Aside from culture, how can the diagnosis of coccidioidomycosis be made?
- Besides giving the patient antifungal agents, what else can be done to improve her ability to fight off this life-threatening infection?
- Why are the lab workers angry at the patient's doctors when they find *Coccidioides* growing in the cultures and had not been warned about the possibility of this organism?

BASIC SCIENCE REVIEW AND DISCUSSION

In a normal host, diffuse pneumonia is usually caused by so-called **atypical agents** such as *Mycoplasma*, *Chlamydia*, or *Legionella*. Respiratory viruses, such as the influenza A and B viruses, parainfluenza viruses, and adenovirus, can also potentially produce this picture. The **endemic fungal infections** such as **coccidioidomycosis, blastomycosis,** and **histoplasmosis** can all cause diffuse infiltrates. *Streptococcus pneumoniae* classically causes lobar infiltrates, although studies have shown that it is difficult to distinguish the causative agent of a pneumonia by radiographic appearance alone.

In the host with compromised **cell-mediated immunity,** such as this transplant patient or a patient with AIDS, the differential diagnosis grows larger and includes *Pneumocystis carinii* pneumonia (PCP) and disseminated viral infections, including VZV and CMV.

Fungal Infections

The endemic fungi have many characteristics in common. All are found in the soil in restricted geographic areas. Infection with these organisms is unlikely if the patient has not spent time in or near these areas. Infections are more common in children and in people who have recently moved to the endemic area.

The infections are usually contracted by breathing in fungi from the soil, although skin can occasionally be inoculated directly. These organisms can cause a wide range of infections. Most patients develop self-limited pneumonia syndromes with fever, cough, and pleuritic chest pain. Other patients, such as the immunocompromised, pregnant women, and certain ethnic groups (African Americans, Native Americans, and Filipinos), can develop life-threatening disseminated infections. One feared site of disseminated infection is the meninges; other common sites include bones, joints, and skin and subcutaneous tissues.

Diagnosis

Diagnosis of *Coccidioides* can occasionally be made by direct culture of sputum or other body fluids. Unlike with other fungi, such as *Candida albicans*, which can be either a colonizer or a pathogen depending on the situation, the presence of *Coccidioides* or any endemic fungus in a patient sample is generally regarded as evidence of infection with that fungus. The endemic fungi, unlike most nonpathogenic fungi, have two forms: they grow as **yeasts** at body temperature and as **molds** at room temperature. This trait can be used to help identify them in the laboratory. The **dimorphic** character can also explain their success as pathogens; the mold form is easily spread through the air to new victims and the yeast form survives well in the body. Classically, *Coccidioides* is diagnosed by finding a **spherule,** which is a round cyst filled with small endospores, either on a pathologic sample or by inducing it to form on special medium. Today, however, biochemical and molecular techniques are more likely to be used for speciation.

Most of the time, *Coccidioides* is diagnosed through serologic means rather than culture. There are two approaches to serologic diagnosis. One test, called **complement fixation,** allows the lab to measure the amount of anti-*Coccidioides* antibody the patient has. If the antibody titer is high, this suggests active, severe infection. The antibody titer should decrease with effective treatment. Patients who do not have active disease will have a negative complement fixation test. A second test, called **immunodiffusion,** measures IgM and IgG antibodies to *Coccidioides* to distinguish between recent and chronic infection, respectively. A fourfold rise in serum IgG titers from acute to convalescent serum can diagnose coccidioidomycosis in retrospect. A skin test, called **coccidioidin,** is not used to diagnose acutely ill patients but rather to determine whether a patient has ever been exposed to *Coccidioides* in the past. It measures a cell-mediated immune response, similar to a PPD test for tuberculosis. It is used primarily for public health surveys.

Treatment and Prognosis

In an immunocompetent patient, *Coccidioides* pneumonia is a self-limited illness that does not require any treatment. Our patient is immunocompromised, with respiratory failure, however, and she requires antifungal treatment. This patient was treated with **amphotericin B,** a systemic antifungal agent of the **polyene** class, which binds to **ergosterol** in the fungal membranes and disrupts cell membrane integrity. This drug is highly toxic, with infusion-related side effects of fevers and rigors as well as nephrotoxicity, including decreased GFR and magnesium and potassium wasting. The drug is still commonly used for severe fungal infections, as clinicians have the most experience with it. Another class of drugs, the **azole** class, prevents synthesis of ergosterol by interfering with P450 enzyme function.

Members of this class, such as fluconazole or itraconazole, are often prescribed for serious fungal infections as well.

In an immunocompromised patient, consideration must also be given to improving the patient's immune function if possible. For example, a patient with deficient **humoral** immunity may be given g-globulin to boost his antibody response. A patient with HIV may be started on antiretroviral therapy to allow her immune system to recover and fight off an opportunistic infection. In this case, the patient's immunosuppression was iatrogenic, and her immunosuppressant medicines were curtailed and eventually held. Doing this risked losing her transplanted kidney to rejection, but it was a necessary risk in the face of life-threatening infection.

As a final note, it is dangerous for laboratory workers to handle any of the endemic fungi, particularly in their mold state, without taking adequate precautions to avoid infection through the respiratory route. Other unusual organisms that can easily infect laboratory workers from routine culture plates in the laboratory include *Brucella, Coxiella burnetii,* and *Francisella tularensis.* Whereas *Mycobacterium tuberculosis* has the potential to infect laboratory workers, routine precautions with AFB cultures usually prevent this from happening.

CASE CONCLUSION

The patient was treated with amphotericin B in a liposomal formulation to avoid harming her transplanted kidney. Her immunosuppressants, FK506 and prednisone, were held. Unfortunately, her infection progressed and involved her eyes, pericardium, skin, and GI tract. Despite stopping her immunosuppressants and trying several new antifungal agents such as caspofungin and voriconazole, the patient died of overwhelming infection.

THUMBNAIL: The Endemic Mycoses

Organism	*Coccidioides immitis*	*Blastomyces dermatitidis*	*Histoplasma capsulatum*
Type of organism	Dimorphic fungus	Dimorphic fungus	Dimorphic fungus
Diseases caused	Self-limited pneumonia; skin nodules; lung cavities; osteomyelitis; meningitis; disseminated disease	Rarely self-limited; cutaneous pneumonia; meningitis; disseminated disease	Self-limited pneumonia; pulmonary mediastinitis; pericarditis meningitis; disseminated disease
Epidemiology/ geography	Arizona; Central Valley of California	Mississippi, Ohio, and Missouri valleys	Tennessee, Ohio, and Mississippi valleys
Soil types	Dry alkaline soil at low elevations; rodent burrows	Decomposing wood	Bat or bird excrement
Diagnosis	Culture; serology (complement fixation and immunodiffusion); may form spherules with endospores at 37°	Culture	Culture; histoplasma urinary antigen
Treatment	Azoles; amphotericin	Itraconazole; amphotericin	Itraconazole; amphotericin

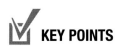

KEY POINTS

- Making the diagnosis of endemic fungal infection requires taking a careful travel history
- These organisms are not always easy to culture, and if suspected, serology and antigen tests are often used to make the diagnosis
- These fungi are dangerous to laboratory personnel and the lab should be warned if they are suspected
- The three major endemic fungi are dimorphic and exist as yeast at body temperature and as molds at room temperature

QUESTIONS

1. A healthy 21-year-old woman moves to the Central Valley region of California and develops signs of an acute pneumonia with fevers, shortness of breath, and cough. Her doctor diagnoses *Coccidioides* pneumonia. What is the recommended treatment for her pneumonia?

   A. Levofloxacin
   B. Fluconazole
   C. Terbinafine
   D. Amphotericin B
   E. None of the above

2. A 34-year-old man has a skin nodule removed. Which morphologic finding on pathology confirms the diagnosis of *Coccidioides*?

   A. Morula
   B. Spherule
   C. Round encapsulated yeast
   D. Acutely branching septate hyphae
   E. Gram-positive cocci in clusters

3. A 25-year-old hiker returns from a hiking trip outside Tucson, Arizona. He notes a large painful nodule on his arm. The nodule is cultured and is found to grow a dimorphic fungus, but final identification is pending. Which is most likely?

   A. *Histoplasma capsulatum*
   B. *Blastomyces dermatitidis*
   C. *Sporothrix schenckii*
   D. *Coccidioides immitis*
   E. *Penicillium marneffei*

HPI: PF is a 23-year-old woman who presents to the emergency department with a chief complaint of fever. She describes fevers, chills, a severe headache, mild abdominal pain, and nausea for the past 3 days. PF had just returned from 6 weeks in Nepal 5 days ago, where she was helping to set up a women's clinic in a rural village over the summer. She took chloroquine prophylaxis for malaria when she was there, was immunized for hepatitis A before she went, and always drank boiled water. She did not have any sexual exposures, nor was she in contact with any animals in Nepal. She does not have any cough, shortness of breath, diarrhea, constipation, or urinary symptoms.

PMH: History of *Chlamydia* STD (sexually transmitted disease) when she was 19; bacterial pneumonia as a child, requiring hospitalization. Takes a multivitamin every day and stopped her chloroquine 5 days ago when she got back. No allergies. Not currently sexually active.

PE: T 38.9°C; HR 115; BP 105/80; RR 18

PF was flushed but in no acute distress. Her lungs were clear and her heart rate was regular, although rapid. Abdominal examination revealed mild diffuse tenderness to palpation with an enlarged spleen. No rashes.

Labs: WBC 4.8 with hematocrit 35.0, platelet count 140,000/μL. Renal and liver function normal.

THOUGHT QUESTIONS

- What is the differential diagnosis for fever in a traveler?
- What are PF's risk factors for developing malaria?
- What is the life cycle of the *Plasmodia* species?
- What are the pathogenesis and clinical manifestations of malaria?
- What are prophylactic and treatment options for malaria?

BASIC SCIENCE REVIEW AND DISCUSSION

Fever in a Traveler

The differential for fever in a traveler depends on the location and activities during travel (insect contact, sexual exposures, animal exposures, food or water exposures, etc.; see Table 1-14).

Malaria

Epidemiology Malaria is one of the most common infectious diseases globally, with 200 to 300 million cases worldwide and 1 to 2 million deaths per year. Malaria is caused by infection with any of four species of the *Plasmodium* protozoa (i.e., *P. falciparum, P. vivax, P. ovale,* and *P. malariae*) and is spread to humans by the female *Anopheles* mosquito. Approximately 500 to 600 cases of imported malaria in civilians are seen in the United States every year, mostly from travelers to Africa, South America, and Asia.

The CDC (Centers for Disease Control and Prevention) performed an analysis of malaria surveillance data on all reported cases in the United States with an onset of illness between August 1, 2000 and December 31, 2000. Two hundred forty-six cases of imported malaria in civilians were seen during that time period; 91.1% of them had prior information regarding the use of chemoprophylaxis to help prevent malaria infection but 53.6% did not take any chemoprophylaxis and 10.7% did not take appropriate prophylaxis, leaving only one third on adequate malaria chemoprophylaxis. As elucidated in the **chemoprophylaxis** section below, our patient PF was taking an ineffective regimen for malaria for her region of travel.

Life Cycle and Pathogenesis Plasmodia species are spread by *Anopheles* mosquitoes. The life cycle of the protozoal organisms is summarized below.

Stages of the life cycle:

1. Female *Anopheles* mosquito bites human (intermediate host), injecting **sporozoite** form of the *Plasmodium* protozoa from mosquito saliva into the bloodstream.
2. **Sporozoites** travel to the liver where they mature and undergo asexual reproduction (**exoerythrocytic schizogony**) to produce **schizonts** within the hepatocytes.
3. A massive number of **merozoites** are released from the **schizonts** within the liver, producing symptomatic infection as they invade and destroy RBCs.
4. In *P. vivax* and *P. ovale* infection, some parasites remain dormant in the liver as **hypnozoites**, which can cause **relapsing malaria** with these two species.
5. **Merozoites** invade RBCs, where **erythrocytic schizogony** occurs: cell division (asexual reproduction) produces *Plasmodia* ring forms (an immature form with the same appearance in all four species), **trophozoites**, and **schizonts**, which contain more merozoites.
6. The schizont-containing RBC eventually bursts, releasing **merozoites** into the bloodstream where they invade new RBCs and the process is continued.
7. After several generations of **erythrocytic schizogony**, some of the **merozoites** develop into male and female **gametocytes** within RBCs, which are subsequently ingested by a mosquito when she takes a blood meal.

Diagnosis The diagnosis of malaria is made by viewing one of the **intra-erythrocytic parasite stages (including gametocyte forms) on thick or thin blood smears** from the patient. *P. falciparum* has a characteristic banana-shaped gametocyte. Figure 1-16 shows the ring forms of *P. falciparum*. The ring forms of each species are indistinguishable, but the appearance of multiple ring forms within the same erythrocyte almost always indicates infection with the rapidly replicating *P. falciparum*.

TABLE 1-14 Fever in a Traveler

Vector-borne:
Malaria, dengue, Lassa fever, typhus, rickettsial diseases, trypanosomiasis, yellow fever

Animal contacts:
Rabies, Q fever, tularemia, brucellosis, echinococcus

Infected person contact:
Hemorrhagic fevers, enteric fevers, meningococcal infection, tuberculosis, sexually transmitted diseases

Food/water-borne:
Enteric infections, trichinosis, tapeworms (cestodes), salmonellosis (nontyphoid and typhoid), shigellosis, *Campylobacter*, hepatitis A, enterovirus, *Aeromonas*, *Plesiomonas*, toxin-mediated illnesses (staphylococcal, *Bacillus cereus*), *Listeria*, *Escherichia coli*

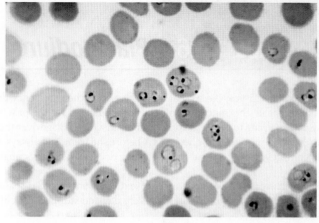

• **Figure 1-16.** Blood smear depicting ring forms of *P. falciparum* inside erythrocytes. The term "ring" is derived from the morphologic appearance of this stage, which includes chromatin (red) and cytoplasm (blue), often arranged in a ring shape around a central vacuole; biologically, the ring is a young trophozoite. (Image in public domain from Centers for Disease and Prevention Control Public Health Image Library, http://phil.cdc.gov/phil/home.asp)

Pathogenesis and Clinical Manifestations Of all the species, **P. falciparum results in the most severe clinical manifestations** because *P. falciparum* can invade RBCs in all stages of maturation and lead to profound degrees of parasitemia (up to 10^6 organisms/mL). *P. vivax* and *P. ovale* can only invade immature RBCs (reticulocytes) and *P. malariae* can only invade older RBCs, limiting the degree of parasitemia to fewer than 10,000 organisms/mL. **The immune response to malaria is not protective,** as there are multiple circulating parasitic stages, as well as antigenic variability among strains and between species. Hence, malaria can be contracted multiple times within a lifetime, although partial immunity conferring limited protection does occur. Disease manifestations are mediated by cytokine production and **obstruction of the microvasculature by peripheral sequestration of the parasitized RBC,** a phenomenon directly proportional to the degree of parasitemia.

The dominant clinical manifestation of malarial infection is **fever** (the oft-quoted cyclical pattern of fevers in malarial illnesses is not sensitive for diagnosis); 98% of imported malaria cases present with fever. Other symptoms include chills, headache, nausea, myalgias, arthralgias, malaise, vomiting, abdominal pain, anorexia, diarrhea, cough, and **dark urine.** Physical findings usually involve a temperature above 38.0°C and may include **splenomegaly** (due to splenic sequestration of infected RBCs), abdominal pain, hepatomegaly, jaundice, or scleral icterus (due to hemolysis of parasitized erythrocytes). Obstruction of the microvasculature by diseased RBCs can cause illness in almost any organ system:

• **Cerebral malaria:** can lead to coma and carries a substantial mortality rate. **Hypoglycemia** contributes to the cerebral manifestations of malaria. Hypoglycemia can be caused by glucose consumption by massive parasitemia, poor glycogen stores in an ill patient, or the release of insulin by pancreatic β cells elicited by quinidine or quinine treatment.

• **Renal malaria:** can see an immune complex-mediated nephrotic syndrome or an acute tubular necrosis caused by the massive amounts of free hemoglobin in the bloodstream from hemolysis (the dark urine from hemoglobinuria has led to the nickname of **blackwater fever** for malaria).

• **Pulmonary:** malaria can cause a **noncardiogenic pulmonary edema,** likely from the protozoal production of cytokines such as TNF-α.

• **Hematologic:** will usually see **anemia** from hemolysis of diseased RBCs and subsequent splenic enlargement (a late complication of *P. vivax* and *P. ovale* infection is splenic rupture); thrombocytopenia is observed in two thirds of patients with malaria.

• **Gastrointestinal:** most likely diarrhea from ischemic compromise of the bowel secondary to microvascular obstruction.

Chemoprophylaxis Prevention of imported cases of malaria in developing world travelers relies on an adequate knowledge of effective chemoprophylactic regimens for malaria by both physicians and patients. Effective regimens include:

• **Chloroquine:** used to be the drug of choice for chemoprophylaxis, but **chloroquine resistance in *P. falciparum*** (and in *P. vivax* to a lesser extent) is burgeoning in Southeast Asia, South America, and Africa (chloroquine resistance is now found in *P. vivax*). Chloroquine prophylaxis is only effective for travelers to malaria-risk areas in Mexico, Haiti, the Dominican Republic, and certain countries in Central America, the Middle East, and Eastern Europe. The regimen is 500 mg orally per week for 1 week prior to travel, during travel, and 4 weeks afterward. Hence, PF failed malaria chemoprophylaxis because there was bound to be chloroquine-resistant *P. falciparum* in Nepal. Furthermore, she did not take the prophylactic medication for the prescribed dosing interval following travel.

• **Mefloquine: used in chloroquine-resistant areas.** Dose is 250 mg orally per week for 1 week prior to travel, during travel, and 4 weeks afterward. **Neurologic symptoms** such as dizziness, confusion, concentration difficulties, anxiety, and even psychosis can occur.

• **Doxycycline:** used in chloroquine-resistant areas. Dose is 100 mg orally every day for the same dosing interval as mefloquine. **Photosensitivity is a common problem** with this medication.

• **Malarone:** new antimalarial combination drug composed of **atovaquone and proguanil** (Malarone). Adult dosage is

1 tablet (250 mg atovaquone/100 mg proguanil) orally every day. Take first dose 1 to 3 days before travel, during travel, and 7 days after travel. **Contraindicated in severe renal impairment, pregnant women, breast-feeding women, and infants less than 24 pounds.** Common side effects are abdominal pain, nausea, vomiting, and headache.

• **Hydroxychloroquine sulfate (Plaquenil):** dose is 400 mg orally every week for the same dosing interval as mefloquine.

Finally, **insect control and pyrethrin-impregnated mosquito bed nets** are essential preventive measures for travelers to regions with high exposure to mosquitoes.

CASE CONCLUSION

PF's thick and thin blood smears revealed multiple RBCs with ring forms of the *Plasmodia* parasite. No other parasitic stage was observed and she was presumed to have chloroquine-resistant *P. falciparum* malaria. Quinine sulfate 650 mg orally every 8 hours for 3 days followed by a single dose of pyrimethamine (for eradication of the liver form of the parasite if *P. vivax* or *P. ovale* was present) was administered. PF defervesced and started to plan her upcoming Uganda trip by asking about mefloquine prophylaxis for malaria.

THUMBNAIL: Malaria

Organisms	*P. falciparum, P. vivax, P. ovale,* and *P. malariae*
Type of organism	Sporozoans (category of protozoan)
Diseases caused	Malaria, including manifestations of fever, neurologic compromise, anemia, hemoglobinemia, and hemoglobinuria (dark urine)
Epidemiology	200 to 300 million cases yearly in developing areas of the world harboring the *Anopheles* mosquito, including areas in South America, Africa, and Asia; approximately 500 imported cases of malaria per year in the United States
Diagnosis	Observation of intra-erythrocytic parasite on thick and thin blood smears
Treatment	Chemoprophylaxis prior to travel; treatment is usually with quinine, although atovaquone-proguanil or mefloquine can be used for treatment; an agent such as primaquine, pyrimethamine, or doxycycline should be administered after the quinine to kill hypnozoites in the liver from *P. vivax* or *P. ovale*

KEY POINTS

■ Cases of imported malaria in the United States often reflect inadequate chemoprophylaxis: mefloquine, doxycycline, hydroxychloroquine sulfate, or atovaquone-proguanil should be used for travel in areas where chloroquine-resistant *P. falciparum* has been reported

■ Malaria is caused by four species (*P. falciparum, P. malaria, P. vivax,* and *P. ovale*), with *P. falciparum* causing the highest morbidity and

mortality and *P. vivax/P. ovale* causing chronic relapses from establishment of an intrahepatic parasitic stage

■ Diagnosis is made by seeing intra-erythrocytic parasites on thick and thin blood smears

QUESTIONS

1. Which of the following enzyme levels in the host should be checked prior to initiating primaquine therapy to eradicate the intrahepatic parasitic stage?

   A. Dihydrofolate reductase
   B. Phenylalanine hydroxylase
   C. Glucose 6-phosphate dehydrogenase
   D. Insulin
   E. Pepsinogen

2. Although PF was thought to have only *P. falciparum* infection, her likelihood of having another *Plasmodia* species in addition to *falciparum* is:

   A. 100%
   B. 75%
   C. 50%
   D. 20%
   E. 5%

PART II

Immunology

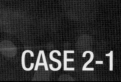

CASE 2-1 | Cell-Mediated Immunity

HPI: IL is a 45-year-old diabetic man **who had a kidney transplant** 2 weeks ago. IL now presents with **shortness of breath, severe hypertension, rapid weight gain,** and **oliguria** (decreased urine production). He has gained 10 pounds over the last 2 days and his blood pressure has increased from 130/85 to the 190s/100s. He has also had a progressive decline in urine output to 500 mL/day. He reports increased shortness of breath with new onset of **orthopnea.** The patient is taking **cyclophosphamide for immunosuppression.**

PE: T 38.0°C; HR 85; BP **190/105;** RR 22; SaO$_2$ 96% on room air

On exam, he is in mild respiratory distress. His exam is significant for diffusely **increased skin turgor, bibasilar crackles** to the mid-chest, a **cardiac flow murmur,** a **distended abdomen** with left lower quadrant tenderness to palpation, and significant lower extremity **pitting edema.**

Labs: He has a normal CBC but an elevated potassium. His serum **creatinine is elevated** at 5.0. UA reveals **3+ protein** and WBCs. Blood cultures are negative.

THOUGHT QUESTIONS

- What is cell-mediated immunity and how does it defend against invading pathogens and foreign cells?
- What is the major histocompatibility complex and its involvement in antigen presentation? What are cytokines and how are they involved?
- How does tolerance to self-antigen develop among T lymphocytes?
- How are foreign cells recognized and eliminated? What implication does this have for allogeneic transplant rejection?
- What is the pathogenesis of the different forms of transplant rejection and their clinical manifestations? How is transplant rejection medically suppressed?

BASIC SCIENCE REVIEW AND DISCUSSION

Cell-mediated immunity, an arm of the adaptive immune system, is involved in the surveillance of not only the extracellular but also the **intracellular compartment** for the elimination of pathogens. Its mediators not only help B cells produce antibodies to neutralize extracellular pathogens but also eliminate intracellular pathogens by killing cells that harbor these pathogens. Targets of cellular immunity include mycobacteria, fungi, and cells viewed as defective or foreign, such as tumor cells and transplanted cells. Like the humoral immune system, the cellular immune system must be capable of (*a*) **specific recognition** of its targets; (*b*) processing and **presenting antigen** to effector cells involved in the immune response; (*c*) activating the most appropriate components of the immune response to optimize **pathogen elimination;** and (*d*) **establishing memory** of these pathogens for more rapid elimination upon re-exposure.

T-Lymphocyte Development

T lymphocytes are the primary effectors of cellular immunity. They arise from lymphoid progenitors in the bone marrow that mature and eventually migrate to the thymus where they undergo further development. Figure 2-1 is a diagram of T-cell development and the key receptors present in each stage.

Antigen recognition in T cells is mediated by the **T-cell receptor (TCR).** The TCR is similar to the B-cell receptor in that it consists of two subunits, α and β, homologous to immunoglobulin heavy and light chains. The α-chain genes include multiple alleles for the V, J, and C regions. The β-chain genes include multiple alleles for the V, D, J, and C regions. The final TCR product consists of recombinations of these alleles within each region of the α- or β-chains. This rearrangement during development allows for the production of an almost infinite array of antigen-recognizing TCRs using relatively few genes.

Following migration to the thymus, T cells undergo a process whereby they develop **the ability to distinguish self from nonself.** Within the thymus, T cells are exposed to thymic epithelial cells and antigen-presenting cells (macrophages and dendritic cells) that expose them to the majority of self-peptides. Immature T cells that recognize self-antigen are destroyed by **negative selection.** Those that successfully recognize foreign antigen and MHC-I or MHC-II receptors undergo **positive selection.** Those that fail to recognize MHC at all die of attrition.

CD4+ T cells become **T-helper cells,** which become restricted to recognizing antigen complexed to **class II MHC.** These cells support T and B cells in orchestrating the adaptive immune response. **CD8+ T cells** become **cytotoxic T cells,** restricted to recognizing antigen bound to **class I MHC** and to the lysis of virus-infected, tumor, or foreign cells. CD4+ and CD8+ T cells are released from the thymus into the bloodstream to mediate cellular immunity.

Cell-Mediated Immunity

Cell-mediated immunity is most easily demonstrated by the process of eliminating viral infection. Viruses have both extracellular and intracellular phases. An antigen-presenting cell (APC) may take up virus in two ways: through **phagocytosis** and through **direct viral infection.** Viruses that are phagocytized are fused with vesicles containing digestive enzymes. Viral peptides are then processed, bound to class II MHC molecules, and presented on the APC surface to CD4+ T lymphocytes. The T cells recognize the antigen-MHC complex via the TCR, stabilized by the CD4 receptor. A **costimulatory signal** between the APC's **B7 receptor** and the T-helper cell's **CD28 receptor**

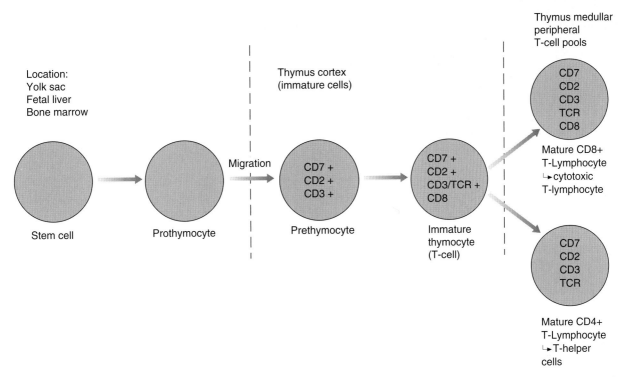

• **Figure 2-1.** T-cell development begins at a primary hematopoietic site such as the bone marrow and ends in the thymus. In the thymus, T cells undergo T-cell antigen receptor (TCR) rearrangement. The T-cell population is then selected for tolerance to self-antigen and for reactivity to self-MHC receptors that will eventually bear foreign antigen. The immature thymocyte expresses TCR as well as CD4 and CD8 concurrently. T cells are fully mature when they express either CD4 or CD8. CD4+ cells differentiate into T-helper cells that orchestrate the adaptive immune response. CD8+ cells develop into cytotoxic T lymphocytes that kill infected cells as well as neoplastic and foreign cells.

is required as a "confirmation" signal for T-cell activation. This up-regulates **CD40 ligand (CD40L)** expression in T-helper cells, which serves to drive B-cell **isotype switching,** a key step in antibody **affinity maturation.**

T-helper cells differentiate and are activated to secrete signaling peptides, or **cytokines,** depending on the nature of the pathogen to be eliminated. T-helper cells universally secrete **IL-2** upon activation, which stimulates proliferation of many immune cells, including B cells, cytotoxic lymphocytes (CTLs), and T-helper cells. T-helper cells differentiate into two types: T_h1 cells and T_h2 cells. T_h**1-cell** differentiation is stimulated by APC-secreted **IL-12.** T_h**1 cells primarily promote immunity against small extracellular pathogens** such as viruses and bacteria, eliminated through phagocytosis and cell killing. Both CD40L and the cytokine **interferon-γ (IFN-γ)** promote B-cell isotype switching toward IgG production. IFN-γ also superactivates macrophage phagocytosis and antigen presentation by up-regulating their oxidative killing machinery and MHC expression, respectively. T_h1 cells also secrete **tumor necrosis factor (TNF),** which activates neutrophil phagocytosis and CTL-mediated elimination of virally infected cells.

T_h**2 cells are differentiated toward eliminating large extracellular pathogens, such as parasites.** T_h2-cell differentiation is driven by **IL-4,** secreted by mast cells and basophils after a parasite encounter. T_h2 cells in turn secrete more cytokines like IL-4 itself, which promotes B-cell isotype switching to IgE, the primary antiparasitic antibody. **IL-5** promotes eosinophil function, the primary parasite killer cell. Eosinophils recognize the Fc portion of IgE via **Fcε receptors,** which activate the

extracellular release of **major basic protein** and other enzymes that attack the parasite's cell membranes (Figs. 2-2 and 2-3).

To initiate intracellular compartment surveillance, APCs take up virus through direct infection. Viral peptides produced during replication are processed differently than those that are phagocytized; intracellularly replicated viral particles are ultimately associated with class I MHC molecules. **This antigen-MHC I complex specifically activates CD8+ T lymphocytes, which are then stimulated to differentiate into CTLs.** One important molecular interaction includes the up-regulated CD40L/CD40 receptors.

The CD40L-CD40 interaction activates CTLs to produce several cell-killing mediators. ***Fas* ligand receptor** surface expression is up-regulated, which binds to ***Fas*** on infected cells and thereby induces cell **apoptosis.** The CD40L-CD40 interaction also promotes the production of **perforin, granzymes,** and **caspases** that kill cells by inserting into the plasma membrane of the infected cell, forming a pore that leads to cell lysis. CTLs recognize virus-infected cells by their TCRs binding to class I MHC molecules, presenting the specific viral peptide to which they are sensitized. This activates the cytotoxic machinery described above. Finally, the T-helper cell's CD40L also binds CD40 on B cells, promoting activation and antibody production.

Immunologic memory to a pathogen is established through the differentiation of a subpopulation of activated T-helper, B, and CD8+ T cells into their own respective memory cells. If the body is re-exposed to the antigen, it will be able to mount a faster, more effective immune response with more efficient elimination of the pathogen, the process we commonly refer to as "immunity."

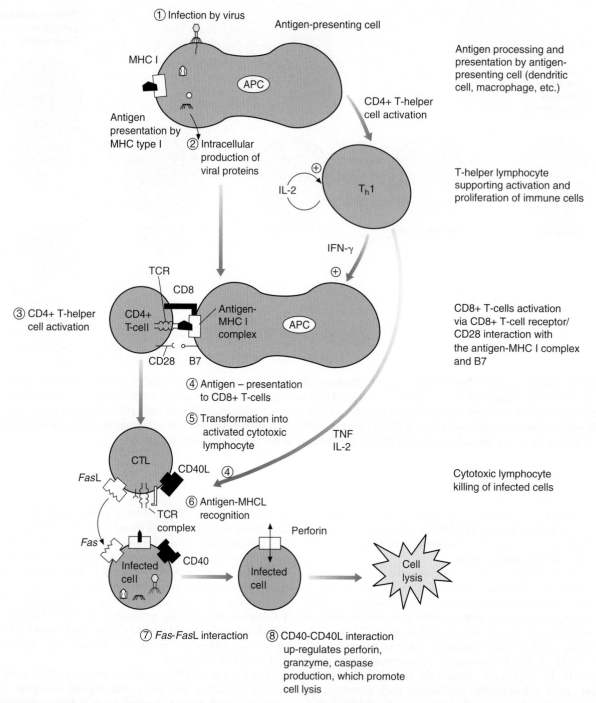

• **Figure 2-2.** Cell-mediated immunity against intracellular pathogens, such as viruses. This pathway uses class I MHC to present antigens that are found in the cytosolic compartment of any cell. CD8+ T lymphocytes are subsequently activated and mature into cytotoxic T cells, which kill infected cells. T-helper cells are also involved in augmenting this immune response. *MHC*, major histocompatibility complex; *IFN-γ*, interferon-γ; *TCR*, T-cell receptor; *TNF*, tumor necrosis factor.

Clinical Discussion

Transplant Rejection There are two types of allograft rejection: humoral (antibody mediated) and cellular (T-lymphocyte mediated). In **humoral rejection,** antibodies are formed by identification of foreign antigen with subsequent B-cell differentiation into antibody-producing plasma cells. These antibodies bind

allograft tissue and activate complement, which leads to platelet aggregation and thrombosis. Ischemic injury and ultimate transplant rejection ensue.

There are two pathways in **cell-mediated allograft rejection:** the direct and indirect pathways. In the **direct pathway,** recipient CD4+ T-helper cells and CD8+ T cells recognize

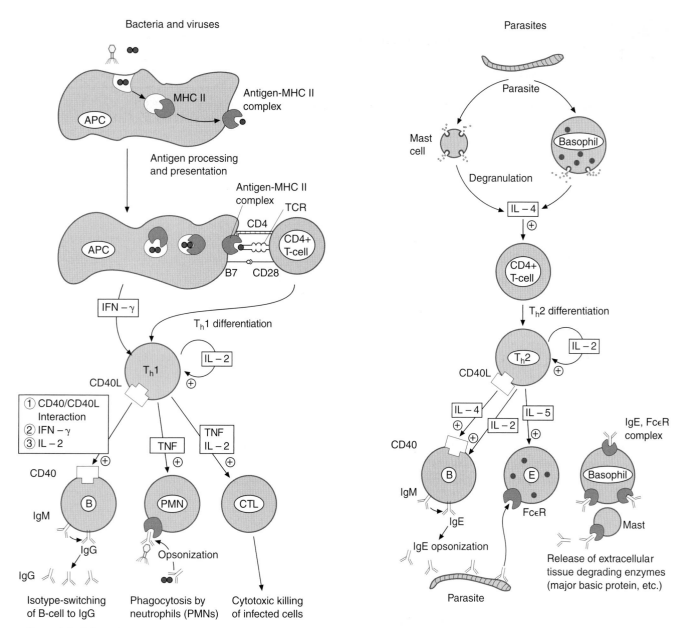

• **Figure 2-3.** Cell-mediated immunity against extracellular pathogens, such as bacteria and fungi. Class II MHC are used to present antigens endocytosed by antigen-presenting cells such as macrophages to CD4+ cells. These cells are activated and mature into T-helper cells that subsequently promote B-lymphocyte maturation, plasma cell antibody production, and the phagocytic activity of macrophages, neutrophils, and eosinophils in the elimination of bacteria and fungi. *MHC*, major histocompatibility complex; *TCR*, T-cell receptor; *APC*, antigen-presenting cell; *IFN-γ*, interferon-γ; *TNF*, tumor necrosis factor; *CTL*, cytotoxic lymphocyte

foreign class II and class I **human leukocyte antigens** (HLA, the MHC in humans), respectively, on **dendritic cells** (APCs) carried in the donor organ. The T cells are then activated and cause a local increase in vascular permeability, lymphocyte and macrophage infiltration, and cell lysis of allograft tissue. In the **indirect pathway,** foreign HLA is processed like any foreign antigen and presented by the host's own APCs to T cells; this eventually leads to transplant rejection.

Therefore, an important clinical issue is **HLA matching** of the donor to the transplant recipient. There are six HLA types to match: HLA-A, HLA-B, and HLA-C (those that contribute to class I HLA) and HLA-DP, HLA-DQ, and HLA-DR (those in class II HLA). Individuals are likely to match with siblings, having a 25% chance of matching. However, the likelihood of matching falls dramatically between unrelated individuals. Matching affords prolonged survival of the graft. With the exception of identical twins, lifelong immunosuppression is necessary to prolong graft survival and is accomplished with such drugs as azathioprine, steroids, cyclosporine, antilymphocyte globulins, and monoclonal anti–T-cell antibodies. Immunosuppression unfortunately also makes the recipient susceptible to opportunistic infections (Table 2-1.)

TABLE 2-1 Types of Rejection and Pathogenesis

Rejection Type	Timing	Pathogenesis
Hyperacute rejection	Minutes to <48 hr	• Classically upon reperfusion of allograft → graft failure • Preformed antibodies to HLA, ABO Ag, and vascular endothelium are in circulation and bind immediately to vasculature, causing complement activation, platelet aggregation, and thrombosis → vasculitis and ischemia
Accelerated rejection	7–10 days	• Humoral: anti-HLA antibodies • Cellular: T-lymphocyte mediated, from prior sensitization • 60% graft loss
Acute rejection	7 days–3 months	• Development of cellular and humoral immunity, often due to inadequate immunosuppression • Signs and symptoms: graft pain, warmth, edema, fever, malaise, fatigue, and signs of specific organ failure
Chronic rejection	Months to years	• Unclear etiology: presumable humoral and cellular • Signs and symptoms of specific organ failure • Diagnosed by biopsy, showing concentric vessel narrowing and ischemic disease of the graft

CASE CONCLUSION

With the suspicion of acute kidney transplant rejection, our patient is started on prednisone and stabilized hemodynamically with diuretics and angiotensin-converting enzyme (ACE) inhibitors. His immunosuppressive dosing regimen is increased and his symptoms eventually resolve. At this time, IL continues to have normal functioning of his kidney allograft.

THUMBNAIL: Cytokines and Their Actions

Cytokine	Cell Origin	Cell Target	Stimulus for Release and Subsequent Actions
Cytokines released from local insult			
IL-1	Macrophages Infected cells	T and B cells Neutrophils Epithelial cells Dendritic cells	Secretion stimulated by infection → • Acts on hypothalamus to induce fever • Stimulates cell growth • T-cell differentiation, IL-2 production
IL-6	Macrophages Neutrophils	Hepatocytes T and B cells	Phagocytosis of microbe stimulates → • Production of acute-phase proteins (e.g., ESR) • Promotes T- and B-cell growth and differentiation
TNF-α	Macrophages Mast cells/basophils Eosinophils NK cells T and B cells	All cells except RBCs	Local tissue damage or infection → • Induces fever, anorexia, shock • Causes capillary leak syndrome • Enhanced cytotoxicity, NK cell function • Acute-phase protein synthesis
TNF-β	T and B cells	All except RBCs	• Cell cytotoxicity, lymph node, and spleen development

(Continued)

THUMBNAIL: Cytokines and Their Actions *(Continued)*

Cytokine	Cell Origin	Cell Target	Stimulus for Release and Subsequent Actions
Cytokines of antiviral immunity			
IFN-α/β	Macrophages Infected cells	All cells, especially neighboring cells	Viral infection → induces antiviral state; antitumor activity • Up-regulates MHC class I antigen expression • ↓ Protein synthesis in infected cell • ↑ RNase expression → degrade viral RNA
Cytokines of T-helper type 1 cells			
IFN-γ	T$_h$1 cells NK cells	Macrophage NK cells B cells Dendritic cells	Bacterial/viral infection → antigen presentation • Promotes T$_h$1-cell differentiation • Regulates macrophage and NK cell activation • Stimulates B-cell growth and IgG isotype switching
IL-2	T$_h$1 cells	T-helper cells CD8+ cells B cells	• Activates all branches of adaptive immunity to proliferate and differentiate (activates cytokine production, effector functions)
IL-12	APC: macrophages, dendritic cells	T-helper cells CD8+ T cells NK cells	• Promotes T$_h$1 proliferation • CTL activation • NK cell activation
Cytokines of T-helper type 2 cells			
IL-4	T$_h$2 cells	B cells T-helper cells	Helminthic infection and allergen exposure → • Stimulates B-cell growth; IgE isotype switching • Recruits eosinophils • Promote T$_h$2 cell proliferation • Inhibits macrophages/delayed-type reaction
IL-5	T$_h$2 cells	B cells Eosinophils	• Activates eosinophils IgE binding via FcεR • Stimulates B-cell differentiation
IL-10	T$_h$2 cells	Macrophages	• Inhibits macrophage activation
Cytokines of mast cells			
Histamine Serotonin Lipid mediators	Mast cells	Vascular endothelium Smooth muscle cells	Helminthic infection and allergen exposure → • Increased vascular permeability → hypotension, edema • Bronchiole contraction → bronchospasm • Intestinal hypermotility → diarrhea

QUESTIONS

1. The following is a series of immunologic events that occurred during the course of IL's transplant rejection. Which step did not occur?

   A. APCs from the donor and the recipient take up HLA protein from the allograft and present it to recipient T-helper cells on class I and class II HLA receptors.

   B. B cells are activated by T$_h$2 cells to proliferate and isotype switch to producing IgG, which bind to allograft vascular endothelium and activate complement, causing thrombosis and ischemic injury to the graft.

   C. Activated T-helper cells secrete IL-2 and thereby promote proliferation and maturation of B cells, CD4+ T cells,

CD8+ T cells, and monocytes into plasma cells, T$_h$1 cells, cytotoxic T lymphocytes, and macrophages, respectively.

   D. TNF-α is released from activated macrophages, creating symptoms such as fever and malaise, promoting allograft edema by increasing local vascular permeability, and promoting allograft rejection by enhancing NK cell cytotoxicity.

   E. The CD40-CD40L interaction between allograft dendritic cells and IL's T-helper cells promotes cytotoxic lymphocyte activity by up-regulating *Fas* ligand receptor expression, which binds *Fas* on infected cells and induces apoptosis of that cell.

2. There is an immunodeficiency of the INF-γ receptor that leads to serious infections caused by the BCG vaccine for *Mycobacteria tuberculosis* and nontuberculous mycobacteria. What immune machinery would be defective in this deficiency?

A. There is a lack of signal to the hypothalamus to induce enough of a febrile reaction to eliminate mycobacterial infection.

B. This deficiency yields a defective mechanism of specific antigen recognition, thereby shielding mycobacterial species from immune recognition.

C. This deficiency prevents the up-regulation of MHC class I and RNase expression, thus preventing intracellular mycobacteria from having their antigen presented to T-helper cells as well as preventing degradation of the pathogen's genomic material.

D. This deficiency prevents the proliferation of subtype 1 T-helper cells and the subsequent activation of oxidative killing by macrophages required to fully eliminate phagocytized mycobacteria.

E. This deficiency prevents the activation of B cells to isotype switch toward IgE production, preventing the elimination of mycobacteria.

HPI: SM is a 25-year-old African American woman who presents with a **fever, "butterfly" facial rash, oral lesions,** and **joint pain.** She began to experience fatigue and malaise 4 weeks ago. She then developed a persistent low-grade fever and painful oral ulcers. She then noticed discomfort in both her wrists and knees, which has worsened over the past week. After a few days of lying in bed, she decided to step outside "to get some sun" and subsequently developed a rash over her nose and cheeks. In addition, she notes sharp **chest pain upon inspiration.** She was previously healthy, taking no medications. She has two aunts who have "some sort of skin disease."

PE: T 38.5°C; HR 86; BP 135/85; RR 20; SaO$_2$ 98%

On exam, SM is ill appearing, in no acute distress. Her exam is significant for an **erythematous, raised rash over her nose and cheeks.** She has multiple **ulcerated lesions on her labia and gingiva** and cervical lymphadenopathy. She has bilaterally symmetric diminished lung movement with diffuse crackles and a palpable spleen tip. She has grossly normal-appearing **wrists and knees with tenderness** upon palpation and passive flexion. No neurologic deficits.

Labs: WBC 3,500/µL; hemoglobin (Hgb) 10.0; Hct 30%; platelets (Plt) 105,000/µL; prothrombin time (PT) 13 seconds, **partial thromboplastin time (PTT) 42 seconds; Coombs test +; ANA +; anti-Sm antibody +; VDRL +.**

THOUGHT QUESTIONS

- What are the fundamental functions of the adaptive immune system?
- What is humoral immunity and what function does it serve in the defense against invading pathogens? How does humoral immunity eliminate such pathogens?
- How do effectors of humoral immunity develop the ability to distinguish between self and nonself?
- What diseases occur when there are derangements in the ability to distinguish between self and nonself? How are these diseases diagnosed and treated?

BASIC SCIENCE REVIEW AND DISCUSSION

Roughly speaking, there are two compartments in the body that require immune surveillance: the extracellular and intracellular space. Extracellular pathogens include bacteria and toxic particles such as exotoxins; intracellular pathogens include viruses and mycobacteria (although these too have an extracellular phase). Because extracellular pathogens float freely outside of the cell, soluble antibodies are required to recognize and attack them. Intracellular pathogens, however, successfully hide from such antibodies. The immune system protects all other cells by sacrificing infected cells in order to eliminate the pathogen within.

Antibodies

Antibodies, or **immunoglobulins (Ig),** are products of antigen-activated B lymphocytes and are the main effectors of humoral immunity. They provide the function of **pathogen recognition** by binding to specific portions of a pathogen's molecular structure, called an **epitope.** Epitopes can include any molecule, such as peptides, carbohydrates, lipids, and nucleic acids. This binding serves to neutralize and tag the particle for final elimination through phagocytosis. Figure 2-4 is a diagram of an IgG antibody.

There are five immunoglobulin isotypes: IgG, IgM, IgE, IgA, and IgD, each with their own functional niche. Upon activation of the humoral immune response, the primary antibody raised against extracellular pathogens is **IgM,** a pentameric molecule that generally has low **affinity** (single molecular binding force)

but high **avidity** (summed binding force from having more points of attachment) to an antigen. This IgM response is followed by the development and proliferation of **IgG,** a monomeric antibody that has high affinity but low avidity (strong binding with fewer points of attachment) to that same antigen. Both IgM and IgG activate the complement cascade and both serve as B-cell surface antigen receptors, which stimulate B-cell proliferation and differentiation into antibody-secreting **plasma cells.**

IgA is the major antibody found in secretions and serves the purpose of protecting mucosal surfaces from invading microorganisms. **IgE** is the major antibody elicited in allergic reactions and antiparasitic humoral immunity. **IgD** is present on mature B-cell surfaces; its role has not yet been elucidated. Table 2-2 lists some of the basic characteristics of the five antibody classes.

B Lymphocytes and Antibody Development

B lymphocytes are the primary cell mediators of humoral immunity. Their primary function is to produce antibodies that neutralize pathogens by recognition of specific antigenic epitopes. B cells arise from pluripotent stem cells that differentiate into lymphoid progenitors in the bone marrow and fetal liver. They recognize the Fc region of IgG as well as opsonizing complement components that facilitate phagocytosis of antigen for subsequent presentation. They also recognize whole, unprocessed extracellular antigen through surface-bound Ig, which serve as B-cell receptors for B-cell activation. To allow for recognition of such a vast diversity of possible epitopes, B cells have developed a mechanism of creating an equally vast and diverse repertoire of antibodies from relatively few genes. This is accomplished through two stages: (a) **antigen-independent rearrangement** of immunoglobulin gene segments and (b) **antigen-dependent somatic mutation** (point mutation) of these genes. In the first stage, heavy chain genes result from a combinatorial rearrangement of the V, D, J, and C segments. Light chains, which are either of the κ or λ subtype, are generated by the rearrangement of V and J segments. Given 10,500 possible heavy chain segments and 320 possible light chain segments, over 3 million possible antibodies can be produced. Somatic mutation of these rearrangements followed by positive selection of B cells that produce antibodies with progressively higher affinity to antigen, a

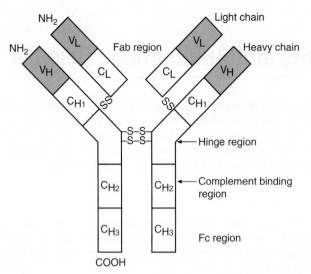

• **Figure 2-4.** Schematic structure of the immunoglobulin G molecule. The basic structure of all antibodies consists of two heavy chains and two light chains covalently linked by disulfide bonds. There is a variable region, which includes both amino termini of the heavy and light chains and serves to *recognize* antigen through specific epitope binding. The constant regions, of which there are three per heavy chain and one per light chain, *communicate* with and thereby activate the rest of the immune system through various mechanisms. The Fc (constant) region includes portions that bind C1q of the classic complement pathway as well as a portion that binds Fc receptors found on macrophages, natural killer cells, B cells, neutrophils, and eosinophils.

strongly binding, highly specific antibody is produced in a process termed **affinity maturation.** This process yields a B cell that produces one antibody type; but, within the population of B cells in an individual, a virtually infinite array of antibodies that recognize almost any molecule can be produced.

Development of Tolerance to Self-Antigen

Random rearrangement and somatic mutation of developing B cells generate self-reactive antibodies that must be changed or eliminated to avoid self-damage. **Central B-cell tolerance** occurs in immature B cells within the bone marrow where they first develop. Those cells that strongly interact with widely expressed self-antigens are **negatively selected** through induction of apoptosis. In addition, self-reacting B cells also undergo **B-cell receptor editing** by reactivating their Ig gene recombination machinery to modify the receptor specificity. This "pruning" process occurs continually in the B-cell population as it expands and refines it ability to differentiate between benign and nonbenign, self and nonself. **Peripheral B-cell tolerance** occurs once mature B cells are released into circulation. Those B cells that repeatedly recognize self-antigen become anergic, or immunologically inactivated.

Antibody-Mediated Immunity

Development of antibody-mediated immunity begins with a new infection by a pathogen, such as a bacterium or parasite. **Pattern-recognized antigens,** such as lipopolysaccharide (LPS) on gram-negative bacteria, or **multivalent (or repeating) antigens,** such as polysaccharides, induce **T-cell–independent activation** of B cells. T cells activate B cells by binding the **B-cell receptor (BCR) complex,** consisting of surface immunoglobulin IgM or IgD, in a pattern- or dose-dependent fashion. This directly induces B-cell proliferation and differentiation into antibody-producing plasma cells.

Most antigens (especially proteins) are neither multivalent nor pattern recognized like LPS. Such antigens require "help" from T-helper cells to produce an antibody response, which is described as **T-cell–dependent activation.** This is accomplished through **antigen presentation,** a process wherein a pathogen is ingested and processed by an APC to produce a small peptide fragment, which is then covalently bound to an **MHC** receptor. An antigen that comes from the extracellular space (like bacteria) is presented on type II MHC to a CD4+ T-helper cell, which "helps" the rest of the immune system to respond effectively to this antigen. APCs include dendritic cells (or Langerhans cells, if in the skin or mucosal), macrophages, follicular dendritic cells in the spleen, B lymphocytes, and microglia in the CNS.

Once an antigen is bound to type II MHC, it is presented to T-helper cells via the **TCR** and the **CD4 receptor.** A "confirmatory" second signaling interaction then occurs between the APC surface protein **B7** and the T cell's **CD28,** which is required for T-helper cell activation. Without this second signal, no activation occurs and the lymphocyte is actually rendered immunologically nonfunctional, or **anergic.** Other interactions include those between the T-helper cell's **CD40L** and **CD40** on B cells, which stimulates B-cell proliferation and antibody production, effects that are also supported by cytokines secreted by T-helper cells.

TABLE 2-2 Properties of Immunoglobulins

Property	IgG	IgA	IgM	IgD	IgE
Structure	Monomer	Monomer/dimer	Monomer/pentamer	Monomer	Monomer
Function	1. Secondary antibody response 2. Complement activation 3. B-cell antigen receptor 4. Placentally transferred Ig	Secretory immunoglobulin preventing microbial attachment to mucous membranes	1. *Primary antibody response* 2. Complement activation 3. B-cell antigen receptor (monomer)	Mature B-cell marker	1. Allergy 2. Antiparasitic response
Relative percentage	80%	10%	9%	0.04%	0.0003%
Binding cells via Fc receptor	1. Macrophages 2. Neutrophils 3. NK cells (LGL)	Lymphocytes	Lymphocytes	None	1. Mast cells 2. Basophils 3. B cells

Finally, the antibodies produced by plasma cells must be "tailored" for optimal elimination of the specific pathogen. The first step is **isotype switching** (or class switching), a process whereby a B cell is stimulated to produce antibodies of a particular isotype (e.g., IgG or IgE). IgGs, which opsonize microbes (tagging them for phagocytosis) provide optimal defense against small extracellular pathogens (e.g., bacteria and viruses). IgE antibodies are more suited for parasite elimination, as they bind to Fcε receptors on eosinophils, the cellular mediators of antiparasitic defense. Activated B cells initially produce IgM, a low-affinity antibody. Once the CD40-CD40L interaction occurs, isotype switching is initiated. Different cytokines direct final antibody isotype production. T-helper cells activated by extracellular bacteria or viruses differentiate into T-helper type 1 cells (T_h1) and those stimulated by parasites differentiate into T-helper type 2 cells (T_h2). **T_h1 cells secrete IFN-γ,** which promotes IgG isotype switching and phagocytic killing. **T_h2 cells secrete IL-4,** which promotes IgE class switching, as well as **IL-5,** which activates eosinophils for parasitic elimination. Similarly, T-helper cells in the respiratory and GI mucosa stimulate IgA class switching. The final step in "tailoring" the humoral immune response is affinity maturation of the antibody, as described above. From this point, most activated B cells differentiate into antibody-producing **plasma cells.** However, a fraction differentiate into **memory B cells,** which circulate for months to years, providing immunologic memory, ready to respond to a pathogen if it were to re-infect the body (see Fig. 2-1 in Case 2-1).

Clinical Discussion

Autoimmune Disease Autoimmune disease results from failure of the immune system to maintain tolerance to self-antigen, causing immune-mediated destruction of the body's own cells and tissues. This results from the production of antibodies against self-antigens or activation of self-reactive T cells, which may be due to either an intrinsic abnormality in lymphocytes or abnormalities in the display of self-antigens. For the most part, autoimmune disease is thought to arise from failures of peripheral tolerance rather than of central tolerance. Autoimmune diseases are associated with specific subtypes of HLA (the name of human MHC), often preceded by infectious prodromes. It is thought that the local innate immune response to tissue infection up-regulates costimulators and cytokines that activate and break anergy of self-reactive T cells. Alternatively, some microbes may have antigens that are similar to self-antigens, a phenomenon termed "molecular mimicry." Antibodies and T cells from such an infection may later cross react with self-antigen, causing an inflammatory response to one's own tissue. This is thought to be the underlying basis of poststreptococcal rheumatic heart disease, in which IgG developed to group A *Streptococcus pyogenes* epitopes cross react with proteins in cardiac muscle tissue. Finally, tissue injury may release antigen normally sequestered from the immune system, causing autoimmune reaction against intracellular self-antigen; this can occur after trauma to immune-protected sites such as the cornea and the testes.

Systemic Lupus Erythematosus Systemic lupus erythematosus (SLE) is a multisystemic autoimmune disease that arises from the failure to maintain tolerance to self-antigen. This results in the presence of a large array of autoantibodies to nuclear and cytoplasmic antigens, particularly **ANA.** These antibodies can react to red cells, platelets, lymphocytes, and phospholipid-associated plasma proteins. These antibodies can mediate a **type II cytotoxic hypersensitivity** reaction resulting in hemolytic anemia, leukopenia, and thrombocytopenia. Tissue injury also results from **immune complex-mediated disease (type III hypersensitivity),** which can lead to glomerulonephritis, arthritis, and vasculitides.

SLE is a common disease, occurring predominantly among women of child-bearing age and is more common and severe among African American women. There is a familial clustering of the disease. SLE presents classically as an acute or chronic, recurrent, and remitting febrile illness with damage to the skin, joints, kidneys, and serosal membranes. For formal diagnosis, the American Rheumatology Association developed the criteria as described in Table 2-3. Symptomatic exacerbations are treated with corticosteroids and immunosuppressant drugs.

TABLE 2-3 Criteria for Diagnosis of Systemic Lupus Erythematosus

Criterion	Description
1. Malar rash	"Butterfly-shaped" rash, flat, erythematous rash of sun-exposed areas
2. Discoid rash	Erythematous raised patches
3. Photosensitivity	Skin rash from sun exposure
4. Oral ulcers	Often painless oral or nasopharyngeal ulceration
5. Arthritis	Nondegenerative arthritis of two or more joints with tenderness, swelling, and effusion
6. Serositis	Pleuritis, pericarditis
7. Renal disorder	Proteinuria, RBC casts
8. Neurologic disorder	Seizures, psychosis
9. Hematologic disorder	Hemolytic anemia, leukopenia, lymphopenia, thrombocytopenia
10. Immunologic disorder	Anti-dsDNA + anti-Sm antibodies; anti-phospholipid Ab (false-positive VDRL)
11. ANA	ANA (in virtually 100% of patients with SLE)

The presence of 4 of 11 criteria is diagnostic of SLE; the presence of both anti-dsDNA and anti-Sm antibodies is virtually diagnostic of SLE.

☑
☑
☑ **CASE CONCLUSION**

SM is diagnosed with SLE. She is treated with the nonsteroidal anti-inflammatory drug (NSAID) naproxen and with a course of prednisone for her exacerbation of symptoms. She is subsequently maintained on low doses of NSAIDs with intermittent steroid tapers. She is currently doing well on this lifelong regimen, monitored regularly by her rheumatologist.

⚙ **THUMBNAIL:** Autoimmune Diseases

Disease	Pathogenesis	Clinical Manifestations
SLE	ANAs and other antibodies cause immune complex disease and hematologic cytotoxicity	Young, female, child-bearing age, African American; rash, arthritis, serosal damage, glomerulonephritis, pancytopenia, neurologic disorders
Sjögren syndrome	Lymphocytic infiltration and destruction of lacrimal and salivary glands	Women, 35–45 years old; dry eyes, dry mouth (xerostomia), parotid gland enlargement
Scleroderma	Unknown etiology; excessive fibrosis throughout the body (skin, GI tract, kidneys, heart, muscles, lungs, and microvasculature) from abnormal immune activation	Women, 50–60 years old; localized or diffuse skin fibrosis; diffuse visceral fibrosis and organ dysfunction; ischemic tissue injury from microvascular disease; CREST syndrome: *c*alcinosis, *R*aynaud phenomenon, *e*sophageal dysmotility, *s*clerodactyly, *t*elangiectasia
Inflammatory myopathies	Dermatomyositis: immune-mediated inflammation of skin and muscle; from damage to capillaries → ischemia	Lilac discoloration of upper eyelids, periorbital edema; rash over knees, knuckles, and elbows; proximal muscle weakness
	Polymyositis: muscle inflammation from cell-mediated injury from CTLs and macrophages	*Symmetric muscle weakness without skin involvement;* inflammatory change in heart, lungs, and blood vessels
	Inclusion-body myositis: muscle inflammation; possible CTL injury	Begins with distal muscle involvement (weakness), especially knee extensors and wrist/finger flexors; asymmetric
Mixed connective tissue disease	High titers of antibodies to ribonucleoprotein (RNP)	SLE + polymyositis + systemic sclerosis
Vasculitides	Necrotizing inflammation of blood vessel walls	Fever, fatigue, weight loss, occlusion of blood vessels, and resulting ischemia

QUESTIONS

1. The following is a list of SM's clinical symptoms, with their underlying immunopathology. Which is *least* likely to be correct?

   A. Arthritis: immune complex deposition in synovial membranes

   B. Malar rash: immunoglobulin- and complement-mediated injury at the dermo-epidermal junction of the skin

   C. Pleuritic chest pain: chronic pleuritis and chronic interstitial fibrosis

   D. Palpable spleen tip: follicular hyperplasia in spleen with abundance of IgG- and IgM-producing plasma cells

   E. Anemia, leukopenia, and thrombocytopenia: immune complex-mediated injury to hematologic components

2. There is a receptor called CTLA-4 that can be up-regulated and acts as an antagonist to costimulatory B7 surface protein. Soluble CTLA-4 protein is in trials for preventing graft-versus-host disease in bone marrow transplant patients. Through what mechanism is this likely to work?

   A. CTLA-4 binds B7, preventing the necessary second signal required to initiate the immune reaction against a certain foreign antigen; it can thus prevent donor bone marrow T lymphocytes and other immune cells from being immunologically activated against host antigen

   B. CTLA-4 binds B7 and inhibits binding of the host antigen to the MHC receptor, thus preventing antigen presentation to donor lymphocytes and subsequently preventing immunologic attack of host tissue

   C. CTLA-4 acts as a general immunosuppressant, preventing activation of T lymphocytes from the donor, preventing damage to host tissue

   D. CTLA-4 prevents the expression of CD40 in APCs, thus preventing the subsequent sensitization of donor T lymphocytes to host tissue

   E. CTLA-4 down-regulates the expression of CD28, thereby preventing the needed second signal

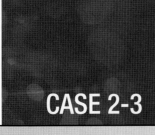

Innate Immunity and the Complement System

HPI: CD is a 4-year-old boy who presents to the ER **lethargic** with a **high fever** and a **diffuse petechial rash.** The child's illness began 3 days ago when he developed a low-grade fever and a sore throat. The next day, he was seen by his pediatrician and was found to be slightly febrile with pharyngitis. His throat was cultured and he was sent home with supportive care. Today he developed a diffuse petechial rash and a fever peaking at 104°F. He complains of a **headache, joint pain, nausea,** and **vomiting** and has become more lethargic.

PMH: An **admission for pneumococcal pneumonia** at the age of 1, which resolved without complication.

PE: T 39.6°C; HR 145; BP 80/50; RR 24; SaO$_2$ 95% on room air

He is **toxic appearing, somnolent** but arousable. His exam is significant for **nuchal rigidity** with positive **Kernig and Brudzinski signs,** diffuse **petechial rash,** and bilateral knee inflammation. He has no focal neurologic deficits.

Labs: WBC 36,000/μL; Hct 40%; Plt 110,000/μL

He is hemodynamically stabilized; 2 blood cultures are sent and IV ceftriaxone is initiated for presumed **meningitis.** Head CT (computed tomography) shows no evidence of a mass lesion. A lumbar puncture is performed, which reveals grossly cloudy CSF with a 1200 opening pressure and increased protein and decreased glucose content. Microscopically, the CSF reveals elevated WBCs with a neutrophil predominance and gram-negative intracellular diplococci. The patient is admitted. At day 2, blood and CSF cultures grow *Neisseria meningitidis.* IgM and IgG levels to meningococcus are elevated.

THOUGHT QUESTIONS

- What is innate immunity? What are its cellular and humoral components?
- What are the major categories of deficiencies in innate immunity?
- What are the clinical manifestations that occur with these immunodeficiencies?
- How are these immunodeficiencies diagnosed and treated?

BASIC SCIENCE REVIEW AND DISCUSSION

The **innate immune system** is the most primitive division of immunity and represents **the first line of defense** against pathogens such as bacteria, foreign cells such as allografts, and tumor cells. These means of immune protection are less specific than that of adaptive immunity and broadly include protective barriers like skin, mucosal epithelium, and stomach acid as well as pattern recognition proteins that recognize and eliminate broad classes of pathogens by binding to commonly expressed molecular patterns like LPS on gram-negative bacteria. **Unlike the adaptive immune system, this branch of immunity does not require prior exposure to a pathogen to be activated and thus is an important line of defense against pathogens to which the body is naïve.** But like adaptive immunity, innate immunity has both a humoral and a cellular component that interact and work synergistically to eliminate pathogens.

The humoral components of innate immunity consist of **antimicrobial peptides,** soluble **pattern recognition proteins,** and **complement proteins.** The antimicrobial peptides include defensins that bind microbes and create pores within their membranes, causing cell lysis. There are also a number of soluble pattern recognition proteins, called **collectins,** capable of binding carbohydrates unique to microbial membranes. These proteins tag extracellular pathogens for phagocytosis and activate the inflammatory response via the complement cascade.

The **complement system** is an important part of innate immunity consisting of several proteins that mediate three main functions: (*a*) **opsonization** of extracellular pathogens, (*b*) **cell lysis** via the formation of the membrane attack complex (MAC), and (*c*) **cell signaling** via by-products of the cascade that activate local inflammation. There are three pathways through which complement is activated: (*a*) **the alternative pathway,** (*b*) **the lectin pathway,** and (*c*) **the classic pathway.** These pathways converge upon the formation of **C3b,** a central component that activates several arms of the immune response. The alternative and lectin pathways rely on pattern recognition proteins and are important for first-time infections where there are no specific antibodies available for opsonization. In contrast, the classic pathway relies on preexisting immunoglobulins for its action. Opsonization neutralizes and tags a pathogen for phagocytosis. This subsequently initiates a cascade of proteolysis and activation of complement proteins. The small peptides released from the cascade (e.g., C2a–C5a) serve as cytokines that promote the inflammatory response by recruiting leukocytes and increasing local vascular permeability to facilitate leukocyte transmigration. In addition, cytokines initiate the adaptive immune response by promoting antibody production to the specific antigens involved. Finally, the terminal complement proteins form the **MAC,** a transmembrane pore that inserts into microbial membranes and thereby promotes leakage of leukocyte-recruiting bacterial proteins, bacterial lysis, and phagocytosis (Fig. 2-5 and Table 2-4).

The cellular arm of innate immunity includes **neutrophils, monocytes-macrophages,** and **natural killer (NK) cells.** Once microorganisms are opsonized and cytokines are released, neutrophils and macrophages are recruited to the site of inflammation.

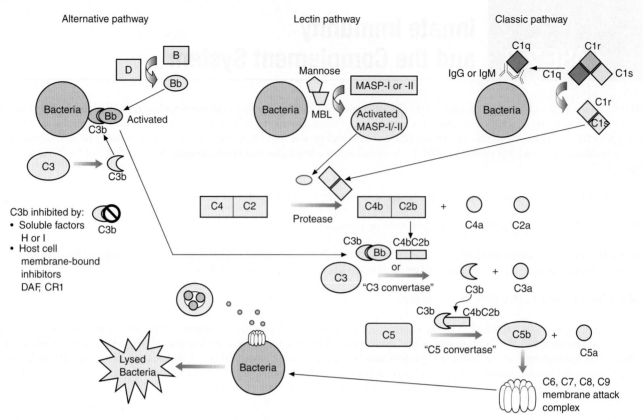

• **Figure 2-5.** The complement cascade. There are three pathways that all converge upon the conversion of C3 to C3b. It is a proteolytic cascade that releases small cytokine fragments and eventually leads to the formation of the membrane attack complex.

TABLE 2-4 Complement Components and Their Actions

Complement Component	Action
C3b	**Opsonin** of the alternative pathway; complexes with Bb to produce C3 convertase
MBL	**Opsonin** of the lectin pathway; binds polysaccharides unique to microorganisms
2 IgG or 1 IgM	**Opsonin** of the classic pathway; binds specific antigen and C1q releasing C1r/C1s
DAF, CR1, MCP	**Cell surface-bound protein** *inhibitors of C3b* that protect host cells
Factor H or I	**Soluble** *inhibitors of C3b;* prevents activation of complement cascade
MASP-I or MASP-II	**Lectin pathway** *protease* that cleaves C4/C2 → C4b/C2b + C4a + C2a
C1r/C1s	**Classic pathway** *protease* that cleaves C4/C2 → C4b/C2b + C4a + C2a
C3bBb	**Alternative pathway** *C3 convertase* that cleaves C3 → C3b + C3a
C4b/C2b	**Classic pathway** *C3 convertase* that cleaves C3 → C3b + C3a
C4a	Weak **anaphylatoxin**; evokes *histamine release* from basophils and mast cells
C3b	1. Complexes with C4b/C2b to form "**C5** convertase": cleaves C5 → C5b + C5a 2. Amplification of alternative pathway loop by producing more C3b to complex with Bb to form C3bBb, the "**C3 convertase complex.**" 3. **Opsonin** for neutralization and tagging of particles for phagocytosis 4. Promotes *immune complex binding* to macrophages and neutrophils 5. Promotes *solubilization of immune complexes* 6. C3b bound to particles *promotes antibody production* to particle antigens

(Continued)

TABLE 2-4 Complement Components and Their Actions *(Continued)*

Complement Component	Action
C3a	1. **Anaphylatoxin;** evokes histamine release from basophils and mast cells 2. Acts on endothelial cells to *promote vascular permeability*
C5b	Binds covalently to microbial membranes (esp. gram-negative bacteria and enveloped viruses) → **nucleates formation of membrane attack complex** with C6, C7, C8, and C9
C5a	1. **Anaphylatoxin;** evokes histamine release from basophils and mast cells 2. Potent *chemoattractant* for monocytes and neutrophils 3. Acts on endothelial cells to *promote vascular permeability*
C5, C6, C7, C8, C9	**Membrane attack complex:** polymerizes to form a transmembrane pore → weakens membrane integrity and allows leakage of immune mediators that promotes leukocyte recruitment for phagocytosis of microorganism

MBL, mannose-binding lectin; *Ig,* immunoglobulin; *MASP,* MBL-associated serine protease; *DAF,* decay accelerating factor; *CR1,* complement receptor 1; *MCP,* membrane cofactor of proteolysis

These cells use pattern recognition receptors to recognize microbial polysaccharide structures and opsonins that facilitate phagocytosis. These cells also do not require prior exposure to a pathogen in order to be activated. Once phagocytized, microorganisms within phagosomes are partially degraded by the digestive enzymes of lysosomes. However, the most effective killing action comes from the reactive oxygen and nitrogen intermediates of NADPH (nicotinamide adenine dinucleotide phosphate, reduced) oxidase and inducible nitric oxide synthase (iNOS), respectively. **NADPH oxidase** products mediate **rapid oxidative killing,** whereas **iNOS products** provide a **slower, more sustained mechanism of killing** of extracellular pathogens. NK cells eliminate intracellular pathogens by attacking cells infected by virus (as well as tumor cells and transplanted cells) via important differences in surface protein expression. They can detect absent or reduced expression of self-MHC class I receptors on foreign cells and infected cells (as many viruses evade cytotoxic T-cell killing by inhibiting MHC expression). They also kill cells with stress-induced expression of surface proteins MIC-A and MIC-B.

Clinical Discussion: Defects in the Complement System

Table 2-5 describes defects of the complement system and their clinical manifestations. The severity of disease reflects the relative importance of each component in their defense against infection.

Diagnosis of Complement Deficiency
- Consider complement deficiency in anyone with recurrent encapsulated bacterial infections
- Consider MAC deficiency in anyone with recurrent or disseminated *Neisseria* infections

TABLE 2-5 Complement Deficiencies

Defect	Disease	Possible Mechanisms
C1q, C1r, C1s, C2, or C4	**Immune complex syndromes:** SLE, discoid lupus, glomerulonephritis, vasculitis; ↑ risk of septicemia in C2 deficiency	*Classic pathway defect* Impaired processing and clearance of immune complexes
C3, H, or I	**Recurrent, *severe* pyogenic infections** with encapsulated bacteria, e.g., pneumococcus, meningococcus → pneumonia, otitis media, sinusitis	*Alternative pathway defect* Inefficient opsonization by C3b may cause susceptibility to infection; inability to dismantle C3 convertase
C5, C6, C7, or C8 MAC deficiency	**Recurrent, disseminated neisserial infections,** commonly meningococcal meningitis; immune complex diseases	**Defective MAC:** bacterial cell lysis may be required for effective killing of this pathogen
C1 esterase inhibitor (INH) protein	**Hereditary angioedema:** episodic, localized, nonpitting edema without pruritus on face or limb in response to trauma/stress; painful bowel edema; life-threatening laryngeal edema	**Uncontrolled C1 activity,** with breakdown of C4 and C2 and release of vasoactive peptide, *kinin,* from C2 causes edema

Diagnostic Tests

- **Total hemolytic complement activity (CH$_{50}$)** → low or undetectable for most complement deficiencies (C1–C8)
- **Serum C3 and C4:** different profiles suggest different complement deficiencies
- **Quantitation of complement factors** to identify specific complement deficiency

Treatment of Complement Deficiency and other Cellular Innate Immunodeficiency

- Acute infection: broad-spectrum IV **antibiotics**
- Chronic/recurrent infection: prophylactic antibiotics, **vaccination** against pneumococcus, meningococcus, and *Haemophilus influenzae*
- **C1 INH (isoniazid) concentrate** infusion for hereditary angioedema: aborts acute attacks; prophylaxis for surgical procedures
- **Gene therapy** for complement deficiencies may have a role in the future

CASE CONCLUSION

CD's meningococcal meningitis and bacteremia resolved with antibiotic therapy. Given his recurrence of major encapsulated bacteria infection, a complement deficiency was suspected. Subsequent CH$_{50}$ testing revealed no detectable activity. C3 and C4 levels were normal. Quantitative testing of complement factors revealed a C5 deficiency. CD's family was subsequently educated on the significance of this disease, the necessity for vaccination against encapsulated bacteria, and the need for immediate medical attention with any signs of infection. CD is doing well otherwise and shows no signs of neurologic sequelae from the meningitis.

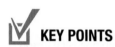

KEY POINTS

- The innate immune system is the more primitive branch of immunity that uses nonspecific means to exclude or eliminate infection
- It uses physical barriers such as skin as well as pattern recognition of molecular structures unique to microorganisms to provide protection from and elimination of infection
- The humoral component consists of several antimicrobial peptides, soluble pattern recognition proteins, and the complement cascade, which directly attack microbes and promote further amplification of the inflammatory response
- The complement system is a central component of humoral innate immunity and provides three functions: (*a*) *opsonization* of pathogens, (*b*) promotion of *cell lysis* via the MAC, and (*c*) *amplification of the innate and adaptive immune responses*

- The cellular components include neutrophils, macrophages, and NK cells, each of which has their own set of receptors that recognize microbial molecular structures, opsonins, or differences in cell surface expression; they eliminate pathogens by phagocytosis followed by lytic and oxidative killing or by killing cells infected with intracellular pathogens
- Deficiencies in complement and cell killing reflect the relative importance of each immune component
- Diagnosis involves measurement of complement activity and quantitative testing for specific complement factors; treatment consists mostly of supportive therapy

QUESTIONS

1. The following is a list of aspects of CD's history and physical exam that would make one suspicious of a complement deficiency. Which is the *least* correct?

   A. Previous history of pneumococcal pneumonia
   B. Current meningococcal pneumonia
   C. Petechial rash
   D. Arthritis
   E. Nuchal rigidity with positive Kernig and Brudzinski signs

2. The following is a list of possible steps in the pathogenesis of meningococcal infection at the onset of CD's illness. Which is *not* expected to happen?

   A. Extracellular pathogens like *N. meningitidis* are recognized by LPS-binding pattern recognition proteins
   B. IgG molecules to *N. meningitidis* bind to specific antigens on the bacteria and activate the complement cascade via the classic pathway
   C. C3b binds the bacterial cell surface and complexes with Bb to form C3 convertase, which cleaves C3 to form C3b and C3a

   D. C3b complexes with C3 convertase to form C5 convertase, which cleaves C5 to form C5b and C5a
   E. Immune complexes form with IgM bound to extracellular meningococci and deposit in joints and end vasculature in the skin to form a diffuse petechial rash
   F. Membrane-associated complex is formed from C5, C6, C7, C8, and C9 and inserts into the bacterial membrane, causing cell leakage promoting cell lysis and phagocytosis

3. Five years later, CD experienced another episode of meningococcal infection with a less severe and more indolent course with symptoms limited to low-grade fever, polyarthritis, petechial rash, and hematuria, but no evidence of meningitis. What may be a possible pathophysiologic explanation for this?

   A. CD has developed a faster, more efficient innate immune response to *N. meningitidis* due to his previous exposure to the bacterium
   B. CD's infection is marked by symptoms of immune complex deposition reflecting the availability of IgG to

meningococcus that can limit the spread of infection via the classic pathway and other mechanisms of adaptive immunity

C. CD has been able to compensate for his lack of C5 protein by up-regulating other proteins of the complement cascade and thereby improve the efficiency of this line of defense

D. CD's natural killer cells, having been previously exposed to meningococcus, can now more efficiently destroy bacteria of this species, thereby limiting spread of infection

E. The reactive intermediates of NADPH oxidase and iNOS limit the infection by providing a rapid as well as slow and sustained oxidative killing of phagocytized bacteria

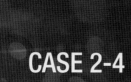

CASE 2-4 Immunodeficiency

HPI: BD is a 12-month-old boy who presents with 1 day of **fever, cough,** and **dyspnea.** The mother recorded a fever of **102.3°F** and notes increased **irritability, rhinorrhea,** frequent **ear pulling, diarrhea,** and **vomiting.** The cough began yesterday and has progressed to rapid breathing. This is his **sixth respiratory tract infection in the last 5 months,** which includes one episode of bronchitis, three episodes of otitis media, and one episode of pneumonia requiring hospitalization.

PE: T 39.4°C; BP 97/52; HR 135; RR 49; SaO_2 95% on room air

On exam, he is in **mild respiratory distress.** His weight is 10% less than that of the last recorded weight, which was in the fifth percentile. His exam is significant for **erythematous and purulent tympanic membranes, thick green sputum in the nasopharynx,** chest retractions, diffuse rhonchi, and diminished capillary refill. His **chest X-ray** showed **diffuse infiltrates.**

He was immediately given oxygen, nebulized albuterol, as well as one dose of prednisone. He was admitted for pneumonia and the immunologist was consulted to investigate the possibility of a primary immunodeficiency.

THOUGHT QUESTIONS

- What are the common forms of primary immunodeficiency?
- What are the underlying defects of such immunodeficiencies?
- What are the clinical manifestations of these diseases?

BASIC SCIENCE DISCUSSION AND REVIEW

There are many primary immunodeficiencies affecting many divisions of the immune system. These immunodeficiencies highlight the importance of each component of immunity.

Immunodeficiencies caused by defects in phagocytic function prevent the immune system from carrying out the final steps in microbial killing (Table 2-6). This leads to persistent microbial infection, which clinically manifests as chronic abscess formation and abnormal wound healing. Immunodeficiencies caused by defects in leukocyte recruitment to sites of infection or injury cause patterns of poor wound healing and inadequate pus formation (the clinical manifestation of adequate neutrophil infiltration).

Most immunodeficiencies of humoral immunity manifest themselves between 6 months and 2 years of life, after protective maternal antibodies clear from circulation in infants. These generally predispose the child to infections by organisms requiring opsonization and phagocytosis for final elimination. These include small extracellular pathogens such as encapsulated bacteria. Individuals with deficiencies in specific immunoglobulin isotypes are susceptible to infections at the sites usually protected by those immunoglobulin isotypes (e.g., IgA deficiencies predispose people to infections of mucosal surfaces, like gastritis) (Table 2-7).

Those persons with deficiencies in cell-mediated immunity from T-lymphocyte abnormalities exhibit poor immune defense against organisms that have a significant intracellular phase requiring antigen presentation by macrophages. These immunodeficiencies are marked by increased susceptibility to viruses, mycobacteria, and fungi (Table 2-8).

There are also a number of immunodeficiencies that arise from defects in both B and T lymphocytes. These diseases cause marked susceptibility to all types of infection (viral, bacterial, and fungal) from dysfunctional antibody-mediated *and* cell-mediated immunity, leading to high rates of morbidity and mortality, often at earlier ages. In addition, affected individuals may have other disease manifestations specific to the underlying genetic defect that caused the immunodeficiency syndrome (Table 2-9).

CASE CONCLUSION

The immunology consultant performs an evaluation on BD and discovers that he has a history of poison ivy contact dermatitis and no prior episodes of thrush. His family history is significant for a granduncle who died of pneumonia as a child. On exam, he has no lymphadenopathy. His CBC with a differential smear reveals lymphopenia with a marked decrease in mature B cells as determined by immunohistochemistry. Serum immunoglobulin levels show marked decreases in all five classes of immunoglobulin. BD is subsequently diagnosed with Bruton X-linked αγ-globulinemia and is treated with immunoglobulin replacement.

TABLE 2-6 Phagocyte Defects

Immunodeficiency	Pathogenesis	Clinical Manifestations
Chronic granulomatous disease	**Deficiency in NADPH oxidase** causing impaired production of reactive oxygen intermediate production → impaired cell killing results in granulomas, which represent an attempt by phagocytes to contain the spread of infection	Commonly X-linked; *defective clearing of a few microbial species*; staphylococcal infections in first months of life; later, groin, cervical, or axillary abscesses, osteomyelitis, lung/liver abscess, colitis; *Serratia* and *Nocardia* infections
Leukocyte adhesion deficiency	**Defect in tight adhesion of neutrophils** to endothelium preventing normal migration to site of infection	*Abnormal wound healing*, progressive neonatal periumbilical necrosis; recurrent surface infections; neutrophilia without adequate pus formation
Chédiak-Higashi syndrome	**Mutation of lysosomal trafficking gene** impairs normal trafficking and release of vesicle contents preventing chemokine release, PMN chemotaxis, and T-cell stimulation; abnormal pigment handling	*Progressive local infections without pus formation*; partial oculocutaneous albinism; late-onset lympho-proliferative disease

TABLE 2-7 Deficiencies of Humoral Immunity (B-Cell Defects)

Immunodeficiency	Pathogenesis	Clinical Manifestations
Bruton X-linked $\alpha\gamma$-globulinemia	**Failure of precursor B cells to differentiate into mature B cells** due to mutations in *Bruton tyrosine kinase;* after heavy chain rearrangement (*no light chains*); X-linked → **immunoglobulin deficiency** causes defect in clearing of organisms requiring phagocytosis; absent or few B cells and plasma cells • All immunoglobulin levels depressed • Underdeveloped lymphoid germinal centers	• Males; after age 6 months • *Recurrent bacterial infections* of the respiratory tract: pharyngitis, sinusitis, otitis media, bronchitis, pneumonia • Common bacteria: *Haemophilus influenza, Streptococcus pneumoniae, Staphylococcus aureus* • Common viruses: enteroviruses → gastritis → encephalitis • *Giardia lamblia:* ↓ IgA; gastritis • *Mycoplasma* infection causes arthritis • Treatment: IV immunoglobulin
Common variable immunodeficiency	**Deficient production of all different antibody classes** due to immature circulating B cells that can recognize antigen, respond, but fail to fully mature to plasma cells → nodular B-cell hyperplasia Treatment: IV immunoglobulin replacement	• Can present during adulthood • *Chronic pulmonary infections,* chronic giardiasis, intestinal malabsorption, atrophic gastritis with pernicious anemia • S/Sx of lymphoid hyperplasia: fever, weight loss, anemia, splenomegaly, lymphadenopathy, thrombocytopenia, lymphocytosis
Isolated IgA deficiency	**Inability to produce IgA antibodies;** associated with congenital intra-uterine infection (toxoplasmosis, rubella, CMV) or following treatment with phenytoin or other medications in genetically susceptible individuals → halted B-cell differentiation	• Caucasian, familial • *Asymptomatic or recurrent respiratory infections, chronic diarrheal disease* • Associated with atopic disease, arthritis, SLE

TABLE 2-8 Deficiencies of Cellular Immunity (T-Cell Defects)

Immunodeficiency	Pathogenesis	Clinical Manifestation
DiGeorge syndrome	Failed development of the 3rd and 4th pharyngeal pouches causing congenitally absent thymus and parathyroids → **loss of T-cell–mediated immunity** and parathyroid function; deletion in chromosome 22q11	• ↓ Circulating T cells → *poor defense against fungal and viral infections* • Congenital heart defects • Facial abnormalities • Hypocalcemic tetany

(Continued)

TABLE 2-8 Deficiencies of Cellular Immunity (T-Cell Defects) *(Continued)*

Immunodeficiency	Pathogenesis	Clinical Manifestation
Hyper-IgM syndrome	**A mutation causes abnormal CD40/CD40L interaction** preventing 1. Activation of CTLs and macrophages → poor cell-mediated immunity 2. B cells from isotype switching from IgM to IgA, IgG, or IgE → poor opsonization (also a humoral immunodeficiency)	• Male: X-linked inheritance • *Recurrent pyogenic infections* (because IgG levels are low) • *Pneumocystis carinii* pneumonia • Autoimmune hemolytic anemia, thrombocytopenia, neutropenia (from IgM antibody reaction)

TABLE 2-9 Combined B- and T-Cell Defects

Immunodeficiency	Pathogenesis	Clinical Manifestations
Severe combined immunodeficiency syndrome	**Impaired humoral and cell-mediated immunity** caused by multiple defects in T, B, and NK cell development, e.g., adenosine deaminase deficiency • RAG-1 and -2 gene mutations impair V(D)J rearrangement • JAK3 protein kinase deficiency	• X-linked or autosomal recessive • *Severe fungal, bacterial, and viral infection* • Affected infants rarely survive beyond 1 year without treatment • Treated with pluripotent hematopoietic stem cell transplant
Wiskott-Aldrich syndrome	**Progressive T-lymphocyte depletion** in circulation and in paracortical (thymus-dependent) areas of lymph nodes → loss of cellular immunity, poor antibody development to polysaccharide and protein antigens; poor IgM levels	• X-linked disease • *Recurrent fungal, bacterial, and viral infection* • Thrombocytopenia • Eczema • Early death
Ataxia telangiectasia	Mutant ATM gene causes **defect in monitoring of DNA repair** and coordination of DNA synthesis in cell division; maldevelopment of the thymus	• *Respiratory tract infections* Cerebellar ataxia: truncal *ataxia* • Oculocutaneous *telangiectasia* • *Lymphomas* and carcinomas
Hyper-IgE syndrome	Mechanism and gene defect unknown → **very high IgE levels,** abnormal neutrophil chemotaxis, diminished antibody responses to immunizations	• *Recurrent skin and lung abscesses* • Staphylococcal infections and other pyogenic infections • Recurrent bone fractures, scoliosis

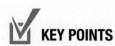

THUMBNAIL: Immunodeficiency

• Defects in phagocytic function prevent final digestion and elimination of many infections with many consequences, including abscess formation
• Defects in humoral immunity lead to infections by small organisms requiring opsonization and phagocytosis for final elimination (extracellular infections)
• Defects in cellular immunity cause susceptibility to infections by mycobacteria, fungi, and viral infection (intracellular infections)

KEY POINTS

■ The specific profiles of susceptibility to different infections illustrate the specific function of the defective immune component of an immunodeficiency

■ Complement deficiencies are marked by susceptibility to infections by bacteria that require the opsonizing activity of complement, particularly encapsulated organisms such as *Neisseria meningitidis*

■ B-lymphocyte immunodeficiencies are marked by susceptibility to organisms that require opsonization by antibodies, especially in the GI mucosa where IgA serves as an important defense

■ T-lymphocyte immunodeficiencies are marked by susceptibility to mycobacterial and fungal infection, both of which require a robust cell-mediated immunity to suppress

QUESTIONS

1. What is the significance of BD's prior history of poison ivy contact dermatitis without history of thrush?

   A. It suggests an abnormal delayed-type hypersensitivity reaction that is associated with his immunodeficiency syndrome.

   B. The contact dermatitis suggests atopic disease, which makes him susceptible to respiratory tract infection and inflammation.

   C. This suggests an autoimmune skin disease activated by recognition of poison ivy antigen acting as a hapten by binding dermal cells, eliciting cell-mediated immunity against BD's cell surface antigens.

   D. Having no prior history of thrush makes the diagnosis of immunodeficiency in the protection of the upper respiratory tract mucous membranes questionable.

   E. This past medical history suggests normal cell-mediated immune function.

2. LE is a 10-year-old boy who presents to an immunology clinic after his sixth hospitalization for diarrhea. His immunoglobulin panel reveals an absence of IgA. What is the immunopathology underlying this immunodeficiency?

   A. The absence of IgA, the first immunoglobulin raised against pathogens, prevents proper neutralization of bacteria, making LE more susceptible to gastritis.

   B. The absence of IgA prevents intravascular clearing of bacteria, making LE susceptible to recurrent gastritis, causing diarrhea.

   C. The absence of IgA prevents the opsonization of intraluminal parasites of the GI tract, making LE susceptible to chronic amebiasis.

   D. The absence of IgA prevents the opsonization of pathogens within the GI tract, thus making LE more susceptible to GI bacteria infection, gastritis, and subsequent diarrhea.

   E. The absence of IgA prevents complement fixation, which is essential for initiating the inflammatory reaction, and opsonizing and eliminating bacteria, thus making LE susceptible to recurrent gastritis.

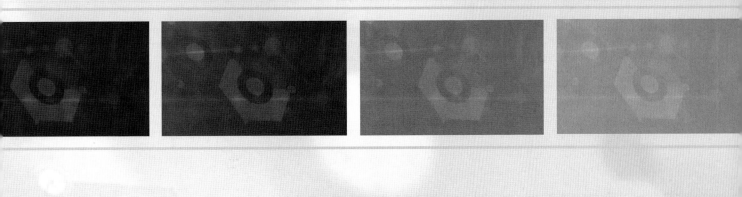

PART III

Pharmacology

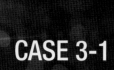

CASE 3-1 Clinical Pharmacokinetics

CASE 3-1A: Presentation 1 HPI: BK is a 72-year-old 60-kg man who is admitted to the hospital for treatment of sepsis. He has a long history of diabetes mellitus for which he has been receiving glipizide. He has a leg wound that is erythematous and tender. Blood cultures and a needle aspirate of the leg ulcer were taken and sent to the laboratory for culture and sensitivity.

Labs: His labs include serum creatinine (Cr) level 2.4 mg/dL; BUN 44 mg/dL; fasting blood glucose (FBG) 85 mg/dL; WBC count 18,000/mL. He is currently febrile at 38.5°C. He has an allergy to penicillin (rash and shortness of breath).

As empiric therapy for sepsis and the leg ulcer, BK is started on vancomycin 1 g IV every 12 hours and tobramycin 100 mg IV every 8 hours.

CASE 3-1B: Presentation 2 HPI: TE is a 62-year-old 75-kg man who is admitted to the hospital for shortness of breath (SOB) and "palpitations." In the past he has experienced short episodes of "chest pounding," but previously it always spontaneously resolved. TE has essentially normal laboratory values. Electrocardiography indicates he is in atrial fibrillation. His previous medical history (PMH) is significant for hypertension treated with hydrochlorothiazide only. He has no known drug allergies (NKDA).

For initial treatment, TE is to be given a 1-mg loading dose of digoxin IV and then started on a maintenance dose of 0.25 mg every morning PO. Following rate control, TE is to be started on amiodarone 400 mg every day PO for 1 month and then the maintenance dose will be reduced to 200 mg each morning PO. He was instructed to continue on the hydrochlorothiazide.

THOUGHT QUESTIONS 1A

- What is BK's renal function?
- Should vancomycin or tobramycin therapy be initiated with a "loading" dose?
- Is the initial maintenance dose appropriate?
- If a decrease in the "dose" is required, would it be more appropriate to decrease the dose and maintain the same interval or to keep the same dose and extend the interval?

THOUGHT QUESTIONS 1B

- Is the loading dose of digoxin appropriate for TE?
- Is TE's maintenance dose appropriate?

BASIC PHARMACOKINETIC PRINCIPLES

Absorption (Bioavailability)

It is assumed that when a drug is given parenterally that the entire dose is available for pharmacologic effect. Following oral administration, not all drugs are completely or even well absorbed (i.e., they have a limited or poor oral bioavailability). Absorption following oral administration is a complex process, and any number of factors can limit absorption, including water versus lipid solubility, stability of the drug in the GI tract, and metabolism by enzymes in the gut wall or liver.

Volume of Distribution

Volume of distribution is the space in which the drug appears to distribute. Volume of distribution is a complex relationship

between water and lipid solubility, drug binding to plasma and tissue proteins, and active transport systems.

Volume of distribution can be used to estimate a loading dose in order to rapidly achieve effective drug concentrations and therapeutic effects. In clinical practice the use of a loading dose is not always necessary. The three most common reasons for not administering a loading dose are (*a*) the first maintenance achieves a therapeutic effect, (*b*) the nonacute clinical setting dictates that immediate effect is not necessary or desirable, and (*c*) the pharmacologic effect is delayed due to a sequence of biologic processes.

Volume of Distribution, Two-Compartment Model

Following rapid IV administration, most drugs have an initial distribution phase wherein the drug is distributing from plasma to the more slowly equilibrating tissues (Fig. 3-1).

The graph in Figure 3-1 depicts plasma drug concentrations following rapid input into the plasma compartment. The initial rapid decline represents a distribution phase wherein the drug is moving into the more slowly equilibrating tissues. The elimination phase represents equilibrium between the rapidly and slowly equilibrating tissues and drug elimination from the body. Because of the potential for an intense and rapid onset of drug effect when the initial drug concentrations are high, the rate at which many drugs are infused into the body must be carefully controlled.

Clearance

Clearance is the term describing how the body eliminates solute from the body. Clearance is the key pharmacokinetic parameter to consider when determining maintenance doses of drugs.

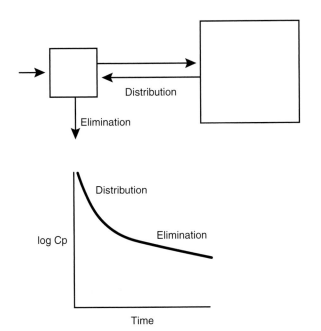

Figure 3-1. Plasma drug concentrations.

For most drugs the two primary routes of clearance or elimination are hepatic and renal, or a combination of these two pathways. As a general rule the maintenance dose of a drug would be reduced in proportion to the patient's decrease in clearance.

Hepatic Clearance

Patients with significant hepatic dysfunction would be expected to have a decreased ability to metabolize or clear drugs. An increase in liver enzymes (AST, ALT, and alkaline phosphatase [Alkphos]) or an increase in bilirubin and prothrombin time, and a decrease in serum albumin usually indicate hepatic dysfunction.

Renal Clearance

Serum creatinine and creatinine clearance (CrCl) rates are the most common measurements of renal function. In adult patients the normal value for serum Cr is 1 mg/dL (range 0.7–1.4), and in the average 70-kg young individual (approximately 20–30 years of age) this serum Cr corresponds to a CrCl rate of approximately 100 mL/min. As a general rule every doubling of the serum Cr represents a halving of a patient's renal function.

The following equation by Cockroft and Gault, which considers age, weight, sex, and serum Cr at steady state, is commonly used to estimate CrCl rate.

$$\text{Creatinine clearace (mL/min)} = \frac{(140 - \text{age in yrs})(\text{weight in kg})}{(72)(\text{Cr in mg/dL})} \ (0.85 \text{ if female})$$

Capacity-Limited Metabolism

For some drugs, clearance changes with the drug concentration. Increases in maintenance doses will result in a disproportionate increase in the steady-state drug concentration. Phenytoin is the classic capacity-limited drug.

Half-Life

The drug half-life (T½) is defined as the time required for the drug to decline by half (Fig. 3-2). The T½ is determined by the drug's volume of distribution and clearance or elimination from

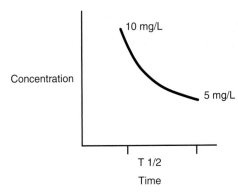

Figure 3-2. Drug half-life.

the body. T½ can be used to determine the rate at which the drug will accumulate once a maintenance regimen is started. In one half-life, a drug will achieve 50% of the final steady-state plateau value; in two half-lives, 75%; in three half-lives, 87.5%; and in 3.3 half-lives, 90% of steady state (Fig. 3-3). Most clinicians use between 3.3 and 5 half-lives as the time required to achieve steady state.

Half-life is also useful in determining the dosing interval. For some drugs the goal is to maintain a relatively constant drug concentration. In these cases the drug should be given as a constant IV infusion, in a sustained oral dosage form, or with a dosing interval that is short compared with the drug T½. In other cases, it is clinically acceptable to have wide swings in the drug concentration within the dosing interval (drugs with a wide therapeutic window or a pharmacologic reason for having the peak concentration much higher than the trough concentration, e.g., aminoglycoside antibiotics, which exhibit a concentration-dependent antibacterial effect). In these cases it would be acceptable to intermittently administer the drug with a dosing interval that is longer than the drug T½.

Plasma Samples for Therapeutic Monitoring

In most cases it is recommended that routine drug plasma samples for therapeutic monitoring be obtained after steady state has been achieved (i.e., 3.3–5 half-lives after starting on a maintenance regimen). In addition, most drug samples are obtained at a specific time within the dosing interval, usually at the drug trough or just before the next scheduled dose. Care should be taken to avoid obtaining drug samples during the distribution phase (i.e., soon after drug administration).

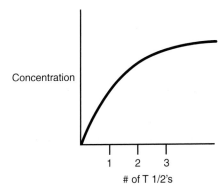

Figure 3-3. Drug half-life.

PRESENTATION 1 CONCLUSION 1A

Both vancomycin and tobramycin are administered with dosing intervals that are longer than the drug's T½. Under these conditions there is little accumulation, and loading doses are not usually administered. Both vancomycin and tobramycin are eliminated from the body primarily by the renal route. BK is a 72-year-old man with a serum Cr level of 2.4 mg/dL. As a first estimate, his renal function would appear to be approximately half of the normal value. Using the equation that accounts for age, body size, sex, and serum Cr, his estimated CrCl rate is expected to be approximately 25 mL/min.

$$\text{CrCl for males (mL/min)} = \frac{(140-\text{age})(\text{weight})}{(72)(\text{Cr})}$$

$$= \frac{(140-72 \text{ yrs})(60 \text{ kg})}{(72)(2.4 \text{ mg/dL})}$$

$$= 23.6 \text{ mL/min} \approx 25 \text{ mL/min}$$

Assuming 100 mL/min to be the "normal" value, BK's renal function is only about one fourth of normal. Clearly, some type of dose adjustment seems warranted for both vancomycin and tobramycin. The question is whether to decrease the dose and maintain the same interval or to keep the same dose and increase the interval. In any case, we would expect to administer the two drugs at about one fourth the usual rate.

Vancomycin exhibits **time-dependent** antibacterial activity; thus, the primary goal is to keep the minimum drug concentration above the minimum inhibitory concentration. Therefore, decreasing the dose would be the proper approach. Administering 250 mg (one fourth the usual dose) every 12 hours (the usual interval) might be appropriate. An alternative might be to administer 500 mg (half the usual dose) every 24 hours (twice the usual interval). These two regimens represent the same rate but the second has the convenience of once-daily dosing.

Tobramycin exhibits **concentration-dependent** antibacterial activity. The higher the drug level, the better the bacterial killing. Achieving high peak concentrations is an important therapeutic goal. Therefore, the most logical approach would be to keep the same dose of 100 mg and extend the interval by a factor of four. Unfortunately, this produces an interval of 32 hours, which would result in an inconsistent time of administration each day and increase the possibility of missing a dose or administering the dose at the wrong time. Most clinicians would probably compromise and give the tobramycin every 24 hours.

PRESENTATION 2 CONCLUSION 1B

Because digoxin has a usual T½ of approximately 2 days, it would take approximately 7 to 10 days (3.3–5 half-lives) for digoxin to accumulate to the final steady-state concentration. To shorten the time required to achieve therapeutic concentrations, it is common to administer a digoxin loading dose. However, this process of loading digoxin is usually restricted to the acute care setting, where the patient can be closely monitored for adverse events. Digoxin is approximately 80% eliminated by the renal route. Although TE has a "normal" serum Cr level (assumed to be approximately 1 mg/dL), he is 62 years of age and would have an expected CrCl rate of approximately 80 mL/min based on the equation of Cockroft and Gault. Although 80 mL/min is slightly below the usually accepted normal of approximately 100 mL/min, TE's renal function would not be considered to be "compromised." At first inspection the initial loading and maintenance dose of digoxin would appear to be reasonable. However, with the addition of amiodarone the digoxin level would be expected to increase. This is because there is a drug–drug interaction such that amiodarone inhibits the body's ability to metabolize and renally eliminate digoxin by a factor of 0.5 (i.e., clearance is half of normal). To prevent the undesired increase in the digoxin concentration, TE should have his digoxin maintenance reduced to about half of the prescribed amount. This could be accomplished by either doubling the interval to 2 days or decreasing the dose to 0.125 mg/day. Because daily dosing is probably more convenient and most likely to result in adherence, the previous regimen would be discontinued and a new digoxin regimen of 0.125 mg each day would be prescribed.

THUMBNAIL: Pharmacokinetics

Absorption/bioavailability: The percentage or fraction of a drug that reaches the systemic circulation. Drugs administered by the parenteral route (IV, IM, or SC) are assumed to have 100% absorption. Some drugs administered orally have very good (>80%) and some very poor (<20%) absorption. The percentage absorption must be taken into account when changing from the parenteral to the oral route. Some drugs have such a low bioavailability that to achieve systemic effects they must be administered parenterally.

Volume of distribution: The space into which the drug appears to distribute. Most important when administering a loading dose.

Loading dose = (volume of distribution) × (plasma concentration)

and

$$\text{Plasma concentration} = \frac{\text{(loading dose)}}{\text{(volume of distribution)}}$$

All drugs when administered by the IV route display two-compartment pharmacokinetics. Therefore, many drugs must have the rate of IV drug input controlled to avoid acute toxicities.

Clearance: Clearance of drugs is almost always either hepatic or renal. Hepatic and renal function as well as the route by which a drug is eliminated must be assessed when determining maintenance doses.

Maintenance dose = (clearance) × (steady − state plasma concentration)

and

$$\text{Steady-state plasma concentration} = \frac{\text{(maintenance dose)}}{\text{(clearance)}}$$

Creatinine clearance: The normal CrCl rate for an adult is approximately 100 mL/min. The most common equation for estimating renal function is:

$$\text{CrCl (mL/min)} = \frac{(140 - \text{age in yrs})(\text{weight in kg})}{(72)(\text{Cr in mg/dL})} \ (\times \ 0.85 \text{ if female})$$

Half-life: The time required for a drug to decline to half its value. (Assumes no drug input and volume of distribution and clearance are constant or "first order" elimination.)

$$T\tfrac{1}{2} = \frac{(0.693)(\text{volume of distribution})}{\text{clearance}}$$

Time to decay: With each half-life a drug concentration will decline by half. After 3.3 half-lives, 90% of the drug will have been eliminated.

Time to steady state: When on a consistent maintenance regimen, 90% of steady state is achieved in 3.3 half-lives. Steady state is assumed after 3.3 to 5 half-lives.

Dosing interval: The time between doses. Usually determined by the $T\tfrac{1}{2}$ of the drug and the desire to maintain a relative constant drug concentration (dosing interval less than the drug $T\tfrac{1}{2}$) or a drug concentration that swings widely within the interval (dosing interval longer than the drug $T\tfrac{1}{2}$).

Time to obtain plasma sample: Most drug samples are obtained as trough concentrations at steady state. If a peak sample is to be obtained, the absorption/distribution phase should be avoided. Recording the time of sampling is important.

QUESTIONS

1. A 55-year-old woman is admitted for treatment of her heart failure. She is experiencing frequent premature ventricular contractions and chest pain. In addition, she has had a recent weight gain of 11 pounds. Her medications include benazepril, digoxin, furosemide, and amiodarone. Her labs are significant for the following: potassium 2.8 mEq/L, digoxin 3.6 µg/L, Cr 2.2 mg/dL. You may assume that the patient has been taking all medications as directed and the T1/2 of digoxin in this patient is approximately 4 days. Which of the following is/are true statement(s):

   A. The potassium value of 2.8 mEq/L is in part responsible for the elevated digoxin level.
   B. The amiodarone is in part responsible for the elevated digoxin level.
   C. The digoxin should be held for 4 days in order for the digoxin level to decline to approximately 1 µg/L.
   D. Digoxin is primarily eliminated by the liver metabolism.
   E. Benazepril reduces the elimination of digoxin and is in part responsible for the elevated digoxin level.

2. HS is an 80-year-old man with a postoperative infection. You are asked to write an order for cefepime. HS weighs 72 kg and has a serum Cr level of 3 mg/dL. The hospital dosing guidelines for cefepime are given in Table 3-1. Which of the following dosing regimens is/are appropriate based on the hospital's dosing guidelines?

   A. 1 g IV Q 12 hr
   B. 2 g IV Q 12 hr
   C. 1 g IV Q 24 hr
   D. 2 g IV Q 24 hr
   E. 0.5 IV g Q 24 hr
   F. 0.25 g IV Q 24 hr
   G. C and E

TABLE 3-1 Dosing Guidelines for Cefepime Based on Renal Function

	Creatinine Clearance			
	>60 mL/min	30–60 mL/min	10–30 mL/min	<10 mL/min
Cefepime dose	1–2 g	1–2 g	0.5–1 g	0.25–0.5 g
Dosing interval	Every 12 hr	Every 24 hr	Every 24 hr	Every 24 hr

CASE 3-2   Nitrates

HPI: TT is a 48-year-old man who presents to the general medicine clinic complaining of recent onset of chest pain (CP) on exertion. He says that he was feeling fine until about a week ago when he started experiencing intermittent CP while mowing the lawn. He also states that the CP subsides after sitting down in the shade and resting for about 5 minutes.

FH: Father who died at age 46 secondary to coronary artery disease (CAD). Smoking History: One pack of cigarettes per week for 20 years.

THOUGHT QUESTIONS

- What are the different types of angina?
- What is the drug of choice for acute chest pain?
- What is nitrate tolerance? How do you minimize tolerance?

BASIC SCIENCE REVIEW AND DISCUSSION

Angina pectoris is a symptom of **ischemic heart disease** that is frequently characterized by chest pain. There are three basic categories of angina: stable (exertional) angina, unstable angina, and vasospastic angina. Both stable and unstable angina reflect underlying **atherosclerotic** narrowing of coronary arteries. Vasospastic angina, or Prinzmetal variant angina, is usually not associated with CAD and is due to coronary spasms that result in decreased myocardial blood flow.

Angina occurs when atherosclerotic plaques obstruct coronary blood flow, therefore decreasing the oxygen supply to myocardial tissues. Atherosclerotic plaques are composed of cholesterol and foam cells (derivatives of macrophages) enclosed within a fibrous capsule. Thrombus formation occurs within the plaque, and as erosion of the endothelium occurs, the thrombus extends into the arterial lumen. Coronary blood flow may become occluded depending on the size of the atherosclerotic plaque and therefore produce symptoms of angina.

Nitrates are the drugs of choice for relieving angina because they decrease preload and myocardial oxygen demand by **venous dilatation.** In addition, nitrates dilate coronary arteries even in the setting of atherosclerosis. The two proposed mechanisms by which nitrates promote venodilatation are stimulation of cyclic guanosine monophosphate (GMP) production and inhibition of thromboxane synthetase.

Short-acting nitrates, such as sublingual (SL) tablets or translingual sprays, are the preparation of choice for quick relief, especially in the setting of exertional angina. Long-acting nitrates (e.g., isosorbide dinitrate [ISDN] and isosorbide mononitrate [ISMO]) become useful when the number, severity, and duration of anginal attacks increase.

When using long-acting nitrates, it is important to schedule a 10- to 12-hour nitrate-free interval to minimize **tolerance.** With continuous exposure to nitrates, tolerance or the loss of antianginal and hemodynamic effects occurs. When exposure is discontinued, symptoms of withdrawal (severe headache, chest pain, or sudden cardiac death) can occur. Short-acting nitrates are not likely to lead to tolerance due to their rapid onset of action and short duration.

CASE CONCLUSION

After the cardiac workup for TT, it was concluded that he had a diagnosis of unstable angina. He was prescribed nitroglycerin SL tablets for chest pain and a beta-blocker to help decrease the workload of the heart and decrease myocardial oxygen demand. His lipid panel revealed elevated cholesterol (250 mg/dL with low-density lipoprotein [LDL] 140 mg/dL and high-density lipoprotein [HDL] 40 mg/dL) and triglycerides (296 mg/dL). He was started on atorvastatin to help lower his cholesterol because it is a component of atherosclerotic plaques. Smoking cessation counseling was given and the patient was advised to start on nicotine patches.

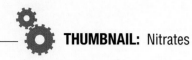

THUMBNAIL: Nitrates

Prototypical agent: Nitroglycerin

Clinical use: Primarily for the management of anginal symptoms of CAD.

MOA: Nitrates cause venous and arterial dilatation. However, venous dilatation is more evident because it increases venous pooling, therefore decreasing preload and reducing myocardial oxygen demand. In addition, nitrates dilate epicardial coronary arteries, consequently decreasing coronary vasospasm.

Adverse reactions: Headache, postural hypotension, and syncope are common. After several days of therapy, tolerance develops and headache and hypotension should resolve. Patients with nitrate-induced syncope should have their doses reduced. Dizziness, facial flushing, nausea, and tachycardia also occur. Methemoglobinemia may develop with large doses of IV nitroglycerin.

Drug interactions: The concurrent use of sildenafil (used for erectile dysfunction) is contraindicated due to potentiation of hypotensive effects of nitrates. Ergot alkaloids (used for migraine headaches) may cause increased blood pressure and decreased anti-anginal effects of nitrates—avoid concurrent use.

QUESTIONS

1. KB is a 59-year-old man who presents to the clinic with unresolved mild chest pain after taking numerous SL nitroglycerin tablets (one every 5 minutes over a total of 30 minutes). He reports that he hasn't used these pills for over a year, but still keeps them by his bedside. He also adds, "Now that I need these pills, they don't work!" Which is the most logical reason for the ineffective SL tablets?

   A. Nitrate tolerance
   B. Expired SL tablets
   C. Took too many tablets
   D. Took the wrong medication
   E. Nitrate intolerance

2. JK is a 70-year-old woman who has had angina for 5 years. She was well controlled on SL nitroglycerin until 3 weeks ago, when she started to note an increase in anginal episodes, ranging from three to five times per week. The attacks usually occurred on the fairways of the local golf course, where she meets and plays golf with friends three times a week. Today's vital signs are BP 119/69 mm Hg, HR 68 beats/min, RR 14 breaths/min. What is the most reasonable therapeutic option?

   A. Isosorbide dinitrate tablets
   B. Atenolol
   C. Verapamil
   D. Nitroglycerin ointment plus SL nitroglycerin
   E. SL isosorbide dinitrate

CASE 3-3 | Beta-Blockers

HPI: AV is a 62-year-old white man with a 6-year history of hypertension (HTN). His current antihypertensive therapy consists of enalapril and hydrochlorothiazide, but AV's BP is still elevated at 165/94 mm Hg.

PMH: Chronic obstructive pulmonary disease (COPD), peptic ulcer disease (PUD), HTN, and chronic back pain.

PE: HR 85, RR 14

Medications: Omeprazole, enalapril, hydrochlorothiazide, acetaminophen. Metoprolol was initiated.

Labs: Serum Cr 1.5 mg/dL, K$^+$ 5.0 mEq/L

THOUGHT QUESTIONS

- What is the primary pharmacology of beta-blockers?
- Which of the beta-blockers are β_1 selective?
- Which beta-blockers provide alpha blockade as well?
- Which beta-blocker is the most lipid soluble?
- What are the advantages and disadvantages of having intrinsic sympathomimetic properties?
- When might a beta-blocker be chosen over some of the other antihypertensives?
- Which beta-blocker is the shortest acting?

BASIC SCIENCE REVIEW AND DISCUSSION

Beta-blockers are one of the antihypertensive agents useful in patients with CAD because they have been shown to reduce morbidity and mortality. Beta-blockers competitively block both β_1 and β_2 but with different selectivity. Blocking β_1 receptors, which are found primarily on cardiac muscle, will lead to negative chronotropic and inotropic effects. In hypertensive patients, this will lower their blood pressure. β_2 receptors are found predominantly on the outer membrane of the smooth muscle cells of the vasculature, bronchioles, and myometrium and regulate the relaxation of these cells. Blockage of this receptor can lead to vasoconstriction and bronchoconstriction.

Some beta-blockers demonstrate β_1 selectivity. At low doses, metoprolol and atenolol predominantly antagonize the receptors on cardiac tissues with less activity on β_2 receptors. Therefore, they are less likely to cause bronchospasm in patients with COPD or asthma. The nonselective beta-blockers also have the disadvantage of masking hypoglycemic symptoms, especially in insulin-dependent diabetics. Blocking β_2 receptors also leaves the alpha-mediated vasoconstriction unopposed and, as a result, may worsen Raynaud disease or peripheral vascular disease. Some beta-blockers, such as labetalol and carvedilol, also possess alpha-blocking properties.

Another important difference among the beta-blockers is their relative lipophilicity. Propranolol is the most lipophilic agent. It undergoes a more extensive first-pass hepatic metabolism than other less lipophilic beta-blockers. Hence, propranolol has more interpatient variability in serum concentrations. More lipophilic beta-blockers also have an extensive volume of distribution, even crossing the blood–brain barrier. Consequently, these agents may have more CNS adverse effects such as drowsiness, nightmares, confusion, and depression. On the other hand, because propranolol penetrates the CNS, it is useful in treating migraines and anxiety. Less lipophilic beta-blockers are excreted more by the kidney and may require dosage adjustments in renal impairment.

Beta-blockers with intrinsic sympathomimetic (ISA) properties are not pure antagonists. These agents partially stimulate the beta-receptors as well. Theoretically, these agents are less likely to cause bradycardia and bronchospasm, increase lipids, decrease cardiac output, and cause peripheral vasoconstriction. However, these agents can still cause bronchospasm or exacerbate heart failure. ISA beta-blockers may have a role in patients who experiences severe bradycardia with non-ISA agents. When these agents are given to someone with a slow heart rate at rest, they may increase the heart rate. Conversely, ISA agents given to someone with exercise-induced tachycardia may decrease the heart rate because the beta-blocking activity predominates. Avoid these agents in patients who are s/p MI (status post myocardial infarction) because the agonistic properties may be detrimental.

In addition to their use as antihypertensive agents, beta-blockers are useful in treating many other conditions. Beta-blockers are considered first-line therapy in the management of chronic stable angina because they decrease the cardiac workload. Patients with a history of MI should receive beta-blockers if they do not have contraindications. Furthermore, they are used as antiarrhythmic agents in supraventricular and ventricular arrhythmias. Propranolol is used in the setting of hyperthyroidism to reduce symptoms and heart rate as well as decrease the conversion of thyroxine (T_4) to triiodothyronine (T_3) and to treat migraines, headaches, anxiety, and essential tremors. The nonselective beta-blockers are also used for hepatic portal HTN in patients with liver cirrhosis. Topical beta-blockers are used in glaucoma to reduce intraocular pressures (Table 3-2).

TABLE 3-2 Beta-Blockers: Selectivity, Activity, and Metabolism

Agent	Selectivity	Lipid Solubility	Metabolism	T1/2	Notes
Acebutolol	β_1	Moderate	Hepatic/renal	3–4 hr	Partial agonist
Atenolol	β_1	Low	Renal	6–7 hr	
Betaxolol	β_1	Low	Hepatic/renal	14–22 hr	Used in glaucoma
Bisoprolol	β_1	Low	Hepatic/renal	9–12 hr	
Carteolol	β_1 and β_2	Low	Hepatic/renal	6 hr	Partial agonist, Used in glaucoma
Carvedilol	β_1, β_2, and α_1	High	Hepatic	6–10 hr	Used mostly for CHF
Esmolol	β_1	Low	RBCs	10 min	Used IV, short-acting
Labetalol	β_1, β_2, and α_1	Moderate	Hepatic/renal	6–8 hr	α-blockade
Metoprolol	β_1	Moderate-high	Hepatic/renal	3–7 hrs	
Nadolol	β_1 and β_2	Low	Renal	20–24 hrs	Long-acting
Penbutolol	β_1 and β_2	High	Hepatic/renal	5 hrs	Partial agonist
Pindolol	β_1 and β_2	Moderate	Hepatic/renal	3–4 hrs	Partial agonist
Propranolol	β_1 and β_2	High	Hepatic	4–6 hrs	
Timolol	β_1 and β_2	Low-moderate	Hepatic/renal	4–5 hrs	Used in glaucoma

CASE CONCLUSION

Although this patient has a history of COPD, a β_1-selective agent may still be used, especially at low doses. In addition, the patient has renal impairment; thus, metoprolol was selected because it is primarily hepatically metabolized.

THUMBNAIL: Pharmacology

Prototypical agent: Propranolol has no beta-receptor selectivity. Metoprolol and atenolol were developed with more β_1 selectivity.

Clinical use: Primarily as an antihypertensive agent. Also used for controlling ventricular rate in atrial fibrillation (AF), post-MI, congestive heart failure (CHF), angina, and hyperthyroidism. Additionally, propranolol may be used for migraine headaches, essential tremors, and anxiety. The nonselective beta-blockers are useful in the treatment of hepatic portal HTN in patients with liver cirrhosis. Topical agents are used to lower intraocular pressures in patients with glaucoma.

MOA: Beta-blockers competitively antagonize beta-receptors, leading to decreased calcium influx into myocardial cells, which in turn leads to both decreased heart rate (chronotropic effect) and cardiac contractility (inotropic effect).

Pharmacokinetics

Absorption: Most are well absorbed orally; however, propranolol undergoes a large first-pass effect by the liver. Increasing the dose may compensate for this effect.

Distribution: Large volumes of distribution. Propranolol crosses the blood–brain barrier.

Elimination: Most are hepatically metabolized. The exceptions are atenolol and nadolol, which are renally excreted unchanged.

(Continued)

THUMBNAIL: Pharmacology *(Continued)*

Adverse reactions: The most important adverse reactions are seen in asthmatics. In asthmatics, beta-blockers may lead to constriction of the airways via smooth muscle contraction. Although β_1-selective agents may have less of an effect, they should still be used cautiously. The most common adverse effects are fatigue, bradycardia, hypotension, dizziness, nausea, diarrhea, and exercise intolerance. They are also associated with increased triglycerides and hyperglycemia. Additionally, beta-blockers can block some of the symptoms normally induced by hypoglycemia, particularly in insulin-dependent diabetics. Other side effects seen are depression, sleep disturbance, and impotence. The more lipophilic agents have more CNS adverse effects, such as drowsiness, nightmares, confusion, and depression. Beta-blockers with α_1-antagonist activity may produce more vasodilation activity and have a higher incidence of postural dizziness, light-headedness, and fatigue.

Warning: If beta-blockers are stopped abruptly, they can cause rebound HTN.

Drug interactions: An interaction at the level of cardiac activity may be seen, particularly with the calcium channel blocker verapamil. This can lead to bradycardia and severely diminished cardiac output.

QUESTIONS

1. A 66-year-old man who has been taking furosemide, atenolol, and loratadine for 5 months ran out of his medication for 1 week. The patient's blood pressure is 173/96 mm Hg compared with 155/90 mm Hg 5 months ago before drug therapy. PMH includes HTN, asthma, and diabetes. What is the most likely reason for the increased BP?

   A. Antihypertensive medication not adequate
   B. Rebound HTN
   C. Loratadine
   D. Hyperglycemia
   E. Asthma

2. An 82-year-old patient presents to the clinic with untreated HTN. PMH includes CAD, MI, COPD, and renal impairment. There is a strong indication for initiating a beta-blocker in this patient. Which one would you select?

   A. Atenolol
   B. Nadolol
   C. Metoprolol
   D. Propranolol
   E. Labetalol

HPI: A 60-year-old woman presents to the clinic for a 6-month follow-up exam for newly diagnosed HTN, which has not been adequately controlled by dietary and lifestyle changes.

PMH: Angina and asthma.

PE: BP 160/99; HR 55

Allergies: Sulfa-based drugs.

Medications: Albuterol inhaler, fluticasone inhaler, and nitroglycerin sublingual tablets.

THOUGHT QUESTIONS

- What are the different mechanisms of actions for calcium channel blockers?
- How do the four types of calcium channel blockers differ?
- What are some indications for calcium channel blocker use?
- What are the common side effects of calcium channel blockers?

BASIC SCIENCE REVIEW AND DISCUSSION

There are 10 calcium channel blockers available today in the United States. As a diverse class of drugs, they have many roles in the treatment of cardiovascular diseases. One calcium channel blocker, **nimodipine,** also has a specific role in treating sub-arachnoid hemorrhages.

Calcium channel blockers inhibit L-type calcium channels in cardiac and smooth muscle. As a result, inhibition of calcium influx into cells occurs, causing a **decrease in myocardial contractility** and rate, resulting in reduced oxygen demand. **Cardiac rate** is slowed by the ability of calcium channel blockers to block electrical conduction through the **atrioventricular (AV) node.** In addition, calcium channel blockers can reduce systemic arterial pressure by relaxing arterial smooth muscle and **decreasing systemic vascular resistance.**

Four categories of calcium channel blockers can be defined based on their chemical structures and actions: diphenylalkylamines, benzothiazepines, dihydropyridines, and bepridil. Both diphenylalkylamines (verapamil) and benzothiazepines (diltiazem) exhibit effects on both cardiac and vascular tissue. With specificity for the heart tissue, these two types of calcium channel blockers can slow conduction through the AV node and are useful in treating arrhythmias. The dihydropyridines (nifedipine is the prototypical agent) are more potent peripheral and coronary artery **vasodilators.** They do not affect cardiac conduction but can dilate coronary arteries. They are particularly useful as antianginal agents. Bepridil is unique in that it blocks both fast sodium channels and calcium channels in the heart. All calcium channel blockers, except nimodipine and bepridil, are effective in treating HTN.

Most side effects of the calcium channel blockers are related to their mechanism of action. Both verapamil and diltiazem can cause **sinus bradycardia** and may worsen CHF. **Constipation** has been associated with verapamil use. The dihydropyridines often cause symptoms associated with vasodilatation, such as facial flushing, peripheral edema, hypotension, and headache. Because dihydropyridines are potent vasodilators, they can cause reflex tachycardia, which may precipitate palpitations, worsening angina, or MI. Lastly, all calcium channel blockers can cause GI complaints and fatigue.

CASE CONCLUSION

Diuretics and beta-blockers are first-line agents for treating HTN. Because this patient has asthma, beta-blockers should be avoided. Calcium channel blockers are favorable therapeutic options in patients with both angina and HTN. Because her heart rate is low, diltiazem and verapamil are not optimal choices because they can slow down AV nodal conduction. A long-acting dihydropyridine, amlodipine, was started.

THUMBNAIL: Calcium Channel Blockers

Agent	Verapamil	Diltiazem	Nifedipine	Bepridil
Clinical use	Angina (vasospastic, chronic stable and unstable), HTN, arrhythmias, migraine prophylaxis	Angina (vasospastic, chronic stable and unstable), HTN, arrhythmias	Vasospastic angina, HTN, nimodipine is used for subarachnoid hemorrhage	Chronic stable angina
MOA	Calcium channel antagonists bind to L-type channels in cardiac and smooth muscle and inhibit influx of calcium into cardiac muscle, which decreases contractility and rate.			
Hemodynamic properties				
AV node conduction	↓↓↓	↓↓	0	↓
Myocardial contractility	↓↓	↓	↓	↓
Peripheral vascular resistance	↓↓	↓	↓↓↓	↓
Pharmacokinetics				
Route of administration	PO, IV	PO, IV	PO	PO
Metabolism	Liver (T½ 3–7 hours)	Liver (T½ 3–7 hours)	Liver (T½ 2–5 hours)	Liver (T½ 24 hours)
Adverse reactions	Sinus bradycardia, constipation, gingival hyperplasia	Sinus bradycardia	Facial flushing, peripheral edema, hypotension, headache, gingival hyperplasia, reflex tachycardia (palpitations, angina, MI)	Agranulocytosis, arrhythmias (torsade de pointes)
Drug interactions	Increased levels of digoxin, carbamazepine, cyclosporine, theophylline; additive AV nodal block with concurrent beta-blockers		Grapefruit juice may increase levels of some dihydropyridine agents	

QUESTIONS

1. A 55-year-old man is hospitalized for observation after an anginal attack. He suddenly develops shortness of breath and fatigue and tells his nurse that his heart feels like its ready to "jump out" of his chest. His ECG monitor shows AF with a ventricular rate of 160 beats/min. PMH: COPD and diabetes. Which of the following medications is best to control his ventricular rate?

   A. Quinidine
   B. Metoprolol
   C. Diltiazem
   D. Amlodipine
   E. Nimodipine

2. A 25-year-old woman with a history of migraine headaches was started on a calcium channel blocker 6 months ago for prophylaxis therapy. She now reveals that she has been having problems with constipation since starting therapy. In addition, she says that her gums are "overgrowing." PMH: Depression and diabetes. Which calcium channel blocker is the most likely cause of her side effects?

   A. Diltiazem
   B. Amlodipine
   C. Bepridil
   D. Verapamil
   E. Nifedipine

CASE 3-5 | Diuretics

HPI: MS is a 64-year-old woman newly diagnosed with HTN.

PMH: Osteoporosis. Her current medications include calcium carbonate, estrogen, and medroxyprogesterone.

PE: T 37.3°C; BP 162/70; HR 65; RR 18

Labs: K^+ 3.7 mEq/L; BUN 18 mg/dL; Cr 1.0 mg/dL

Medications: Hydrochlorothiazide was started to lower her blood pressure.

THOUGHT QUESTIONS

- What are the three main classes of diuretics?
- Why choose thiazide diuretics over other diuretics for the treatment of HTN?
- Discuss the differences in pharmacology between the classes.

BASIC SCIENCE REVIEW AND DISCUSSION

The three main diuretic classes are **thiazide, loop,** and **potassium-sparing diuretics.** Thiazide diuretics are considered one of the first-line agents for the treatment of HTN. Acutely, thiazide diuretics lower blood pressure by inhibiting sodium chloride cotransporters in the ascending loop of Henle and distal tubule, increasing sodium excretion and causing diuresis. The reduction in plasma volume decreases cardiac output and consequently reduces blood pressure. However, with continued therapy, the plasma volume returns to pretreatment levels and there is a decrease in peripheral vascular resistance, which is responsible for the long-term antihypertensive effects. The most common indication for thiazide diuretics is HTN.

The loop diuretics, including furosemide, bumetanide, torsemide, and ethacrynic acid, are the most potent diuretics available. They inhibit sodium and chloride channels in the thick ascending limb of the loop of Henle and prevent sodium reabsorption, leading to diuresis. In general, they do not reduce peripheral vasodilatation to the same extent as thiazide diuretics; therefore, they do not consistently or as effectively lower blood pressure. Loop diuretics are more potent than thiazides for diuresis and are most commonly used in patients with fluid overload.

Spironolactone, triamterene, and amiloride are potassium-sparing diuretics. They inhibit sodium reabsorption in the distal and collecting tubules and decrease potassium excretion through different modes. Spironolactone is a competitive aldosterone antagonist in the distal tubule and prevents the formation of protein important in sodium transport. It is indicated in the management of CHF for its mortality benefits and in patients with hyperaldosteronism (e.g., patients with hepatic cirrhosis and ascites). Triamterene and amiloride reduce the passage of sodium ions by directly acting on the sodium and potassium transporters in the distal and collecting tubule. The natriuretic activity of potassium-sparing diuretics is limited compared with thiazide and loop diuretics. For this reason, they are usually given in combination with thiazide or loop diuretics in HTN to reduce the potassium loss.

CASE CONCLUSION

According to the Sixth Report of the Joint National Committee on Prevention, Detection, Evaluation, and Treatment of High Blood Pressure (JNC VI),[1] diuretics are the preferred first-line agents in patients with isolated systolic hypertension (ISH). Studies have shown significant reduction in strokes, heart attacks, and mortality with diuretics and dihydropyridine calcium channel blockers in the treatment of ISH. Because this patient has ISH and adequate renal function, a thiazide diuretic is appropriate as initial treatment.

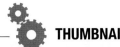

THUMBNAIL

	Thiazide	Loop	Potassium-Sparing
Clinical use	HTN, adjunct to loop diuretics for edema	Edema HTN in patients with CrCl <30–50 mL/min	HTN Spironolactone: systolic heart failure & hepatic cirrhosis

MOA	Inhibits reabsorption of NaCl in the ascending loop of Henle and the early distal tubules	Inhibits reabsorption of NaCl in the ascending loop of Henle and distal tubule	Spironolactone blocks aldosterone
			  receptors in the distal renal tubules
			Triamterene and amiloride interfere
			  with K^+/Na^+ exchange in the distal
			  and collecting tubule

Pharmacokinetics			
Absorption	Good absorption, except for chlorothiazide (mostly given IV)	Well absorbed; in heart failure patients with edematous bowels, IV diuretics may be required	Well absorbed
Distribution	Protein binding varies among different agents, but most have large volumes of distribution	Highly protein bound and small volumes of distribution	Spironolactone is highly protein bound Triamterene has moderate protein binding Amiloride has insignificant protein binding and a very large volume of distribution
Elimination	Renally excreted unchanged	Hepatically, except for furosemide	Spironolactone is metabolized by the liver to an active metabolite, canrenone Triamterene is hepatically cleared Amiloride is renally excreted
Adverse reactions	Electrolyte imbalances; $\downarrow K^+$, $\downarrow Mg^{2+}$, $\downarrow Na^+$, $\downarrow Cl^-$ $\uparrow$, uric acid reabsorption in the proximal tubules can precipitate gouty attacks; other side effects include rash, $\uparrow$ glucose, dizziness, photosensitivity, $\downarrow$ BP, headache, $\uparrow$ lipids	Similar to thiazide diuretics, except may also cause hypocalcemia	$\downarrow$ BP, $\uparrow K^+$, constipation, and nausea; gynecomastia can occur with spironolactone
Comments	Electrolytes, blood glucose, and lipids need to be monitored periodically	Ototoxicity may occur with furosemide at high infusion rates	$\uparrow K^+$ most often occurs in patients with renal impairment or in combination with ACE-I (acetylcholinesterase inhibitor)

QUESTIONS

1. SL is an 82-year-old man admitted to the hospital 3 days ago for pulmonary edema and received nitroglycerin and a diuretic. Now he complains of decreased hearing. Which diuretic most likely caused the ototoxicity?

   A. Hydrochlorothiazide
   B. Furosemide
   C. Bumetanide
   D. Torsemide
   E. None of the above

2. LC is a 56-year-old woman with HTN and renal insufficiency (CrCl 20 mL/min) who presents to the clinic. Her BP is elevated at 150/92 mm Hg. Which diuretic is probably not effective in this patient?

   A. Furosemide
   B. Hydrochlorothiazide
   C. Bumetanide
   D. Torsemide
   E. A, C, and D

REFERENCE

1. Joint National Committee on Detection, Evaluation, and Treatment of High Blood Pressure. The Sixth Report of the Joint National Committee on Detection, Evaluation and Treatment of High Blood Pressure. Arch Intern Med 1997;157:2413–2446.

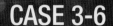

CASE 3-6 Angiotensin-Converting Enzyme Inhibitors

HPI: MM is 64-year-old Asian man who presents to the clinic for an HTN follow-up exam after starting hydrochlorothiazide 6 months ago. He denies chest pain, shortness of breath, dizziness, or headache. His past medical history is significant for diabetes and HTN. He is currently only receiving hydrochlorothiazide. His BP remains elevated above goal (130/85), and an ACE inhibitor is begun.

PE: T 37.5°C; BP 154/92; HR 82; RR 16.

Urinalysis (UA): 3+ protein

Labs: K⁺ 4.3 mEq/L; BUN 26 mg/dL; Cr 1.4 mg/dL

THOUGHT QUESTIONS

- What is the pharmacology of ACE inhibitors (ACE-Is)?
- When would an ACE-I be preferred over other antihypertensive medications?
- Which ACE–I has the shortest half-life?

BASIC SCIENCE REVIEW AND DISCUSSION

ACE-Is block the conversion of angiotensin I to angiotensin II, which causes vasoconstriction and stimulates the production of aldosterone synthesis. Thus, ACE-Is promote vasodilatation and decrease sodium retention, consequently lowering blood pressure. The inhibition of angiotensin-converting enzymes also blocks the breakdown of bradykinins. The increase in bradykinin level leads to additional vasodilatation effects. However, the increase in bradykinin is also responsible for adverse effects such as cough and angioedema.

In addition, ACE-Is are particularly useful in treating patients with **diabetic nephropathy.** In these patients, ACE-Is can decrease proteinuria and stabilize renal function independent of their antihypertensive effects. The benefits are attributed to their effects on renal hemodynamics. Angiotensin II may adversely affect the kidney by increasing the glomerular efferent arteriole resistance. Hence, the decrease in production of angiotensin II results in vasodilatation of the efferent arteriole and lowering intraglomerular capillary pressure. These agents also have favorable effects in patients with CHF and post-MI. ACE-Is have been shown to reduce mortality to preserve left ventricular function by reducing remodeling of the myocardium in these patients.

Captopril is the shortest and fastest-acting oral ACE-I (Table 3-3). Because of these properties, it is used to titrate patients to the desired response and prior to conversion to a longer-acting ACE-I.

TABLE 3-3 Comparison of Currently Available ACE Inhibitors

Agent	Onset (min)	Duration (hr)	T½ (hr)	Elimination
Captopril	15–30	10–12	2	Renal
Enalapril	60	24	11	Renal
Lisinopril	60	24	12	Renal
Ramipril	60–120	24	13–17	Renal
Benazepril	30–60	24	10–11	Renal
Fosinopril	60	24	12	Renal + hepatic
Quinapril	60	24	2	Renal
Moexipril	90	24	2–9	Renal + hepatic
Trandolapril	240	24	10	Renal

CASE CONCLUSION

A 24-hour urine collection is performed, which reveals 780 mg of protein and a CrCl rate of 58 mL/min. Thus, this patient has chronic renal disease, most likely diabetic nephropathy. Therefore, an ACE-I would be a good choice for this patient.

THUMBNAIL: Pharmacology

Prototypical agent: Captopril, shortest-acting ACE-I. Additional agents have been developed with longer durations of action, allowing for once-daily dosing.

Clinical use: ACE-I are most commonly used for HTN, diabetic nephropathy, CHF, and post-MI.

MOA: ACE-Is block the conversion of angiotensin I to angiotensin II, promoting vasodilatation and decreasing sodium retention.

Pharmacokinetics

Absorption: Most are well absorbed, but food may reduce the absorption of captopril, moexipril, quinapril, and trandolapril.

Distribution: The distribution greatly varies depending on the protein binding of the agent: moexipril > lisinopril > captopril > trandolapril > benazepril, fosinopril.

Elimination: Most ACE-Is are renally eliminated.

Adverse reactions: The most common adverse effects are hypotension, headache, fatigue, dizziness, **hyperkalemia,** and **cough.** The incidence of ACE-I–induced cough ranges from 1 to 10%. The onset may occur within a couple of weeks to months after initiation. The cough is dry, nonproductive, and not responsive to cough suppressants. It should resolve 1 to 4 days after discontinuing the ACE-I. Less common side effects are dysgeusia, rash, **agranulocytosis,** and **angioedema.** The incidence of angioedema is less than 1% and may occur anytime during therapy. The swelling is usually confined to the face, lips, tongue, glottis, and larynx. Patients should not be rechallenged with an ACE-I if they have a history of angioedema.

Warning: The use of ACE-Is during the second and third trimesters of pregnancy can cause injury or death to the developing fetus.

QUESTIONS

1. A 63-year-old man presents to the clinic complaining of dizziness and light-headedness. The patient's BP is 95/62 mm Hg and HR 110 beats/min. He was recently started on benazepril 10 days ago. His PMH is notable for HTN and osteoarthritis. He is currently taking furosemide and ibuprofen. Stat labs include $Na^+ < 128$ mEq/L, K^+ 4.6 mEq/L, and Cr 1.1 mg/dL. What is(are) the risk factor(s) for ACE-I–induced hypotension?

   A. Hyponatremia (serum sodium <130 mEq/L)
   B. Concurrent diuretic use
   C. Concurrent NSAID use
   D. Tachycardia
   E. A and B

2. A 72-year-old woman with an anterior MI was admitted to the hospital 7 days ago and has developed swelling of her lips and tongue, and bradycardia. She also complains of flushing and hallucinations. During the hospital course, the patient was started on metoprolol, captopril, isosorbide dinitrate, aspirin, and morphine. Which of the following adverse drug reactions is mostly likely caused by captopril?

   A. Bradycardia
   B. Swelling of lips and tongue
   C. Flushing
   D. Hallucinations
   E. None of the above

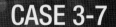

CASE 3-7 | Angiotensin Receptor Blockers

HPI: Six weeks after starting lisinopril for HTN, MM develops a dry, nonproductive cough. After ruling out other causes of the cough, he was switched to losartan.

PE: T 36.8°C; BP 145/85; HR 80; RR 16. Lungs clear to auscultation.

Medications: Hydrochlorothiazide and lisinopril

UA: Positive protein

Labs: K$^+$ 4.7 mEq/L, BUN 24 mg/dL, Cr 1.2 mg/dL

THOUGHT QUESTIONS

- What is the primary pharmacology of angiotensin receptor blockers (ARBs)?
- When are ARBs indicated?
- What are the advantages of ARBs over ACE-Is?

BASIC SCIENCE REVIEW AND DISCUSSION

ARBs are selective and competitive **angiotensin II receptor antagonists** (Table 3-4). They block vasoconstriction and aldosterone-secreting effects similar to ACE-Is. However, because ARBs do not block the metabolism and increase the levels of bradykinin, they are less likely to be associated with non–renin-angiotensin effects such as cough and angioedema.

Angiotensin II antagonists share the hemodynamic effects of ACE-Is and therefore have similar indications such as HTN, CHF, and diabetic nephropathy. However, ARBs have not been shown to be superior to ACE-Is and are more expensive. There is also an absence of data documenting comparable long-term cardiovascular benefits. Therefore, ARBs should be reserved principally for patients in whom ACE-Is are indicated but who are unable to tolerate the medication.

CASE CONCLUSION

The patient was switched to an ARB because he was experiencing cough, a possible side effect of ACE-Is. It is important to rule out other causes of cough before discontinuing the ACE-I. The incidence of ACE-I–induced cough may vary, ranging from 1 to 10%, and occurs less frequently with ARBs because ARBs do not inhibit the breakdown of bradykinins. ACE-I–induced cough may occur within a couple of weeks to months after initiation of therapy. After discontinuing the ACE-I, the cough should resolve within 1 to 4 days.

TABLE 3-4 Comparison of Currently Available Angiotensin Receptor Blockers

Agent	Onset (min)	Duration (hr)	T½ (hr)	Elimination
Losartan	60–90	24	2–9	Hepatic + renal
Valsartan	120	24	6	Hepatic
Irbesartan	60–120	24	11–15	Hepatic
Candesartan	120–240	24	9	Hepatic + renal
Telmisartan	60–180	24	24	Hepatic

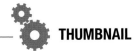

THUMBNAIL

Prototypical agent: Losartan

Clinical use: ARBs have indications similar to those for ACE-Is, but they are mainly used in patients who are unable to tolerate ACE-Is.

MOA: Angiotensin II receptor antagonist, which prevents vasoconstriction and aldosterone-secreting effects of angiotensin II.

Pharmacokinetics

Absorption: The absorption greatly varies depending on the agent: irbesartan > telmisartan > losartan, valsartan > candesartan.

Distribution: Variable depending on the protein binding of the agent.

Elimination: ARBs are predominantly eliminated through hepatic metabolism.

Adverse reactions: Similar to ACE-Is. The most common side effects are **cough,** hypotension, headache, fatigue, dizziness, and **hyperkalemia.** The less common adverse reactions include dysgeusia, rash, diarrhea, **agranulocytosis,** and **angioedema.** Cough and angioedema occur less frequently than with ACE-Is, but precautions should be taken when initiating ARBs in someone who experienced angioedema with an ACE–I because there is some cross-reactivity.

Warning: Use during the second and third trimesters can cause injury or death to the developing fetus.

QUESTIONS

1. A 57-year-old woman is admitted to the hospital for CHF. Losartan was started, and 2 days later her renal function began declining rapidly over the ensuing few days. PMH: asthma, AV block, CHF, diabetes, and bilateral renal stenosis. Why are ARBs contraindicated in this patient?

   A. Bilateral renal stenosis
   B. CHF
   C. Asthma
   D. AV block
   E. None of the above

2. A 63-year-old man was recently started on valsartan for HTN. What should be monitored upon initiation of ARBs?

   A. Serum creatinine
   B. Blood pressure
   C. Serum potassium
   D. Blood urea nitrogen
   E. All of the above

HPI: AF is a 55-year-old woman who is scheduled to undergo left hip replacement surgery. While in the operating room and postanesthesia care unit (PACU), she has on thromboembolic deterrent (TED) stockings and sequential compression devices (SCDs). On postoperative day 1, the SCDs are discontinued, and she is started on enoxaparin for deep vein thrombosis (DVT) prophylaxis. On postoperative day 7, as AF is getting ready for discharge, she becomes acutely short of breath and develops a painful and swollen left leg.

Labs: Cr 1.2 mg/dL, INR 1.1, activated partial thromboplastin time (aPTT) 35 seconds, Hct 38%, platelets 247,000/mm³. Doppler ultrasound: Partial noncompressibility of the left popliteal vein, nonocclusive clot. Ventilation-perfusion scintigraphy: High probability for acute pulmonary embolism. Unmatched ventilation perfusion defect is seen in the left lower lobe.

THOUGHT QUESTIONS

- What are some of the risk factors for venous thromboembolism?
- How does factor X contribute to clotting?
- What are the contraindications for low molecular-weight heparins (LMWH)?
- What are some of the disadvantages of warfarin-based therapy?

BASIC SCIENCE REVIEW AND DISCUSSION

Patients with a high risk for clotting require thromboprophylaxis. Some risk factors for venous thromboembolism include age greater than 40 years, prolonged immobility, history of prior venous thromboembolism (DVT, pulmonary embolism [PE]), cancer, major surgery (abdominal, pelvic, or lower extremity), fracture (pelvis, hip, or leg), CHF, MI, stroke, obesity, and high-dose estrogen use.

The coagulation pathway can be activated by one of two pathways: the **extrinsic** (tissue factor) pathway or the **intrinsic** (contact activation) pathway (Fig. 3-4). The main coagulation pathway in vivo is the tissue factor pathway. Tissue factor is exposed by damaged endothelium. This exposed tissue factor binds and activates factor VII, which, in turn, activates factor X. Factor Xa results in the generation of a thrombin (factor IIa) burst. Thrombin, in turn, activates factors XI, VIII, and V, leading to the further generation of thrombin and clottable fibrin. Additionally, the tissue factor VIIa complex activates factor IX, which further contributes to the activation of factor X.

Heparins inhibit factors Xa and IIa through their interaction with antithrombin, a naturally occurring anticoagulant. **Unfractionated heparin** (UFH) is a parenteral agent that requires monitoring of the aPTT. Complications with UFH include osteoporosis, heparin-induced thrombocytopenia (HIT), and mineralocorticoid deficiency. There are two types of HIT. HIT type I involves a transient decrease in platelets, which resolves even with continued use of UFH. HIT type II is observed in 1 to 5% of patients and characteristically occurs after 5 to 10 days of heparin exposure. It is characterized by a significant reduction in platelet count, often falling to the 30,000 to 80,000 cells/mm³ range or to a level less than 50% of baseline. The pathogenesis of HIT type II is immune mediated, resulting from antibodies that activate platelets in the presence of heparin.

Low molecular-weight heparins, such as enoxaparin, dalteparin, and tinzaparin, were introduced in 1982. These are parenteral agents that have fixed or weight-adjusted dosing, involve less monitoring, and are easier to administer. The half-lives of LMWHs are longer than that of UFH. Because LMWHs are metabolized renally and because of a 90% cross-reactivity to HIT antibodies, they are contraindicated in patients with poor renal function and in patients with HIT. In rare instances, antifactor Xa levels are measured. This peak level is drawn 4 hours after the third dose (prophylaxis 0.2–0.4 units/mL; treatment 0.5–1.0 units/mL).

Vitamin K antagonists, such as **warfarin,** interfere with gamma-carboxylation of vitamin K-dependent clotting proteins: factors II, VII, IX, and X and proteins C and S. Because warfarin affects the natural anticoagulants and proteins C and S, and takes 4 to 5 days to become fully established, it should be overlapped with heparin. Although factor VII is quickly depleted and an initial prolongation of the prothrombin time is seen in 8 to 12 hours, maximum anticoagulation is not approached for about 4 days as the other factors are depleted and the drug achieves steady state. Its therapeutic index is narrow, so INRs need to be monitored closely. There are also many food and drug interactions with warfarin, and it is contraindicated in pregnant patients. Warfarin is metabolized by cytochrome P450 (CYP450) enzymes in the liver. Medications that are potent inhibitors (amiodarone, fluconazole, metronidazole, TMP-SMX, etc.) or potent inducers (carbamazepine, rifampin, phenobarbital, etc.) of the CYP450 system can dramatically increase or decrease warfarin effect, respectively. Concomitant illnesses, such as liver disease and hyperthyroidism, can affect the patient's response to warfarin therapy as well. This is dependent on the synthesis of the vitamin K-dependent coagulation factors and the rate of decay.

CASE CONCLUSION

AF was started on enoxaparin 60 mg subcutaneously (SC) every 12 hours, followed by warfarin 5 mg PO at bedtime. The patient's goal INR was 2 to 3. She was discharged with warfarin and enoxaparin after being clinically stable, follow-up appointments were obtained, and the patient was taught how to give SC injections to herself. Once the warfarin dosing was therapeutic, the enoxaparin was discontinued and the patient was continued on warfarin, with monthly monitoring, for 6 months.

CASE 3-8 / Anticoagulant Agents

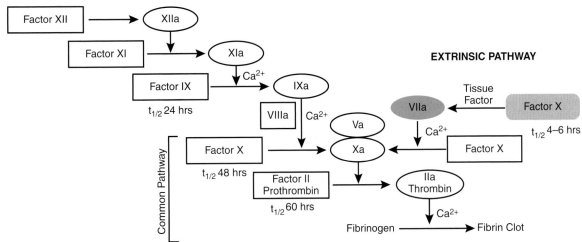

• **Figure 3-4.** Extrinsic and intrinsic pathway.

THUMBNAIL

Drug	Unfractionated Heparin	LMWHS (Dalteparin, Enoxaparin, Tinzaparin)	Warfarin
Clinical indications	Prophylaxis and treatment of venous thrombosis; PE; peripheral arterial embolism; AF	Prevention of DVT and other thromboembolic complications; treatment of acute DVT with or without PE	Prophylaxis and treatment of venous thrombosis and its extension; PE and thromboembolic complications associated with AF
Mechanism of action	Potentiates the action of antithrombin III and thereby inactivates thrombin (as well as factors IXa, Xa, XIa, XIIa, and plasmin); prevents the conversion of fibrinogen to fibrin; molecular weights of heparin vary from 300 to 30,000 daltons	Enhances the inhibition of factor Xa and thrombin by binding to and accelerating antithrombin III activity; molecular weights vary from 2000 to 9000 daltons	Interferes with the hepatic synthesis of vitamin K-dependent clotting (factors VII, IX, X, and II); anticoagulant effects are dependent on the T½ of these clotting factors
Absorption/distribution	Must be given IV or SC (not absorbed PO); IV bolus results in immediate anticoagulant effects; peak plasma levels of heparin are achieved in 2–4 hr following SC use; once absorbed, heparin is distributed in plasma and is extensively and nonspecifically protein bound	Bioavailability of SC injection is about 90%; the onset of anticoagulant effect is approximately 4 hrs	Rapidly and completely absorbed; highly bound to plasma proteins, primarily albumin
Metabolism/elimination	Rapidly cleared from plasma with an average T½ of 30–180 min; the T½ is dose dependent and nonlinear (may be prolonged at higher doses); heparin is partially metabolized by liver heparinase and the reticuloendothelial system	Metabolized by the kidneys	Metabolized by hepatic microsomal enzymes and is excreted primarily in the urine as inactive metabolites
Adverse reactions	Hemorrhage; other side effects include thrombocytopenia, osteoporosis, cutaneous necrosis	Similar to UFH; incidences of HIT may occur but are rare	Hemorrhage; some complications may present as paralysis, headache, chest or joint pain, shortness of breath, and difficulty breathing or swallowing
Drug interactions			Co-trimoxazole Erythromycin Metronidazole Rifampin Amiodarone
Contraindications	Allergy to heparin; uncontrolled bleeding	Allergy to heparin; avoid in patients with CrCl of <30 mL/min; use with caution in patients with low body weights	Pregnancy; hemorrhagic tendencies

QUESTIONS

1. A patient with a mechanical prosthetic mitral valve is seen in the clinic. He has been stable on 5 mg of warfarin taken every evening. His INRs have been ranging from 2.5 to 2.7 for the past 6 months. He was started on amiodarone 2 weeks ago for an arrhythmia. Today his INR is 5.1 and thyroid-stimulating hormone (TSH) level is 2.1 mIU/L. How does amiodarone play a part in this patient's anticoagulation therapy?

   A. Decrease warfarin absorption
   B. Increase metabolism of vitamin K-dependent clotting factors
   C. Additive or synergistic anticoagulant effects
   D. Decrease warfarin metabolism

2. An 80-year-old woman is admitted to the hospital with pneumonia. She has AF and takes warfarin 2.5 mg PO every morning. She reports a slight nosebleed last night. Her appetite has been poor this past week and she has had a fever for the past 2 days. Her INR is 9.1. How would you manage this patient?

   A. Give one dose of vitamin K 2.5 mg PO, hold warfarin, and recheck INR tomorrow
   B. Give vitamin K 10 mg SC for three doses, hold warfarin, and recheck INR tomorrow
   C. Give vitamin K 5 mg IV, hold warfarin, and recheck INR tomorrow
   D. Hold patient's warfarin dosage and recheck INR tomorrow

HPI: LG is a 28-year-old man brought into the ED by ambulance after a motor vehicle accident.

PE: On physical exam, his vital signs were T 38.2°C, BP 140/80, HR 87, and RR 22; lungs are clear. LG has sustained extensive contusions and superficial lacerations to the left lower extremity. The left leg is edematous, and radiography reveals a tibial fracture. The leg is initially placed in a splint while the swelling subsides. LG is complaining of severe, unremitting pain, described as sharp and throbbing. He rates the pain as an 8 on a scale of 10.

THOUGHT QUESTIONS

- How can LG's pain be classified?
- What is the pharmacology of opioids?
- What are the differences between the various opioid agents?
- What are common adverse effects of opioid treatment?

BASIC SCIENCE REVIEW AND DISCUSSION

Pain is defined as an unpleasant sensory and emotional experience associated with actual or potential tissue damage. The nerves that transmit pain are of two types, the A-delta and C. The **A-delta** fibers are myelinated, rapidly conducting fibers that are primarily responsible for well-localized, sharp, stabbing pain, otherwise know as "first pain." **C fibers** are unmyelinated fibers that respond to noxious mechanical, thermal, and chemical stimuli at a much slower rate and mediate "second pain." Acute pain is attributable to direct injury of the tissues due to physical trauma or invasive procedures. It is generally self-limiting, but inadequate relief can impair the healing process. Acute pain is treated aggressively with opioids and nonnarcotic analgesics. Chronic malignant and nonmalignant pain have musculoskeletal and neurologic origins. Chronic nonmalignant pain is associated with a traumatic event or a chronic disease.

Opioids are both natural and synthetic compounds that target endogenous opioid receptors: mu, kappa, and delta. These receptors are further subdivided into mu_1 and mu_2, $kappa_1$, $kappa_2$, and $kappa_3$, and $delta_1$ and $delta_2$. Endogenous opioid peptides—endorphins, enkephalins, and dynorphins—act on these receptors to mediate analgesia. Opioids mimic the activity of endogenous peptides at these receptors and act on excitatory neurotransmitters such as N-methyl-D-aspartate (NMDA) and substance P to modulate pain perception.

Severity of pain, route of administration, and patient history of opioid use should guide the selection of an appropriate opioid. Morphine is the prototypical pure agonist to which other agents are compared. Pure agonists do not exhibit a ceiling to the analgesic effects. Hence, as the dose of a pure agonist is increased, a corresponding log-linear increase in analgesia is seen. The dose may be increased until adequate analgesia is achieved or until dose-limiting adverse effects occur. Codeine, hydrocodone, and propoxyphene are less potent agents. These agents are formulated with adjunctive agents such as acetaminophen or aspirin and are used primarily for mild to moderate pain. Morphine, methadone, hydromorphone, meperidine, and fentanyl are used for moderate to severe pain. With the exception of methadone, all have short durations of action, permitting frequent titration of dose (Table 3-5). The transdermal form of fentanyl has a long onset time and lasts for 72 hours, making titration with the patch difficult. Hence, it is reserved for chronic, stable pain.

Opioid use can be limited by intolerable side effects. CNS effects include **somnolence,** cognitive impairment, and mood alterations. Opioid receptors throughout the GI system mediate the slowing of gut peristalsis, causing **constipation.** Use of stool softeners and stimulant laxatives may provide prophylaxis for constipation. Nausea and vomiting, affecting 10 to 40% of patients, are produced through direct stimulation of the medullary chemoreceptor trigger zone, enhanced vestibular sensitivity, and increased gastric antral tone. **Myoclonus** is a dose-related effect that can occur with high doses of any opioid, but the incidence is higher with meperidine. Normeperidine, the active metabolite of meperidine, has twice the seizure potential of the parent compound. **Respiratory depression,** through direct effects on the chemoreceptors of the respiratory centers in the brainstem, is the most dangerous adverse effect of opioids. The threshold for respiratory depression is above the threshold for sedation, which itself is above that for analgesia. Opioids also cause **pruritus** due to histamine release, hypotension, addiction, and miosis. **Tolerance** can develop to all side effects with the exception of constipation and miosis. Excess sedation or respiratory depression can be reversed with the opioid antagonist **naloxone,** given IV. Orally administered naloxone, which is 3% absorbed, may be given for refractory constipation without reversing systemic analgesic effects.

CASE CONCLUSION

In the ED, the patient was given IV morphine with adequate pain control. After an overnight hospital stay for observation and casting of the left leg, LG was discharged to home with a prescription for hydrocodone/acetaminophen tablets, to be taken as needed for pain.

TABLE 3-5 Comparison of Opioid Analgesics

	Metabolites	Duration of Action	Adverse Effects	Comments
Morphine	Morphine-6-glucuronide is more potent than morphine sulfate; renally cleared	3–4 hrs	Sedation, nausea, decreased BP, constipation, pruritus	Gold standard starting agent
Codeine	10% is converted to morphine sulfate	3–4 hrs	Frequent nausea	Similar to morphine, less potent
Hydrocodone	Metabolized to hydromorphone	3–4 hrs	Less nausea/constipation than codeine	Similar to morphine
Oxycodone	Metabolized to oxymorphone	3–4 hrs	Less nausea/constipation than codeine	Rapid CNS dysphoria or euphoria
Hydromorphone	No active metabolites	3–4 hrs	Less emesis and fewer CNS effects than morphine	3–6 times more potent than morphine
Fentanyl	No active metabolites	1–2 hrs (IV); 3 days	Fewer effects on BP, no histamine release (transdermal patch)	Patch has slow onset; prolonged drug absorption after patch removal
Meperidine	Normeperidine has half the analgesic activity but twice the seizure potential; renally cleared	3–4 hrs; normeperidine T1/2 15–30 hrs	Most potent CNS irritant	Active metabolite may accumulate
Methadone	No active metabolite	6–8 hrs; increases with chronic dosing secondary to accumulation	Less sedation than morphine	No cross-reactivity with morphine or meperidine
Propoxyphene	Norpropoxyphene has greater CNS depressant effects	3–4 hrs		Less potent than other opioids; no antitussive activity

THUMBNAIL: Opioids

Prototypical agent: Morphine, a naturally occurring opioid, is derived from the poppy plant. Other natural, semisynthetic, and synthetic opioids include codeine, hydrocodone, oxycodone, methadone, fentanyl, and hydromorphone, among others.

Clinical usage: Primarily used as an analgesic for relief of moderate to severe acute and chronic pain. Morphine is used in MI for analgesia, venodilation, and reduction in preload and oxygen requirements. Fentanyl and sufentanil are used as general anesthesia due to their short duration and minimal effects on the cardiovascular system. Codeine is used as an antitussive and in cough associated with pulmonary edema. Diarrhea may be alleviated with diphenoxylate. Methadone is used in maintenance programs for addiction.

MOA: Binds primarily to endogenous mu, kappa, and delta receptors in the central and peripheral nervous system, altering pain perception.

Pharmacokinetics

Absorption: Oral bioavailability is variable depending on drug and formulation (morphine < hydrocodone and oxycodone < methadone). The exception is fentanyl, which is very poorly absorbed and hence is only available in IV, transdermal, and transmucosal formulations.

Distribution: Opioids are widely distributed in tissue and particularly in highly perfused organs, such as the liver, lungs, kidney, and spleen. Opioids also distribute into and accumulate in fatty tissue.

Elimination: Opioids are hepatically metabolized via the CYP2D6 enzyme into metabolites that are renally eliminated. The exception is methadone, which is metabolized via the CYP3A4 enzyme.

(Continued)

THUMBNAIL: Opioids *(Continued)*

Adverse reactions: Sedation, respiratory depression, constipation, myoclonus, nausea, vomiting, flushing, itching, miosis, hypotension, and hallucinations. Tolerance develops to all side effects with the exception of constipation and miosis. **Physical dependence** may develop within 5 days of opioid use.

Drug interactions: Drugs utilizing the CYP2D6 (i.e., fluoxetine, cimetidine) or the CYP3A4 (i.e., macrolides, antiretrovirals) pathways may inhibit opioid metabolism and potentiate side effects. Drugs such as benzodiazepines and barbiturates should be used cautiously in combination with opioids, as they may potentiate respiratory depression or sedative effects.

QUESTIONS

1. A 76-year-old man is admitted to the hospital with severe abdominal pain and a progressive inability to swallow solid foods. He can tolerate a soft diet of pureed foods and liquid. Further workup reveals a large, inoperable, esophageal tumor obstructing the fundus. A gastric tube (GT) is placed for medication administration and feeding. The patient continues to have severe pain, requiring opioid analgesics. Which of the following would not be a good choice for treatment of this patient's pain?

    A. Hydrocodone/acetaminophen extra-strength tablets per GT (PGT)
    B. Sustained-release oxycodone PGT
    C. Morphine sulfate elixir PGT
    D. IV hydromorphone
    E. Acetaminophen with codeine tablets PGT

2. A 62-year-old man with a history of diabetes and severe osteoarthritis of the knees undergoes a right knee replacement. He has been placed on a hydromorphone PCA (patient-controlled analgesia) and must be transitioned to an oral regimen in preparation for discharge. Labs are normal with the exception of increased BUN 32 mg/dL and serum Cr 2.4 mg/dL. Which of the following would be an appropriate pain medication on which to start this patient?

    A. Morphine tablets
    B. Morphine elixir
    C. Fentanyl patch
    D. Meperidine tablets
    E. Oxycodone/acetaminophen tablets

CASE 3-10 Anticonvulsants

HPI: JJ is a 50-year-old woman with metastatic lung cancer, s/p frontal-temporal craniotomy for resection of a metastatic brain lesion 2 days ago. JJ is complaining of a pruritic, erythematous rash on her back and arms that she denies having prior to admission.

PMH: Metastatic lung cancer s/p chemotherapy and radiation therapy 6 months prior. Presented 3 weeks prior to admission with a new-onset generalized tonic-clonic **seizure.**

PE: Vitals: T 37.8°C; BP 124/74; HR 80; RR 18 breaths/min

Medications: Phenytoin (started 3 weeks ago), dexamethasone, famotidine. Patient has NKDA.

Labs: Slightly elevated transaminases (AST 78 Iu/L; ALT 201 Iu/L; AlkPhos 176 Iu/L; total bilirubin [Tbili] 0.9 mg/dL)

THOUGHT QUESTIONS

- Which **antiepileptics** are indicated for which types of seizures?
- What are the most common signs of **anticonvulsant hypersensitivity?**
- What other antiepileptics can be used in a patient who is thought to have a hypersensitivity reaction to phenytoin?

BASIC SCIENCE REVIEW AND DISCUSSION

Choosing an antiepileptic agent for treatment of seizures depends on the diagnosis and classification of the seizure type. One of the first antiepileptics discovered was phenobarbital, which is used for **generalized tonic-clonic seizures** and **status epilepticus.** Phenytoin (also known as diphenylhydantoin, or DPH) is used in the treatment of partial, focal, and generalized seizures and status epilepticus. Carbamazepine and valproic acid were found to be effective in partial and generalized tonic-clonic seizures. A dozen other agents are now also being used as adjunctive treatment for generalized seizures and as adjunctive therapy and monotherapy for **absence** and **partial seizures.** Treatment should generally start with one agent to minimize adverse effects and enhance compliance.

Many of the anticonvulsants can cause **rash,** which can range in severity from benign (resolving with dose reduction or discontinuation of therapy) to severe hypersensitivity reactions necessitating a change in therapy. Phenytoin is known to cause **hypersensitivity** reactions, most often presenting as a rash that generally occurs 2 weeks to 2 months after initiation of therapy. The rash is often described as morbilliform, although it can present in a variety of forms (scarlatiniform, maculopapular, urticarial). The rash is often pruritic and distributed on the trunk, arms, and chest. Facial edema also has been observed. Reactions are often accompanied by fever, lymphadenopathy, elevated transaminases, leukocytosis, and eosinophilia. These rashes can progress to more severe, potentially fatal reactions, such as erythema multiforme, exfoliative dermatitis, or toxic epidermal necrolysis. Thus, if phenytoin is suspected as the etiology of the reaction, it should be discontinued immediately and an alternative anticonvulsant started if necessary. Corticosteroid therapy may mask some of the signs and symptoms of a hypersensitivity reaction, and patients on concomitant corticosteroids should be evaluated carefully for any symptoms resembling a hypersensitivity reaction.

True hypersensitivity reactions to phenytoin are related to the "aromatic" anticonvulsants. Thus, in patients in whom a reaction is suspected, other arene anticonvulsants such as carbamazepine, oxcarbazepine, phenobarbital, or primidone should be avoided, as there is a high rate of cross-reactivity (estimated as high as 80%). Valproic acid is an agent that can be safely used as an alternative anticonvulsant in such patients.

CASE CONCLUSION

Phenytoin was discontinued and JJ was started on valproic acid. She received an initial IV dose, followed by oral maintenance therapy of divalproex sodium. She was monitored closely for resolution of her reaction, which took several weeks.

THUMBNAIL: Anticonvulsants

Drug	Phenytoin (DPH)	Carbamazepine (CBZ)	Valproic Acid (VPA) and Divalproex Sodium	Phenobarbital (PB)
Clinical indications	Status epilepticus, generalized tonic-clonic, complex partial, focal motor seizures Not effective for absence seizures	Partial, generalized tonic-clonic seizures Pain associated with trigeminal neuralgia	Complex partial, absent, generalized tonic-clonic, myoclonic seizures Migraine headache prophylaxis, mania associated with bipolar disorder	Status epilepticus, partial, generalized tonic-clonic seizures Sedative hypnotic
MOA	Appears to block posttetanic potentiation of synaptic transmission; with effects on sodium channels	Thought to be similar to phenytoin, and reduces polysynaptic responses	Not established; may be related to increased brain concentrations of gamma-aminobutyric acid (GABA)	Sodium effects similar to phenytoin, with effects on calcium and GABA
Absorption/distribution	Absorption: very good; use only extended-release capsule for once-daily dosing IM not recommended Enteral feedings bind phenytoin	Absorption: good; no parenteral form available Distribution: CSF, 15–22% of serum concentration	Absorption: excellent; conversion between the oral and parenteral dosage forms are equivalent Distribution: plasma and extracellular water; CSF, 10% of serum concentrations	Absorption: excellent Distribution: all tissues, high concentrations in the brain
Metabolism/elimination	Primarily hepatic metabolism; saturable metabolism (small dosage increases can result in large serum level fluctuations)	Hepatic metabolism (CYP450); initially induces own metabolism; monitor closely, dosage adjustment when initiating therapy	Primarily hepatic metabolism; saturable protein binding; serum concentrations not proportional to dosage changes	Primarily hepatic metabolism; 25–50% of dose eliminated unchanged
Adverse reactions	Infusion related (hypotension, cardiovascular collapse, CNS depression) Dose related (nystagmus, ataxia, slurred speech) Diplopia, nausea/vomiting (N/V), gingival hyperplasia, hepatotoxicity Hypersensitivity reactions, hematologic abnormalities	Idiosyncratic aplastic anemia and agranulocytosis (can be fatal) Leukopenia (usually mild; monitor closely) Dose related: GI upset, ataxia, diplopia, dizziness, drowsiness Hypersensitivity reactions	Hepatic failure (monitor liver function tests [LFTs] prior to initiation and frequently thereafter), pancreatitis Dose related: N/V, abdominal pain Tremor, somnolence, dizziness, asthenia, weight gain, alopecia, thrombocytopenia, and hyperammonemia	Infusion related: hypotension (administer slowly), somnolence, CNS depression, ataxia Hypersensitivity reactions Paradoxic excitation
Contraindications	Allergy to phenytoin or other hydantoins	History of bone marrow suppression, hypersensitivity to carbamazepine (CBZ) or tricyclic antidepressants (chemically related)	Hepatic disease; hypersensitivity to drug; known urea cycle disorders	Hypersensitivity to barbiturates, hepatic dysfunction, porphyria, severe respiratory disease
Drug interactions	Decreased levels with CBZ, rifampin, chronic alcohol ingestion Increased levels with amiodarone, sulfonamides, isoniazid, fluconazole Unpredictable effects with valproic acid (VPA) and phenobarbital (PB) Decreased effectiveness of warfarin, CBZ, doxycycline, estrogens	Decreased levels with CYP450 enzyme inducers: DPH, PB Increased levels with erythromycin, itraconazole, propoxyphene, VPA Decreased effectiveness of DPH, VPA, warfarin, oral contraceptives	Decreased levels with enzyme inducers: DPH, CBZ, PB CYP450 enzyme inhibitors (i.e., antidepressants) expected to have little effect Increased levels of ethosuximide, lamotrigine, PB	Decreased levels with enzyme inducers (rifampin) Increased levels with VPA Increased sedation with other CNS depressants Decreased effectiveness of warfarin, CBZ, metronidazole, oral contraceptives

QUESTIONS

1. A 65-year-old 60-kg woman presents to the ambulatory care clinic 2 weeks after a frontotemporal craniotomy (for resection of a glioblastoma) for removal of her staples. She was started on phenytoin extended-release capsules 300 mg orally at bedtime, after receiving 1 g of phenytoin IV during her surgery. She has no history of seizures. Today, her LFTs were normal (AST 29 Iu/L, ALT 30 Iu/L, AlkPhos 40 Iu/L, Tbili 1.0 mg/dL). Labs drawn yesterday afternoon: phenytoin = 5 μg/mL, albumin = 2.8 g/dL. She denies missing any doses of medication. A decision is made to increase her maintenance dosage of phenytoin. What most likely influenced this decision to change her phenytoin regimen?

A. Her compliance
B. Accounting for the albumin level when evaluating the phenytoin level
C. Her phenytoin level was drawn at the wrong time
D. Her LFTs
E. Phenytoin levels in patients without a history of seizures have a lower targeted range (< 10 mcg/ml)

2. KM is a 20-year-old woman with a history of epilepsy and scoliosis. Her seizures have been controlled on a maintenance dosage of divalproex sodium. She is scheduled to undergo a spinal fusion and will not be taking anything by mouth (NPO) for several days. Which factor should be taken into consideration for her postsurgical care?

A. Avoid propoxyphene napsylate for pain relief as it can interact with her valproic acid therapy.
B. Change her antiepileptic regimen to phenytoin immediately postoperatively, as phenytoin can be given IV.
C. Convert her oral divalproex regimen to an equivalent IV regimen of valproic acid while she is NPO.
D. Monitor peak levels of valproic acid postoperatively to evaluate whether additional doses are needed.
E. Avoid doxycycline as it has decreased effectiveness when given with valproic acid.

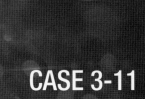

CASE 3-11   Agents Used for Anxiety Disorders

HPI: CV is a 52-year-old woman brought into the ED by her husband complaining of chest pain, dizziness, SOB, and sweating. This is her third visit to the ED for chest pain in the past 2 years. On two previous visits it was concluded that she did not suffer an MI.

SHx: Works full-time as an office manager in the business district, but has been on medical leave for the past 4 weeks for "mental exhaustion" and is due to return to work in 2 days. Married for 25 years with two adult children living on the opposite side of the country. Drinks one to two cups of coffee daily and one large gin and tonic nightly; does not exercise.

PMH: Postmenopausal for 5 years. Migraine headaches (averages one per month; has had three in the past month); HTN.

General: Anxious-appearing female in obvious distress; sweating profusely; alert and coherent. Expresses fear of returning to work and shares that she has been reluctant to leave the house for the past year. Denies sadness or anhedonia. Admits to mid-nocturnal insomnia, increased weight (17 pounds in 2 months), low energy. Denies paranoia or hallucinations.

ECG: Sinus tachycardia; normal rhythm.

Medications: Hydrochlorothiazide/triamterene; diphenhydramine for sleep.

PE: T 37.3°C; HR 108; RR 22; BP 145/92

Labs: Within normal limits (WNL)

THOUGHT QUESTIONS

- What pharmacologic agents are used in maintenance treatment of anxiety disorders?
- What medications can be used for acute relief of anxiety or panic attacks?
- What pharmacologic options are available for patients with a history of substance abuse?

BASIC SCIENCE REVIEW AND DISCUSSION

The pharmacologic management of **generalized anxiety disorder (GAD)** and **panic disorder** often features the use of **benzodiazepines** and/or **selective serotonin reuptake inhibitor (SSRI)** antidepressants. While tricyclic antidepressants (TCAs) and monoamine (MAO) inhibitors were once popular for the long-term management of anxiety, their clinical utility has been overshadowed by the greater tolerability and acceptance of SSRIs. At the present time, SSRIs have received FDA approval for the treatment of GAD, panic disorder, obsessive-compulsive disorder (OCD), posttraumatic stress disorder (PTSD), and social phobia. Although not all agents are FDA approved for these disorders, all SSRIs are believed to be therapeutically effective for each of these indications. In general, clinicians have found that the SSRI should be started at relatively low doses to improve tolerability, but that

the eventual effective dose may actually be slightly higher than average doses prescribed for major depression.

For the acute relief of anxiety or panic attacks, benzodiazepines are often useful, usually on an as-needed basis. Many clinicians are reluctant to prescribe these medications for an extended period of time (due to risks associated with **physiologic dependence,** withdrawal, or abuse), but for the relief of acute symptoms, benzodiazepines are a valuable therapeutic modality. Although a wide variety of benzodiazepines are currently available, they are all qualitatively similar in terms of their pharmacologic effects and side effect potential. Clonazepam and alprazolam are the two benzodiazepines used most commonly to treat anxiety disorders.

An additional psychotropic medication that may be worth considering specifically for GAD is buspirone. One major benefit of buspirone can be found in the virtual absence of dependence and abuse liability. Although it is not effective for the acute relief of anxiety or panic disorders (anxiolytic effects may take up to a week to be established), buspirone may be indicated for patients with a history of alcohol abuse or among those who fear physiologic and psychological dependence with benzodiazepines.

In summary, the pharmacologic management of GAD and panic disorder usually features maintenance with an SSRI and acute symptom relief with benzodiazepines (if necessary). The duration of maintenance treatment is highly variable with pharmacologic management, but it should be remembered that in most patients GAD and panic disorders will be chronic and recurrent conditions.

CASE CONCLUSION

After beginning another rule-out MI protocol, CV was given an IM injection of lorazepam to acutely control her anxiety and related somatic complaints. She was seen by her primary care provider the next day and ultimately diagnosed with panic disorder and agoraphobia. She was started on daily paroxetine therapy and instructed that she could use clonazepam as needed for extreme anxiety. In addition, she was counseled to diminish the use of alcohol to self-medicate. A referral for psychological counseling was given as well.

THUMBNAIL: Agents Used for Anxiety Disorders

	Benzodiazepines	SSRIs	Buspirone
Prototypic agent	Diazepam (D)	Fluoxetine (F)	Buspirone
Other agents	Clonazepam (C) Alprazolam (A) Lorazepam (L)	Paroxetine (P) Sertraline (S) Citalopram (C)	
MOA	Bind to components of $GABA_A$ receptors → facilitate inhibitory actions of GABA in CNS	Inhibit reuptake of serotonin	Partial agonist at $5HT_{1A}$ brain receptors; anxiolytic action unknown
Indications	Anxiety disorders (especially A and C for panic and phobic disorders); sedation; seizure disorders; muscle relaxants (D); management of alcohol withdrawal	Depression, anxiety disorders (OCD, panic attacks, social phobias, etc.)	Anxiety disorders (GAD)
Pharmacokinetics	Potency: C > A > L > D T½: L = A < C < D Hepatic metabolism	PO only; hepatic metabolism	PO only; hepatic metabolism
Adverse reactions	Cognitive impairment, sedation, amnesia, diminished motor skills	Sedation or insomnia; headache, nausea, appetite and weight changes, sexual dysfunction	Dizziness, headache, nausea
Warnings/precautions	Additive sedative effects with other CNS depressants (ethanol); tolerance and dependence may develop with prolonged use	**Serotonin syndrome** may occur with other serotonergic drugs (i.e., MAO inhibitors); SSRIs may inhibit CYP450 liver enzymes	

QUESTIONS

1. RM is a 25-year-old professional football player who was recently diagnosed with social phobic disorder. Although he has never missed a football game for this condition, he has experienced extreme anxiety in other public situations, failing to appear for numerous press conferences and community events. He is not interested in psychotherapy ("I don't have the time") and doesn't want to take any medication that may cause weight gain or addiction. What would be the best treatment option?

   A. Sertraline
   B. Paroxetine
   C. Buspirone
   D. Clonazepam
   E. Propranolol

2. JF is a 41-year-old man suffering from PTSD for the past 3 years, after his near death in an automobile accident. During this time, he has suffered from nightmares, jitteriness, irritability, and avoidance behavior, which has only been partially relieved for the last 3 months with a combination of trazodone and clonazepam. Tired of "feeling like a zombie" with the clonazepam, JF decides to abruptly discontinue this agent. What is the most likely consequence of this treatment action?

   A. Extreme sluggishness and ataxia within 24 hours
   B. Restlessness, blurred vision within 2 to 3 days
   C. Muscle tension and irritability within 5 to 6 days
   D. Grand mal seizures within 2 to 3 days
   E. Dizziness and paresthesias within 2 to 3 days

HPI: PM is a 39-year-old woman who arrives today at her gynecologist's office for her annual exam. When asked how she has been feeling, PM mentions that she's been "kind of down in the dumps" for the past month. She says that she feels very sad, particularly when she wakes up in the morning, and has missed 3 days of work during this time frame. ("I just don't have the energy to get up out of bed some days and I don't know why.") She also says that even when she does go to work, her concentration is poor and she has a hard time making decisions. PM also complains of occasional stress headaches and has noticed that she has returned to her old habit of binging on snack foods (she has gained approximately 7 pounds in the past month). She denies suicidality but does feel like giving up sometimes. Her PMH is significant for an acute episode of depression following the breakup of a long-term relationship 1 year ago. PM was previously successfully treated with sertraline but discontinued the medication 3 months ago because "it was interfering with my sex life."

THOUGHT QUESTIONS

- What are the treatment options for depression?
- What are the main adverse effects of the various antidepressants?

BASIC SCIENCE REVIEW AND DISCUSSION

From a pathophysiologic perspective, a decrease in certain neurotransmitters (serotonin, norepinephrine, and possibly dopamine) has been causally associated with depression through the indirect evidence that all approved antidepressants will increase the activity of one or more of these chemical messengers.

All of the current antidepressant agents are equally effective in the general depressed population, generating a therapeutic response in 60 to 70% of patients given a therapeutic trial. Generally, symptoms begin to improve within the first 2 weeks of treatment, and 4 weeks (or more) are required to observe optimal treatment outcomes.

SSRIs are the most popular treatment option due to safety in overdose situations, low side effect burden, and ease of administration (i.e., once-daily dosing with minimal titration required). SSRIs are also effective treatment for the management of anxiety disorders, a common psychiatric comorbidity among the depressed.

In general, SSRIs are regarded as "activating antidepressants" less likely to induce sedation or sluggishness than tricyclic antidepressants or trazodone. Many patients experience mild nausea or light sleep when they first start taking an SSRI, but these side effects usually abate after a few days of continued treatment. Sexual dysfunction, most commonly presenting as a difficulty achieving orgasm, is more problematic and frequently leads to discontinuation, particularly if the patient is uncomfortable discussing this condition with his or her physician. Sweating is another common and dose-dependent phenomenon, and bruxism may present on occasion as well.

The potential of SSRIs to inhibit liver enzymes and cause drug interactions is relatively well known, but there are important differences among the SSRIs in this regard. Paroxetine and fluoxetine have a particularly strong affinity for the CYP450 2D6 isoenzyme, elevating plasma concentrations of drugs such as narcotics and beta-blockers that are metabolized via this route. Fluvoxamine and norfluoxetine (the principal metabolite of fluoxetine) have a high affinity for the CYP450 3A4 isoenzyme, responsible for the metabolism of calcium channel blockers, antifungals, certain benzodiazepines (alprazolam and triazolam), and estrogen. Although it is true that sertraline and citalopram have a lower likelihood than other SSRIs of causing drug interactions, these reactions are somewhat unpredictable, and caution should be exercised whenever other medications are prescribed with an SSRI.

Because 25% of patients will stop SSRIs due to side effects and an additional 30 to 40% will fail to achieve a therapeutic response, other antidepressant alternatives are of great importance. Venlafaxine is a dual-action antidepressant that enhances serotonin activity at low doses and norepinephrine at higher doses. Preliminary evidence suggests that these multiple actions on neurotransmitters may confer therapeutic superiority over SSRIs for the management of severe or melancholic depression, but the risk of HTN with high-dose venlafaxine should not be overlooked.

Bupropion is another second-line agent, particularly for patients who are wary of the SSRIs' negative impact on sexual dysfunction. Because it appears to relieve depression through a completely different mechanism than SSRIs, enhancing norepinephrine or dopamine, it is often administered to patients who fail SSRIs or exhibit a partial response. The most common side effects encountered with bupropion are insomnia, jitteriness, and nausea. Bupropion is contraindicated in patients with a history of seizures or eating disorders.

Mirtazapine is another antidepressant with a unique mechanism of action, enhancing serotonin and norepinephrine in a manner quite complex and distinct from venlafaxine or tricyclics. Like venlafaxine, it may be effective for severe or treatment-resistant depression, though its widespread use has been hampered by a high incidence of sedation and weight gain. Similarly, the popularity of trazodone and nefazodone has been limited by the potent sedating properties of these agents. In addition, nefazodone has been implicated rarely with the development of liver failure and it is also a potent inhibitor of the CYP450 3A4 isoenzyme.

CASE CONCLUSION

Given her favorable response to an SSRI in the past, sertraline would appear to be a logical choice for treatment of her latest episode, but her complaint of sexual dysfunction should be taken seriously, as this commonly leads to medication noncompliance. As all SSRIs and venlafaxine are capable of inducing this side effect, bupropion is initiated and slowly titrated to effect. The activating properties of bupropion proved to be a notable benefit for this patient as her symptoms resolved within the first 3 weeks of receiving a therapeutic dose.

THUMBNAIL: Adverse Effects of Antidepressant Medications

Medication	Sedation	Agitation/ Insomnia	Anticholinergic Effects	Orthostasis	GI Effects (nausea/diarrhea)	Sexual Dysfunction	Weight Gain
SSRI							
Fluoxetine	+	++++	0/+	0/+	++++	++++	+
Sertraline	+	+++	0/+	0	+++	+++	+
Paroxetine	++	++	+	0	+++	++++	++
Citalopram	++	++	0/+	0	+++	++	+
Tricyclics							
Desipramine	++	+	++	+++	0/+	+	++
Nortriptyline	++	+	++	++	0/+	+	++
Amitriptyline	++++	0/+	++++	++++	0/+	++	+++
Imipramine	+++	0/+	+++	++++	0/+	++	++
Doxepin	++++	0/+	++++	++++	0/+	++	++
Others							
Bupropion	0	+++	+	0	+	0/+	0
Venlafaxine	++	++	+	0	+++	+++	+
Nefazodone	+++	+	+	++	++	0/+	0/+
Mirtazapine	++++	0	++	0/+	+	0/+	+++

0, negligible; +, very low; ++, low; +++, moderate; ++++, high.

QUESTIONS

1. RH is a 48-year-old man who enjoyed an excellent response to paroxetine. Two months after starting the antidepressant, he mentions that he is no longer able to ejaculate and, though he has no interest in stopping the SSRI, wonders what can be done to preserve his marital relations. Which would be the best option at the present time?

   A. Change his paroxetine to sertraline
   B. Reduce his paroxetine dose
   C. Add bupropion
   D. Add sildenafil
   E. Encourage marital counseling

2. EV is a 21-year-old college student suffering from an acute episode of major depressive disorder with severe symptomatology. Although her symptoms went into remission after 8 weeks of venlafaxine, she now complains of sudden dizziness, anxiety, and shooting pains in her legs. What is the most likely explanation for these complaints?

   A. Eosinophilia myalgia syndrome
   B. Serotonin syndrome
   C. SSRI withdrawal syndrome
   D. Stroke (cerebrovascular accident)
   E. Neuroleptic malignant syndrome

CASE 3-13 Agents for Schizophrenia

HPI: SH is a 32-year-old, moderately obese man brought into the ED by the police after attempting to cut himself with a piece of glass from his bathroom mirror. He said he had to cut himself in order to "let the evil out!" In the exam room, SH looked suspiciously at the interviewer and was muttering to himself. His PMH is significant for chronic schizophrenia, HTN, hyperlipidemia, and major depressive disorder. Medications include thioridazine, benztropine, paroxetine, atorvastatin, and metoprolol, although SH states he discontinued all his medications 3 weeks ago for fear he was being poisoned.

PE: On physical exam, he has noticeable cuts on his hands. During the interview, he demonstrated noticeable facial grimacing and lip smacking, a stooped posture, and sluggish gait.

THOUGHT QUESTIONS

- What are the mechanisms of action of neuroleptics and atypical antipsychotics and how do they affect the positive and negative symptoms of schizophrenia?
- How are neuroleptics and atypical antipsychotics classified and how do they differ in potency, dosing range, and adverse effects?
- What are **extrapyramidal symptoms** (EPS) and what are the predisposing risk factors? What is the recommended treatment of choice?
- What is **neuroleptic malignancy syndrome** (NMS) and what are the predisposing risk factors? What is the recommended treatment of choice?

BASIC SCIENCE REVIEW AND DISCUSSION

Traditional **antipsychotics** or **neuroleptics** block the D_2 dopamine receptor and alleviate the positive symptoms of schizophrenia (e.g., hallucinations, delusions, thought dysfunction). These positive symptoms are due to excess dopamine in the mesolimbic pathway while the negative symptoms are due to deficiency of dopamine in the mesocortical pathway and frontal cortex (regulated by serotonin). Negative symptoms can include affective blunting, avolition, anhedonia, and memory impairment. Traditional neuroleptics have little effect on controlling negative symptoms or cognitive dysfunction associated with schizophrenia. Neuroleptics also block dopamine receptors in the nigrostriatal and tuberoinfundibular pathway in the brain and result in adverse effects such as movement disorders and hyperprolactinemia, respectively.

Atypical antipsychotic agents or "newer" agents alleviate both positive and negative symptoms. The atypical antipsychotics also improve cognitive deficits associated with schizophrenia. Although these agents are much safer, they have added cost and have been associated with their own class of adverse effects.

Traditional neuroleptics are classified in terms of potency or how strongly they bind to D_2 receptors. Low-potency agents have less affinity for D_2 receptors and therefore require high dosages to have equal effect as high-potency agents. They are, as a class, poorly tolerated because of unfavorable side effect profiles. They are associated with EPS and **tardive dyskinesia** (TD) as well as muscarinic (M_1), histaminergic (H_1), and adrenergic (α_1- and α_2) side effects.

Extrapyramidal symptoms are common adverse effects of traditional neuroleptics, although they may still occur with atypical agents. Pseudoparkinsonism, akathisia, and acute dystonic reactions are the three early-onset types of EPS, whereas TD, tardive dystonia, and tardive akathisia are late-onset EPS types that occur 6 months to 1 year after initiating treatment. High-potency antipsychotics at high dosages have the greatest risk for inducing EPS. Atypical agents have a low risk for inducing EPS, and clozapine has been shown in limited cases to improve TD. The management of early-onset EPS symptoms includes drug discontinuation, dosage reduction of the antipsychotic agent, or switching to an agent with less risk for inducing EPS. Anticholinergic agents (diphenhydramine, benztropine) can be used to treat acute dystonic reactions, parkinsonism, and akathisia. Other agents such as amantadine, benzodiazepines, and propranolol also have been used.

Neuroleptic malignant syndrome is a rare but potentially fatal reaction associated with antipsychotic therapy. NMS can occur within hours or months after initiation of the drug and has a high mortality rate. The four cardinal features of NMS include (*a*) hyperthermia, (*b*) muscular rigidity (lead pipe rigidity), (*c*) autonomic instability, and (*d*) altered consciousness. Leukocytosis with or without a left shift, elevated creatinine phosphokinase, and metabolic acidosis may be present. Drug discontinuation, hydration, oxygenation, and fever reduction are key measures to reduce morbidity and mortality. Many pharmacologic agents (amantadine, bromocriptine, dantrolene) have been used for treatment of NMS with conflicting results.

CASE CONCLUSION

SH's symptoms are consistent with the diagnosis of uncontrolled chronic schizophrenia (paranoid type). Because SH is experiencing positive and negative symptoms and has evidence of EPS, he should be switched to an atypical antipsychotic agent. Clozapine is traditionally reserved for treatment-resistant patients and is not a first-line agent because of the risk of agranulocytosis. Olanzapine and quetiapine can be problematic due to weight gain and potential insulin resistance (if the patient has a family history of diabetes mellitus type 2). Risperidone is also associated with a higher incidence of EPS symptoms compared with other atypical agents. In addition, SH is also taking paroxetine that can significantly elevate levels of risperidone. Therefore, ziprasidone would be the best choice for this patient.

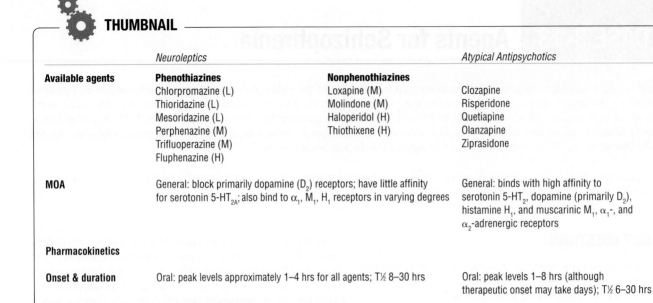

THUMBNAIL

	Neuroleptics		Atypical Antipsychotics
Available agents	**Phenothiazines** Chlorpromazine (L) Thioridazine (L) Mesoridazine (L) Perphenazine (M) Trifluoperazine (M) Fluphenazine (H)	**Nonphenothiazines** Loxapine (M) Molindone (M) Haloperidol (H) Thiothixene (H)	Clozapine Risperidone Quetiapine Olanzapine Ziprasidone
MOA	General: block primarily dopamine (D_2) receptors; have little affinity for serotonin 5-HT_{2A}; also bind to α_1, M_1, H_1 receptors in varying degrees		General: binds with high affinity to serotonin 5-HT_2, dopamine (primarily D_2), histamine H_1, and muscarinic M_1, α_1-, and α_2-adrenergic receptors
Pharmacokinetics			
Onset & duration	Oral: peak levels approximately 1–4 hrs for all agents; T½ 8–30 hrs		Oral: peak levels 1–8 hrs (although therapeutic onset may take days); T½ 6–30 hrs
Elimination	Extensively metabolized by liver with minimal amount of drug excreted in urine unchanged		Metabolized by CYP450 via different isoenzymes; use caution in hepatic impairment and the elderly
Adverse effects	Low potency agents: sedation, anticholinergic effects, orthostasis, ECG changes (QT_c prolongation, T wave flattening, QRS widening) High potency: EPS, hyperprolactinemia Overall, any of the side effects can occur in both low- and high-potency agents Thioridazine: retinal pigmentation at high doses, sexual dysfunction		EPS, TD, and NMS rare; all agents have potential to cause orthostasis, sedation, and weight gain Clozapine: agranulocytosis, seizures, anticholinergic effects, constipation, sialorrhea Risperidone: highest risk for inducing EPS among atypical agents; hyperprolactinemia Olanzapine: glucose intolerance Quetiapine: dizziness, cataracts, mild transient transaminase elevations Ziprasidone: QT_c prolongation, nausea
Drug interactions	Use caution when coadministered with drugs metabolized via the CYP450 system Avoid concomitant use with drugs that have similar side effect profiles Mesoridazine: contraindicated with drugs known to prolong QT_c interval		Use caution when coadministered with drugs metabolized via the CYP450 system Avoid concomitant use with drugs that have similar side effect profiles

H, high potency; *M*, medium potency; *L*, low potency.

QUESTIONS

1. A 20-year-old woman admitted to the inpatient psychiatric unit has been receiving an atypical antipsychotic for her chronic schizophrenia. She is unable to recollect the name of the medication but she does complain of galactorrhea. Which one of the following medications is most likely to cause galactorrhea?

   A. Olanzapine
   B. Quetiapine
   C. Risperidone
   D. Ziprasidone
   E. Clozapine

2. One of your patients comes to your clinic with complaints of insomnia. She has been stable on haloperidol for schizophrenia for the past 5 years and asks you to recommend something for sleep. Which one of the following hypnotic medications would interact with the efficacy of haloperidol in controlling her psychotic symptoms?

   A. Zaleplon
   B. Diphenhydramine
   C. Diazepam
   D. Zolpidem
   E. Trazodone

CASE 3-14 Agents for Hyperthyroidism

HPI: HP is a 32-year-old white woman who reports profuse sweating, irritability, and a rapid heart beat. HP has been unable to exercise over the past few weeks, complaining of tachycardia and decreased exercise tolerance. She also reports diaphoresis, which contributes to frequent nocturnal awakenings.

PE: BP 130/84; HR 120; weight 125 lbs (143 lbs at last visit)

THOUGHT QUESTIONS

- What treatment options are available for Graves hyperthyroidism?
- What are the pharmacologic differences between each treatment approach?
- What side effects are associated with the use of **thioamides**?

BASIC SCIENCE REVIEW AND DISCUSSION

Hyperthyroidism results in a **hypermetabolic state** due to an excess of thyroid hormones. Hyperthyroidism is more common in women (2%) than in men (0.1%). Graves disease is an autoimmune disorder that leads to hyperthyroidism, diffuse goiter, ophthalmopathy, dermopathy, and acropachy. Graves disease is the most common cause of hyperthyroidism, more common than multinodular or uninodular goiters.

Hyperthyroidism treatment involves partial or complete thyroidectomy, radioactive iodine (RAI) treatment, or thioamide therapy. There is no one best approach because treatment is often individualized.

The thioamides are often used as primary therapy for hyperthyroidism. They are also used as adjunctive therapy to achieve euthyroidism in patients prior to surgery or RAI therapy. The thioamides primarily inhibit thyroid hormone synthesis but do not affect existing thyroid hormone stores (which last approximately 30 days). Therefore, hyperthyroid symptoms may continue for 4 to 6 weeks after thioamide initiation. Other agents such as beta-blockers and iodides are used short term for symptomatic relief. Beta-blockers are used for 2 to 3 weeks or until cardiac symptoms have resolved. Thioamide treatment is typically continued for 12 months or longer to induce long-term spontaneous remission once the drug is discontinued. Because the thioamides do not alter the course of the disease process, spontaneous remission is often poor, and many patients require long-term thioamide therapy, often for many years.

During the hyperthyroid state, other drugs that are metabolized by the liver or eliminated renally may need to be adjusted because metabolism may be increased. Patients using drugs with a narrow therapeutic index, such as digoxin, warfarin, and phenytoin, should be monitored carefully because dosing adjustments will be necessary as the hyperthyroidism or hypermetabolic state resolves.

Other treatment options, besides thioamide therapy, involve RAI. The iodine-131 isotope is taken up by the thyroid gland and the radioactivity destroys the gland. RAI is safe, pain free, easy to administer, and very effective. RAI may result in euthyroidism but more frequently results in hypothyroidism, requiring lifelong levothyroxine supplementation. RAI should never be given during pregnancy since it crosses the placenta.

CASE CONCLUSION

HP began methimazole therapy for her Graves hyperthyroidism. She also began propranolol to help control her tachycardia and tremor. During this time HP should avoid excessive exercise or other sympathomimetic drugs until her symptoms of tachycardia have subsided. HP will return to the clinic for follow-up in 4 weeks. At that time, methimazole dose, tolerability, compliance, and thyroid function tests will be reassessed.

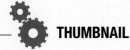

THUMBNAIL

Available agents: Propylthiouracil (PTU) and methimazole.

MOA: Thioamides inhibit the synthesis of thyroid hormones by inhibiting thyroid peroxidase-catalyzed reactions to block iodine organification. Thioamides also block coupling of mono-iodothyronine and diiodothyronine. PTU also inhibits the peripheral conversion of T_4 to T_3.

Pharmacokinetics: PTU is rapidly absorbed. The oral bioavailability of 50 to 80% may be due to a large hepatic first-pass effect. Methimazole is completely absorbed. The duration of action for PTU is approximately 7 hours and therefore requires multiple daily doses (every 6–8 hours).

Adverse reactions: The most common adverse effect is maculopapular rash. Rarely, hepatitis, vasculitis, urticarial rash, and arthralgia have been observed. **Agranulocytosis** can occur in 0.3 to 0.6% of patients. Patients who develop agranulocytosis with one thioamide should not be switched to the alternate thioamide because there is a 50% cross-reactivity between the agents. Methimazole is contraindicated during pregnancy because scalp defects have been observed in infants born to mothers using methimazole.

Drug interactions: The thioamides do not directly interact with other drugs. Because the thioamides can affect thyroid hormone synthesis and therefore decrease clotting factor turnover, the thioamides may increase anticoagulant activity.

QUESTIONS

1. MJ is a 42-year-old woman who was recently diagnosed with Graves disease and will be started on a thioamide and a beta-blocker. Which of the following characteristics regarding thioamides are true?

   A. Methimazole has a long T½ and may be dosed once daily.
   B. PTU can cause pretibial myxedema.
   C. Methimazole interacts with amiodarone therapy.
   D. PTU therapy typically induces spontaneous remission within 12 months.

2. JC is a 31-year-old woman with Graves disease in her first trimester of pregnancy. Which of the following statements regarding PTU are true?

   A. PTU can increase the peripheral conversion of T_4 to T_3.
   B. PTU is safe to use in pregnancy since it is not teratogenic.
   C. PTU is used following surgery to prevent complications.
   D. PTU can be used during myxedema coma.

HPI: AJ is a 27-year-old woman with type 1 diabetes diagnosed at age 11. She has not been seen by a healthcare provider for 3 years. She is 5 feet 6 inches tall and weighs 60 kg. She takes 70/30 insulin twice daily, before breakfast and dinner. She self-monitors her blood glucose once a day; her FBG range is 200 to 250 mg/dL.

Labs: Upon completing her laboratory work, you learn her HgbA1c is 9.5%.

THOUGHT QUESTIONS

- What is your assessment of AJ's blood glucose control?
- What is the difference between the various insulin preparations?
- What insulin therapy would you consider for AJ to intensify her glucose control?

BASIC SCIENCES REVIEW AND DISCUSSION

Type 1 diabetes is characterized by a near-absolute insulin deficiency at diagnosis or soon thereafter. The beta cells of the pancreas no are longer are able to secrete **insulin** due to autoimmune destruction. Therefore, people with type 1 diabetes require exogenous administration of insulin for survival. People with **type 2 diabetes** may require insulin therapy when diet, exercise, and the oral agents are no longer enough to provide adequate glucose control. At this point, a person with type 2 diabetes is experiencing beta-cell failure.

The insulin molecule consists of 51 amino acids arranged in two chains, an A chain (21 amino acids) and a B chain (30 amino acids), that are linked by two disulfide bonds. **Proinsulin** is the insulin precursor that is first processed in the Golgi apparatus of the beta cell, where it is processed and packaged into granules. Proinsulin, a single-chain 86-amino acid peptide, is cleaved into insulin and **C-peptide,** a connecting peptide. These are secreted in equimolar portions from the beta cell upon stimulation from glucose and other insulin secretagogues. C-peptide has no known physiologic function. Insulin exerts its effect on glucose metabolism by binding to insulin receptors throughout the body. Upon binding, insulin promotes the cellular uptake of glucose into fat and skeletal muscle and inhibits **hepatic glucose output,** thus lowering the blood glucose.

Normal, endogenous insulin secretion is characterized by a continuous basal insulin release and food-stimulated bursts of insulin. Exogenous insulin regimens should mimic physiologic insulin release as best as possible. Basal insulin secretion is about 50% of the body's total daily insulin requirement and prandial insulin, approximately 40 to 60% (10–20% of daily insulin at each meal). This is referred to as the "basal/bolus" concept. The rapid and short-acting insulins serve as prandial insulin replacement, while the intermediate and long-acting insulins serve as basal insulin replacement. There are numerous types of insulin regimens, from one to two injections a day, to multiple daily injections or a continuous SC insulin infusion with an insulin pump. The sources of commercially available insulins are pork, human, and human analogues and are injected subcutaneously. The only exception is regular insulin, which can be used intravenously for hospitalized patients or for patients on insulin infusions. Pork insulin is rarely used. The strength of commercially available insulins is 100 units per 1 mL (U-100).

CASE CONCLUSION

AJ is not in good glycemic control. Her HgbA1c and FBG are well above goal. For a patient with type 1 diabetes, generally it is not possible to achieve good glycemic control with a daily regimen of one to two injections. To achieve better glycemic control, a daily regimen of three to four injections should be initiated. This can be accomplished by using a short- or rapid-acting insulin before each meal (e.g., insulin lispro or aspart or regular insulin) and a longer-acting insulin (e.g., ultralente or insulin glargine) as basal insulin. AJ should also be instructed to self-monitor her blood glucose more frequently, at least three to four times a day (e.g., premeal and bedtime with occasional 2-hour postmeal monitoring), to properly adjust her insulin regimen and detect any hypoglycemia. Because AJ has not been seen in the healthcare system for 3 years, she also should be assessed for the standards of care set forth by the American Diabetes Association (ADA).

THUMBNAIL

Insulin	Onset (hr)	Peak (hr)	Duration (hr)
Rapid-acting			
Insulin lispro	Within 15 min	½–1½	3–5
Insulin aspart	Within 10 min	1–3	3–5
Short-acting			
Regular	½–1	2–4	5–8
Intermediate-acting			
NPH	1–2	6–14	12+
Lente	1–3	6–14	12+
Long-acting			
Ultralente	6	18–24	24+
Insulin glargine	1.5	Flat	24

QUESTIONS

1. RC is a 40-year-old woman with type 1 diabetes for 25 years. She takes four injections daily: insulin lispro before each meal and insulin glargine at bedtime. She states that she feels jittery, sweaty, and disoriented in the mid-afternoon two to three times a week; her blood glucose when she feels like this is 50 to 55 mg/dl. Her HgbA1c is 7.1%. Which of the following actions regarding her insulin regimen would be most appropriate?

   A. Do nothing. Her HgbA1c represents good glycemic control.
   B. Switch her to a twice-daily insulin regimen with 70/30 insulin.
   C. Increase her insulin glargine dose.
   D. Decrease her lunchtime insulin lispro dose.
   E. Increase her breakfast insulin lispro dose.

2. Which of the following are factors that can affect insulin absorption?

   A. Massage of injection site
   B. Exercise
   C. Heat
   D. Lipohypertrophy
   E. All of the above

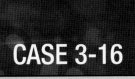

CASE 3-16   Agents for Diabetes: Oral Agents

HPI: DK is a 62-year-old woman with type 2 diabetes for 5 years. She has been treated with glyburide for 4 years. She follows dietary recommendations (low fat; distributes carbohydrates throughout her three meals a day) to the best of her ability and walks 30 minutes three times weekly. At a routine visit with her primary care provider, her FBG is 180 mg/dL. She does not monitor her blood glucose at home and does not have a glucose meter. She is a nonsmoker and her father has type 2 diabetes. Her only long-term diabetes complication is background diabetic retinopathy.

PE: BP 138/84; 5'4"; 157 lbs; body mass index (BMI) 27

Labs: HgbA1c 9.0%; Cr 0.9 mg/dL; LFTs WNL

THOUGHT QUESTIONS

- What is your assessment of DK's blood glucose control?
- What are the pharmacologic options for her diabetes management?
- What are the contraindications to the various diabetes medications?

BASIC SCIENCE REVIEW AND DISCUSSION

Nearly 17 million Americans have diabetes, representing approximately 6% of the population. The majority of people with diabetes have type 2 diabetes, whereas approximately 1 million have type 1 diabetes. It is estimated that one third of people with type 2 diabetes are undiagnosed. Type 2 diabetes is a metabolic disorder involving a defect in insulin secretion and insulin action (i.e., insulin resistance), whereas type 1 diabetes is an autoimmune disorder associated with an absolute insulin deficiency.

The diagnostic criteria for diabetes are (*a*) symptoms of diabetes plus a casual plasma glucose concentration of ≥200 mg/dL (casual means any time of day without regard to meals); (*b*) FBG concentration of ≥126 mg/dL; or (*c*) 2-hour plasma glucose concentration of ≥200 mg/dL during an oral glucose tolerance test. All criteria must be confirmed on a subsequent day. The FBG is the most common criterion used due to its simplicity in measuring. Symptoms of hyperglycemia include polyuria, polydipsia, polyphagia, unexplained weight loss, blurred vision, and increased fatigue. A normal FBG concentration is <110 mg/dL and an FBG concentration >110 mg/dL or <126 mg/dL is defined as impaired fasting glucose (IFG).

The glycemic goals recommended by the ADA include the following: (*a*) premeal blood glucose of 80 to 120 mg/dL; (*b*) bedtime blood glucose of 100 to 140 mg/dL; and (*c*) HgbA1c of <7% (the American Association of Clinical Endocrinologists recommends an HgbA1c of <6.5%). The HgbA1c is the glycosylated hemoglobin, which represents the average blood glucose over the past 2 to 3 months. The United Kingdom Prospective Diabetes Study (UKPDS) demonstrated that improved glycemic control lowers the risk for developing microvascular complications. In this landmark, multicenter trial of newly diagnosed type 2 diabetes patients, for every 1% decrease in the HgbA1c there was a 35% reduction in the risk of microvascular complications of diabetes (e.g., nephropathy, neuropathy, and retinopathy). The study demonstrated a trend in reducing cardiovascular events, but it was not statistically significant.

The current approach used by many clinicians for glycemic control in the management of diabetes is a stepped-care approach.

The first step is lifestyle changes (e.g., diet and exercise). When diet and exercise are no longer enough to control the blood glucose, pharmacologic therapy is added. Monotherapy with oral antidiabetic agents is added to the diet and exercise plan as the second step. Six classes of oral agents for type 2 diabetes medications are available. In an overweight patient with type 2 diabetes, metformin is often considered the first-line agent because it does not cause hypoglycemia when used alone. Metformin decreases **hepatic glucose output** and does not cause weight gain, an advantage in an overweight patient with type 2 diabetes. However, sulfonylureas are still often used as oral monotherapy because they are still some of the most potent antidiabetic medications available. On the beta cell, insulin secretagogues (e.g., sulfonylureas) cause closure of the potassium channels, which results in a depolarization of the cell membrane and subsequent opening of the calcium channels. The increase in intracellular calcium leads to insulin secretion.

When a single oral agent is no longer enough to achieve the target glucose levels, combination oral therapy is used. The key to combination oral therapy is to add a second agent that has a different mechanism of action. Some patients may eventually require three oral agents and/or the initiation of insulin therapy to achieve glucose goals. The UKPDS demonstrated that 3 years and 9 years after diagnosis of diabetes, 50% and 75% of patients will require combination therapy, respectively, which is consistent with the progressive decline in beta-cell function.

CASE CONCLUSION

DK's HgbA1c of 9% and FBG of 180 mg/dL are both above the target glycemic goals set forth by the ADA. Because she has been on glyburide for 4 years and follows a diet/exercise plan, addition of a second oral agent would be indicated in this patient to lower her blood glucose. Metformin would be an appropriate choice in this overweight patient. Reinforcement of the diet and exercise plan is also important at this point. It is important to provide this patient with diabetes self-management education so that she can achieve her target metabolic goals. Self-monitoring of blood glucose should be incorporated, especially since she is on a regimen that could cause hypoglycemia.

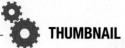

THUMBNAIL

	Sulfonylureas	Meglitinides	Amino Acid Derivatives	Biguanides	Thiazolidinediones	Alpha-Glucosidase Inhibitors
Available agents	Acetohexamide Chlorpropamide Tolazamide Tolbutamide Glimepiride Glipizide Glyburide	Repaglinide	Nateglinide	Metformin	Pioglitazone Rosiglitazone	Acarbose Miglitol
Primary MOA	Stimulate insulin secretion	Stimulate insulin secretion	Stimulate insulin secretion	Decreased hepatic glucose output	Decreased insulin resistance[a]	Delayed carbohydrate absorption
Efficacy as monotherapy (HgbA1c ↓)	1.5–2%	1.7%	0.5%	1.5–2%	0.6–1.5%	0.5–1%
Pharmacokinetics						
Metabolism/ elimination	Acetohexamide, chlorpropamide, tolazamide, glyburide, glimepiride: weakly active metabolites Glipizide, tolbutamide: inactive metabolites	Inactive metabolites	Predominantly inactive metabolites	Excreted unchanged in urine	Extensively metabolized in liver to metabolites	Acarbose: inactive metabolites Miglitol: excreted unchanged in urine
Adverse reactions	Hypoglycemia; weight gain	Hypoglycemia; weight gain	Hypoglycemia; weight gain	GI (nausea, cramping, diarrhea); lactic acidosis[b]	Fluid retention; anemia; weight gain	Abdominal pain; diarrhea; flatulence
Contraindications	Hepatic impairment; renal impairment (use caution; glipizide/tolbutamide preferred agents in renal impairment)	Hepatic impairment	Hepatic impairment	Renal impairment; CHF requiring drug therapy	Hepatic impairment (require bimonthly LFT monitoring for first year; periodically thereafter)	Hepatic impairment; intestinal obstruction; other chronic intestinal diseases

[a]Due to delay in onset of effect, assessment of response should be at 3 months (using HgbA1c).
[b]Very rare side effect (~1 in 30,000 people). Metformin should be temporarily withheld prior to any surgical procedure; it should be withheld at the time of (or prior to) a radiologic study involving the use of intravascular iodinated contrast dye and withheld 48 hours after the study and restarted after renal function has been found to be normal.

QUESTIONS

1. AK is a 55-year-old man diagnosed with diabetes 2 years ago. He has been following a diet and exercise program, but his HgbA1c is now 8.5%. BMI 202. Labs: Cr 1.6 mg/dL; LFTs WNL. Which of the following oral agents is most appropriate to initiate in this patient to obtain an HgbA1c of less than 7%?

A. Metformin
B. Glipizide
C. Nateglinide
D. Chlorpropamide
E. Acarbose

2. RJ has had type 2 diabetes for 10 years. His other medical problems include dyslipidemia, HTN, and retinopathy. He takes benazepril, simvastatin, and metformin. His BP is 120/70 mm Hg; LDL cholesterol 137 mg/dL; HgbA1c 7.8%. He had a dilated retinal eye exam 1.5 years ago. He has not had a pneumococcal vaccination and has never brought a urine sample into the lab. Which of the standards of care is in compliance according to the ADA guidelines?

A. Blood pressure
B. Eye exam visit
C. LDL cholesterol
D. HgbA1c
E. Pneumococcal vaccination
F. Microalbuminuria test

HPI: JL is a 55-year-old man s/p MI 3 years ago. He was placed on cholesterol-lowering therapy following his MI. He currently takes simvastatin to control his cholesterol. He finds it difficult to incorporate any physical activity into his daily routine and does not attempt to reduce his cholesterol/fat intake. His most recent lipid panel is total cholesterol 206 mg/dL; triglycerides 180 mg/dL; HDL 35 mg/dL; LDL 135 mg/dL.

THOUGHT QUESTIONS

- What is your assessment of JL's lipid profile?
- Would you modify his current lipid-lowering therapy? If so, how?
- What are the common side effects associated with lipid-lowering medications?
- What are the common drug interactions with lipid-lowering medications?

BASIC SCIENCE REVIEW AND DISCUSSION

Coronary heart disease (CHD) is one of the leading causes of morbidity and mortality in the United States. Hyperlipidemia is a major risk factor for atherosclerosis and CHD. Hyperlipidemia is defined as an elevation in blood cholesterol or triglycerides (TGs). Lipids are primarily transported in the body by three major lipoproteins: **LDL, very low-density (VLDL), and HDL.** Cholesteryl esters and TGs are carried by the lipoproteins, which vary in size and composition of cholesterol and TGs. Cholesterol is used to form cell membranes and is the precursor to bile acids and steroid hormones.

Although several lipoproteins are considered to play a role in atherogenesis [VLDL, LDL and Lp(a)], LDL cholesterol (LDL-C) is the primary target of therapy. The risk of CHD is inversely related to levels of HDL, because HDL is responsible for reverse cholesterol transport. Lipoprotein disorders can involve abnormalities in lipid metabolism (e.g., synthesis, transport, and catabolism). Attainment of a lipid profile must be made after a 9- to 12-hour fast.

In addition to the level of LDL-C, the following are major risk factors for CHD: (*a*) cigarette smoking; (*b*) HTN (BP ≥140/90 mm Hg or on antihypertensive medication); (*c*) low HDL-C (<40 mg/dL); (*d*) family history of premature CHD (CHD in male first-degree relative <55 years of age or CHD in female first-degree relative <65 years of age); and (*e*) age (men ≥45 years, women ≥55 years).

Four main classes of lipid-lowering medications are available: HMG CoA reductase inhibitors (otherwise known as statins), bile acid sequestrants, nicotinic acid, and fibric acids.

CASE CONCLUSION

Because JL already has CHD (s/p MI) and his LDL-C goal is more than 100 mg/dL, his current therapy is inadequate. Lifestyles changes should be emphasized to him, including reduction of saturated fat and cholesterol and physical activity as tolerated. Physical activity will be beneficial in raising the HDL-C in this patient. In addition, his simvastatin dose should be increased. LDL-C reduction with statins is dose dependent. In general, a doubling of the dose will result in an additional 6% lowering of the LDL-C. If he is already taking the maximum dose, combination drug therapy should be instituted.

THUMBNAIL

Drug Class	MOA	Lipid Effects	Adverse Reactions	Metabolism	Drug Interactions	Contraindications/ Precautions
HMG CoA reductase inhibitors (statins) Atorvastatin Fluvastatin Lovastatin Pravastatin Simvastatin	Inhibit rate-limiting step in cholesterol synthesis	LDL ↓ 18–55% HDL ↑ 5–15% TGs ↓ 7–30%	Myopathy (rare) ↑ LFTs (rare)	All via CYP450, although the specific isoenzyme is drug specific	Macrolide antibiotics Cyclosporine Digoxin Nefazodone Azole antifungals HIV protease inhibitors Amiodarone Warfarin Fibric acids Niacin	Liver disease; pregnancy and lactation

(Continued)

THUMBNAIL *(Continued)*

Drug Class	MOA	Lipid Effects	Adverse Reactions	Metabolism	Drug Interactions	Contraindications/ Precautions
Bile acid sequestrants Cholestyramine Colestipol Colesevelam	Bind to bile acids in gut	LDL ↓ 15–30% HDL ↑ 30% TGs no change or ↑	GI: constipation, bloating, abdominal pain	None (not systemically absorbed)	↓ bioavailability of coadministered drugs; separate other drugs at least 1 hr before or 4–6 hr after	Complete biliary obstruction; severely elevated TGs
Nicotinic acid	Inhibit VLDL secretion	LDL ↓ 5–25% HDL ↑ 15–35% TGs ↓ 20–50%	Flushing; ↑ blood sugar and uric acid; GI upset; liver toxicity	88% excreted as unchanged drug and nicotinuric acid	Statins	Liver disease; active PUD; arterial bleeding; caution use in diabetes; gout
Fibric acids Clofibrate Gemfibrozil Fenofibrate	Increase VLDL catabolism; PPAR$_\alpha$ agonist	LDL ↓ 5–20% HDL ↑ 10–20% TGs ↓ 20–50%	GI upset, dyspepsia, gallstones, ↑ LFTs, myopathy	Non-CYP450 metabolism	Warfarin Cyclosporine Statins	Liver or severe renal disease; primary biliary cirrhosis; preexisting gallbladder disease

PPAR$_\alpha$: peroxisome proliferator activated receptor

QUESTIONS

1. RM had his dose of lovastatin increased since his LDL-C was above his goal. How soon should his response to the higher dose be assessed?
   A. 1 week
   B. 2 weeks
   C. 3 weeks
   D. 4 weeks
   E. 6 weeks

2. PJ is a 60-year-old woman with a history of an abdominal aortic aneurysm who is taking niacin for her dyslipidemia. Her LDL-C is 120 mg/dL, so a statin is added to her therapy. Which of the following are true for statins?

   A. Baseline LFTs should be checked prior to initiation.
   B. Generally taken at dinner or bedtime.
   C. Statins interact with cyclosporine.
   D. Statins interact with azole antifungals.
   E. Statins interact with niacin and fibrates.
   F. All of the above.

CASE 3-18   Agents for Asthma

HPI: KG is a 39-year-old woman with asthma on fluticasone and albuterol complaining of SOB associated with exercise. Three months ago she started an aerobic exercise program that has been hampered by chest tightness and SOB shortly after she begins running. She admits to poor compliance with her corticosteroid inhaler and requests an oral medication to control her asthma symptoms. Her PMH is significant for mild, persistent asthma for 35 years and allergic rhinitis. Her medications include fluticasone and albuterol inhalers and fexofenadine. Pulmonary function tests (PFTs) reveal her forced expiratory volume in the first second (FEV_1) = 89% of predicted.

THOUGHT QUESTIONS

- What general classes of medications are appropriate for the treatment of mild persistent asthma?
- Which medications are effective for exercise-induced bronchospasm (EIB)?
- What adverse effects are associated with inhaled corticosteroid therapy?

BASIC SCIENCE REVIEW AND DISCUSSION

Asthma is a chronic inflammatory disease of the airways afflicting an estimated 15 million people in the United States (approximately 6% of the population), nearly 5 million of whom are younger than age 18 years. Symptoms of asthma include recurrent wheezing, difficulty breathing, chest tightness, and cough (particularly at night). Pharmacotherapy for asthma consists of quick-relief (rescue) and long-term control (maintenance) medications. Quick-relief medications are used to provide rapid relief of asthma symptoms (wheezing, cough, and SOB) and include short-acting inhaled β_2-agonists and systemic corticosteroids. Long-term control medications are taken on a daily basis to achieve and maintain control of persistent asthma and include antiinflammatory agents (inhaled corticosteroids, mast cell stabilizers), long-acting β_2-agonists, methylxanthines, and leukotriene modifiers.

The goal of EIB treatment is to allow patients to exercise (including vigorous activities) without experiencing symptoms of bronchospasm. Recommended treatments consist of medications taken as needed just prior to exercise to prevent symptoms or those taken long term on a daily basis to decrease inflammation and airway hyperresponsiveness. Medications taken immediately before exercise include β_2-agonists and mast cell stabilizing agents. Inhaled β_2-agonists are the mainstay of treatment and are more than 80% effective in preventing EIB if administered prophylactically. Short-acting inhaled β_2-agonists (albuterol, bitolterol, pirbuterol) administered 5 to 15 minutes before exercise are generally effective for 2 to 3 hours. Long-acting agents (salmeterol, formoterol) offer protection for up to 12 hours. The mast cell stabilizing agents (cromolyn, nedocromil) when taken 10 to 15 minutes before exercise are also effective alternatives.

Patients who experience symptoms more than twice weekly have persistent asthma and should be managed with a long-term control medication with antiinflammatory activity. In general, inhaled corticosteroids are well tolerated. Local reactions including cough, dysphonia (hoarseness), and oral candidiasis (thrush) are the most commonly observed adverse effects. These can be minimized by administering the drug with a spacer device and by rinsing the oral cavity with water after inhalation. Systemic adverse effects associated with corticosteroids (adrenal suppression, osteoporosis, growth suppression, ocular toxicity, dermal thinning, easy bruising) are significantly less likely to occur with the inhaled route of administration. Although higher doses of inhaled corticosteroids increase the risk for systemic adverse effects, these risks are far less than would be seen with oral administration of corticosteroids. When prescribed at the recommended doses, the superior effectiveness of inhaled corticosteroids outweighs the minimal risks for serious adverse effects.

CASE CONCLUSION

Because KG is poorly compliant with her inhaled corticosteroid therapy, she is started on daily montelukast to control her mild persistent asthma and EIB. She is also instructed to use her albuterol inhaler 15 minutes before exercise to provide additional protection against EIB.

THUMBNAIL: Agents for Asthma

Class/specific Agent	MOA	Adverse Reactions	Comments
β₂-agonists (inhaled): administered prior to exercise to prevent EIB			
Short-acting • Albuterol • Bitolterol • Pirbuterol	β₂-selective adrenergic agonists that induce bronchodilation through activation of adenylate cyclase, causing an increase in cyclic AMP levels and resulting in smooth muscle relaxation in the airways	Tachycardia, skeletal muscle tremor, hypokalemia, prolonged QT$_c$ interval (in overdose)	**Onset of action:** 5–15 min **Duration of action:** 2–3 hr Nonselective agents (epinephrine, isoproterenol, metaproterenol) are not recommended due to their potential for excessive cardiac stimulation Oral agents are less preferred due to the slower onset of action (30–60 min) and higher incidence of systemic side effects
Long-acting • Formoterol • Salmeterol			**Onset of action:** 15 min (formoterol); 15–30 min (salmeterol) **Duration of action:** 12 hr
Mast cell stabilizers (inhaled): administered prior to exercise to prevent EIB			
• Cromolyn • Nedocromil	Work topically on lung mucosa. Block early and late reaction to allergen. Stabilize mast cell membranes and inhibit activation and release of inflammatory mediators from eosinophils and epithelial cells, inhibiting broncho-constriction caused by exercise and cold dry air	Poorly absorbed so adverse effects usually localized: cough, mouth dryness, throat irritation, metallic taste (15–20%) with nedocromil	**Onset of action:** 10–15 min **Duration of action:** 1–2 hr
Corticosteroids (inhaled): administered on a daily basis to control airway hyperresponsiveness and prevent EIB			
• Beclomethasone • Budesonide • Flunisolide • Fluticasone • Triamcinolone	Block late reaction to allergen and reduce airway hyperresponsiveness; inhibit production of cytokines responsible for initiation of inflammatory cascade	Cough, dysphonia, oral candidiasis (thrush); high doses may cause systemic effects (e.g., adrenal and growth suppression, osteoporosis, skin thinning, and cataracts)	**Onset of action:** 7–14 days; full effect may not be realized for 6–8 wks Adverse effects minimized by administering with a spacer and by rinsing the oral cavity with water after inhalation
Leukotriene modifiers: administered on a daily basis to control airway hyperresponsiveness and prevent EIB			
Leukotriene receptor antagonists • Montelukast • Zafirlukast	Selective, competitive inhibitor of the leukotriene D₄ (LTD₄) receptor; inhibition of LTD₄ reduces broncho-constriction, airway hyperresponsiveness, mucosal edema, and mucus production	Headache, abdominal pain, hepatotoxicity (≤2%), Churg-Strauss syndrome (rare)	Oral medications administered once (montelukast) or twice (zafirlukast) daily
5-lipoxygenase inhibitor • Zileuton	Inhibitor of the 5-lipoxygenase enzyme necessary for the biosynthesis of leukotrienes, including LTD₄	Headache, hepatotoxicity (12%) Abdominal pain, nausea, Churg-Strauss syndrome (rare)	Oral medication administered four times daily; regular monitoring for hepatotoxicity is necessary

QUESTIONS

1. JC is a 14-year-old boy with a 7-year history of mild intermittent asthma who complains of SOB, cough, and poor endurance during football practice. Other than this EIB, his asthma has been well controlled for the past several years with only "as needed" β₂-agonist therapy for asthma symptoms. He has not needed to use his rescue inhaler (albuterol) for nearly a year. PFTs reveal his FEV₁ = 95% of predicted. Which of the following is the best treatment for JC?

A. Administer albuterol aerosol 5 to 15 minutes before exercise.

B. Administer oral albuterol 5 to 15 minutes before exercise.

C. Administer albuterol aerosol every 6 hours during football season.

D. Administer epinephrine aerosol 5 to 15 minutes before exercise.

E. Initiate high-dose inhaled corticosteroid therapy.

2. A 32-year-old woman receiving beclomethasone, eight puffs twice daily, for moderate persistent asthma complains of white spots on her tongue and hard palate and pain on swallowing. Her asthma control has been excellent and she has no other medical problems. The most appropriate change in her asthma therapy would be to:

A. Discontinue beclomethasone.
B. Change the beclomethasone inhaler to two puffs four times daily.
C. Change the beclomethasone inhaler to a flunisolide inhaler.
D. Instruct the patient to use the beclomethasone inhaler with a spacer.
E. Change the beclomethasone inhaler to oral prednisone.

HPI: JL is a 23-year-old woman who complains of severe abdominal cramping, heavy menstrual flow, headache, and irritability during the first few days of her menstrual cycle. Last month her doctor started her on a 21-day monophasic combined oral contraceptive (COC) containing ethinyl estradiol (EE), and levonorgestrel (LNG). After completing two cycles she states that her cramping and flow have improved, but she is experiencing break-through bleeding (BTB) around day 17 of her cycle, her acne has worsened, and she is considering stopping her pills. Her PMH is significant for a seizure disorder.

THOUGHT QUESTIONS

- How do monophasic and triphasic COCs differ?
- Aside from COC pills, what other formulations are available?
- What drugs and disease states would preclude the use of a particular contraceptive?
- What are some possible reasons that JL is having BTB?

BASIC SCIENCE REVIEW AND DISCUSSION

Monophasic formulations contain a constant dose of estrogen and progestin. **Triphasic** formulations contain varying doses of progestin (generally increasing) every 7 days, and either a stable or a variable amount of estrogen every 7 days. Typically, the total progestin amount per cycle in monophasics is greater than that in triphasics. Estrogen content per cycle is similar between the two.

Patients who have contraindications to estrogen or who experience intolerable side effects are good candidates for progestin-only contraceptives. Progestin-only pills are less effective than COC pills and are associated with a greater incidence of dysmenorrhea, amenorrhea, irregular menses, and BTB. Use of nonoral formulations may be desirable in individuals who forget to take their pills on a daily basis or who are noncompliant. Options include an intramuscular (IM) injectable (depo-medroxyprogesterone acetate [DMPA], Depo-Provera), a surgically placed subdermal implant (LNG, Norplant), and a surgically placed intrauterine system (LNG, Mirena). DMPA has been linked to reversible bone loss. Estrogen is also available as a transdermal patch, a vaginal ring, and a monthly IM injectable. These nonoral routes allow for lower doses of hormones to be used and bypass first-pass metabolism, thereby limiting the production of factors produced by the liver (e.g., fibrinogen, C-reactive protein).

Contraceptive efficacy can be decreased when taken concurrently with drugs that increase the metabolism of hormones (e.g., CYP450 inducers). Similarly, drugs that reduce enterohepatic recycling of COCs (e.g., tetracycline, penicillins) can also reduce efficacy.

There are a variety of contraindications to contraceptive use. A family history of breast cancer does not preclude the use of COCs. In general, COC use does not increase the risk for breast cancer and may diminish the risk for endometrial, colorectal, and ovarian cancer. COC use is not recommended, however, in patients who have a current or past history of breast, hepatic, or cervical cancer. COC use may increase the risk for cervical dysplasia and cancer with more than 1 year of use. It also may increase the risk for hepatic cancer and gallbladder disease. Benefits of short-term COC use may include improved cycle regularity, less dysmenorrhea, fewer premenstrual symptoms, less irregular bleeding and blood loss, reduced risk for ectopic pregnancy and functional ovarian cysts, and possible reduction in acne. Long-term benefits of COC use may include a reduced risk for pelvic inflammatory disease (PID) and benign breast disease and improved bone mineral density and lipid profile ($\uparrow$ HDL).

Once initiated, patients should be monitored for side effects of COCs. BTB is a common reason for drug discontinuation. Generally, spotting and BTB diminish after the third cycle of use. BTB that extends beyond the third cycle may be due to patient noncompliance, insufficient estrogen dose (if occurring between days 1 and 9), insufficient progestin dose (if occurring between days 10 and 21), or a drug interaction that is reducing the amount of circulating estrogen/progestin. Newer COCs that employ very low doses of hormones are associated with fewer side effects overall but may increase the risk for BTB due to endometrial instability.

CASE CONCLUSION

JL is experiencing BTB during days 10 to 21 of her cycle, which may be due to progestin deficiency. Her acne also has worsened, which is most likely due to the high androgenicity of LNG. Although she has completed only two cycles of pills, and BTB tends to diminish after three cycles, she can be switched to another pill with more progestational/less androgenic activity.

THUMBNAIL: Oral Contraception

MOA

COCs decrease ovulation, sperm and egg transport, and implantation. The estrogen component alters FSH (follicle-stimulating hormone) and LH (leuteinizing hormone) release, accelerates egg transport, and alters the endometrium so that it is unsuitable for implantation. Progestins alter FSH and LH release, thicken cervical mucus to reduce sperm and egg transport, inhibit enzymes necessary for fertilization, and also alter the endometrium so that it is unsuitable for implantation.

Common Estrogenic Side Effects	Common Progestational Side Effects
Estrogen excess:	**Progestin excess (also see androgenic effects):**
Nausea, vomiting	Dysmenorrhea, amenorrhea
Fluid retention, weight gain, edema	Hypertension
↑ breast size or tenderness	Candida vaginitis
Skin discoloration (chloasma)	Breast tenderness
White or yellowish vaginal discharge	
Hypertension	**Androgenic Side Effects (Excess):**
Cyclic headache	↑ LDL, ↓ HDL cholesterol
Heavy flow, hypermenorrhea	↑ appetite, weight gain
Increased risk thrombus, blood clot	↑ acne, oily skin, hirsutism, hair loss
	↑ tenderness
Estrogen Deficiency:	↑ depression, fatigue
BTB days 1–9	↓ libido
Vasomotor symptoms	
Nervousness, irritability	**Progestin Deficiency:**
Decreased libido	BTB days 10–21
Atrophic vaginitis	Amenorrhea
	Heavy flow/clots

QUESTIONS

1. RM is a 35-year-old woman who severely tore her anterior cruciate ligament in a skiing accident and is having major surgery in 2 months, followed by an additional 2 months of bed rest and reduced mobility. She has been taking COC pills for the past 4 years. Which of the following would be good advice for RM?

   A. Initiate aspirin 1 month prior to surgery.
   B. Initiate warfarin 1 month prior to surgery.
   C. Maintain COC use before and after the surgery.
   D. Discontinue COC use 1 month prior to surgery and re-initiate immediately after.
   E. Discontinue COC use 1 month prior to surgery and re-initiate after the patient is able to ambulate.

2. LN would like to initiate a contraceptive for the next 2 years. Her only specification is that she would like to use a contraceptive method that does not delay her fertility once she discontinues its use. A prolonged delay in fertility postdiscontinuation has been observed with which of the following?

   A. COC pills
   B. Depo-Provera (progestin injectable every 3 months)
   C. Norplant (progestin subdermal implant)
   D. Minera (progestin IUD)
   E. Vaginal ring

CASE 3-20 Agents for Peptic Ulcer Disease

HPI: OF is a 42-year-old white man who presents to the acute care clinic with severe mid-epigastric pain. OF has been working long hours and is under a great deal of stress at work. OF drinks one to two beers per night, and has smoked one pack of cigarettes per day for the past 10 years. He has lost 10 pounds in the past 2 months.

PE: Endoscopy reveals a 4-cm gastric ulcer (antral), which tests positive for *Helicobacter pylori*.

THOUGHT QUESTIONS

- What are the risk factors for gastroduodenal ulcers?
- What treatment options are available for gastric ulcers?
- What are the pharmacologic differences between each treatment approach?
- What side effects are associated with the use of *H. pylori* treatment regimens?

BASIC SCIENCE REVIEW AND DISCUSSION

Dyspepsia is a chronic or recurrent discomfort/pain in the upper abdomen. The causes for dyspepsia involve gastroduodenal ulcer, atypical gastroesophageal reflux, and gastric cancer. Classic symptoms related to gastroduodenal ulcers, such as postprandial epigastric pain or pain relieved by eating, are common. More importantly, dyspepsia may be associated with certain alarm features such as recurrent vomiting, weight loss, dysphagia, bleeding, or anemia.

Helicobacter pylori is a gram-negative spiral bacterium that has been implicated in the pathogenesis of gastroduodenal ulcers.

H. pylori has been found in nearly 90% of patients with duodenal ulcers and nearly 70% of patients with gastric ulcers. Eradication of *H. pylori* has been shown to decrease the recurrence rate and accelerate the ulcer healing process.

In cases of *H. pylori*-positive dyspepsia, treatment is aimed at eradicating bacteria as well as alleviating symptoms. In cases of *H. pylori*-negative dyspepsia, empiric antisecretory drugs or pro-kinetic agents are often initiated. If treatment with these agents fails, the patient should be referred for endoscopy to rule out chronic ulceration or other causes.

Patients with documented *H. pylori* cultures and active ulceration should be treated with **antisecretory agents** and combination antibiotics. Treatment regimens are individualized and may include one, two, or three of the following antimicrobials: amoxicillin, clarithromycin, metronidazole, tetracycline, and bismuth subsalicylate. Treatment regimens can be taken together at the same time, without regard to meals or drug interactions among the regimens. This is because systemic blood levels are not necessary; rather, the goal of therapy is local GI antimicrobial activity.

 CASE CONCLUSION

OF began combination antisecretory and antimicrobial therapy for his *H. pylori*-positive gastric ulcer. He has completed a 2-week course of therapy with a four-drug regimen without side effects or other complications. He reports no gastric pain or other symptoms associated with gastric ulcers. OF has also began a smoking cessation program because smoking has been shown to decrease ulcer healing.

THUMBNAIL: H₂-Receptor Antagonists

Available agents: Cimetidine, ranitidine, nizatidine, famotidine

Clinical use: Treatment of dyspepsia, gastroduodenal ulcers, gastroesophageal reflux disease (GERD), and Zollinger-Ellison syndrome

MOA: Competitively and selectively inhibit the action of histamine on H$_2$ receptors of the parietal cells

Pharmacokinetics: All oral H$_2$-receptor antagonists are rapidly absorbed within 1 to 3 hours. Oral bioavailability is lower for ranitidine, cimetidine, and famotidine than for nizatidine. This is because ranitidine, cimetidine, and famotidine are incompletely absorbed and undergo first-pass hepatic metabolism. All of the H$_2$-receptor antagonists are eliminated via renal filtration and secretion. For this reason, the H$_2$-receptor antagonist T½ may be increased in patients with renal dysfunction.

(Continued)

THUMBNAIL: H$_2$-Receptor Antagonists *(Continued)*

Adverse reactions: All H$_2$-receptor antagonists are generally well tolerated with few adverse effects. The most common H$_2$-receptor antagonist adverse effects include confusion, dizziness, headache, constipation, and diarrhea. Rarely, reversible thrombocytopenia has been reported with the H$_2$-receptor antagonist class. High doses of cimetidine for prolonged periods may lead to dose-dependent elevation in serum prolactin activity and possible alterations in estrogen metabolism. These changes have led to reversible gynecomastia and breast tenderness in males. Famotidine and ranitidine have been associated with headache and CNS changes, specifically in patients with decreased renal function.

Drug interactions: Cimetidine is a CYP450 inhibitor and can inhibit the metabolism of phenytoin, warfarin, and theophylline. Famotidine, nizatidine, and ranitidine are unlikely to cause clinically significant drug interactions. All H$_2$ antagonists have the potential to interact with other drugs that require gastric acid for absorption (e.g., ketoconazole, itraconazole).

QUESTIONS

1. CT is a 47-year-old man who is about to be started on combination therapy for his *H. pylori*-positive ulcer with antibiotics and either a proton pump inhibitor (PPI) or an H$_2$-receptor antagonist. Although PPIs and H$_2$-receptor antagonists are well tolerated, which of the following drug side effect combinations is most likely to occur during therapy?

   A. Famotidine/headache
   B. Omeprazole/insomnia
   C. Lansoprazole/rash
   D. Cimetidine/seizure

2. CT is going to be started on omeprazole plus two antimicrobials. Which of the following antimicrobials has activity against *H. pylori*?

   A. Doxycycline
   B. Ampicillin
   C. Tetracycline
   D. Miconazole

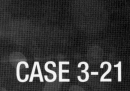

Agents for Gastroesophageal Reflux Disease

HPI: ST is a 60-year-old man who presents to the clinic with increasing daytime heartburn, episodes of postprandial heartburn, and regurgitation. ST has been using over-the-counter (OTC) H$_2$-receptor antagonists and antacids with no relief. He reports a bitter taste in his mouth and mild chest pain. ST recently sustained a compound fracture of his left knee from a motor vehicle accident. He has been immobile for 2 months and has been working long hours on his computer from home. ST drinks alcohol occasionally on the weekends, and smokes half a pack of cigarettes per week. He has gained 15 pounds in the past 2 months.

THOUGHT QUESTIONS

- What are the risk factors for gastroesophageal reflux disease (GERD)?
- What treatment options are available for GERD?
- What side effects are associated with the use of GERD treatment regimens?

BASIC SCIENCE REVIEW AND DISCUSSION

GERD results from an imbalance between aggressive factors (acid and pepsin) and defensive factors (antireflux barriers, esophageal clearance, and mucosal resistance). Specifically, GERD causes the reflux of acidic gastric contents into the esophagus. The hallmark symptoms of GERD involve esophagitis and esophageal complications (esophageal stricture, hemorrhage, Barrett esophagus, and, rarely, esophageal cancer). Unfortunately, the frequency or severity of GERD is not predictive of esophageal damage.

The **lower esophageal sphincter** (LES) is the major barrier to reflux. Spontaneous and transient relaxation of the LES can occur in healthy adults. Patients with GERD experience more frequent relaxation of the LES, resulting in GERD symptoms. Other protective mechanisms, including gravity, saliva, and peristalsis, help to reduce the contact time of gastric acid with the esophagus. These mechanisms, however, may not be active in patients who are supine or lying down.

Treatment of GERD is aimed at relieving symptoms, promoting healing, preventing recurrence, and reducing complications.

The most important treatment approach is to incorporate diet and lifestyle changes. The staged approach to GERD facilitates treatment; however, an individualized approach to therapy is preferred. Stage I GERD is classified as mild or infrequent heartburn occurring less than two to three times per week. Stage I GERD consists of intermittent heartburn, which typically resolves with lifestyle modification, antacids, and OTC H$_2$-receptor antagonists. Stage II GERD involves frequent or consistent episodes of heartburn unrelieved by antacids or H$_2$-receptor antagonists. This stage of disease requires PPIs; if no response is observed, the use of promotility agents may be considered. Stage III GERD commonly involves warning symptoms or erosive GERD (cough, dysphagia, odynophagia, weight loss, laryngitis, hematemesis, anemia). Patients with these symptoms should undergo upper endoscopy to identify morphologic or histologic changes in the esophagus (ulceration, erosive esophagitis, cancer, Barrett esophagus). These patients will typically require long-term therapy with PPIs.

PPIs are considered the drugs of choice for patients with stage II or III GERD. PPIs accelerate esophageal healing and are effective in relieving symptoms. In some patients with chronic symptoms, long-term maintenance therapy with PPIs (3–6 months) can help control symptoms and prevent complications. Patients with severe symptoms or atypical GERD (stage II) will require high-dose PPIs along with promotility agents. Promotility agents facilitate gastric emptying by increasing LES pressure and therefore decrease the chance of regurgitation.

CASE CONCLUSION

ST was started on a PPI for the treatment of his stage II moderate-to-severe GERD symptoms. He will need treatment for at least 4 to 8 weeks. ST's recent immobility has led to his weight gain and possibly his worsening symptoms. ST was also counseled on nondrug therapies to help relieve his GERD symptoms.

THUMBNAIL: Agents for Gastroesophageal Reflux Disease

	PPIs	Prokinetic Agents
Available agents	Omeprazole Lansoprazole Pantoprazole Rabeprazole Esomeprazole	Metoclopramide Cisapride

(Continued)

THUMBNAIL: Agents for Gastroesophageal Reflux Disease *(Continued)*

	PPIs	*Prokinetic Agents*
Clinical use	Short-term treatment of gastroduodenal disorders, GERD, and for pathologic secretory conditions such as Zollinger-Ellison syndrome. The PPIs are superior to H_2-receptor antagonists in patients with stage III erosive GERD.	Used in patients with severe symptoms or in those with atypical GERD symptoms. Typically reserved for patients who fail high-dose PPIs. Desired most in patients who also report nausea, constipation, or other related symptoms.
MOA	PPIs are substituted benzimidazoles that irreversibly inhibit gastric parietal cell release of acid. PPIs are prodrugs that must be activated in the acidic environment of the secretory canaliculus located in the parietal cell. PPIs inhibit the H+/K+ ATPase pump and can inhibit nearly 100% of the gastric acid secretion.	Promotility agents increase LES tone and accelerate gastric emptying.
Pharmacokinetics	All oral PPIs are rapidly absorbed and undergo hepatic metabolism. The bioavailability of the oral PPIs ranges from 30 to 85%. All of the PPIs have a short elimination T½ (<2 hr), but this has minimal effect on the duration of antisecretory action due to irreversible binding to the proton pump.	Both cisapride and metoclopramide have a rapid onset of action, <1 hr. Both agents have a similar oral bioavailability: 50–80% and are extensively metabolized by the liver to inactive metabolites.
Adverse reactions	PPIs are very well tolerated. Rarely, headache, diarrhea, constipation, nausea, and pruritus have been observed.	Metoclopramide is associated with CNS side effects, especially in the elderly or in those with decreased renal function. Metoclopramide also leads to drowsiness, diarrhea, abdominal cramps, and **extrapyramidal reactions.** Cisapride, at high doses, is associated with QT segment prolongation. When used at the recommended doses in patients with normal renal and hepatic function, cardiac effects are rare.
Drug interactions	The PPIs differ in their ability to inhibit CYP450. Omeprazole may inhibit the metabolism of diazepam, phenytoin, and warfarin. All PPIs have the potential to interact with other drugs that require gastric acid for absorption (e.g., ketoconazole, itraconazole).	Fatal cardiac arrhythmias have been reported when cisapride was combined with drugs that are metabolized by the CYP450 system. Most of the interactions involved antifungal and antimicrobial agents. For this reason, cisapride is available on a limited access basis in the United States.
Comments	PPIs are most effective when taken 30 min before a meal. PPIs should not be taken with H_2-receptor antagonists since this puts the parietal cell in a resting state. Because consistent gastric acid suppression is desired for healing, the PPIs should not be used for GERD on an as-needed basis.	Cisapride is effective in providing both symptomatic relief and in promoting healing.

QUESTIONS

1. SL is a 56-year-old man who was recently diagnosed with stage II GERD. In addition to lifestyle modification, SL is started on a PPI. SL should be counseled to take his PPI:

   A. 30 minutes before breakfast
   B. Together with an H_2 antagonist
   C. With food to decrease stomach upset
   D. On an as-needed basis
   E. All of the above

2. MJ is a 45-year-old man diagnosed with stage III GERD by endoscopy. He is started on a PPI and a promotility agent, cisapride. Cisapride can cause which of the following side effects?

   A. Dry cough
   B. Excessive nausea
   C. Microcytic anemia
   D. Severe constipation
   E. Cardiac arrhythmias

Penicillins

HPI: JB is a 21-year-old man who presents to the ED with a 3-day history of worsening pain, redness, and swelling on his right leg, which occurred after falling off his mountain bike. Exam reveals a swollen, warm, and extremely tender leg. JB appears quite ill.

PE: T 39.2°C; BP 112/69; HR 80; RR 24. He has NKDA.

THOUGHT QUESTIONS

- Which organisms cause cellulitis?
- Which antibiotics are appropriate for the treatment of cellulitis?
- What is the mechanism of resistance to penicillins?

BASIC SCIENCE REVIEW AND DISCUSSION

Cellulitis results when the integrity of the skin is broken due to an abrasion, ulceration, skin puncture, or surgical wound. Moderate to severe infections can progress to more serious infections such as **osteomyelitis** if not adequately treated. Cellulitis is most commonly caused by group A β-hemolytic streptococci (*Streptococcus pyogenes*) and *Staphylococcus aureus*. Wound cultures have a very low yield and rarely identify the causative pathogen. Thus, cultures are rarely done and therapy is usually presumptive.

Nafcillin, an antistaphylococcal penicillin, is an appropriate IV antibiotic for the treatment of cellulitis requiring hospitalization. Appropriate alternatives would include cefazolin or clindamycin. Second- and third-generation cephalosporins offer no advantage over the listed regimens since they are broader in spectrum and more expensive. While gram-negative organisms such as *Escherichia coli*, *Pseudomonas aeruginosa*, and *Klebsiella pneumoniae* can cause cellulitis, they should only be considered in patients who either fail first-line regimens or are immunocompromised. For those patients with severe penicillin allergies, alternative regimens include clindamycin or vancomycin.

Penicillins are classified into several groups depending on their chemical structure: **penicillins,** extended-spectrum penicillins or **aminopenicillins,** and **antistaphylococcal penicillins.** Penicillins inhibit bacterial cell wall synthesis by attaching to **penicillin-binding proteins** (PBPs), thereby inhibiting bacterial growth. Although penicillin and ampicillin have activity against *Streptococcus pyogenes*, they lack activity against *Staphylococcus aureus*. *Staphylococcus aureus* produces an enzyme, **penicillinase,** which breaks down penicillin and ampicillin, rendering them ineffective. Nafcillin is unique because it is stable in the presence of penicillinase. Another common mechanism of resistance to penicillins is through modification of PBPs. Penicillin-resistant *Streptococcus pneumoniae* is an example of an organism that produces modified PBPs.

In general, penicillins are very well tolerated. The most common adverse effects are **hypersensitivity reactions.** While skin rash is the most common manifestation, **anaphylaxis** rarely can occur. In those patients who have experienced an anaphylactic reaction to penicillin, a non–β-lactam antibiotic should be used.

CASE CONCLUSION

The patient is admitted to the hospital and diagnosed with cellulitis. No cultures are done and nafcillin is prescribed. After 3 days of nafcillin, JB was switched to oral dicloxacillin and discharged home to complete his course of therapy.

THUMBNAIL: Penicillins

Antibiotic	Penicillins	Aminopenicillins	Antistaphylococcal Penicillins
Available agents	Penicillin (IV/IM/PO)	Ampicillin (IV) Amoxicillin (PO)	Dicloxacillin (PO) Nafcillin (IV) Oxacillin (PO/IV)
Clinical usage	Drug of choice for the treatment of infections caused by streptococci, meningococci, penicillin-susceptible pneumococci, and for the treatment of syphilis. The oral form of penicillin is indicated for minor infections only.	Ampicillin is primarily indicated for the treatment of infections due to enterococcus and streptococcal species. Amoxicillin is primarily used for the treatment of upper and lower respiratory tract infections due to streptococcal species or non–β-lactamase-producing *H. influenzae*.	These agents are primarily used for the treatment of infections caused by β-lactamase–producing staphylococci. Antistaphylococcal penicillins also are active against penicillin-susceptible strains of streptococci.

(Continued)

THUMBNAIL: Penicillins *(Continued)*

Antibiotic	Penicillins	Aminopenicillins	Antistaphylococcal Penicillins
Activity	Primarily gram-positive organisms: streptococcal species, enterococcus, penicillin-susceptible pneumococci, *Treponema pallidum*. Few gram-negative anaerobic organisms and *Clostridium* species.	Primarily gram-positive organisms such as streptococcal species, enterococcus, penicillin-susceptible pneumococci, *Treponema pallidum*. Compared with penicillin, aminopenicillins have greater gram-negative activity. *H. influenzae* (non–β-lactamase producing).	Methicillin-susceptible staphylococci, penicillin-susceptible strains of streptococci and pneumococci.
Absorption	Oral penicillin has poor bioavailability.	Amoxicillin has very good bioavailability.	Dicloxacillin has good bioavailability.
Distribution	Penicillins are widely distributed throughout the body. Penicillins penetrate poorly into CSF. However, in the presence of inflamed meninges, CSF concentrations are adequate to treat bacterial meningitis due to susceptible organisms.		
Elimination	Penicillin and ampicillin are excreted by the kidneys into the urine. Dose adjustments are required in the setting of renal dysfunction.		Nafcillin is primarily cleared by biliary excretion while dicloxacillin is eliminated by both kidney and biliary excretion. No dose adjustments are needed in the setting of renal or hepatic dysfunction.
Adverse reactions	Overall, the penicillins are well tolerated. The most common adverse effects are due to hypersensitivity reactions. Hypersensitivity reactions can be simply categorized as immediate reactions (type 1) or late reactions. Type 1 reactions are IgE mediated and are often associated with systemic manifestations, such as diffuse erythema, pruritus, urticaria, angioedema, and bronchospasm. The most severe yet rare IgE-mediated side effect is anaphylaxis (0.05%). Type 1 reactions usually occur within 72 hrs of administration. Late reactions usually occur 72 hrs after drug administration. The most common late reactions include skin rashes characterized as maculopapular or morbilliform rashes. Rarely, nafcillin may cause **neutropenia.** Seizures in high doses, vaginal moniliasis, and *Clostridium difficile* infection also can occur with all penicillins.		
Drug interactions	In general, there are no clinically significant drug interactions associated with the penicillins. Dicloxacillin may increase the effects of warfarin.		

QUESTIONS

1. A 42-year-old woman presents to her primary care provider with a 3-day history of redness, swelling, and increasing pain in her right arm after falling off her ladder while washing her windows. The area is warm to the touch with a defined erythematous border. She has NKDA. She has a temperature of 38.5°C. The presumptive diagnosis is cellulitis. What would be an appropriate empiric outpatient regimen?

   A. Clarithromycin
   B. Nafcillin
   C. Penicillin
   D. Cephalexin
   E. Ciprofloxacin

2. A 32-year-old woman is admitted to the hospital with cellulitis after being bitten by a spider 5 days ago. She is empirically started on nafcillin; however, 10 hours later the patient develops hives and difficulty breathing. What alternatives should be considered?

   A. Cefazolin
   B. Ampicillin
   C. Ceftriaxone
   D. Clindamycin
   E. Gentamicin

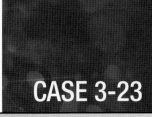

CASE 3-23 Cephalosporins

HPI: AL is a 42-year-old febrile and unresponsive man who is brought to the ED by a friend. Over the past several days he was experiencing fever, chills, and a worsening productive cough.

PE: He has a temperature of 40.1°C; BP 85/55; RR 25; and HR 115. Crackles were heard throughout both lung fields.

Labs: Lab tests revealed a WBC count of 22,000/µL (98% PMNs) and Cr of 2.0 mg/dL. Results of lumbar puncture showed the following: WBC count 4,000/µL, protein 120 mg/dL, and glucose 35 mg/dL. Results of studies on blood, CSF, sputum cultures, and Gram stains are pending. AL has NKDA.

THOUGHT QUESTIONS

- What are the most common organisms associated with adult meningitis?
- Which cephalosporins are appropriate for the treatment of meningitis?
- What adverse effects are associated with cephalosporins?

BASIC SCIENCE REVIEW AND DISCUSSION

The etiology of bacterial meningitis is highly dependent on the patient's age and underlying medical conditions. The most common causes of bacterial meningitis in an immunocompetent adult is *Streptococcus pneumoniae* and *Neisseria meningitidis*. In contrast, the most likely causes of bacterial meningitis in a neonate are group B *Streptococcus*, *Escherichia coli*, and *Listeria monocytogenes*. Bacterial meningitis is a life-threatening infection that necessitates prompt antibiotic administration. Predisposing factors for meningitis in adults include alcohol abuse, splenectomy, chronic obstructive airway disease, and upper respiratory tract infections. The treatment of bacterial meningitis is challenging because antibiotics must cross the blood–brain barrier to reach the CSF. There are a limited number of antibiotics that have adequate penetration into the CSF. Historically, *N. meningitidis* and *Streptococcus pneumoniae* have been susceptible to penicillin G. However, over the past several years in the United States strains of *Streptococcus pneumoniae* demonstrating intermediate and high-level penicillin resistance have emerged, making treatment even more challenging. Third-generation cephalosporins are a mainstay in the management of bacterial meningitis because these agents are active against *N. meningitidis* and *Streptococcus pneumoniae*.

Cephalosporins are divided into four classes: first, second, third, and fourth generations. This nomenclature delineates when these agents were developed and, more importantly, their spectrum of activity. In general, the cephalosporins are a heterogeneous group of drugs with differences in spectrum of activity and pharmacokinetics. In general, as the generation increases from first to fourth, the amount of gram-negative coverage increases while gram-positive coverage decreases.

More specifically, first-generation cephalosporins are very active against *Staphylococcus aureus* and *Streptococcus* species, whereas gram-negative activity is limited to *Proteus mirabilis*, *E. coli*, and *Klebsiella pneumoniae*, which can easily be remembered by the pneumonic **PEK.** The second-generation cephalosporins

are less active than the first-generation cephalosporins against gram-positive bacteria but have increased gram-negative activity that includes *Haemophilus influenzae* and *N. meningitidis* as well as the **PEK** organisms **(HNPEK).** Among gram-negative bacteria, the third-generation cephalosporins are also active against *Serratia* species; therefore, they cover the **HNPEKS** organisms. Finally the activity of fourth-generation cephalosporins is expanded to include *Enterobacter* species and *Citrobacter* species **(HENPECKS).**

Of note, ceftazidime and cefepime are the only two cephalosporins active against *Pseudomonas aeruginosa*. The third- and fourth-generation cephalosporins are active against most staphylococci but less so than the first-generation cephalosporins. However, ceftazidime has very weak antistaphylococcal activity. Cephalosporins are available in both PO and IV formulations. The pharmacologic properties of the cephalosporins are relatively similar, with a few exceptions. The cephalosporins distribute well into most tissues except for the CSF, prostate, and eye. However, the third- and fourth-generation cephalosporins have adequate CSF concentrations in the setting of inflamed meninges. The majority of the cephalosporins are excreted renally via active tubular secretion, except for ceftriaxone. Since ceftriaxone has nonrenal elimination, there is no need to adjust the dose in patients with renal insufficiency. The elimination T½ for most of the cephalosporins is 1 to 2 hours, except for cefotetan (3 hours), cefixime (4 hours), and ceftriaxone (8 hours).

Overall, the cephalosporins are remarkably well tolerated. The most common adverse effects are **hypersensitivity** reactions such as skin rashes, fever, and hemolytic anemia. Cross-reactivity between penicillins and cephalosporins ranges from 5 to 10%. Even though some patients with a history of penicillin allergy may tolerate cephalosporins, patients with a history of anaphylaxis to penicillin should not receive cephalosporins.

Ceftriaxone is associated with biliary sludging or **pseudocholelithiasis** due to precipitation of the drug in bile. This occurs when its solubility in bile is exceeded when used in high doses. Ceftriaxone and cefotaxime are the preferred third-generation cephalosporins for the empiric treatment of bacterial meningitis since these agents are the most active cephalosporins against *Streptococcus pneumoniae*. Cefotetan has a methylthiotetrazole group that may inhibit vitamin K synthesis and cause **hypoprothrombinemia** and bleeding disorders. In addition, **disulfiram-like reactions** can occur if coadministered with alcohol-containing medications.

CASE CONCLUSION

Because the etiology of bacterial meningitis in AL is most likely attributable to *Streptococcus pneumoniae* or *N. meningitidis*, ceftriaxone, a third-generation cephalosporin, is started empirically. Ceftriaxone will also treat his potential community-acquired pneumonia. Even though the patient has some degree of renal insufficiency (Cr 2.0 mg/dL), the dose of ceftriaxone does not need to be adjusted since it is hepatically eliminated.

THUMBNAIL: Cephalosporins

	First Generation	Second Generation	Third Generation	Fourth Generation
Available agents	PO: Cephradine Cephalexin Cefadroxil IV: Cefazolin	PO: Cefuroxime Axetil Cefprozil IV: Cefuroxime Cefotetan Cefoxitin	PO: Cefixime Cefpodoxime Cefdinir Cefditoren IV: Ceftriaxone Ceftazidime Cefotaxime Ceftizoxime	IV: Cefepime
MOA	Inhibition of cell wall synthesis. **Bactericidal.**			
Activity	*S. aureus, Streptococcus* species, *P. mirabilis, E. coli, K. pneumoniae*	*S. aureus, Streptococcus* species, *H. influenzae* (including β-lactamase–producing), *N. gonorrhoea, P. mirabilis, E. coli, K. pneumoniae.* Cefoxitin and cefotetan have good activity against *Bacteroides fragilis.*	*S. aureus* (not as active compared with 1st generation), *Streptococcus* species, *H. influenzae* (including β-lactamase–producing), *N. gonorrhoea, P. mirabilis, E. coli, K. pneumoniae, Serratia marcescens, P. aeruginosa* (ceftazidime only)	*S. aureus, Streptococcus* species, *H. influenzae* (including beta-lactamase producing), *Enterobacter* species, *N. gonorrhea, P. mirabilis, E. coli, Citrobacter* species, *K. pneumoniae, Serratia marcescens, Acinetobacter* species, *P. aeruginosa*
Bioavailability	All oral cephalosporins have good absorption.			
Distribution	Widely distributed, except to the prostate, CSF, and eye. In the presence of inflamed meninges, adequate CSF concentrations are achieved by the third- and fourth-generation cephalosporins.			
Elimination	Renally eliminated (>70%) via active tubular secretion and glomerular filtration, except ceftriaxone, which has nonrenal clearance (biliary). All renally eliminated cephalosporins require dosage adjustment in renal insufficiency.			
Adverse effects	**Hypersensitivity reactions:** Incidence is 5–10% in patients with history of penicillin allergy vs. 1–2.5% of patients with no penicillin allergy history. Diarrhea: most common with ceftriaxone and oral agents. Pseudomembranous colitis can occur with any cephalosporin. Pseudocholelithiasis (biliary sludging) can occur with ceftriaxone in high doses. Cefotetan can cause hypoprothrombinemia and, if coadministered with alcohol, disulfiram reactions.			
Drug interactions	No clinically significant drug interaction			

QUESTIONS

1. JK is a 32-year-old man who was diagnosed with cellulitis. A detailed medication history taken by the medical student reveals that JK experienced anaphylaxis after receiving amoxicillin about a year ago. Which of the following antibiotics would you avoid prescribing in JK?

A. Cefuroxime
B. Clarithromycin
C. Penicillin
D. Clindamycin
E. A and C

2. MN is a 54-year-old man who was diagnosed with an intra-abdominal abscess after sustaining a stab wound. He is started on a 21-day course of cefotetan. His social history includes drinking two beers per night. His PMH is significant for PUD, HTN, and seasonal allergies. His medications include omeprazole, enalapril, and cetirizine. Which of the following statements are correct?

A. While on cefotetan, MN will have to increase his omeprazole dose.

B. While on cefotetan, MN will have to increase his enalapril dose.

C. While on cefotetan, MN will have to stop drinking alcohol.

D. While on cefotetan, MN may resume his current medications and lifestyle.

E. None of the above.

HPI: MT is a 63-year-old man who presents to the clinic complaining of sudden onset of fever, headache, malaise, and a sore throat. He says he has been feeling ill since taking care of his sick granddaughter, who had group A streptococcal pharyngitis. He has a history of AF and is currently being treated with digoxin and warfarin. He has a history of an allergic reaction to penicillin, which resulted in laryngeal edema, and he has a 30-pack per year tobacco history. A chest radiograph done in the clinic is clear. A rapid antigen detection test is positive for group A *Streptococcus*.

PE: T 39.1°C; BP 120/60; HR 130 (irreg); RR 24

THOUGHT QUESTIONS

- What is the spectrum of activity of the macrolides?
- Which macrolide has poor *Haemophilus influenzae* coverage?
- What is the MOA of macrolides?
- Which macrolide (erythromycin, clarithromycin, or azithromycin) may cause drug interactions with his current medications?
- Which of the three macrolides is most likely to cause GI upset?

BASIC SCIENCE REVIEW AND DISCUSSION

Macrolides are appropriate antibiotics for the management of respiratory tract infections because they are active against *Streptococcus pneumoniae*, *Streptococcus pyogenes* (group A streptococci), and atypical organisms such as *Legionella pneumophila*, *Mycoplasma pneumoniae*, and *Chlamydia pneumoniae*. The newer generation macrolides such as clarithromycin and the **azalide** azithromycin also have reliable coverage against *H. influenzae*, unlike erythromycin. However, macrolide-resistant *Streptococcus* is becoming an increasingly important issue in the outpatient treatment of respiratory tract infections such as community-acquired pneumonia. Thus, selection of appropriate antibiotics should be based on local resistance patterns.

Erythromycin inhibits RNA-dependent protein synthesis by binding to the bacterial 50S ribosomal RNA, by blocking aminoacyl translocation reactions, and by blocking formation of the initiation complex. It is also a strong inhibitor of hepatic **cytochrome P450** (CYP450) and will increase the serum concentration of warfarin, prolonging the INR. Erythromycin increases the bioavailability of digoxin, also leading to increased serum concentrations. Clarithromycin, although not as strong an inhibitor against CYP450, may still increase digoxin and warfarin levels. Azithromycin does not inhibit CYP450 and will be least likely to cause drug-drug interactions in this patient. Erythromycin is a **motilin** receptor agonist and can cause abdominal cramping and diarrhea. Incidentally, erythromycin is often used in patients with diabetic gastroparesis to stimulate GI motility.

CASE CONCLUSION

The treatment of choice for group A streptococcal pharyngitis is penicillin. However, due to MT's hypersensitivity reaction to penicillins, macrolides are an appropriate alternative choice. Because erythromycin may increase digoxin and warfarin levels, azithromycin is started for MT's pharyngitis.

⚙ THUMBNAIL: Macrolides

Prototypical agent: Erythromycin. Clarithromycin and azithromycin developed to overcome limitations of erythromycin: poor bioavailability, poor GI tolerability, need for frequent dosing (short T½) and limited *H. influenzae* coverage.

Clinical usage: Primarily as an antibacterial agent for the treatment of respiratory tract infections and sexually transmitted diseases. Also used for treatment of PUD in combination with other agents. Erythromycin is considered the drug of choice for whooping cough.

MOA: Block protein synthesis at 50S ribosomal subunit. The antibacterial action of the macrolides is bacteriostatic.

Activity: Macrolides are active against gram-positive organisms, particularly pneumococci, streptococci, and staphylococci. Some gram-negative organisms, such as *Neisseria* species and *Bordetella pertussis* (whooping cough), are also covered. Other organisms covered include some *Mycobacterium*, *Legionella*, *Mycoplasma*, and *Chlamydia* species. Although azithromycin and clarithromycin are active against *H. influenzae* and *Moraxella catarrhalis*, erythromycin is less active. Clarithromycin also has activity against *Helicobacter pylori*.

(Continued)

THUMBNAIL: Macrolides *(Continued)*

Pharmacokinetics

Absorption: Erythromycin is poorly absorbed orally and is readily broken down by stomach acid. Thus, erythromycin is enteric coated to increase absorption.

Distribution: Macrolides widely distribute into tissue and obtain high intracellular levels.

Elimination: All macrolides are hepatically eliminated. Clarithromycin is hepatically activated to the 14-OH metabolite. T½: erythromycin < clarithromycin < azithromycin.

Adverse reactions: Erythromycin can cause nausea, vomiting, diarrhea, and abdominal cramping. GI intolerance due to erythromycin is due to direct stimulation of the motilin receptor, leading to increased GI motility. This occurs with both the IV and PO formulation. Although rare, all macrolides can cause hepatotoxicity. The estolate formulation of erythromycin has been associated with cholestatic hepatitis in pregnant women. In high doses, all macrolides can cause **tinnitus.**

Drug interactions: Erythromycin is a strong inhibitor of CYP450. CYP450 inhibition decreases with the newer macrolides. Thus, clarithromycin is a mild inhibitor, and azithromycin has no effect on CYP450.

QUESTIONS

1. CT is a 3-year-old boy brought in by his mother to see the pediatrician for a follow-up appointment. CT was started on high-dose amoxicillin 3 days ago for acute otitis media. CT continues to be febrile with no clinical improvement on amoxicillin. Tympanocentesis reveals gram-negative coccobacilli on Gram stain. What is the most appropriate treatment for CT at this time?

A. Amoxicillin + clavulanate
B. Levofloxacin
C. Doxycycline
D. Continue amoxicillin
E. Erythromycin

Tetracyclines

HPI: VD, a 23-year-old man about to leave for a Caribbean cruise, complains of mild dysuria with 3 days of painless urethral discharge that started about 2 weeks after his last intercourse. He has been sexually active with his girlfriend for the past 2 to 3 months but admits to being promiscuous. He denies fever.

PE: On exam he has no lymphadenopathy or penile lesions. Exam is remarkable for a white urethral discharge. Gram stain and culture for *Neisseria gonorrhoeae* were negative. A presumptive diagnosis of nongonococcal urethritis (NGU) is made.

THOUGHT QUESTIONS

- What is the most common cause of NGU?
- Which tetracycline is preferred for the treatment of NGU?
- What are the adverse effects associated with the tetracyclines?

BASIC SCIENCE REVIEW AND DISCUSSION

Chlamydia trachomatis is the primary cause of NGU, followed by *Ureaplasma urealyticum*. Doxycycline is the tetracycline of choice for the treatment of NGU because it has activity against both organisms. There are three tetracyclines that are primarily used for the treatment of infections: tetracycline, doxycycline, and minocycline. Demeclocycline is primarily used for the treatment of chronic syndrome of inappropriate secretion of antidiuretic hormone (SIADH). Doxycycline and minocycline have the advantage of twice-daily dosing, whereas tetracycline is dosed four times daily. An alternative to doxycycline for the treatment of NGU is a single 1-g dose of azithromycin. Although azithromycin is an expensive alternative, it may be useful in patients with poor compliance. Both regimens have been shown to be equally effective.

Doxycycline can cause nausea, vomiting, and diarrhea. The bioavailability of doxycycline is reduced if coadministered with multivalent ions such as iron or magnesium. However, unlike tetracycline, it can be administered with food and dairy products. In addition, patients taking tetracyclines may experience **photosensitivity,** especially if they are fair skinned. Patients taking tetracyclines should avoid prolonged exposure to sunlight.

CASE CONCLUSION

VD is started on doxycycline for 7 days. The patient is instructed to avoid prolonged exposure to sunlight and to avoid concomitant dosing with antacids or any other medications that may contain multivalent cations.

THUMBNAIL: Tetracyclines

Available agents: Tetracycline, doxycycline, minocycline

Clinical usage: Tetracyclines are effective for sexually transmitted diseases caused by chlamydia and syphilis. They are also commonly used for the treatment of community-acquired pneumonia, Lyme disease, and Rocky Mountain spotted fever and in combination with other agents for *Helicobacter pylori.*

MOA: Tetracyclines inhibit protein synthesis by binding with the 30S and 50S ribosomal subunits of bacteria. The antibacterial action of the tetracyclines is **bacteriostatic.**

Activity: Tetracyclines are active against gram-positive organisms, such as pneumococci, *Staphylococcus aureus,* and gram-negative organisms such as *Haemophilus influenzae, H. ducreyi, Yersinia pestis, Bartonella* species, and *Klebsiella* species. Other organisms covered include *Legionella, Mycoplasma,* and *Chlamydia* species, *Borrelia burgdorferi,* and some mycobacteria.

Pharmacokinetics

Absorption: Tetracyclines are well absorbed after oral administration; however, absorption is impaired by food, by multivalent cations (Ca^{+2}, Mg^{+2}, Fe^{+2}, or Al^{+3}), and by dairy products.

Distribution: Tetracyclines widely distribute into tissue and body fluids except CSF.

Elimination: Tetracycline and minocycline are excreted mainly in bile and urine. Doxycycline is eliminated by nonrenal mechanisms. Doxycycline is the tetracycline of choice in patients with renal insufficiency. T½ doxycycline = minocycline > tetracycline.

(Continued)

THUMBNAIL: Tetracyclines *(Continued)*

Rarely, the tetracyclines can cause esophageal ulcers. Patients with esophageal obstruction may be at increased risk. Demeclocycline can cause diabetes insipidus.

Adverse reactions: Tetracyclines can cause nausea, vomiting, and diarrhea. Administering doxycycline with food can minimize these effects. The use of tetracyclines during pregnancy or in children younger than age 8 years is contraindicated because it can cause discoloration of teeth and inhibit normal bone growth. The tetracyclines may cause photosensitivity, so patients should avoid prolonged exposure to sunlight. Doxycycline and minocycline can cause dizziness, vertigo, and nausea. Tetracycline and minocycline should be avoided in patients with renal insufficiency because toxic levels may accumulate. *Clostridium difficile* infections and monilia also can occur.

Drug interactions: The bioavailability of tetracyclines is significantly decreased when administered with antacids containing aluminum, calcium, or magnesium, with iron-containing products, or with food. Food or dairy products do not affect the bioavailability of doxycycline or minocycline.

QUESTIONS

1. A 32-year-old woman in her first trimester of pregnancy presents with a mucopurulent vaginal discharge and dysuria. She is diagnosed with NGU. Which of the following antibiotics should be avoided?

   A. Azithromycin
   B. Doxycycline
   C. Penicillin
   D. Cefuroxime
   E. Ceftriaxone

2. A 46-year-old woman is prescribed doxycycline for a diagnosis of community-acquired pneumonia. Her PMH is significant for iron-deficient anemia, PUD, HTN, a recent DVT, and headaches. Her current medications include ferrous sulfate, ibuprofen, enalapril, acetaminophen, famotidine, and warfarin. Which of her following medications is most likely to result in decreased levels of doxycycline?

   A. Acetaminophen
   B. Warfarin
   C. Ferrous sulfate
   D. Famotidine
   E. Ibuprofen

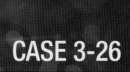

CASE 3-26

Fluoroquinolones and Trimethoprim-Sulfamethoxazole

HPI: LD is a 19-year-old female college sophomore who presents to the student health clinic with a 3-day history of dysuria. Mild suprapubic tenderness with no flank pain was revealed on physical exam. No vaginal discharge or lesions were seen. LD's last menstrual period was 2 weeks ago. She is sexually active and uses a diaphragm with spermicide for birth control. Her medications include ferrous sulfate and acetaminophen. She has NKDA. A clean-catch midstream urine sample shows gram-negative rods on Gram stain.

PE: T 37.9°; BP 120/78; HR 80; RR 15

THOUGHT QUESTIONS

- What are the leading organisms that cause UTIs?
- What are some of LD's risk factors for a UTI?
- Which agents achieve high urinary concentrations?

BASIC SCIENCE REVIEW AND DISCUSSION

UTIs can be classified by anatomic site of involvement into lower and upper UTIs. Lower UTIs include cystitis, urethritis, prostatitis, and epididymitis, whereas upper urinary tract infections include pyelonephritis. UTIs can be further classified as complicated or uncomplicated. In females with a structurally normal urinary tract, both cystitis and pyelonephritis are considered uncomplicated UTIs. UTIs in men, elderly individuals, pregnant women, or patients with in-dwelling catheters or anatomic or functional abnormalities are considered complicated UTIs.

Escherichia coli is the causative pathogen in 80% of infections. Other organisms that can cause UTIs include *Staphylococcus saprophyticus* and *Enterococcus* species.

The antimicrobial agents most commonly used to treat uncomplicated UTIs include TMP-SMX, trimethoprim alone, β-lactams, fluoroquinolones, nitrofurantoin, and fosfomycin. These agents are used primarily due to their tolerability, spectrum of activity against the suspected uropathogens, and favorable pharmacokinetic profiles. All the antimicrobial agents approved for the treatment of UTIs achieve inhibitory urinary concentrations that significantly exceed serum levels. Because most uncomplicated UTIs are treated empirically, therapy should be based on local resistance patterns in the community to ensure that the most appropriate antimicrobial agent is used.

CASE CONCLUSION

LD was treated with a 3-day course of TMP-SMX with total resolution of her symptoms (Table 3-6).

TABLE 3-6 Quinolone Activity by Generation

	First Generation	Second Generation	Third Generation
Agents	Nalidixic acid Cinoxacin Norfloxacin Enoxacin	Ciprofloxacin Ofloxacin	Levofloxacin Moxifloxacin Gatifloxacin
Spectrum of activity	**Gram-negative** *Proteus* species ***E. coli*** *Klebsiella* species *Citrobacter* species *Acinetobacter* species *Pseudomonas aeruginosa* *Enterobacter* species *Serratia marcescens* **Intestinal pathogens** *Shigella* species *Campylobacter jejuni* *Salmonella* species	**Same as first generation** ***Plus*:** **Gram-positive** *Staphylococcus aureus* *Staphylococcus epidermidis* **Respiratory pathogens** *Haemophilus influenzae* *Moraxella catarrhalis* *Legionella* species **Genital pathogens** *Neisseria gonorrhoeae* *Chlamydia trachomatis*	**Same as first and second generation** ***Plus*:** **Gram-positive** *Streptococcus pneumoniae* **Atypicals** *Chlamydia pneumoniae* *Mycoplasma pneumoniae* *Mycobacterium* species **Anaerobes** *Bacteroides fragilis* (moxifloxacin)

THUMBNAIL: Fluoroquinolones and Trimethoprim-Sulfamethoxazole

	Fluoroquinolones	*TMP-SMX*
Clinical usage	Quinolones are divided into "generations" based on their spectrum of activity. The higher the generation, the broader the spectrum of activity. First generation: UTIs Second and third generations: UTIs, prostatitis, respiratory tract infections, sinusitis, infectious diarrhea, uncomplicated skin and skin structure infections, traveler's diarrhea	UTIs Prostatitis Acute otitis media Exacerbations of chronic bronchitis Treatment and prophylaxis of *Pneumocystis carinii* infections Traveler's diarrhea
MOA	Inhibition of topoisomerase II (DNA-gyrase) and topoisomerase IV. Inhibition of topoisomerases disrupts DNA replication and transcription, resulting in bacterial cell death.	SMX interferes with bacterial folic acid syntheses via inhibition of dihydrofolic acid formation from para-aminobenzoic acid. TMP inhibits dihydrofolic acid reduction to tetrahydrofolate, resulting in sequential inhibition of enzymes of the folic acid pathway. TMP and SMX are synergistic when used together.
Activity	Bactericidal with varying activity against gram-positive, gram-negative, and anaerobic organisms based on generation. Excellent activity against Enterobacteriaceae (such as *E. coli*). Moderate activity against *Enterococcus* species for systemic infections, but the high urinary concentrations are adequate to successfully eradicate the organism in UTIs. Moxifloxacin and gatifloxacin have expanded spectrums of activity that include improved gram-positive (*Streptococcus pneumoniae*) and anaerobic activity (*Bacteroides fragilis*).	Bactericidal with varying activity against gram-positive, gram-negative, and anaerobic organisms based on generation. Gram-positive organisms, particularly *Staphylococcus aureus* Gram-negative organisms: *Haemophilus influenzae, E. coli, Listeria monocytogenes, Moraxella catarrhalis,* and *Salmonella* species Other organisms: *Pneumocystis carinii, Toxoplasma gondii, Nocardia* species, and *Stenotrophomonas maltophilia*
Pharmacokinetics		
Absorption	High Ciprofloxacin < levofloxacin = gatifloxacin = moxifloxacin	High (PO dose equivalent to IV)
Distribution	Wide distribution into body fluids and tissues, including the prostate	
Metabolism	Hepatic Ciprofloxacin = moxifloxacin > levofloxacin = gatifloxacin	Hepatic
Elimination	Renal Gatifloxacin = levofloxacin > ciprofloxacin > moxifloxacin	Renal elimination as metabolites and unchanged drug
Adverse effects	Well tolerated Common adverse effects: CNS side effects (dizziness, headache, insomnia), rash, nausea, vomiting, photosensitivity, elevated transaminases and tremor Rare side effects: cartilage toxicity, tendon rupture and QT_c prolongation. An increase in QT_c prolongation and torsade de pointes has been associated with the use of fluoroquinolones, particularly the newer generations.	Well tolerated Common adverse effects: rash, nausea, vomiting and photosensitivity. Rare: hepatotoxicity (increased transaminases), anemia, leukopenia, and Stevens-Johnson syndrome. TMP-SMX should be used with caution in patients with G6PD deficiency since this can cause hemolytic anemia.
Drug interactions	Cytochrome interactions: CYP450 inhibitors Norfloxacin > ciprofloxacin > moxifloxacin > levofloxacin = gatifloxacin Warfarin: The exact warfarin-quinolone drug interaction is unknown. Reduction of intestinal flora responsible for vitamin K production by antibiotics is probable, as are decreased metabolism and clearance of warfarin due to CYP450 inhibition by the quinolones. Metal cations such as aluminum, magnesium, calcium, iron, zinc, and multivitamins with minerals may chelate with fluoroquinolones and decrease the oral absorption if administered concurrently.	TMP-SMX is a known inhibitor of CYP450 and can substantially increase warfarin plasma concentrations and hypoprothrombinemic response.

QUESTIONS

1. HG is a 65-year-old man diagnosed with acute prostatitis. He has an allergy to sulfa drugs, which give him urticaria. Which of the following agents would be the most appropriate option for his prostatitis?

    A. Cephalexin
    B. TMP-SMX
    C. Ciprofloxacin
    D. Amoxicillin
    E. Nitrofurantoin

2. JP is a 35-year-old woman who presents with an uncomplicated UTI. She has a history of cardiac arrhythmias for which she takes amiodarone and digoxin. Her allergies include anaphylaxis to sulfa medications. Which of the following medications would be the best choice to treat her UTI?

    A. Gatifloxacin
    B. Moxifloxacin
    C. TMP-SMX
    D. TMP

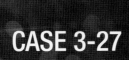

CASE 3-27 | Aminoglycosides

HPI: After 2 days of treatment for her UTI, LD now returns to the clinic complaining of chills, fever, nausea, flank pain, and increased lower tract symptoms (frequency, dysuria, and urgency).

THOUGHT QUESTIONS

- What are the most likely organisms to be causing LD's pyelonephritis?
- What are appropriate antibiotics that can be used for the treatment of pyelonephritis?
- What toxicities are associated with aminoglycosides?
- What dosing regimens are available for aminoglycosides?

BASIC SCIENCE REVIEW AND DISCUSSION

The infecting organisms causing pyelonephritis are typically similar to the infecting pathogens responsible for lower UTIs. In uncomplicated cases, antibiotics used for treatment of lower tract infections also can be used for the treatment of upper tract infections. These agents typically include fluoroquinolones and TMP-SMX. In more serious cases, pyelonephritis may be accompanied by bacteremia, warranting hospitalization and parenteral therapy.

Aminoglycosides are parenteral antibiotics most widely used in the treatment of infections due to enteric gram-negative bacteria. However, aminoglycosides are often used in combination with cell wall-active agents such as β-lactams or vancomycin for treatment of endocarditis. Aminoglycosides initially diffuse passively across the bacterial outer membrane and are then actively transported into the cytoplasm. This active transport is inhibited in low pH or anaerobic conditions. Once inside the cytoplasm, aminoglycosides inhibit protein synthesis by binding to the bacterial 30S ribosomal subunit and preventing the formation of the initiation complex and interfering with the accuracy of translation and translocation. Because aminoglycosides are inhibited in acidic or anaerobic conditions, aminoglycosides are not active against anaerobic bacteria or in low pH conditions such as abscesses or necrotic tissue.

Aminoglycosides are most notably associated with **ototoxicity** and **nephrotoxicity** and have a narrow therapeutic window. Risk factors include prolonged therapy, preexisting renal dysfunction, elderly patients, and concurrent use of other ototoxic or nephrotoxic agents. Ototoxicity typically presents as cochlear (tinnitus, high-frequency hearing loss) and, not as commonly, vestibular toxicity (vertigo, ataxia). Nephrotoxicity due to aminoglycosides typically presents as an increase in serum creatinine or a decrease in creatinine clearance. Rarely, in high doses, aminoglycosides can cause neuromuscular paralysis due to a concentration-dependent inhibition of presynaptic release and postsynaptic binding of acetylcholine. This can lead to tingling, muscle paralysis, and apnea.

There are two dosing regimens used for aminoglycosides: once daily and conventional (three times daily). Because aminoglycosides exhibit **concentration-dependent killing,** increasing concentrations kill an increasing proportion of bacteria. In addition, aminoglycosides exhibit a **postantibiotic effect.** Thus, antibacterial activity persists even when the drug falls below levels that are detectable in serum. By dosing aminoglycosides once daily, higher peak concentrations are achieved, leading to a more rapid bactericidal effect and longer postantibiotic effect. The less frequent dosing of once-daily aminoglycosides leads to lower or nondetectable trough concentrations and may lead to less nephrotoxicity.

CASE CONCLUSION

LD is admitted to the hospital for treatment of her pyelonephritis. On admission, blood and urine cultures are drawn and LD is empirically started on ampicillin and gentamicin for coverage for *Enterococcus* species and gram-negative organisms pending culture results. Parenteral therapy is used because LD is nauseated and is exhibiting signs of a systemic infection. Two days later, cultures return positive for *Escherichia coli*.

THUMBNAIL: Aminoglycosides

Available agents: Gentamicin, tobramycin, amikacin, streptomycin, neomycin

MOA: Irreversible protein synthesis inhibitor that binds to the 30S subunit of bacterial ribosomes; prevents the formation of the initiation complex, interferes with the translational accuracy of the mRNA, and inhibits translocation.

Activity: Aerobic bacteria only. Primary activity is against aerobic gram-negative bacilli. Tobramycin is more active against *Pseudomonas aeruginosa*. Can be used in combination with cell wall-active agents for treatment of infections due to staphylococcal or enterococcal species. Streptomycin is used for infections due to mycobacteria.

Pharmacokinetics

Absorption: Poorly absorbed orally, thus limited to parenteral use; however, neomycin can be used for GI decontamination.

Distribution: Requires aerobic environment for activity. Effectiveness is reduced in low pH or anaerobic environments, such as abscess fluid or necrotic tissue. Does not cross the blood–brain barrier. Treatment of CNS infections requires intraventricular or intrathecal administration.

Elimination: Renal. Excretion occurs via glomerular filtration and is directly proportional to creatinine clearance. Dose adjustment is needed in renal impairment.

Adverse reactions: Irreversible ototoxicity (cochlear and vestibular) in 0.5 to 5% of patients. High-frequency hearing is affected first and can progress to low-frequency hearing loss. Reversible nephrotoxicity is seen in up to 25% of patients, particularly in patients receiving aminoglycosides for more than 7 days. Rarely, neuromuscular paralysis (curare-like effect) can occur.

QUESTIONS

1. KC is a 45-year-old man receiving ampicillin and gentamicin for endocarditis due to *Enterococcus faecalis*. He has a baseline serum Cr of 1.5 mg/dL secondary to uncontrolled diabetes mellitus. His other medications include furosemide, aspirin, and captopril. During his second week of therapy, KC complains of ringing in his ears and a sensation of fullness. Risk factors for ototoxicity in KC include:

A. Age
B. Preexisting renal dysfunction
C. Prolonged therapy
D. Furosemide
E. Ampicillin
F. Captopril
G. A, B, and C
H. B, C, and D
I. All of the above

2. CJ is a 7-year-old boy with neuroblastoma receiving chemotherapy. He is currently neutropenic and is febrile at 38.2°C. His physicians would like to empirically cover him for *Pseudomonas aeruginosa* with two agents and he is started on cefepime and an aminoglycoside. Which aminoglycoside would be the best choice?

A. Gentamicin
B. Streptomycin
C. Tobramycin
D. Amikacin
E. Neomycin

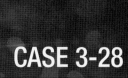

CASE 3-28   Vancomycin

HPI: KS is a 25-year-old woman with acute lymphocytic leukemia (ALL) who presents to the oncology clinic complaining that she has had fevers and chills for the past day. KM receives chemotherapy via a peripherally inserted central catheter (PICC) inserted in her left antecubital vein, last dose 3 weeks ago.

PE: T 39.6°C; BP 100/60; HR 110; RR; lungs are clear. Her PICC appears hot and erythematous.

Labs: WBC 3500/μL; Hgb 14 gm/dL; Hct 40%; Plt 178,000 mm³; Cr 0.7; BUN 20 mg/dL

THOUGHT QUESTIONS

- What is the most likely organism to cause a catheter-related infection in KM?
- What are common side effects of vancomycin?
- How is toxicity or efficacy of vancomycin assessed?

BASIC SCIENCE REVIEW AND DISCUSSION

Coagulase-negative staphylococci, such as *Staphylococcus epidermidis*, are the most common causes of catheter-related infections due to their ability to adhere to prosthetic material. *Staphylococcus aureus*, aerobic gram-negative bacilli, and *Candida albicans* are also common causes of catheter-related infections. Depending on local susceptibility patterns, MRSA may represent up to 20% of all isolates. In contrast, upward of 80% of *Staphylococcus epidermidis* are methicillin resistant (MRSE).

In the past, side effects attributed to vancomycin were most likely due to impurities in the earlier preparations. Today, the majority of side effects due to vancomycin are minor and include **"red man"** or **"red neck"** syndrome, rash, or chemical **phlebitis** at the infusion site. The potential for vancomycin to cause **nephrotoxicity** and **ototoxicity** remains controversial. Early reports of vancomycin-induced nephrotoxicity and ototoxicity may be exaggerated. In patients who receive vancomycin alone, nephrotoxicity and ototoxicity appears to be rare. However, nephrotoxicity can be enhanced when given in combination with an agent known to cause nephrotoxicity, such as an aminoglycoside. Similarly, ototoxicity can occur when vancomycin is given in combination with a known ototoxic agent, such as erythromycin or an aminoglycoside. When given for prolonged periods, vancomycin can cause **neutropenia** in rare cases.

Serum monitoring of vancomycin levels should be done in patients receiving prolonged courses of vancomycin, particularly in the setting of preexisting renal insufficiency. However, elevated trough levels have been poorly correlated with the development of nephrotoxicity. Similarly, a relationship between vancomycin levels and ototoxicity has not been well established. Trough levels are typically used to evaluate efficacy because vancomycin exhibits **time-dependent killing.** Therapeutic trough levels range from 5 to 15 μg/mL. Higher trough levels may be indicated in the setting of meningitis, due to poor penetration across the blood–brain barrier. In general, peak concentrations are not routinely measured.

CASE CONCLUSION

KM is admitted to the hospital and two sets of blood cultures are drawn. Vancomycin is started empirically. The next day, the 2/2 blood cultures return positive for MRSE. KS is continued on vancomycin for 10 days.

THUMBNAIL: Vancomycin

Clinical usage: IV vancomycin is primarily indicated for the treatment of infections due to methicillin-resistant staphylococci such as sepsis, endocarditis, and meningitis secondary to penicillin-resistant *Streptococcus pneumoniae.* Vancomycin is also indicated in patients with hypersensitivity reactions to β-lactams. Oral vancomycin is used for the treatment of antibiotic-associated colitis secondary to *Clostridium difficile.*

MOA: Glycopeptide antibiotic that inhibits cell wall synthesis by binding to the D-Ala-D-Ala terminus of the peptidoglycan pentapeptide. This prevents elongation and cross-linking of the cell wall, leading to the inability to form a rigid cell wall and, ultimately, cell lysis. Vancomycin exhibits time-dependent killing.

Activity: Vancomycin is bactericidal against most gram-positive organisms such as streptococci and staphylococci (including those that are methicillin resistant). Vancomycin is bacteriostatic against *Enterococcus* species, and is usually given in combination with an aminoglycoside to achieve a bactericidal effect. Other bacteria include gram-positive bacilli such as *Bacillus* species, corynebacteria, and *Lactobacillus* and most *Clostridium* species, including *Clostridium difficile.*

(Continued)

THUMBNAIL: Vancomycin *(Continued)*

Pharmacokinetics

Absorption: Vancomycin is poorly absorbed orally; thus, oral vancomycin is used only for the treatment of antibiotic-associated enterocolitis due to *Clostridium difficile*.

Distribution: Vancomycin is widely distributed. Vancomycin penetrates poorly into CSF. However, in the presence of inflamed meninges, CSF vancomycin concentrations range from 7 to 21% of simultaneous serum concentrations.

Elimination: Eighty-five to ninety percent of vancomycin is excreted unchanged in the urine. Dose adjustments are necessary in the setting of renal dysfunction. The T½ of vancomycin ranges from 5 to 10 hours and is prolonged in patients with renal insufficiency. In patients with end-stage renal disease, the T½ can approach 7 days.

Therapeutic range: Recommended trough concentrations range from 5 to 15 μg/mL. Recommended peak concentrations range from 20 to 50 μg/mL, although it is not routinely recommended to check peak levels.

Adverse reactions: Although long thought to be nephrotoxic and ototoxic, the incidence of nephrotoxicity and ototoxicity secondary to vancomycin is rare, yet may occur when given in combination with other nephrotoxic or ototoxic agents. Peak levels of greater than 60 to 80 μg/mL may be associated with an increased risk of ototoxicity. Flushing, rash, and hypotension (i.e., red man syndrome) may occur during IV infusion and are mediated by histamine.

QUESTIONS

1. TM is a 56-year-old man who is dialysis dependent secondary to diabetes mellitus. Upon arrival for his thrice-weekly hemodialysis, TM is found to be febrile at 39°C. TM has NKDA. Which of the following is the best course of treatment for TM?

   A. Draw two sets of blood cultures and wait for culture results.
   B. Draw two sets of blood cultures and start nafcillin IV.
   C. Draw two sets of blood cultures and start vancomycin IV.
   D. Start vancomycin PO.
   E. Start vancomycin IV.
   F. A and C
   G. A and D

2. TM is given a single dose of vancomycin. Ten minutes into the infusion, TM's BP suddenly drops to 80/60 mm Hg and he feels "hot and flushed." What is the best course of action for TM's red man syndrome?

   A. Discontinue the infusion, start nafcillin.
   B. Discontinue the infusion, give vancomycin PO.
   C. Slow down the infusion.
   D. Give diphenhydramine.
   E. Give epinephrine.
   F. C and D
   G. D and E

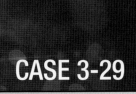

CASE 3-29 Antianaerobic Agents

HPI: While on duty, FD, a 42-year-old policeman, sustains a gunshot wound to the stomach and colon. He is admitted to the hospital and within 1 hour he undergoes an emergency laparotomy. During surgery there is spillage of GI contents into his peritoneal cavity.

PE: BP 90/65; HR 100; T 39.7°C; WBC 20,000/μL. **Allergy:** anaphylaxis to penicillin.

THOUGHT QUESTIONS

- Which bacteria should be considered as potential pathogens in intraabdominal infections?
- What are the common adverse effects associated with metronidazole and clindamycin?

BASIC SCIENCE REVIEW AND DISCUSSION

Normal GI flora sparsely populate the stomach, whereas the large bowel contains a high bacterial inoculum of *Bacteroides* species, particularly *Bacteroides fragilis* and gram-negative organisms such as *Escherichia coli*, *Klebsiella*, and *Enterobacter* species. Since the colon has significantly more bacteria than does the stomach, it is much more likely to be associated with infections if ruptured. Thus, *B. fragilis* is the most common anaerobe isolated, and *E. coli*, *Klebsiella*, and *Enterobacter* are the most common gram-negative bacteria associated with intraabdominal infections.

Metronidazole and clindamycin are **protein synthesis inhibitors** that inhibit bacteria by interacting with the DNA to cause a loss of helical DNA structure and strand breakage. This results in inhibition of protein synthesis and cell death. Metronidazole and clindamycin are commonly used in the treatment of intraabdominal infections. Metronidazole has excellent activity against gram-negative anaerobes, whereas clindamycin has activity against both gram-positive and gram-negative anaerobes. The expression, "clindamycin for above the belt and metronidazole for below the belt" highlights the fact that metronidazole does not have good activity against gram-positive anaerobes found in the mouth, whereas clindamycin does. Metronidazole is also an antiprotozoan drug and is the treatment of choice for amebiasis, giardiasis, and trichomoniasis. The most troublesome side effect associated with metronidazole is GI intolerance. Metronidazole can cause a **disulfiram-like** reaction in patients who consume ethanol, due to inhibition of aldehyde dehydrogenase.

The most notable adverse effect associated with clindamycin is **antibiotic-associated colitis** secondary to toxigenic *Clostridium difficile*. This organism usually overgrows in the GI tract in the presence of antibiotics due to the inhibition of normal GI flora. Ironically, the drug of choice for the treatment of antibiotic-associated colitis is metronidazole. Clindamycin also can cause diarrhea that is not related to *C. difficile*.

CASE CONCLUSION

Because the etiology of intraabdominal infections is most often polymicrobial (gram-negative and anaerobic bacteria) and the patient has an allergy to penicillin, FD can be treated empirically with tobramycin and metronidazole or clindamycin. This regimen provides adequate empiric coverage of the most noteworthy pathogens associated with intraabdominal infections.

THUMBNAIL: Antianaerobic Agents

	Metronidazole	Clindamycin
MOA	Inhibits bacteria by interacting with the DNA to cause a loss of helical DNA structure and strand breakage, resulting in inhibition of protein synthesis and cell death.	Reversibly binds to 50S ribosomal subunits, thereby inhibiting bacterial protein synthesis.
Activity	*Bacteroides* species, *C. difficile*, *C. perfringens*, *Gardnerella vaginalis* (a common cause of bacterial vaginosis in women), *Trichomonas vaginalis*, *Entamoeba histolytica*, *Giardia lamblia*, *Helicobacter pylori*.	*Bacteroides* species, *Streptococcus* species, *Staphylococcus aureus* (not MRSA), anaerobic streptococci (i.e., Peptostreptococcus), *C. perfringens*. Other noteworthy pathogens: *Pneumocystis carinii*, *Toxoplasma gondii*.

(Continued)

THUMBNAIL: Antianaerobic Agents *(Continued)*

	Metronidazole	Clindamycin
Pharmacokinetics		
Bioavailability	High	Moderate absorption (70%)
Distribution	Widely distributed; readily crosses the blood–brain barrier	Widely distributed; minimal levels achieved in CSF
Elimination	Hepatic	Hepatic
Adverse effects	Metallic taste, anorexia, nausea, vomiting (administering with food or milk can reduce GI side effects) Neurologic: vertigo, headache Dark urine due to azo metabolite in some patients	Diarrhea, nausea and vomiting (2–20%) Pseudomembranous colitis (0.1–10%) is a result of *C. difficile* overgrowth in the stool
Drug interactions concomitantly	Can cause a disulfiram-like reaction in patients who consume ethanol due to inhibition of aldehyde dehydrogenase Metronidazole prolongs the prothrombin time in patients taking warfarin	No clinically significant drug interactions

QUESTIONS

1. MB is a 39-year-old man who is diagnosed with cellulitis. Since he has an allergy to penicillins (urticarial rash), he is prescribed clindamycin for 10 days. Nine days into therapy he develops diarrhea. A stool culture detects *C. difficile* toxin. What is the best treatment for MB's diarrhea?

   A. Cefotetan
   B. Metronidazole
   C. No treatment necessary
   D. Oral vancomycin
   E. Penicillin

2. GQ is 33-year-old alcoholic who is placed on metronidazole, clarithromycin, and omeprazole for a recently diagnosed peptic ulcer. A urease breath test is positive for *H. pylori*. His other medications include ibuprofen, lisinopril, and meclizine. Which of the following is most likely to interact with GQ's metronidazole?

   A. Omeprazole
   B. Ibuprofen
   C. Alcohol
   D. Meclizine
   E. None of the above

CASE 3-30　Antiviral Agents for Herpes Viruses

HPI: SL is a 35-year-old female lawyer who is complaining of itching and burning in her genital area. She states that she has had these symptoms in the past, particularly when she is under a lot of stress.

THOUGHT QUESTIONS

- What is the difference between primary herpes and recurrent herpes?
- When should therapy for genital herpes be started?
- What is the MOA of acyclovir?
- Which of the antiviral agents are active against herpes simplex virus (HSV)?

BASIC SCIENCES REVIEW AND DISCUSSION

Herpes simplex virus is divided into HSV-1 and HSV-2. Genital herpes is usually caused by HSV-2, whereas oral herpes is caused by HSV-1. **Primary herpes** refers to the first outbreak of infection, whereas **recurrent herpes** refers to subsequent infections. With each outbreak, patients typically experience symptoms 2 to 10 days after the initial infection. Symptoms may include a "prodrome" of burning or itching, followed by the appearance of blisters and open sores within a few days. Other symptoms such as fever, headache, muscle aches, painful urination, or vaginal discharge are also common. In general, recurrent outbreaks are usually mild and shorter in duration.

Because viral replication occurs prior to the onset of symptoms, initiation of early therapy is imperative for optimum clinical efficacy. Thus, treatment must be initiated at the first signs and symptoms of infection, typically during the prodrome period.

Acyclovir is an acyclic guanosine derivative that requires three phosphorylation steps for activation. Conversion to the monophosphate is carried out by the virus thymidine kinase, and conversion to the diphosphate and triphosphate is carried out by host kinases. The active nucleotide triphosphate inhibits viral replication by competing with the viral deoxy-GTP for the viral DNA polymerase. Thus, acyclovir triphosphate is inserted into the growing viral DNA, leading to irreversible chain termination. Reduced susceptibility to acyclovir is due to altered viral thymidine kinase. Because the MOA of ganciclovir is similar to that of acyclovir, HSV that is resistant to acyclovir is also resistant to ganciclovir.

Although acyclovir is considered the drug of choice for the treatment of HSV infection, ganciclovir, foscarnet, and cidofovir also have in vitro activity against HSV, but these agents are most commonly used for the treatment of infections due to CMV. Valacyclovir is the L-valyl ester of acyclovir and was developed to overcome the poor bioavailability of acyclovir. Famciclovir is the ester prodrug of penciclovir, an acyclovir analogue. Although the serum T½ of penciclovir is similar to that of acyclovir, the intracellular T½ of penciclovir is extended. Penciclovir is not available as an oral agent, but only as a cream.

CASE CONCLUSION

SL is experiencing a recurrent genital herpes outbreak. The treatment of choice is either acyclovir or one of the acyclovir analogues. The duration of symptoms may be shortened because SL was able to identify and seek treatment for her outbreak early.

THUMBNAIL: Antiviral Agents for Herpes Viruses

	Acyclovir	Ganciclovir	Foscarnet	Cidofovir
MOA	Monophosphorylation by viral kinases and dephosphorylation and triphosphorylation via host kinases; inhibition of viral DNA polymerase; insertion into forming DNA, leading to chain termination		Inorganic pyrophosphate compound that inhibits viral DNA and RNA polymerase; does not require phosphorylation for activity	Cytosine nucleotide analogue phosphorylated by host kinase; inhibition of viral DNA polymerase, insertion into forming DNA, leading to chain termination

(Continued)

THUMBNAIL: Antiviral Agents for Herpes Viruses *(Continued)*

	Acyclovir	Ganciclovir	Foscarnet	Cidofovir
Activity	HSV-1, HSV-2, VZV Weak activity against EBV, CMV	HSV-1, HSV-2, VZV, CMV, EBV, human herpes virus (HHV)-8	HSV-1, HSV-2, VZV, CMV, EBV, HHV-6, HHV-8; may be used for treatment of resistant HSV or CMV	
Pharmacokinetics				
Absorption	Poor oral absorption (10–30%)	Poor oral absorption (5%)	IV only	IV and intravitreal
Distribution	Distributes widely, including CSF			
Elimination	Renal, via glomerular filtration and tubular secretion. Dose adjustment needed in renal insufficiency.			
T½	3–4 hrs	2–4 hrs	6–8 hrs	2 hrs; intracellular T½ 17–60 hrs
Adverse reactions	Thrombophlebitis from IV administration, headache, crystal nephropathy, concentration dependent neurotoxicity (lethargy, coma, seizure, tremor, hallucinations)	Bone marrow suppression: neutropenia (40%), thrombocytopenia, anemia, GI symptoms with oral formulation, teratogenic, carcinogenic	Thrombophlebitis, nephrotoxicity (acute tubular necrosis, crystalluria, interstitial nephritis), anemia, electrolyte disturbances ($\downarrow$ Ca, $\downarrow$ Mg, $\uparrow$/$\downarrow$ PO$_4$) neurotoxicity	Nephrotoxicity, teratogenic, carcinogenic With intraocular administration: hypotony, iritis, vitreitis
Comments	Valacyclovir, famciclovir formulated to improve bioavailability; penciclovir only available topically	Oral valganciclovir formulated to improve bioavailability	Risk factors for nephrotoxicity include dehydration, high doses, rapid infusion	IV prehydration and administration with probenecid necessary to prevent nephrotoxicity

QUESTIONS

1. SL is a 34-year-old HIV-positive man with CMV who is receiving his second week of induction therapy with ganciclovir. His current labs are Cr 1.8 mg/dL (previously 1.0 mg/dL), WBC 800/μL, Plt 89,000 mm³. How would you treat SL?

   A. Decrease the dose of ganciclovir
   B. Administer filgrastim
   C. Discontinue ganciclovir and switch to cidofovir
   D. Discontinue ganciclovir and switch to foscarnet
   E. A and B
   F. B and C
   G. C and D

2. LY is a 32-year-old woman s/p liver transplantation who is being started on foscarnet for treatment of ganciclovir-resistant CMV. Side effects of foscarnet include:

   A. Hypocalcemia
   B. Hyperphosphatemia
   C. Hypophosphatemia
   D. Thrombophlebitis
   E. Acute tubular necrosis
   F. All of the above

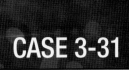

CASE 3-31 Antifungal Agents

HPI: CJ is a 32-year-old man with AIDS (CD4$^+$ cell count 160 cells/mm^3, viral load 35,000 copies/mL) who presents to the clinic with altered taste sensation and difficulty swallowing. CJ is noted to have white plaques on his tongue and upper oral pharynx that are easily scraped off with a tongue depressor. PMH is significant for renal insufficiency secondary to his HIV. His antiretroviral regimen includes stavudine, lamivudine, and lopinavir/ritonavir and he is receiving TMP-SMX for *Pneumocystis carinii* pneumonia (PCP) prophylaxis. He has NKDA.

Labs: Cr 2.0 mg/dL; BUN 43 mg/dL

THOUGHT QUESTIONS

- What are risk factors for developing candidal infections?
- What are options for the treatment of CJ's esophageal candidiasis?
- What are the pharmacologic differences among the azole antifungals?
- What are the toxicities associated with amphotericin B?

BASIC SCIENCE REVIEW AND DISCUSSION

Candida organisms are common inhabitants of the GI tract, skin, and female genital tract. Patients at risk for invasive candidal infections include those who are immunocompromised or diabetic. Iatrogenic risk factors, such as prolonged hospitalization, use of indwelling catheters, parenteral nutrition, and antibiotics, have all been identified as risk factors for developing candidiasis. In patients infected with HIV, the rate of candidal infections increases as the CD4$^+$ lymphocyte count decreases. Since the introduction of highly active antiretroviral therapy (HAART), the incidence of opportunistic infections in patients with HIV has significantly declined.

The two main classes of systemic antifungals that are used in the treatment of candidiasis are **azoles** and **amphotericin B.**

Azole antifungals include systemic agents, such as ketoconazole, fluconazole, itraconazole, and voriconazole. Topical agents used for the treatment of vaginal candidiasis and thrush include miconazole and clotrimazole. The pharmacologic properties of the systemic azoles differ considerably. Ketoconazole, the first oral azole developed, has poor bioavailability and requires an acidic environment for enhanced absorption. Thus, initial studies required ketoconazole to be administered with a cola to increase bioavailability. Fluconazole, unlike itraconazole and ketoconazole, is hydrophilic and has increased penetration across the blood–brain barrier. Fluconazole is also the only azole that is renally eliminated.

Amphotericin B, sometimes referred to as "amphoterrible," is associated with multiple **infusion-related reactions** and adverse effects on the kidneys. Chills, rigors, fevers, and hypotension are common during amphotericin administration. Thus, patients are typically premedicated with diphenhydramine and acetaminophen or NSAIDs prior to infusion. Meperidine can be given in response to rigors. Renal toxicity is also commonly associated with amphotericin and can be irreversible. Renal toxicity may present as azotemia, renal tubular acidosis, or electrolyte wasting. Almost all patients receiving amphotericin will experience some degree of renal insufficiency.

CASE CONCLUSION

Because esophageal candidiasis is most often attributable to *Candida albicans*, CJ can be given either IV amphotericin or an azole antifungal. However, itraconazole, ketoconazole, and voriconazole are potent CYP450 inhibitors and will thus interact with his protease inhibitors. Amphotericin B is also not a good choice because of his preexisting renal insufficiency. Fluconazole is chosen for treatment of his esophageal candidiasis because it is less likely to interact with his protease inhibitors and will not negatively impact his renal function.

THUMBNAIL: Antifungal Agents

	Azoles		Amphotericin B

Available agents	Systemic:
	    Ketoconazole
	    Itraconazole
	    Fluconazole
	    Voriconazole
		Topical:
		    Butaconazole
		    Clotrimazole
		    Econazole
		    Ketoconazole
		    Miconazole
		    Terconazole
			Lipid-based formulations created to attenuate the renal toxicity associated with conventional amphotericin B

(Continued)

THUMBNAIL: Antifungal Agents *(Continued)*

	Azoles	Amphotericin B
MOA	Inhibition of ergosterol synthesis by binding to fungal CYP450 **Fungistatic**	Binds to ergosterol, altering fungal cell membrane permeability, leading to cell lysis **Fungicidal**
Activity	*Candida* species, *Cryptococcus neoformans, Blastomyces dermatitis, Coccidioides immitis*, dermatophytes; itraconazole and voriconazole are the only azoles active against *Aspergillus* species	*Candida* species (except *C. lusitaniae*), *Cryptococcus neoformans, Histoplasma capsulatum, Blastomyces dermatitis, Coccidioides immitis*; molds include *Aspergillus* species and mucor
Pharmacokinetics		
Bioavailability	Ketoconazole: low Itraconazole: low Fluconazole: high Voriconazole: high	Poorly absorbed; IV only
Distribution	Widely distributed; fluconazole readily crosses the blood–brain barrier	Widely distributed; minimal levels achieved in CSF
Elimination	Ketoconazole, itraconazole, voriconazole: hepatic Fluconazole: renal	Minimal excretion in the urine
Adverse reactions	All azoles can cause GI upset and hepatotoxicity Ketoconazole can cause gynecomastia and oligospermia in men and menstrual irregularities in women due to inhibition of gonadal steroid production Voriconazole can cause reversible visual disturbances such as blurred vision, photophobia, altered color perception, and enhanced light perception; most common during 1st month of therapy; photosensitivity with long-term use	Renal dysfunction common Electrolyte wasting, including hypokalemia, hypomagnesemia Infusion-related toxicities include fever, chills, and rigors and hypotension
Drug interactions	Ketoconazole and itraconazole absorption decreased with agents that increase gastric pH All azoles are CYP450 inhibitors and can increase serum levels of drugs metabolized through this pathway. Voriconazole > itraconazole = ketoconazole >> fluconazole	Increased renal toxicity used in combination with other nephrotoxic agents such as cyclosporine, tacrolimus, or aminoglycosides

QUESTIONS

1. PJ is a 23-year-old man with ALL hospitalized for induction chemotherapy. He is scheduled to receive amphotericin B tonight as part of his prophylactic regimen against opportunistic infections. His premedications for amphotericin should include the following:

   A. Diphenhydramine
   B. Acetaminophen
   C. Meperidine
   D. 1 liter of normal saline
   E. A and B only
   F. A, B, and C
   G. A, B, and D
   H. All of the above

2. GM is a 43-year-old woman with poorly controlled insulin-dependent diabetes mellitus. She is complaining of vaginal itching and a thick, "cottage cheese"-appearing vaginal discharge. Her PMH includes GERD, for which she is taking omeprazole. What is the best treatment for GM's vulvovaginal candidiasis?

   A. Ketoconazole
   B. Clotrimazole
   C. Itraconazole
   D. Amphotericin
   E. No treatment necessary

CASE 3-32　Anthracyclines

HPI: DS is a 48-year-old woman recently diagnosed with treatment-induced acute myelogenous leukemia (AML). She was successfully treated for breast cancer 4 years prior after receiving six cycles of AC chemotherapy (doxorubicin [Adriamycin] and cyclophosphamide). Her total cumulative dose of doxorubicin was 360 mg/m². Her current oncologist would like to begin induction chemotherapy for her AML with the goal of achieving remission. He recommends a regimen consisting of high-dose cytarabine and daunorubicin. She is otherwise in good health.

THOUGHT QUESTIONS

- Describe the pharmacology and major side effects of anthracycline agents.
- What special precautions should be considered when administering anthracyclines?
- What labs might be helpful to evaluate prior to proceeding with anthracycline therapy?
- Is this patient at risk for anthracycline-induced cardiotoxicity? How should she be monitored?

BASIC SCIENCE REVIEW AND DISCUSSION

The **anthracyclines** (doxorubicin, daunorubicin, idarubicin, epirubicin) are antineoplastic antibiotics with a broad range of clinical uses. Doxorubicin has activity against a number of solid tumors (such as sarcomas, adenocarcinomas) and hematologic malignancies (leukemia, lymphoma, multiple myeloma). Compared with doxorubicin, daunorubicin and idarubicin are much less active against solid tumors but highly effective against leukemia.

Anthracyclines have several modes of action leading to anticancer activity. They intercalate between base pairs in DNA, interfering with nucleic acid synthesis. Anthracyclines also inhibit DNA topoisomerases I and II, which leads to DNA double-strand breaks. In addition, doxorubicin and daunorubicin may form complexes with metals such as iron. Although these metal-anthracycline complexes result in oxygen free radical formation, which may contribute to antitumor activity, membrane damage incurred from the free radicals is thought to be the mechanism responsible for **cardiotoxicity.** Free radical generation may be less prominent with idarubicin compared with other anthracyclines. Anthracyclines can be cytotoxic in all phases of the cell cycle and are not considered to be cell cycle phase-specific.

Administration and Metabolism

All of the anthracyclines are administered parenterally because oral absorption is poor. Anthracyclines can cause severe tissue damage if **extravasated,** so it is recommended that they be administered via central venous catheters or as a short IV push over 1 to 2 minutes. Anthracyclines are primarily eliminated via hepatic metabolism. Patients with **cholestasis** have impaired clearance and experience greater toxicity. It is recommended that patients receiving anthracyclines have LFTs monitored prior to administration, and that dose reductions be considered if total bilirubin is elevated.

Toxicities

Anthracyclines have a number of significant toxicities. They may result in **myelosuppression,** which is considered the acute dose-limiting toxicity. Leukopenia has a nadir of approximately 10 to 14 days but recovery is usually quick following the nadir. The most significant delayed adverse effect of anthracyclines is **cardiotoxicity.** It may manifest as acute toxicity (arrhythmias) or delayed cardiomyopathy, which is related to total cumulative lifetime exposure. The cardiomyopathy syndrome classically presents as CHF, and it may be irreversible. Patients may be at increased risk for anthracycline-induced cardiomyopathy if they have been exposed to cumulative doses of doxorubicin greater than 550 mg/m² (or equivalent for other anthracyclines), prior mediastinal irradiation, are older than 70 years of age, or have preexisting cardiovascular disease. It is recommended to obtain baseline cardiac function evaluations prior to commencing anthracycline therapy.

CASE CONCLUSION

Given that DS's prior doxorubicin exposure was 360 mg/m² and the current regimen will expose her to an additional 180 mg/m² of anthracycline, it was decided safe to proceed with treatment. After induction therapy, she will have been exposed to 540 mg/m² anthracycline and should be monitored carefully for the potential development of cardiomyopathy.

THUMBNAIL: Anthracyclines

Prototype drug: Doxorubicin (Adriamycin) Other examples in class: daunorubicin, idarubicin, epirubicin, liposomal doxorubicin, liposomal daunorubicin

Clinical uses: Leukemia, lymphoma, multiple myeloma, sarcomas, germ cell tumors of the ovaries or testes, head and neck cancer, lung cancer, Wilms tumor, breast cancer, stomach cancer, pancreatic cancer, liver cancer, ovarian cancer, bladder cancer, uterine cancer, neuroblastoma

MOA: Intercalation into DNA, which leads to blockade of DNA and RNA synthesis; DNA strand breaks; free radical formation

Pharmacokinetics

Absorption: Poor oral absorption (<50%), given intravenously

Distribution: Rapidly distributes into liver, spleen, kidney, lung, and heart; poor penetration into CNS

Metabolism/elimination: Triphasic elimination (primarily in liver); adjust dose or withhold use in patients with increased total bilirubin levels

Adverse reactions: Cardiotoxicity (increased risk when lifetime cumulative dose equivalent to doxorubicin 400–550 mg/m^2 is exceeded), alopecia, vesicant, nausea/vomiting (moderate to high emetogenic potential for doses >60 mg), mucositis, myelosuppression (primarily leukopenia, nadir 10–14 days)

Drug interactions: CYP450 enzyme substrate and inhibitor; unclear clinical significance

QUESTIONS

1. AR is a 48-year-old woman who was treated for Hodgkin disease 15 years ago with ABVD (doxorubicin, bleomycin, vinblastine, dacarbazine). She now presents with breast cancer and her oncologist feels that chemotherapy with FAC (fluorouracil, doxorubicin [Adriamycin], and cyclophosphamide) is the most appropriate regimen. Her previous chemotherapy included a total of 300 mg/m^2 doxorubicin exposure. Which of the following agents may be utilized to reduce risk of cardiotoxicity associated with the anthracycline therapy she is about to receive?

   A. Leucovorin
   B. Mesna
   C. Amifostine
   D. Dexrazoxane
   E. N-acetylcysteine

2. MT is a 49-year-old man admitted for his first cycle of chemotherapy for multiple myeloma. He is scheduled to receive VAD therapy (vincristine, doxorubicin [Adriamycin], and dexamethasone). Past medical history includes asthma and diabetes. Admission laboratory values include WBC count 3400 mm^3, platelets 9500 mm^3 (low), Cr 1.8 mg/dL (high), bilirubin 2.4 mg/dL (high). Which of the following factors may lead you to consider dose modification of doxorubicin?

   A. Diabetes
   B. Asthma
   C. Plt count
   D. Cr
   E. Bilirubin

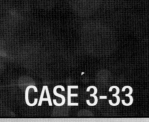

CASE 3-33 | Alkylating Agents

HPI: GH is a 48-year-old woman who presents with stage III epithelial adenocarcinoma of the ovaries. She has received three cycles of cisplatin and paclitaxel, but now the cancer has progressed. Her course has been complicated by severe side effects, including numbness of her feet, persistent N/V, severe neutropenia, and renal dysfunction (serum Cr 1.5 mg/dL). Her physician is considering switching to an alternative regimen consisting of ifosfamide and etoposide. She is reluctant due to her poor tolerability of her previous therapy.

THOUGHT QUESTIONS

- What issues should be considered when selecting an alternative regimen?
- Which agents caused her complications?
- What can be done to minimize toxicities with her alternative regimen?

BASIC SCIENCE REVIEW AND DISCUSSION

Poor response or tolerability is often the rationale for switching chemotherapy regimens. Cisplatin, a platinum **alkylating agent,** and paclitaxel, a **taxane,** are two of the most effective drugs for ovarian cancer. Cisplatin is known to be the most **emetogenic** chemotherapy agent. It is also known to cause **neuropathy, nephrotoxicity, myelosuppression,** electrolyte wasting, and **ototoxicity.** Switching to another platinum alkylating agent, such as carboplatin, may help with nausea, vomiting, nephrotoxicity, and neurotoxicity, but since GH is having a poor response, it may not be the best choice. Paclitaxel may also cause neurotoxicity and myelosuppression, and may have additive toxic effects to the cisplatin (see Case 3-36 for discussion of taxanes).

Cisplatin acts as an alkylating agent to react with cellular DNA, forming both intrastrand and interstrand cross-links, which results in DNA conformational changes and disruption of DNA replication. Alkylating agents are generally considered to be non–cell cycle-specific; however, they exhibit the most activity in cells that are rapidly dividing. Cisplatin metabolites also may react with thiol groups on proteins, and some cisplatin toxicity (ototoxicity, nephrotoxicity, and neurotoxicity) may result from these interactions. **Amifostine** is metabolized to a free thiol product and may be used to bind and detoxify reactive metabolites of cisplatin.

Ifosfamide is an alkylating agent related to cyclophosphamide. It is often used as a second-line agent for ovarian cancer. Its main side effect is **hemorrhagic cystitis.** Hemorrhagic cystitis is caused by the acrolein metabolite, which binds to the bladder and causes irritation and tissue damage. Aggressive hydration and the use of the chemoprotective agent **mesna** are necessary for safe administration. Mesna tends to have a shorter T½ than ifosfamide, so it is imperative that the dose be given for at least 8 to 12 hours after the end of the ifosfamide infusion.

CASE CONCLUSION

GH had a measured 24-hour CrCl rate of 55 mL/min. This was considered adequate for her to proceed with the proposed alternative regimen without dose modification. She was given aggressive hydration and mesna with her ifosfamide. She tolerated the etoposide with minimal problems. Compared with her previous regimen, she had less N/V, although she still experienced 7 days of neutropenia.

THUMBNAIL: Alkylating Agents

Drug Class	Platinum Analogues	Nitrogen Mustards	Nitrosoureas	Other
Agents	Cisplatin Carboplatin	Mechlorethamine Cyclophosphamide Ifosfamide	Carmustine Lomustine Streptozocin	Busulfan Dacarbazine
Clinical uses	Cancer of the testes, ovaries, bladder, lung, head and neck, cervix, and endometrium; sarcomas	Mechlorethamine: lymphoma Cyclophosphamide: leukemia, lymphoma, cancer of the breast, lung, sarcoma Ifosfamide: ovarian and breast cancers, sarcomas	Carmustine and lomustine: lymphomas, brain tumors Streptozocin: pancreatic cancer, insulinoma	Busulfan: leukemia Dacarbazine: melanoma, Hodgkin lymphoma, soft tissue sarcomas

(Continued)

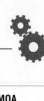

THUMBNAIL: Alkylating Agents *(Continued)*

	Platinum Analogues	Nitrogen Mustards	Nitrosoureas	Other
MOA	Form intrastrand and interstrand cross-links in DNA, which interferes with DNA replication; usually considered cell cycle nonspecific, but do work best when cells are rapidly multiplying			
Pharmacokinetics	Only available as IV injection; predominantly renally excreted	Mechlorethamine: IV only; undergoes rapid chemical transformation Cyclophosphamide and ifosfamide: biotransformed by the liver to active compounds; requires dose adjustment for both hepatic and renal impairment; usually IV, but can be taken orally	Carmustine: renally cleared, readily crosses blood–brain barrier Lomustine: extensive metabolism by the liver to active metabolites; oral only	Busulfan: may give IV or PO; hepatic metabolism, readily distributes to CNS Dacarbazine: hepatic metabolism, but prolonged elimination in the presence of renal dysfunction; IV only
Adverse reactions	Cisplatin: severe N/V, neuropathy, nephrotoxicity, ototoxicity, electrolyte wasting, myelosuppression Carboplatin: thrombocytopenia, leukopenia, less N/V, renal, and neurotoxicity than cisplatin	Mechlorethamine: vesicant, myelosuppression, N/V, skin rash Cyclophosphamide and ifosfamide: hemorrhagic cystitis, SIADH, acute and delayed N/V, myelosuppression	Myelosuppression Carmustine: pulmonary fibrosis with high dose	Myelosuppression, N/V Busulfan: pulmonary fibrosis, hepatic dysfunction, hyperpigmentation Dacarbazine: severe N/V, fatigue, hepatic dysfunction, flu-like symptoms
Special precautions	Amifostine may be used to reduce cumulative renal toxicity associated with repeated cisplatin therapy	Mesna to prevent hemorrhagic cystitis		

QUESTIONS

1. WD is a 24-year-old woman with metastatic melanoma, who is being treated with cisplatin, dacarbazine, IL-2, and interferon-α. What precautions should be taken while she is being treated?

   A. Monitor magnesium and potassium levels
   B. Premedicate with antiemetics, including a serotonin antagonist
   C. Monitor pulmonary function tests
   D. A and B only
   E. All of the above

2. GF is a 43-year-old man with Burkitt lymphoma who is about to receive high-dose cyclophosphamide (4000 mg/m² for one dose) for stem cell mobilization. Which of the following factors should be considered prior to administration?

   A. Prehydration with normal saline
   B. Use in combination with mesna
   C. Use of a serotonin antagonist for acute N/V
   D. Use of antiemetic regimen including dexamethasone for delayed N/V
   E. All of the above

CASE 3-34 Antimetabolites

HPI: TB is a 46-year-old woman with osteosarcoma who is admitted for treatment with very high-dose methotrexate. All of her admit laboratory values were within normal limits. She is given 1000 mL normal saline (NS) IV over 2 hours, then started on D5W with 2 amps (100 mEq) sodium bicarbonate/liter to run at 250 mL/hr. Her urine pH is checked hourly. Once her urine pH is sufficiently alkaline and her urine output is considered adequate, methotrexate is administered IV over 4 hours. Twenty-four hours after the methotrexate infusion, leucovorin "rescue" is begun.

THOUGHT QUESTIONS

- What is the pharmacology of methotrexate and what are the main side effects?
- What is the role of hydration in this patient?
- How does leucovorin work in this case and when should it be stopped?
- What other factors should be considered in patients receiving high-dose methotrexate?
- What are other antimetabolites used in cancer treatment and what are their principal side effects?

BASIC SCIENCE REVIEW AND DISCUSSION

Methotrexate is an antineoplastic folic acid analogue that blocks the conversion of dihydrofolate (FH_2) to tetrahydrofolate (FH_4) by binding to **dihydrofolate reductase** (DHFR) enzyme. Folate is essential for the normal synthesis of purines and pyrimidines and therefore DNA and RNA. In order for folate to function as a cofactor, it must be reduced to FH_4 by DHFR. Methotrexate binds to DHFR, prevents the conversion of FH_2 to FH_4, and, consequently, inhibits purine and pyrimidine synthesis. The **antimetabolites** are considered cell cycle-specific, with most activity for cells in the S (synthesis) phase. With high-dose methotrexate, **leucovorin** rescue often is used to prevent severe toxicity to normal body tissues. Leucovorin (folinic acid) is a reduced form of folate (similar to FH_4) that does not require the use of DHFR. Leucovorin is transported into healthy cells and is utilized for DNA and RNA synthesis. Tumor cells tend to have impaired transport mechanisms and usually cannot use leucovorin. Leucovorin is usually started within 24 to 36 hours of high-dose methotrexate administration and continues until methotrexate serum levels are below nontoxic levels (0.1–0.05 mol/L).

Common side effects seen with methotrexate include **mucositis, leukopenia, thrombocytopenia,** and anemia. At normal doses, methotrexate is primarily excreted unchanged in the urine. Adequate renal function is essential for safe administration of methotrexate. At high doses, methotrexate is partially metabolized to 7-hydroxymethotrexate, which is slightly soluble in acidic environments, so alkalinization of the urine with sodium bicarbonate will help prevent precipitation in the renal tubules. Some drugs (trimethoprim, penicillins, NSAIDs, aspirin, probenecid) may compete with methotrexate for renal elimination, and concurrent use may lead to methotrexate toxicity. Drugs that create an acidic environment in the kidneys also may reduce the rate of methotrexate excretion. Methotrexate is extensively distributed in body water. Patients with fluid accumulations such as **pleural effusions** or **ascites** may have significant difficulty with methotrexate elimination.

Other antimetabolites used in cancer therapy include pyrimidine analogues and purine analogues. Pyrimidine analogues such as **fluorouracil** are used extensively for gastric and colorectal cancers. Fluorouracil is converted to a monophosphate nucleotide (F-UMP), which is reduced to a deoxynucleotide (F-dUMP). With a folate coenzyme, F-dUMP will bind to and inactivate thymidylate synthetase, and therefore inhibit DNA synthesis. Significant side effects include mucositis, **myelosuppression,** and alopecia. **Capecitabine** is an oral prodrug that is converted to fluorouracil intracellularly. It is used in the treatment of metastatic breast cancer and has been associated with severe **diarrhea** and **hand-foot syndrome** (chemotherapy-induced acral erythema) as side effects. **Cytarabine** is a pyrimidine analogue used primarily in the treatment of leukemias. In high doses, this agent is associated with myelosuppression, **rash** (which may be severe), chemical conjunctivitis, and cerebellar dysfunction (especially when used in the presence of renal dysfunction).

Purine analogues include **cladribine** and **fludarabine** and are used to treat a variety of leukemias. Compared with the pyrimidine analogues, these agents are associated with a lower incidence of significant mucositis; however, **neutropenia** tends to be prolonged (4 weeks compared with 2 weeks).

CASE CONCLUSION

TB tolerated her high-dose methotrexate and leucovorin rescue. She received leucovorin rescue for 4 days until her methotrexate levels became nontoxic. Her neutrophil count dropped around day 6, but she did not become neutropenic (ANC <500). She had no evidence of mucositis.

THUMBNAIL: Antimetabolites

Drug Class	Folate Antagonists	Purine Analogues	Pyrimidine Analogues
Agents	Methotrexate	Thioguanine Cladribine Fludarabine Mercaptopurine	Cytarabine (Ara-C) Fluorouracil (5FU) Capecitabine
Clinical uses	Leukemia, lymphoma, sarcoma, cancers of the lung, breast, ovaries, head and neck	Thioguanine: leukemia Cladribine: hairy cell leukemia Fludarabine: chronic lymphocytic leukemia Mercaptopurine: ALL	Cytarabine: leukemias Fluorouracil: gastric, colon, bladder, breast, head and neck cancers Capecitabine: metastatic breast cancer
MOA	Inhibits DHFR enzyme, preventing reduction of FH_2 to FH_4; inhibits purine and pyrimidine synthesis necessary for DNA and RNA synthesis; cell cycle-specific (S phase)	Metabolized to a false purine analogue that will act as a competitive inhibitor after incorporation into cellular DNA	Metabolized to a false pyrimidine analogue that will act as a competitive inhibitor after incorporation into cellular DNA
Pharmacokinetics	Predominantly renally excreted (partially metabolized at high doses) Widely distributed into body fluids At high doses, will penetrate CNS; may be given intrathecally Oral administration is rapid, but often incomplete	Thioguanine: oral only, eliminated renally, poor CNS penetration Cladribine: IV only; rapid plasma clearance Fludarabine: IV only Mercaptopurine: oral only, poor absorption	Cytarabine: extensive hepatic metabolism, but active metabolite is renally cleared; adequate CNS levels may be achieved with high doses; may be given intrathecally; not absorbed orally Fluorouracil: distributes rapidly and is extensively metabolized; oral absorption is erratic but can be given orally as prodrug (capecitabine)
Adverse reactions	Renal dysfunction, myelosuppression, mucositis, hepatotoxicity	Rash, neutropenia, diarrhea	Cytarabine: rash, fever, conjunctivitis, myelosuppression, cerebellar dysfunction if given with renal impairment Fluorouracil: rash, fever, mucositis, alopecia, hyperpigmentation, myelosuppression, neurotoxicity
Special precautions	NSAIDs, penicillins, and other drugs may interfere with methotrexate clearance Consider leucovorin rescue with high-dose methotrexate		Steroid eye drops may help prevent conjunctivitis; increased CNS toxicity with renal impairment Leucovorin is sometimes added to fluorouracil therapy for added cytotoxic effects

QUESTIONS

1. HG is a 68-year-old man with AML. He is to receive induction chemotherapy consisting of high-dose cytarabine and daunorubicin. Which condition(s) should be evaluated in this patient prior to and during treatment with high-dose cytarabine?

   A. Renal function
   B. Conjunctivitis
   C. Rash
   D. Fever
   E. All of the above

2. PO is a 58-year-old Asian man with colorectal cancer. He is on a regimen consisting of fluorouracil and leucovorin over 1 week, every 28 days. What is the role of leucovorin in this case?

   A. Rescues normal cells like it does for methotrexate toxicity
   B. Enhances the cytotoxicity of fluorouracil
   C. Has antitumor activity on its own
   D. Is an antiemetic agent
   E. Is used to prevent hypersensitivity

CASE 3-35 Vinca Alkaloids

HPI: RE is a 26-year-old woman recently diagnosed with ALL. She was admitted for induction therapy consisting of daunorubicin daily for 3 days (on days 1 through 3), vincristine once weekly for four doses (days 1, 8, 15, and 22), prednisone daily for 28 days (days 1 through 28), and asparaginase daily on days 17 through 28. She has no past medical history.

She is currently day 15 and due for her third dose of vincristine. Her main complaints consist of mild numbness in her fingertips and severe constipation (no bowel movement for 4 days).

Labs: Laboratory parameters are generally within normal limits, with the exception of neutropenia (neutrophil count 40 mm³) and elevated bilirubin (1.5 mg/dL).

THOUGHT QUESTIONS

- What is the most likely drug that is causing her complaints?
- Describe the pharmacology and major side effects of vinca alkaloids.
- What should be done?
- Could another vinca alkaloid be substituted?

BASIC SCIENCE REVIEW AND DISCUSSION

The patient's symptoms are most likely due to her vincristine therapy. Vinca alkaloids exert antineoplastic effects by binding to tubulin and thereby inhibiting assembly of microtubules. This results in the dissolution of the mitotic spindle apparatus, and cell arrest occurs in the mitosis (M) phase of the cell cycle. Vinca alkaloids are used for a variety of hematologic malignancies and solid tumors, such as lung, testicular, and breast cancers. The most common vinca alkaloids include vincristine, vinblastine, and vinorelbine.

All of the vinca alkaloids exhibit very poor oral absorption and are given parenterally. Vinca alkaloids are predominantly excreted through the **biliary tract** or by hepatic metabolism. Generally, for patients with mild elevations in bilirubin (serum bilirubin 1.5–3 mg/dL), the dose of these agents should be reduced. For patients with severely abnormal bilirubin levels (>5 mg/dL), the use of vinca alkaloids should be avoided.

Compared with vincristine, vinblastine and vinorelbine are more likely to cause **myelosuppression** (considered to be the dose-limiting toxicity of these agents). In addition, vincristine has very low **emetogenic potential** compared with vinblastine and vinorelbine, which present a more moderate risk.

Vincristine and the vinca alkaloids are known to cause **neuropathy.** Neuropathy may be related to nerve conduction alteration due to microtubule arrest. Although neuropathy is most often seen as finger numbness, it can also manifest as an ileus or **constipation.** Effects are usually reversible, and therapy should be delayed if symptoms are disabling. Use of concomitant drugs that may cause constipation (i.e., opiates) should be avoided if possible, and patients receiving vinca alkaloids should be managed with an aggressive bowel regimen to prevent these complications.

All the vinca alkaloids cause peripheral neuropathy, although a lower incidence of neuropathy is associated with vinorelbine. Vinorelbine, however, does not have an indication for leukemia and therefore should not be substituted for the vincristine.

CASE CONCLUSION

RE was given lactulose to help her constipation, and after three doses she had a bowel movement. Due to her elevated bilirubin, RE's vincristine dose was lowered by 50%. Her finger numbness improved slightly. Her neutrophils remained low until day 23. A repeat bone marrow biopsy performed after recovery demonstrated remission of her ALL.

THUMBNAIL: Vinca Alkaloids

	Vincristine	Vinblastine	Vinorelbine
Clinical uses	Leukemia, sarcoma, lymphoma	Lymphoma, testicular, bladder, renal cancers	Lung, breast, ovarian cancers, lymphoma
MOA	Inhibit polymerization of tubulin, which is necessary for the formation of mitotic spindles for mitosis. Cell cycle-specific for M phase of cell cycle.		
Pharmacokinetics	Poor oral absorption (given IV); predominantly hepatic elimination, slow clearance due to extensive tissue binding		
Adverse reactions	Peripheral neuropathy (may be dose limiting), ileus, low emetogenic potential, low risk for severe myelosuppression	Peripheral neuropathy, ileus, dose-limiting myelosuppression (neutropenia and thrombocytopenia), moderate emetogenic potential	Peripheral neuropathy, ileus, moderate emetogenic potential, moderate risk for severe myelosuppression
Special precautions	All vinca alkaloids are considered vesicants, and extravasations should be avoided. All vinca alkaloids may be **fatal if given intrathecally.**		

QUESTIONS

1. TR is a 24-year-old man with testicular cancer who is about to receive a combination of cisplatin, etoposide, and vinblastine. Which factor(s) should be considered prior to administration of the vinblastine?

   A. LFTs
   B. Bowel movements
   C. WBC counts
   D. Venous access
   E. All of the above

2. LS is a 57-year-old woman with multiple myeloma being treated with VAD chemotherapy, a regimen consisting of a 4-day continuous infusion of vincristine and doxorubicin (Adriamycin) plus oral dexamethasone. Both vincristine and doxorubicin are vesicants. Which of the following precautions should be taken?

   A. Administer via a peripheral line.
   B. Administer via a central line.
   C. Use warm compresses on the skin in the area prior to administration.
   D. Premedicate with hyaluronidase.
   E. All of the above.

CASE 3-36 Taxanes

HPI: ML is a 57-year-old woman with advanced ovarian cancer. She has recently recovered from debulking surgery and presents to receive her first course of adjuvant chemotherapy with carboplatin and paclitaxel. Past medical history is noncontributory and she has no known drug allergies. She receives an antiemetic (ondansetron) as premedication. Ten minutes into the paclitaxel infusion, ML develops dyspnea and urticaria. The infusion is stopped and supportive care is given.

THOUGHT QUESTIONS

- What is the mechanism of action of taxane antineoplastic agents?
- What are some clinical uses for taxanes?
- What precautions should be taken when administering taxanes?
- What pretreatment regimens can be used to minimize adverse reactions to taxanes?

BASIC SCIENCE REVIEW AND DISCUSSION

The taxane antineoplastic agents (paclitaxel and docetaxel) act by promoting formation and stabilization of microtubules. Accumulation of these polymerized microtubules may lead to mitotic arrest and cell death from nonfunctional tubules. They are considered to be cell cycle-specific agents (acting with greatest activity on cells in gap 2 [G_2] and M phases).

Paclitaxel is indicated for the treatment of various solid malignancies. It is considered first-line therapy (usually in combination with a platinum analogue such as cisplatin) for advanced **ovarian cancer.** It is also useful in breast cancer, non-small cell lung cancer (in combination with cisplatin), and as second-line therapy for AIDS-related Kaposi sarcoma. Docetaxel is indicated for the treatment of patients with locally advanced or metastatic breast cancer and non-small cell lung cancer.

Both paclitaxel and docetaxel may result in **anaphylactoid** or severe **hypersensitivity** reactions manifested by dyspnea, bronchospasm, angioedema, hypotension (occasionally HTN), and urticarial skin reactions. The reaction may be due to the active drug itself or to the vehicle (Cremophor or polysorbate 80). Additionally, patients receiving docetaxel may experience serious or life-threatening **fluid retention.** This syndrome is characterized by poorly tolerated peripheral or generalized edema, pleural effusion, dyspnea, ascites, and cardiac tamponade.

It is recommended that all patients receiving paclitaxel receive **pretreatment** with corticosteroids (such as dexamethasone) and antihistamines, both H_1 (diphenhydramine) and H_2 (cimetidine or ranitidine) antagonists. All patients must be premedicated with corticosteroids prior to receiving each cycle of docetaxel to reduce the incidence and severity of hypersensitivity reactions or fluid retention. Patients who experience severe hypersensitivity reactions should not be rechallenged.

CASE CONCLUSION

ML quickly recovered from her mild hypersensitivity reaction to the paclitaxel. For the remaining cycles of chemotherapy, she was pretreated with steroids and antihistamines and tolerated the paclitaxel without further reaction. After six cycles of chemotherapy, her CA-125 marker level was normal, her abdominal CT scan appeared normal, and she appeared to have a complete clinical response.

THUMBNAIL: Taxanes

Prototype drug: Paclitaxel

Other examples in class: Docetaxel

Clinical uses: Advanced ovarian carcinoma, node-positive breast cancer (adjuvant), metastatic breast cancer, non-small cell lung cancer, cervical, bladder, head and neck cancer, AIDS-related Kaposi sarcoma (second line)

MOA: Inhibits mitosis by promoting and maintaining assembly of microtubules. Cell cycle-specific (G2 and M phases). May also lead to chromosome breakage by distorting mitotic spindle apparatus.

(Continued)

THUMBNAIL: Taxanes *(Continued)*

Pharmacokinetics

Absorption: Administered intravenously

Distribution: Highly protein bound

Metabolism/elimination: Hepatic metabolism

Adverse reactions: Alopecia, N/V and diarrhea, **myelosuppression** (dose limiting, granulocytopenia, and thrombocytopenia), hepatic toxicity, peripheral neuropathy, hypersensitivity reactions, myalgias/arthralgias, rare cardiovascular events, fluid retention/pulmonary edema (docetaxel)

Precautions: Doses may be modified or therapy delayed for toxicity (myelosuppression). Adjust dose for hepatic impairment. Avoid use of docetaxel in patients with elevated bilirubin. Corticosteroids and antihistamines (i.e., cimetidine and diphenhydramine) are recommended to lessen risk for anaphylactoid reactions with paclitaxel. Pretreatment with steroids is *required* for docetaxel to minimize risk for fluid retention and hypersensitivity.

QUESTIONS

1. A 65-year-old man is about to receive his first course of paclitaxel therapy for refractory non-small cell lung cancer. Past medical history includes HTN and depression. He has NKDA. Which of the following pretreatment regimens would you recommend prior to infusing the paclitaxel?

   A. Dexamethasone alone
   B. Diphenhydramine alone
   C. Dexamethasone + diphenhydramine + ranitidine
   D. Dexamethasone + diphenhydramine + omeprazole
   E. Omeprazole alone

2. A 48-year-old woman presents for her third cycle of docetaxel therapy for her metastatic breast cancer. Which of the following laboratory parameters are necessary to evaluate prior to administering the docetaxel?

   A. Absolute neutrophil count
   B. Total bilirubin
   C. AST
   D. Alkaline phosphatase
   E. All of the above

PART IV
Biochemistry

HPI: HA is a 2½-year-old boy brought in for a routine visit to his pediatrician. On review of systems, his parents report that he has been increasingly fatigued over the past few months. He tires easily when playing outside and gets short of breath when roughhousing with his older brother. There has been no recent illness and he has no other significant medical history.

PE: He is slightly tachycardic and notably pale. He has no gross jaundice but a mild scleral icterus. The exam of the lungs and heart shows no abnormalities; however, on abdominal exam, he has an enlarged spleen.

Labs: A CBC count reveals a normocytic anemia, with a hematocrit of 23. On inspection of the erythrocytes on peripheral smear, they are noted to be spiculated with an increase in reticulocytes.

THOUGHT QUESTIONS

- What enzyme deficiency in glycolysis will most commonly lead to this clinical scenario?
- What other enzymes in this pathway may be deficient and lead to similar clinical outcomes?
- Why are erythrocytes particularly susceptible to pyruvate kinase (PK) deficiency?
- Why would PK deficiency lead to hemolytic anemia?

BASIC SCIENCE REVIEW AND DISCUSSION

PK is involved in the conversion of **phosphoenolpyruvate to enolpyruvate,** one of the two steps of glycolysis that generates ATP by hydrolyzing a phosphate bound to the initial molecule. A review of the steps of glycolysis is shown in Figure 4-1. During glycolysis, which occurs in the cytosol, two steps require ATP: the addition of phosphate moieties by **hexokinase and phosphofructokinase** (PFK). Further on, glycolysis generates ATP during the release of phosphate by phosphoglycerate kinase and PK. Thus, it might seem that there should be an even trade-off during glycolysis, but the latter two reactions occur after glycolysis has cleaved glucose into two 3-carbon molecules, glyceraldehyde 3-phosphate and dihydroxyacetone phosphate, which are isomers. Because each of these molecules goes through the latter half of glycolysis, there is a net production of two ATP molecules from each molecule of glucose. There is also a net production of two reduced nicotinamide adenine dinucleotide **(NADH)** molecules, which will normally generate three **ATP** molecules under aerobic conditions. However, this is seen primarily in birds, which use the **malate shuttle** to move NADH to the mitochondria, whereas most mammals use the **glycerol phosphate shuttle,** which generates only two ATP molecules per NADH molecule generated in the cytosol.

Glycolysis is regulated primarily by control of PFK-1 and secondarily at hexokinase and PK. Generally, when there exists an abundance of high-energy molecules such as ATP, the activity of these enzymes is decreased. Conversely, when levels of ATP are low, the activity of these enzymes is increased. When levels of ATP and citrate are high, PFK-1 is inhibited; and, with accumulation of adenosine monophosphate (AMP), PFK-1 is activated. Similarly, PK is inhibited by ATP and acetyl-coenzyme A (acetyl-CoA) and activated by increased amounts of fructose 1,6-bisphosphate.

Bioenergetics

The molecule **pyruvate** is the final product from glycolysis. It can undergo a variety of transformations, including (*a*) conversion to **lactate** in the cytosol under anaerobic conditions; (*b*) conversion to **alanine** in the skeletal muscle; (*c*) conversion to **acetyl-CoA,** which enters the tricarboxylic acid (TCA) cycle and is oxidized, generating NADH and reduced-form flavin adenine dinucleotide ($FADH_2$) molecules; and (*d*) carboxylation to **oxaloacetate,** which can be used in the TCA cycle or in gluconeogenesis. If pyruvate is converted to acetyl-CoA, it generates an NADH molecule, then by undergoing oxidation in the TCA cycle under aerobic conditions, it generates three more NADH molecules, an $FADH_2$ molecule, and a guanosine triphosphate (GTP) molecule. After undergoing the electron transport chain (ETC), the net equivalent is 15 ATP molecules per each molecule of pyruvate, or 36 ATP molecules per glucose.

Pyruvate Kinase Deficiency

Because glycolysis is a primary source for ATP and it generates molecules that enter the TCA cycle and ETC during aerobic conditions, decreased enzyme activity throughout glycolysis can be problematic, and dysfunctional and nonfunctional enzymes in glycolysis such as phosphoglucoisomerase, hexokinase, PFK, and others have been identified. PK deficiency is one of the more common enzymatic defects in glycolysis that has been identified and can present with a clinical spectrum. Commonly, the enzyme defect is not lethal and is most detrimental to erythrocytes because they have no mitochondria and are entirely dependent on glycolysis for the generation of ATP. The ATP is required for the erythrocytes to maintain the biconcave shape. The abnormal erythrocyte shape worsens in the spleen, which is particularly anaerobic, leading to increased clearance of these cells by the spleen. Thus, patients present with hemolytic anemia of varying severity. Most commonly, patients present in early childhood with anemia, splenomegaly, and icterus. On the peripheral smear, spiculated RBCs are seen with an increase in reticulocytes.

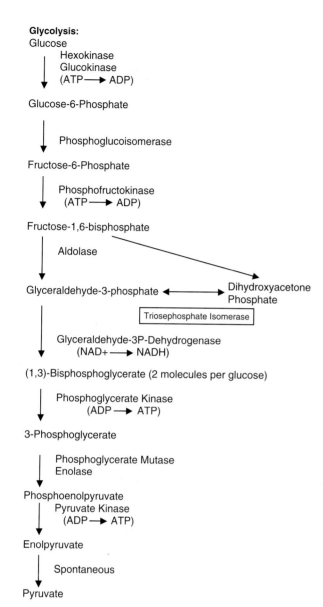

Glycolysis:
Glucose

Hexokinase
Glucokinase
(ATP → ADP)

Glucose-6-Phosphate

Phosphoglucoisomerase

Fructose-6-Phosphate

Phosphofructokinase
(ATP → ADP)

Fructose-1,6-bisphosphate

Aldolase

Glyceraldehyde-3-phosphate ← → Dihydroxyacetone Phosphate

Triosephosphate Isomerase

Glyceraldehyde-3P-Dehydrogenase
(NAD+ → NADH)

(1,3)-Bisphosphoglycerate (2 molecules per glucose)

Phosphoglycerate Kinase
(ADP → ATP)

3-Phosphoglycerate

Phosphoglycerate Mutase
Enolase

Phosphoenolpyruvate

Pyruvate Kinase
(ADP → ATP)

Enolpyruvate

Spontaneous

Pyruvate

• Figure 4-1. The steps of glycolysis and the enzymes that catalyze these steps. *ATP*, adenosine triphosphate; *ADP*, adenosine diphosphate; *NADH*, nicotinamide adenine dinucleotide

CASE CONCLUSION

HA is given a blood transfusion, and after a lengthy discussion with his parents, the decision is made to manage him medically with daily folic acid supplementation. However, he presents with hemolytic anemia twice more in the next year and the decision is made to proceed with a splenectomy. This is effective and he maintains a normal hematocrit level over the following year.

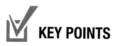

THUMBNAIL: Glycolysis

Glycolysis is a series of enzymatic reactions that convert glucose under differing conditions:

Aerobic conditions: glucose + 2 adenosine diphosphate (ADP) → 2 lactate + 2 ATP

Anaerobic conditions: glucose + 2 ADP + 2 NAD^+ → 2 pyruvate + 2 ATP + 2 NADH

KEY POINTS

■ Regulation of glycolysis is primarily maintained by inhibition of PFK-1, PK, and hexokinase, which are generally activated by a low-energy state with accumulation of AMP or precursors such as fructose-2,6-bisphosphate and inhibited by a high-energy state with accumulation of ATP or molecules such as citrate (PFK-1) or acetyl-CoA (PK)

■ PK deficiency leads to diminished activity of glycolysis, which is particularly detrimental in RBCs, which lack mitochondria and are therefore unable to generate ATP any other way

QUESTIONS

1. In a patient without any enzyme deficiencies who undergoes glycolysis and has normal cytosol and mitochondria, how many molecules of NADH are generated from each molecule of glucose?

A. 4
B. 5
C. 6
D. 8
E. 10

2. In the case presented, PK deficiency leads to hemolytic anemia. However, deficiencies in other enzymes in glycolysis do not necessarily lead to hemolytic anemia. Deficiency of which of the following enzymes does not lead to hemolytic anemia?

A. Glucose-6-phosphate dehydrogenase (G6PD)
B. Hexokinase
C. Aldolase
D. Pyruvate dehydrogenase
E. Phosphoglycerate kinase

HPI: GS is a 9-month-old male infant. He is brought to his primary pediatrician's office for his 9-month checkup. His parents note that although GS eats well and his face and abdomen seem to be growing normally, he does not have the chubby arms and legs that his 11-month-old cousin has.

PE: His head and abdomen are at the fiftieth percentile, but his overall weight and height are below the fifth percentile. He has some yellow plaques on his lower extremities and buttocks. Of note, he has a protuberant abdomen, secondary to an enlarged liver, and consistent with his parents' history, his arms and legs are thin.

Labs: Tests reveal hypoglycemia, with a blood glucose level of 25 mg/dL, increased serum lactate, and both hypertriglyceridemia and hyperuricemia. His CBC count is normal.

THOUGHT QUESTIONS

- What are the pathways of glycogen synthesis and degradation?
- How is glycogen used differently in the liver and skeletal muscle?
- What are the different enzyme deficiencies in the various glycogen storage diseases?

BASIC SCIENCE REVIEW AND DISCUSSION

Glycogen is a highly branched molecule composed of glucose molecules linked primarily by α-1,4-glycosidic bonds, but with α-1,6-glycosidic bonds at the branch points. These branch points require a different enzymatic pathway during synthesis and during degradation, which can make glycogen metabolism seem a bit confusing. Essentially, depending on the driving forces in the body, either the storage or the release of glucose is the most important factor.

Glycogen Synthesis

There are two ways for a glucose molecule to be added to a glycogen molecule: either by lengthening a chain by forming an **α-1,4-glycosidic linkage** or by branching by forming an **α-1,6 bond.** Before their addition to an enlarging glycogen molecule, a glucose molecule must be energized. This process involves the formation of G6P (by glucokinase in the liver and hexokinase elsewhere). The G6P is converted to glucose-1-phosphate (G1P) by **phosphoglucomutase** and the G1P is converted to **uridine diphosphate glucose** (UDP glucose), catalyzed by **UDP glucose pyrophosphorylase.**

This activated glucose molecule, UDP glucose, can donate a glucose molecule to a glycogen chain with an α-1,4 linkage by the enzyme **glycogen synthase.** A branch point is created after approximately 10 glucose molecules have been added by the enzyme **α-1,4- α-1,6-glucan transferase.** This enzyme breaks an α-1,4 bond and moves the glucose to the α-1,6 site, forming a branch point. Glycogen synthase can then add glucose molecules to this newly formed chain.

Glycogen Degradation

Glycogenolysis requires release of G1P units from the ends of glycogen chains and at the branch points. **Glycogen phosphorylase** catalyzes the phosphorolysis of the α-1,4 bond by addition of a phosphate molecule that releases a G1P molecule. This is the rate-limiting step of glycogen degradation and the principal site

of regulation. Once a chain has been broken down to the point where it is approximately four molecules beyond a branch point, **α-1,4- α-1,4-glucan transferase** moves all the glucose molecules from the partially degraded chain, except for the branch point molecule, to the end of the immediate chain to which it is connected. Then the branch point glucose molecule has its α-1,6-glycosidic bond cleaved by α-1,6-glucosidase. These two enzymes working together are considered the debranching enzymes, or debranching system. The G1P molecule can be converted back to G6P by phosphoglucomutase. The G6P can be used by muscle cells in glycolysis; however, in the liver, the G6P is broken down to glucose plus phosphate by G6Pase. The free glucose can then be transported out of the hepatic cells into the serum.

Regulation of Glycogenesis and Glycogenolysis

Glycogen phosphorylase is activated by phosphorylation of a serine side chain. This activation is precipitated by glucagon in the liver or epinephrine in muscle cells, both leading to increased intracellular cyclic AMP (cAMP). Through a cascade mechanism, cAMP-dependent protein kinase A phosphorylates and activates phosphorylase kinase, which, in turn, phosphorylates glycogen phosphorylase. The active form of glycogen phosphorylase can be allosterically inhibited by ATP and glucose and activated by AMP.

In contrast, glycogen synthase is deactivated by phosphorylation that occurs through a similar pathway to the phosphorylation of glycogen phosphorylase. In this way, the same initiating steps of epinephrine or glucagon leading to activation of protein kinase A result in the opposite effect on these two enzymes. Glycogen synthase can be allosterically activated by G6P.

Glycogen Usage in Different Tissues

Glycogen is primarily stored, synthesized, and catabolized in the liver and skeletal muscle. In the liver, glycogen is used primarily to regulate blood glucose levels. After meals with increased levels of blood glucose, glycogenesis is initiated and the excess glucose is stored in the form of glycogen. As blood glucose levels decrease, glycogenolysis can be initiated and can provide glucose for up to 12 hours. While the liver is maintaining glucose levels for the entire body, glycogen storage in skeletal muscle is used to maintain a local fuel source for the highly metabolic cells. Fast-twitch (white) muscle cells release glucose from glycogen and generate ATP via glycolysis, with the end product being lactic acid. Slow-twitch (red) muscle cells, which are mitochondria rich, use the TCA cycle to generate many-fold more ATP from each glucose molecule.

Glycogen Storage Diseases

There are a number of primary glycogen storage diseases, which each have an enzyme deficiency in either the synthesis or the degradation of glycogen. These diseases can range in presentation from hypoglycemia and muscle cramps to severe hypotonia and infant or early childhood death. The most common disease types and enzyme deficiencies are denoted in Table 4-1.

von Gierke Disease

GS in the case presentation is found to have von Gierke disease. This is an autosomal recessive (AR) disease resulting in a deficiency of G6Pase. Without G6Pase in the liver, the final step of glycogen breakdown to glucose cannot occur. This leads to increased levels of G6P and G1P and thus increased levels of glycogen stores in the liver. The G6P can enter glycolysis in the liver, and the end product, lactate, enters the serum. The decreased amount of circulating glucose for bioenergetics leads to increased lipid and protein metabolism. Hyperuricemia develops from both decreased renal clearance and increased production. Long term, these problems can lead to renal failure, growth disturbances, platelet dysfunction, and anemia. Diagnosis is commonly made by liver biopsy, which reveals increased glycogen in the cytoplasm and lipid vacuoles. Type IA disease is confirmed by testing for G6Pase enzyme activity in the biopsy tissue.

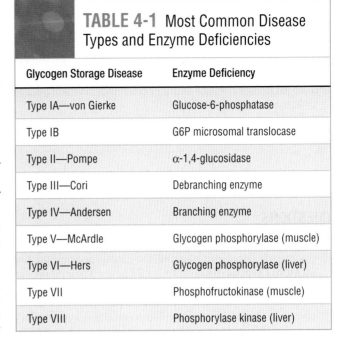

TABLE 4-1 Most Common Disease Types and Enzyme Deficiencies

Glycogen Storage Disease	Enzyme Deficiency
Type IA—von Gierke	Glucose-6-phosphatase
Type IB	G6P microsomal translocase
Type II—Pompe	α-1,4-glucosidase
Type III—Cori	Debranching enzyme
Type IV—Andersen	Branching enzyme
Type V—McArdle	Glycogen phosphorylase (muscle)
Type VI—Hers	Glycogen phosphorylase (liver)
Type VII	Phosphofructokinase (muscle)
Type VIII	Phosphorylase kinase (liver)

CASE CONCLUSION

GS's pediatrician is able to put the constellation of symptoms and laboratory findings together to suspect a glycogen storage disease. He obtains a metabolic consult and a liver biopsy is arranged. This biopsy confirms what is suspected and a diagnosis of von Gierke disease is made. The primary treatment for this disease is frequent feeding, often in the form of continuous tube feeds at night with a mixture of 60% carbohydrates. Cornstarch is commonly used as the primary source of carbohydrates for these patients. GS begins on this dietary regimen provided by his vigilant parents and continues to achieve his developmental milestones over the ensuing year.

THUMBNAIL: Glycogen Synthesis and Degradation

Important Steps in Glycogen Metabolism

Glycogen synthesis:

Step in pathway	Enzyme
Glucose → G6P	Glucokinase (liver) Hexokinase (muscle)
G6P → G1P	Phosphoglucomutase
G1P + uridine triphosphate (UTP) → UDPglucose + PPi	UDPglucose pyrophosphorylase
(Glucose)$_n$ + UDPglucose → (Glucose)$_{n+1}$ + UDP	Glycogen synthase
Glycogen chain → branched chain	α-1,4- α-1,6-glucan transferase

Glycogen degradation:

Step in pathway	Enzyme
(Glucose)$_n$ → (Glucose)$_{n-1}$ + G1P	Glycogen phosphorylase
α-1,4 in branch → α-1,4 linkage in chain	α-1,4- α-1,4-glucan transferase
α-1,6 branch → glycogen chain + glucose	α-1,6-glucosidase

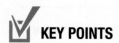

KEY POINTS

■ Glycogen metabolism in the liver is used to maintain serum glucose levels

■ Glycogen storage in muscle cells provides a ready source of glucose for fiber contractions

■ Glycogen metabolism is regulated by activating and deactivating two key enzymes, glycogen phosphorylase and glycogen synthase

■ Glycogen storage diseases result from the inability to either store or break down glycogen. The resulting signs and symptoms are dependent on the severity of the lack of glucose stores.

QUESTIONS

1. An 11-month-old infant presents to the ED with likely gastroenteritis. Because of vomiting, the parents do not think the infant has kept anything down for 24 hours. Their infant has been extremely lethargic and difficult to arouse. On exam, he has a protuberant abdomen. Laboratory tests reveal hypoglycemia, elevated lactate, hyperuricemia, and hypertriglyceridemia. After he is stabilized for several days, a liver biopsy is performed and his G6Pase activity is normal. His most likely diagnosis is which of the following?

   A. Type IA, von Gierke disease
   B. Type IB, G6P microsomal translocase deficiency
   C. Type III, Cori disease
   D. Type VI, Hers disease
   E. Type V, McArdle disease

2. A 17-year-old male presents with complaints of severe muscle cramps and weakness after running. He notes that he has had mild cramping after running for several years, but as he increased the distance run over the last few months, he has had increased severity of symptoms. He has attempted to treat the cramps with potassium supplementation to no avail. He is most likely to have which of the following glycogen storage diseases?

   A. Type I, von Gierke disease
   B. Type II, Pompe disease
   C. Type III, Cori disease
   D. Type IV, Andersen disease
   E. Type V, McArdle disease

3. The patient in question 2 is suspected of having one of the glycogen storage diseases. By what intervention will the diagnosis be made?

   A. Liver biopsy and assessing phosphorylase kinase activity
   B. Liver biopsy and assessing glycogen phosphorylase activity
   C. Muscle biopsy and assessing glycogen phosphorylase activity
   D. Genetic testing for mutation on chromosome arm 6
   E. Body CT to measure muscle versus hepatic mass

HPI: LA is a 13-year-old boy who is brought by his mother to an optometrist. He has had rapid deterioration in his vision over the past 2 months. At first, he noticed the vision in his left eye was blurry and his mother noticed him rubbing this eye frequently. After several weeks, the vision in his right eye also became blurry, and he now notices that colors "don't look right."

PE: He has noticeable nystagmus. On exam, he has papilledema and circumpapillary telangiectatic microangiopathy. His optometrist sends him to an ophthalmologist, who among other things orders a serum lactate.

THOUGHT QUESTIONS

- Of what diagnoses are the optometrist and ophthalmologist suspicious?
- What are the steps of the ETC?
- How does the ETC produce ATP?
- How is this process regulated?

BASIC SCIENCE REVIEW AND DISCUSSION

Leber hereditary optic neuropathy (LHON) results from mitochondrial mutations that lead to disruptions in complexes I and III of the **ETC**. For example, more than 50% of individuals have a point mutation at nucleotide position 11,778, which leads to a substitution of histidine for arginine in complex I. This leads to a disruption in ATP production and a buildup of NADH. The lack of ATP can lead to damage to the optic nerve and a buildup of lactic acid secondary to inhibition of pyruvate dehydrogenase from NADH buildup. To better understand how LHON can affect bioenergetics, we need to review the ETC and oxidative phosphorylation.

ATP Production from Oxidative Phosphorylation

The ETC converts the NADH and $FADH_2$ produced in glycolysis, the TCA cycle, and oxidation of fatty acids back into their oxidized states. This is done in a sequence of steps, and energy produced by several of these steps is used to produce ATP via oxidative phosphorylation. Although this process is not particularly efficient (only 40% of the energy produced is used to make ATP), without it, ATP production from catabolism is decreased dramatically.

NADH Shuttles

The NADH produced in the cytoplasm needs to be brought into the mitochondria to undergo oxidative phosphorylation. There are two shuttles, the **malate shuttle** and the **α-glycerol phosphate shuttle.** NADH can be oxidized in the production of malate from oxaloacetate, and malate is then shuttled across the mitochondrial membrane. Once inside, malate regenerates both the NADH and the oxaloacetate. The latter is converted to aspartate and shuttled back into the cytosol. The NADH can then enter the ETC. Dihydroxyacetone phosphate conversion to α-glycerol phosphate also oxidizes NADH, and then α-glycerol phosphate can be shuttled across the mitochondrial membrane. However, once inside, the regeneration of dihydroxyacetone

phosphate produces an $FADH_2$ molecule instead of an NADH. This leads to one less ATP per molecule shuttled from the α-glycerol phosphate as compared with the malate shuttle.

Electron Transport Chain

There are four enzyme complexes and two sole enzymes (coenzyme Q [CoQ] and cytochrome *c*) that compose the ETC. NADH enters the ETC via complex I and in so doing produces one ATP. Succinate enters the ETC via complex II (which is succinate dehydrogenase from TCA cycle fame), which does not produce an ATP. CoQ is the common entry site for NADH after complex I, succinate after complex II (because it produces an $FADH_2$), and $FADH_2$. All three can then go on to complex III, cytochrome *c*, and complex IV in sequence. This latter process generates two ATPs, and the reduced oxygen produces H_2O.

ATP Synthase

It has been proposed that ATP is produced via a proton motive force secondary to the proton gradient produced by the ETC. Thus, because complex II does not produce protons, it cannot produce ATP. However, complexes I, III, and IV each produce protons that create a gradient across the inner mitochondrial membrane. ATP synthase, or complex V, couples with this proton gradient at the inner mitochondrial membrane and uses the chemiosmotic energy to produce ATP. ATP synthase is composed of two subunits, a proton channel (F0) and an enzyme that catalyzes ADP to ATP (F1) in the presence of a proton gradient.

Leber Hereditary Optic Neuropathy

Although it was described 100 years ago, the genetic etiology of LHON has just recently been determined. Point mutations in the mitochondrial DNA (mtDNA) lead to either single amino acid substitutions or the disruption of a stop codon, which fundamentally changes the polypeptide produced. This disrupts the enzymes in the ETC, leading to decreased ATP production and buildup of NADH in particular. Exactly how these changes lead to LHON is not entirely clear. Because the mtDNA is in the mitochondria, which are derived solely from the mother (passed from ova to offspring), inheritance is via mitochondrial inheritance. Interestingly, men are affected at a much higher rate than women. However, the LHON mtDNA mutations have reduced penetrance, with only approximately 50% of men and 15% of women who possess a primary LHON mtDNA mutation developing blindness.

CASE CONCLUSION

LA's vision proceeded to worsen over the ensuing 2 years, and he developed a large central scotoma. Because of this, he is legally blind and unable to drive. However, he is still able to ambulate and even read with the aid of corrective lenses.

THUMBNAIL: Oxidative Phosphorylation

NADH and FADH$_2$ in the ETC

NADH

Sources: NADH from TCA, oxidation of fatty acids, malate shuttle from cytosol

NADH $\Rightarrow$ Complex I (ATP) $\Rightarrow$ CoQ $\Rightarrow$ Complex III (ATP) $\Rightarrow$ Complex IV (ATP)

Net production of three ATP molecules per NADH molecule

FADH$_2$

Sources: FADH$_2$ from TCA, fatty acid oxidation, α-glycerol phosphate shuttle from cytosol

FADH$_2$ $\Rightarrow$ CoQ $\Rightarrow$ Complex III (ATP) $\Rightarrow$ Complex IV (ATP)

Net production of two ATP per FADH$_2$ molecule

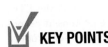

KEY POINTS

- Not all NADH molecules are created equal; for that produced in the cytosol that uses the α-glycerol phosphate shuttle, only three ATPs are generated as compared with the malate shuttle

- Oxidative phosphorylation involves the transfer of electrons to oxygen, producing H$_2$O and ATP

- Oxidative phosphorylation is accomplished by a series of enzyme complexes, coenzymes, and cytochromes

QUESTIONS

1. A catabolic process produces two NADHs in the cytosol that enter the mitochondria via the α-glycerol phosphate shuttle and a pyruvate that enters the mitochondria and leads to one turn of the TCA cycle. How many ATP molecules will be produced?

   A. 14
   B. 16
   C. 18
   D. 19
   E. 21

2. The mother of LA, the patient from this case, understands that LHON is a genetic disease. She is concerned about the risk to LA's children (her grandchildren). What is the chance that LA's children will be affected (assuming his future wife has no mutations)?

   A. 0%
   B. 25%
   C. 33%
   D. 50%
   E. 100%

3. A patient has an enzyme deficiency that leads to a disruption in the α-glycerol phosphate shuttle. In this patient, how many ATPs will be produced for each molecule of glucose catabolized?

   A. 2
   B. 6
   C. 12
   D. 22
   E. 32

CASE 4-4 Fatty Acid Metabolism

HPI: FA is a 7-month-old infant who has been increasingly lethargic over the past month. Her anxious parents bring her to the ED because when they went to wake her this morning for her feeding after sleeping for 8 hours straight, she was difficult to awaken. After being awake for several minutes, she had some twitching and jerking of her arms and legs and was even more difficult to awaken over the next 30 minutes. Her parents report that her pregnancy and birth were entirely normal, and that her weight gain has been within normal limits over the past 7 months. They are particularly anxious because their first child died of sudden infant death syndrome (SIDS) at age 9 months.

PE: She is afebrile with normal vital signs. HEENT, thoracic, cardiac, and pulmonary exams show no abnormalities. Of note, she has a protuberant abdomen secondary to an enlarged liver.

Labs: Hypoglycemia, with a blood glucose level of 28 mg/dL, metabolic acidosis with increased anion gap, but low ketone bodies. Uric acid is elevated, but her ALT and AST levels are normal. Her urine reveals no ketones and increased medium-chain dicarboxylic acids. Her CBC count is normal.

THOUGHT QUESTIONS

- What does FA most likely have, and what are the key elements of this disease?
- How are fatty acids synthesized?
- What are the key steps in β-oxidation of fatty acids?
- How are fatty acid synthesis and oxidation controlled?

BASIC SCIENCE REVIEW AND DISCUSSION

Medium-chain acyl-CoA dehydrogenase (MCAD) deficiency is a disease that is caused by an inability to use the fatty acid stores of the body as a fuel source. In particular, because there are short-, medium-, and long-chain fatty acids, MCAD is necessary for C4-to-C14 fatty acid oxidation. Because the long-chain fatty acids need to go through these chain lengths, this diminishes the amount of energy that can be realized from storage as medium- or long-chain fatty acids. To better understand the syndrome, we present a brief overview of fatty acid synthesis and oxidation.

Fatty Acids

Fatty acids are amphiphilic molecules (both polar and nonpolar) composed of a hydrocarbon chain with a carboxyl group at one terminus. In humans, the important fatty acids generally have an even number of carbons, except propionic acid, which has three. Saturated fatty acids have no double bonds, monounsaturated fatty acids contain one double bond, and polyunsaturated fatty acids contain two or more double bonds. Although many fatty acids can be synthesized, some are considered essential fatty acids, such as linoleic acid (C6 = C3 = C8 − COOH, where the double bonds are indicated by an equal sign), and can only be obtained from the diet. Fatty acids are primarily stored as triacylglycerols, which are glycerol (C3) backbones with ester linkage to three fatty acids.

Fatty Acid Synthesis

The synthesis of fatty acids takes place in the cytosol, but its major fuel, acetyl-CoA, is created inside mitochondria. Because the mitochondrial membrane is impermeable to acetyl-CoA, it is shuttled across with the citrate shuttle. This involves the entrance step of the TCA cycle where citrate is made from acetyl-CoA and oxaloacetate. The citrate molecule then is able to cross the mitochondrial membrane. Once in the cytosol, it can decompose into oxaloacetate and acetyl-CoA. The oxaloacetate further decomposes to pyruvate, which crosses back inside the mitochondria, but the acetyl-CoA molecule can enter into fatty acid synthesis. The first step of this is catalyzed by **acetyl-CoA carboxylase**, which converts acetyl-CoA to **malonyl-CoA** by the addition of a carboxyl group from bicarbonate. Malonyl-CoA then acts to donate two carbon units during the elongation step of fatty acid synthesis. **Fatty acid synthase** acts to catalyze the rest of fatty acid synthesis. It is a multienzyme complex that cycles through four distinct steps in order to donate two carbon units from malonyl-CoA to an elongating fatty acid chain. Acetyl-CoA is bound to the synthase component and added to malonyl-S-acyl carrier protein (ACP) via **condensation to form acetoacetyl-S-ACP**. This then undergoes reduction, dehydration, and a second reduction to become butyryl-S-ACP (butyric acid is a four-carbon fatty acid). The butyryl-CoA can then be transferred to the synthase component and condensed with another malonyl-CoA to elongate the chain. This is generally repeated until the saturated fatty acid palmitoyl-CoA is formed. Palmitoyl-CoA can continue synthesis of longer fatty acids in the endoplasmic reticulum using acetyl-CoA and malonyl-CoA as carbon donors. Unsaturated fats can be synthesized in the endoplasmic reticulum by undergoing desaturation reactions.

Oxidation of Fatty Acids

Unlike synthesis, fatty acid oxidation takes place primarily in the mitochondria. Fatty acids are transported into the mitochondria from the cytosol via the carnitine shuttle. This involves two enzymes and a transporter. Carnitine acyltransferase-I (CAT-I) combines fatty acyl-CoA with carnitine to form fatty acylcarnitine. Carnitine translocase then transports fatty acylcarnitine into the mitochondria. Finally, CAT-II re-forms the activated fatty acyl-CoA in the mitochondria.

Once inside the mitochondria, the fatty acid can undergo β-oxidation of fatty acids, which sequentially removes two carbon fragments from the carboxyl end of the molecule. β-Oxidation involves a cycle of four steps, and the net result from each turn of the cycle is an acetyl-CoA, NADH, and FADH$_2$. The steps (illustrated here) are as follows:

R − C − C − C(=O) − S−CoA (fatty acyl-CoA) → R − C = C − C(=O) − S−CoA (enoyl-CoA) + $FADH_2$

Dehydrogenation: Formation of a double bond between the α and β carbon generates $FADH_2$.

R − C =C − C(=O) − S-CoA + H_2O → R − C(OH) − C − C(=O) − S-CoA (β-hydroxyacyl-CoA)

Hydration: Adds H_2O to the double bond, and OH to the β carbon.

R − C(OH) − C − C(=O) − S-CoA → R − C(=O) − C − C(=O) − S-CoA (β-ketoacyl-CoA) + NADH

Dehydrogenation: Converts OH to =O and NADH.

R − C(=O) − C − C(=O) − S-CoA + CoASH → R − C(=O) − S-CoA + C − C(=O) − S-CoA (acetyl-CoA)

Thiolytic cleavage: Adds CoA-SH to the β carbon and releases acetyl-CoA.

The end result of β-oxidation of fatty acids with an odd number of carbons is propionyl-CoA, which can be converted first to methylmalonyl-CoA and then succinyl-CoA, which can enter into the TCA cycle. For a fatty acid with an even number of carbons, $2n$, the net production of acetyl-CoA molecules is n and the number of NADH and $FADH_2$ is $(n − 1)$ each. So for a fatty acid with 16 carbons, 8 acetyl-CoA, 7 NADH, and 7 $FADH_2$ would be produced. Each acetyl-CoA then can enter the TCA cycle and generate 12 ATPs. Because the fatty acid requires two ATPs to undergo activation, the addition of the high-energy thiol ester bond to CoASH, the net production is then $5*(n) +12*(n−1) − 2$ for a fatty acid with $2n$ carbons.

Regulation of Fatty Acid Metabolism

In fatty acid synthesis, the enzyme that catalyzes the first step, acetyl-CoA carboxylase, is the prime point of control. It is activated by citrate, insulin, and increased carbohydrate availability, and it is inhibited by glucagon and increased fatty acid availability. Its synthesis is actually induced by insulin. β-Oxidation of fatty acids is controlled primarily by controlling the flow of fatty acids across the mitochondrial membrane. CAT-I, which is responsible for bringing fatty acids into the mitochondria, is inhibited by malonyl-CoA. Generally, fatty acid oxidation will be decreased by insulin and increased by glucagon.

MCAD Deficiency

The gene for MCAD is located on chromosome arm 1p31. Many MCAD gene variants have been reported, but one, the K304E MCAD mutation, accounts for the majority of MCAD mutations identified to date. MCAD is an AR disorder; therefore, individuals who are homozygous or compound heterozygous for an MCAD mutation may have abnormal protein product and subsequent insufficient enzymatic activity to metabolize medium-chain fatty acids. The carrier frequency for the K304E MCAD mutation is between 1:40 to 1:100. Whites of northern European descent exhibit the highest frequency of MCAD-deficient genotypes.

Clinical Manifestations

MCAD-deficient patients are at risk for the following outcomes: hypoglycemia, vomiting, lethargy, encephalopathy, respiratory arrest, hepatomegaly, seizures, apnea, cardiac arrest, coma, and sudden death. Long-term outcomes may include developmental and behavioral disability, chronic muscle weakness, failure to thrive, cerebral palsy, and attention deficit disorder (ADD). Although there are a number of different gene mutations, the different phenotypic presentations of these mutations has not been determined. Furthermore, the penetrance of MCAD mutations is unclear because there are a number of patients who have the same MCAD deficiency as their symptomatic siblings yet do not develop the same clinical symptoms in type or severity. Often, a precipitating factor is needed for clinical symptoms to develop, particularly stress secondary to fasting, increased activity, or illness such as infection, in which metabolic demands are higher.

There has been much concern regarding the risk of SIDS in both homozygotes and heterozygote carriers of the MCAD deficiency mutation, particularly the most common K304E mutation. Recent studies suggest that although there is an increase in the incidence of SIDS in homozygotic patients, there does not seem to be an increase in the prevalence of MCAD mutation carriers among infants with SIDS.

Diagnosis

MCAD mutations can be identified through DNA-based tests using PCR and therefore can be detected in patients by DNA analysis. When identification of the K304E mutation is used for diagnostic purposes, detection of homozygosity confirms diagnosis of MCAD deficiency; those heterozygotic for K304E will need confirmation of a second MCAD allelic variant. Mass screening for MCAD deficiency, however, is generally conducted with the detection of abnormal metabolites in urine or blood by tandem mass spectrometry (MS/MS). Typically, MS/MS is used as an initial screening modality followed by confirmation of MCAD deficiency with a urine organic acid profile or DNA mutation analysis.

Treatment and Prognosis

Treatment of MCAD deficiency is primarily by both timing and content of diet. In infants and children, whose metabolic demands are higher, it is important for them to have regular meals, with generally no more than 6 to 8 hours between meals. This issue is more important when they undergo a period of metabolic stress, such as an illness. As with other fatty acid deficiencies, supplementation of the diet with carnitine is also instituted. If the disease is identified early before too many hypoglycemic events have caused brain injury, treatment with diet can lead to a much improved prognosis. Others may unfortunately experience developmental delay, behavioral disorders, and cerebral palsy.

CASE CONCLUSION

FA is started on frequent feedings, including cornstarch before nighttime sleep and carnitine supplementation. Her lethargy improves and she has no further seizure activity. By age 2 years, she is walking, speaking words and short phrases, and appears well.

THUMBNAIL: Fatty Acid Metabolism

Important Steps in Fatty Acid Metabolism
Fatty acid synthesis

Step in pathway	Enzyme	Bioenergetics
Acetyl-CoA + HCO_3^- → malonyl-CoA	Acetyl-CoA carboxylase	Requires one ATP
C2n-S-ACP + malonyl-CoA → C2(n+1)−S-ACP	Fatty acid synthase	Requires two NADPH
Total		
8 acetyl-CoA + HCO_3^- → palmitoyl-CoA (C16)		Requires 7 ATP + 14 NADPH

Fatty acid oxidation

Step in pathway	Enzyme	Bioenergetics
Activation, adding CoASH, and using ATP → AMP + PPi → AMP + 2 Pi	Fatty acyl-CoA synthetase	Two ATP equivalents used
Transfer to mitochondria		
Fatty acyl-CoA + carnitine → fatty acylcarnitine	CAT-I	None
Fatty acylcarnitine into the mitochondria	Carnitine translocase	None
Fatty acylcarnitine → fatty acyl-CoA + carnitine	CAT-II	None
β-Oxidation of fatty acids		
Dehydrogenation forms enoyl-CoA	Fatty acyl-CoA dehydrogenases	$FADH_2$ generated
Hydration forms → β-Hydroxyacyl-CoA		
Dehydrogenation forms β-ketoacyl-CoA		NADH generated
Thiolytic cleavage forms shorter fatty acyl-CoA plus acetyl-CoA		

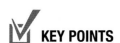

KEY POINTS

- Fatty acids are used both in synthesis of other biologically important molecules and as a source of fuel
- The oxidation of fatty acids yields acetyl-CoA, which can enter the TCA cycle
- MCAD deficiency is the result of a mutation in the fatty acyl-CoA dehydrogenase enzyme responsible for the first step of β-oxidation of fatty acids

QUESTIONS

1. In the setting of MCAD deficiency, one of the aspects of treatment is carnitine dietary supplementation, which is important to overcome which of the following?

   A. A total body deficiency of carnitine seen in these patients
   B. A carnitine deficiency in the mitochondria
   C. A carnitine deficiency in the cytosol
   D. The down-regulation of fatty acyl-CoA activity in the cytosol
   E. The decreased acetyl-CoA for the TCA cycle, by entering into TCA at a later step

2. A total of 81% of MCAD-deficient individuals are homozygous for the K304E mutation, 18% are heterozygous for the K304E mutation, and 1% of MCAD-deficient patients do not have the K304E mutation. Given this information, using Hardy-Weinberg formulations, what percentage of MCAD gene mutations are the non-K304E mutation?

   A. 10%
   B. 20%
   C. 30%
   D. 40%
   E. 50%

3. A patient with type I diabetes presents for a visit with her primary care provider. While waiting in the reception area, the patient gives herself an insulin shot and eats her lunch with 45 g of carbohydrates. If her physician sent labs, which of the following would be the correct change secondary to insulin's activity?

   A. Increased fatty acyl-CoA synthetase activity
   B. Decreased CAT-I activity
   C. Increased CAT-II activity
   D. Decreased acetyl-CoA carboxylase synthesis
   E. Increased protein catabolism

CASE 4-5　Steroid Biosynthesis

HPI: AG is a newborn infant who presents with fused labia majora and clitoromegaly. AG is the product of a normal, full-term pregnancy to a 29-year-old white mother. On day 3 of life while still hospitalized for evaluation of these anomalies, AG becomes listless and exhibits the classic "failure to thrive" syndrome.

PE: AG weighs 3050 g, 350 g less than birth weight, and has a normal BP. While being evaluated for these signs, AG is placed on an IV drip and laboratory tests are sent.

Labs: The immediate lab results reveal low serum sodium and potassium levels, high urinary fractional excretion of sodium (FeNa) level, and elevated serum 17α-hydroxyprogesterone, but decreased 11-deoxycortisol. Serum adrenocorticotropic hormone (ACTH) level and karyotype are pending.

THOUGHT QUESTIONS

- What are the pathways of steroid biosynthesis?
- What organs produce steroid hormones?
- What enzyme deficiencies can lead to congenital adrenal hyperplasia (CAH)?
- In CAH, what hormones need to be replaced?

BASIC SCIENCE REVIEW AND DISCUSSION

Steroid biosynthesis occurs in the ovaries, testes, and adrenal cortex. All of the steroid hormones are derived from a single precursor, cholesterol. **Cholesterol** is converted to **pregnenolone** by an enzyme known as either **20,22-desmolase** or cholesterol side-chain cleavage enzyme. Pregnenolone can then be converted either to **progesterone** or to **17β-hydroxypregnenolone** depending on what pathway the precursor is entering.

Mineralocorticoid Biosynthesis

In mineralocorticoid synthesis, pregnenolone is converted to progesterone by **3β-hydroxysteroid dehydrogenase.** This occurs in the adrenal cortex in the outer region known as the zona glomerulosa. The next two steps in this pathway are catalyzed by enzymes common to glucocorticoid synthesis, **21-hydroxylase** and **11β-hydroxylase** (Fig. 4-2). The final two steps (which rarely have enzymatic deficiencies) are carried out to produce aldosterone.

Glucocorticoid Biosynthesis

Cortisol, the final product from glucocorticoid synthesis, can be produced from either progesterone or 17α-hydroxypregnenolone in the zona fasciculata. **17β-Hydroxylase** can catalyze the production of 17α-hydroxypregnenolone from pregnenolone or 17α-hydroxyprogesterone from progesterone. 17α-Hydroxyprogesterone can also be produced from 17α-hydroxypregnenolone by 3β-hydroxysteroid dehydrogenase. 21-Hydroxylase and 11β-hydroxylase then convert 17α-hydroxyprogesterone to **cortisol.**

Sex Hormone Biosynthesis

Sex hormones are synthesized in the adrenal cortex in the zona reticularis or in the ovaries or testes. The enzyme **17,20-desmolase** can covert either 17α-hydroxypregnenolone or 17α-hydroxyprogesterone to androgenic precursors. The androgenic hormones testosterone and androstenedione can be converted to estrone and estradiol, respectively, by aromatase. However, aromatase is present only in the ovaries.

Congenital Adrenal Hyperplasia

As can be seen in the steroid biosynthetic pathways, if there is a lack of one of the enzymes that lead pregnenolone toward mineralocorticoid or glucocorticoid synthesis, the precursors can be converted to androgens. In women, a small amount of these androgens will be converted to estrogens, but the great majority end up in the peripheral circulation. This leads to the phenotypic findings of virilization seen in this case. In addition, the lack of glucocorticoids and mineralocorticoids can have a disastrous effect, essentially an Addisonian crisis at several days of life. The severity of these findings is associated with the particular enzyme deficiency.

The most common enzyme deficiency leading to **CAH** is that of 21α-hydroxylase. Patients will have symptoms similar to those of AG, and about half will exhibit salt wasting like AG. The diagnosis can be confirmed by the elevation of 17α-hydroxyprogesterone without an elevation in 11-deoxycortisol. If the deficient enzyme is 11β-hydroxylase, then 11-deoxycortisol will be elevated.

Patients with CAH need treatment both to replace their missing hormones and to guard against the effects of the excess androgens. Replacement is most commonly with hydrocortisone or prednisone, and patients with salt wasting will also need a mineralocorticoid such as fludrocortisone. The steroid replacement then acts to both replace missing hormones and produce a negative feedback on ACTH production, diminishing the amount of excess androgens. Females with virilization may require surgical therapy, but often mild effects may reverse with medical therapy.

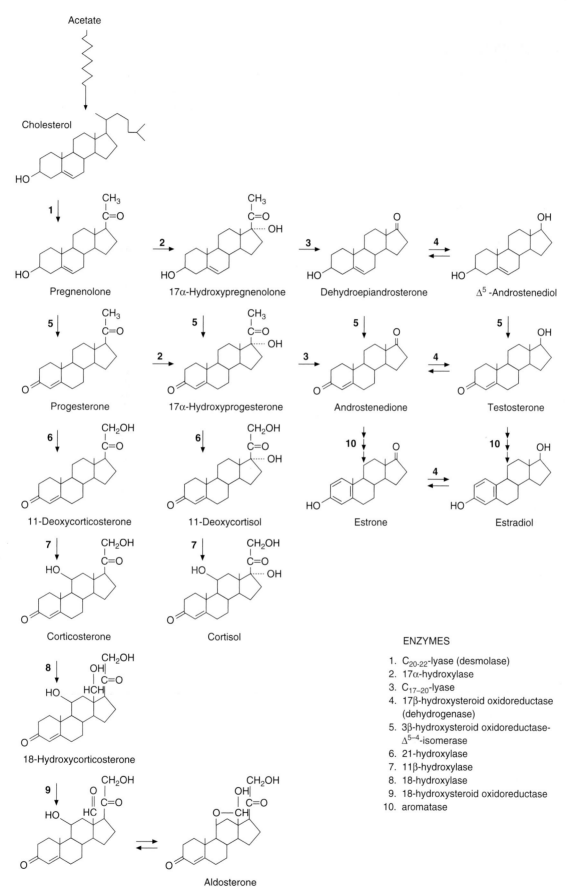

• **Figure 4-2.** The steps in the biosynthesis of the steroid hormones using three primary pathways to generate glucocorticoids, mineralocorticoids, and the sex steroids. (Reproduced with permission from Mishell DR, Davajan V, Lobo RA, et al. Infertility, Contraception, and Reproductive Endocrinology. 3rd ed. Malden: Blackwell Science, 1991.)

ENZYMES

1. C_{20-22}-lyase (desmolase)
2. 17α-hydroxylase
3. C_{17-20}-lyase
4. 17β-hydroxysteroid oxidoreductase (dehydrogenase)
5. 3β-hydroxysteroid oxidoreductase-Δ^{5-4}-isomerase
6. 21-hydroxylase
7. 11β-hydroxylase
8. 18-hydroxylase
9. 18-hydroxysteroid oxidoreductase
10. aromatase

CASE CONCLUSION

AG's karyotype comes back as 46,XX, which reassures her parents that she is indeed a baby girl. Her ACTH level is quite elevated, as are her androstenedione levels. She is given both hydrocortisone and fludrocortisone, and these levels diminish over the next few weeks. An estrogen cream is placed topically on her labia, and over the next few months, the thin adhesions keeping the labia together resolve, as does her clitoromegaly.

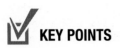

THUMBNAIL: Steroid Biosynthesis

Important Steps in Steroid Synthesis

Enzyme	Pathway	Precursor	Product
20,22-Desmolase	Common	Cholesterol	Pregnenolone
21-Hydroxylase	Mineralocorticoid Glucocorticoid	Progesterone 17α-Hydroxyprogesterone	11-Deoxycortisone 11-Deoxycortisol
11β-Hydroxylase	Mineralocorticoid Glucocorticoid	11-Deoxycorticosterone 11-Deoxycortisol	Corticosterone Cortisol
17α-Hydroxylase	Gluco, sex hormone	Pregnenolone Progesterone	17α-hydroxypregnenolone 17α-hydroxyprogesterone
17,20-Desmolase	Sex hormone	17α-Hydroxypregnenolone 17α-Hydroxyprogesterone	Dehydroepiandrosterone Androstenedione

KEY POINTS

- Cholesterol is the common precursor of all the steroid hormones
- A missing enzyme in these biosynthetic pathways leads to both an absence of one hormone and an excess of another
- The most common enzyme deficiency leading to CAH is 21-hydroxylase

QUESTIONS

1. A 10-day-old boy is diagnosed with a variant of CAH. He is missing the activity of the 11β-hydroxylase enzyme. Which of the following will be elevated?

   A. Cholesterol, pregnenolone, 11-deoxycorticosterone
   B. Cholesterol, pregnenolone, 11-deoxycortisol
   C. Pregnenolone, 11-deoxycortisol, 11-deoxycorticosterone
   D. 11-Deoxycortisol, 11-deoxycorticosterone, estrone
   E. 11-Deoxycortisol, 11-deoxycorticosterone, androstenedione

2. When considering the classic presenting signs, symptoms, and lab abnormalities of CAH, which of the following enzyme deficiencies is likely to cause CAH?

   A. 20,22-Desmolase
   B. 17,20-Desmolase
   C. 3β-Hydroxysteroid dehydrogenase
   D. 18-Hydroxylase
   E. 18-Hydroxysteroid dehydrogenase

HPI: CS is 1-month-old female infant who was born with several congenital anomalies. These include an extra finger on each hand, a cleft lip and palate, and Hirschsprung disease. Over the past month, she has seen several plastic surgeons regarding repair of these congenital anomalies, and now she is being seen by a genetic specialist because her primary pediatrician is concerned that in addition to these congenital anomalies, she is not feeding well or gaining weight.

PE: The geneticist notes the aforementioned anomalies, in addition to low-set ears, drooping eyelids, and a small upturned nose.

Labs: Concerned for a genetic abnormality, she orders a test for a 7-dehydrocholesterol (7-DHC) level, among other tests.

THOUGHT QUESTIONS

- What diagnosis is the geneticist concerned about?
- How will the 7-DHC level help in diagnosis?
- What are the key steps on the pathway of biosynthesis of cholesterol?

BASIC SCIENCE REVIEW AND DISCUSSION

One of the leading diagnoses with this constellation of findings is Smith-Lemli-Opitz syndrome (SLOS). This syndrome is due to a genetic defect in the synthesis of cholesterol; thus, we begin with a review of cholesterol biosynthesis.

Cholesterol Synthesis

The key first steps in **cholesterol synthesis** include two acetyl-CoA molecules combining to make **acetoacetyl-CoA,** which further combines with a third acetyl-CoA to make **hydroxymethylglutaryl-CoA (HMG-CoA)** (Fig. 4-3). A step that is both highly regulated and a primary target for cholesterol-lowering agents is catalyzed by HMG-CoA reductase, which reduces HMG-CoA to **mevalonate** (Fig. 4-4). HMG-CoA reductase inhibitors are first-line agents in cholesterol reduction.

Three ATPs are then required to take mevalonate to **isopentenylpyrophosphate** in three steps. Isopentenylpyrophosphate is the first of several compounds in the pathway that are referred to as isoprenoids. Isopentenylpyrophosphate isomerase interconverts isopentenylpyrophosphate and dimethylallylpyrophosphate. **Prenyl transferase** catalyzes head-to-tail condensations of dimethylallylpyrophosphate with isopentenylpyrophosphate several times to form farnesyl pyrophosphate. Squalene synthase then performs head-to-head condensation of two farnesyl pyrophosphate molecules to form **squalene.** Squalene epoxidase catalyzes oxidation of squalene to form 2,3-oxidosqualene, requiring NADPH as a reductant. Squalene oxidocyclase catalyzes a series of cyclization reactions, producing the sterol **lanosterol** (Fig. 4-5).

The conversion of lanosterol to cholesterol then requires 19 steps. The final step is the conversion of 7-DHC to cholesterol. This is catalyzed by **7-dehydrocholesterol-δ-7-reductase (DHCR7).** A defect in this gene is the etiology of SLOS.

Clinical Correlation

SLOS is a genetic disorder that was first described in 1964 in three boys with poor growth, developmental delay, and a common pattern of congenital malformations including cleft palate, genital malformations, and polydactyly (extra fingers and toes). It was not until 1993 that SLOS was determined to be an AR genetic condition caused by deficiency of the enzyme 7-dehydrocholesterol-δ-7-reductase (also known as 3β-hydroxysterol-δ-7-reductase), the final enzyme in the sterol synthetic pathway that converts 7-DHC to cholesterol. This defect in cholesterol production results in a wide variety of congenital anomalies, as well as developmental delay. The incidence of SLOS may be as high as 1 of 20,000 to 1 of 40,000 births, with a carrier frequency of approximately 1 in 30 individuals.

Currently, the reason defects in cholesterol synthesis cause congenital malformations is not understood. Several disparate lines of research have led to our recent understanding of the critical and somewhat unexpected role of cholesterol in early human development. Cholesterol is important in cell membranes, serves as the precursor for steroid hormones and bile acids, and is a major component in myelin. Cholesterol is covalently bound to the embryonic signaling protein **Sonic hedgehog** (Shh) in a necessary step of the autoprocessing of the precursor to the active form, occurring at about day 0 to 7 estimated gestational age in humans.

Shh plays a critical role in several embryologic fields relevant to SLOS (e.g., brain, face, heart, and limbs). Therefore, cholesterol is an essential triggering agent in the early developmental program of the human. Because 7-DHC also can activate Shh, cholesterol deficiency leading to decreased activation of Shh probably is not the sole explanation for congenital malformations in this syndrome. Abnormalities in the Shh-patched signaling cascade presumably play a role. Membrane instability and dysmyelination from cholesterol deficiency and accumulation of 7-DHC and other potentially toxic cholesterol precursors may also contribute to the SLOS phenotype.

Diagnosis and Treatment

SLOS is most commonly diagnosed postnatally, but certain congenital anomalies that can be seen on ultrasound (US) may raise suspicion for SLOS prenatally. These include polydactyly, cleft palate, hypospadias, cataracts, cardiac anomalies, pyloric stenosis, and microcephaly. Many of these anomalies are missed on a routine US, but others, including low-set ears, abnormal palmar creases, micrognathia, foreshortened thumbs, and Hirschsprung disease, will be missed even on level II US exams. In addition, these anomalies can be seen in other syndromes, thereby making a specific diagnosis quite difficult. Postnatally, the diagnosis becomes easier in the setting of one or more of these anomalies with an elevated 7-DHC level. Prenatal screening for SLOS is conducted in many states with second trimester maternal serum

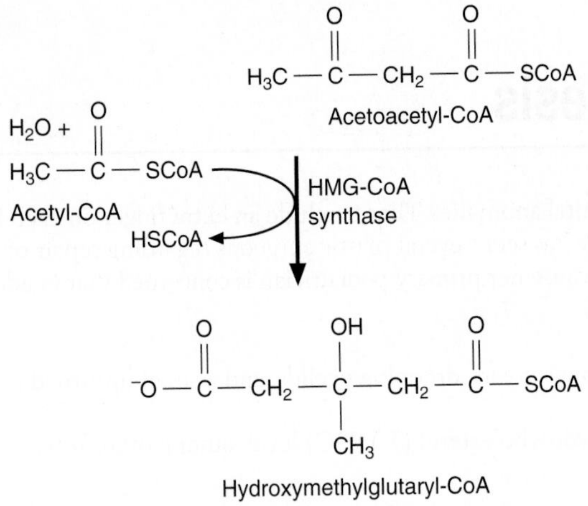

• Figure 4-3. Key regulation step in cholesterol synthesis.

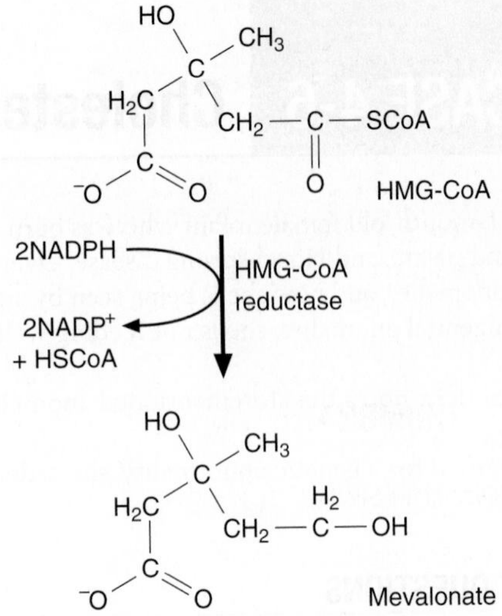

• Figure 4-4. Key pharmacologic target, action of HMG-CoA reductase.

screening. The pattern of analytes suspicious for SLOS is low concentrations of unconjugated estriol, hCG, and alpha-fetoprotein. Carrier detection can be undertaken with biochemical testing of fibroblasts or molecular genetic analysis of known mutations. In addition to elevated levels of 7-DHC, the diagnosis of SLOS can be confirmed by sequence analysis for point mutations in the DHCR7 gene or targeted mutation analysis if a family's mutations are known.

Given the ongoing problem with cholesterol synthesis associated with SLOS, there is hope that treatment can be accomplished with dietary cholesterol supplementation. As a result, many children and adults with SLOS are being given supplementary cholesterol, either in a natural form, such as egg yolks and cream, or in the form of purified cholesterol given as part of several research protocols. Because the accumulation of 7-DHC may contribute to some of the effects of SLOS, HMG-CoA reductase inhibitors are beginning to be used to decrease its production in clinical trials, along with cholesterol supplementation. At this point, curative treatments such as gene therapy are purely theoretical.

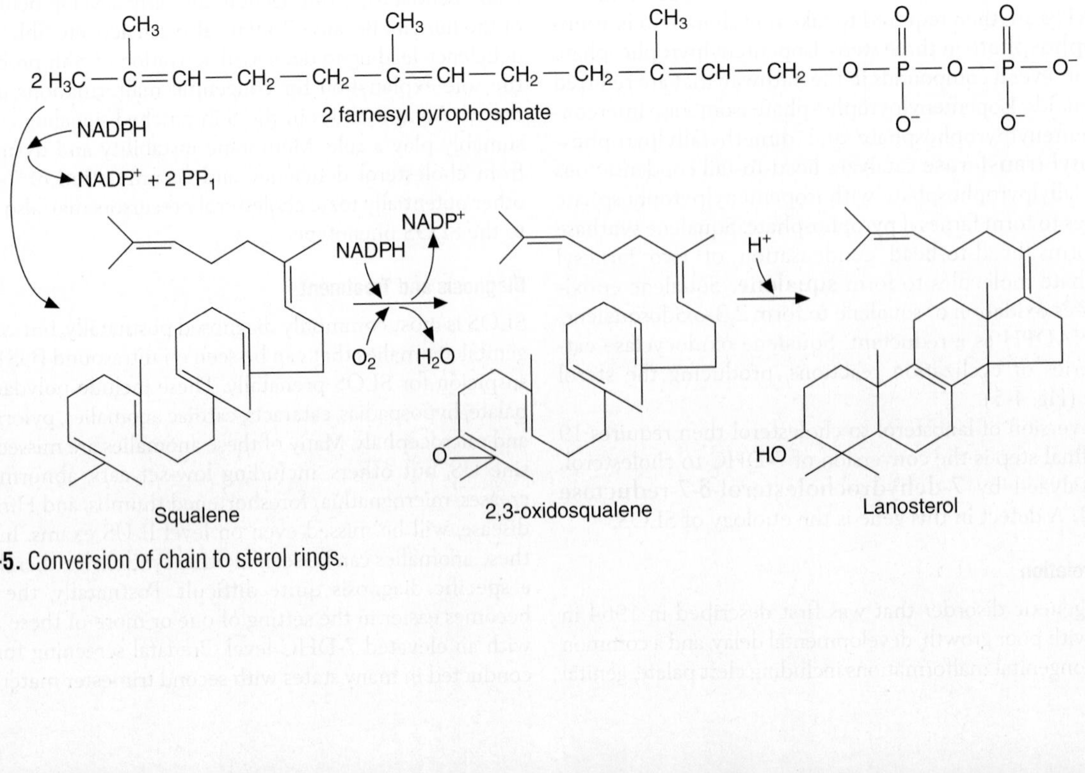

• Figure 4-5. Conversion of chain to sterol rings.

CASE CONCLUSION

CS's lab results reveal an elevated 7-DHC level. She is diagnosed with SLOS and her parents are educated about what this diagnosis means for their daughter and future pregnancies. She begins cholesterol supplementation, and the geneticist and parents begin to look for a clinical trial using HMG-CoA reductase inhibitors in which to enroll CS.

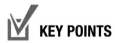

THUMBNAIL: Cholesterol Synthesis

Important Steps in the Synthetic Pathway

Acetyl-CoA + acetyl-CoA → acetoacetyl-CoA

Acetoacetyl-CoA + acetyl-CoA → HMG-CoA

HMG-CoA → mevalonate (catalyzed by HMG-CoA reductase)

Mevalonate →→→ isopentenylpyrophosphate (requires three ATPs)

Isopentenylpyrophosphate and → dimethylallylpyrophosphate isopentenylpyrophosphate isomerase

Isopentenylpyrophosphate and dimethylallylpyrophosphate → farnesyl pyrophosphate

Farnesyl pyrophosphate + farnesyl pyrophosphate → squalene

Squalene → 2,3-oxidosqualene (squalene epoxidase requires NADPH)

2,3-Oxidosqualene →→ lanosterol (squalene oxidocyclase in a series of cyclization steps)

Lanosterol → 18 steps → 7-dehydrocholesterol

7-Dehydrocholesterol → cholesterol (7-dehydrocholesterol-δ-7-reductase)

KEY POINTS

- The key regulation step in cholesterol synthesis is catalyzed by HMG-CoA reductase
- This step is also a key pharmacologic site for cholesterol-lowering agents
- Cholesterol synthesis requires three ATP molecules and an NADPH molecule for each molecule synthesized
- SLOS results from a defect in 7-dehydrocholesterol-δ-7-reductase, which catalyzes the final step in cholesterol synthesis

QUESTIONS

1. Compared with patients with SLOS, patients on enormously high quantities of HMG-CoA reductase inhibitors would have which of the following?

   A. Lower levels of 7-DHC
   B. The same amount of 7-DHC
   C. Greater levels of 7-DHC
   D. Greater levels of mevalonate
   E. Lower levels of HMG-CoA

2. Without reviewing the steps in the thumbnail, the key regulatory step in cholesterol synthesis is which of the following?

   A. Acetyl-CoA to acetoacetyl-CoA
   B. Acetoacetyl-CoA to HMG-CoA
   C. HMG-CoA to mevalonate
   D. Mevalonate to isopentenylpyrophosphate
   E. 7-DHC to cholesterol

HPI: CP is a 29-year-old white man who presents to the ED with chest pain that radiates down his left arm and tingling in his jaw. The symptoms have come and gone at times of stress and exercise for the past year, but the current episode is far worse. His family history includes a deceased maternal grandfather from a heart attack at age 43, as well as a maternal uncle who died of a heart attack at age 38.

PE: Chest and abdominal exams show no abnormalities. Inspection of his ankles reveals nodular swellings on his Achilles tendon. An ECG shows evidence of an acute inferior myocardial infarction (IMI).

Labs: Results are pending.

THOUGHT QUESTIONS

- What genetic diagnoses should the ED doctor consider?
- What key findings help make this diagnosis?
- What are the key elements of lipid digestion, absorption, and transport?
- What is the enterohepatic cycle?

BASIC SCIENCE REVIEW AND DISCUSSION

In patients who do indeed have an MI before the age of 40, **hypercholesterolemia** and **hyperlipidemia** should always be considered in the differential diagnosis. Further strengthening the diagnosis in this patient are the likely **xanthomas** on his tendons, which is seen classically in familial hypercholesterolemia. Before the clinical discussion of these diseases, a brief review of lipid digestion, metabolism, and transport is presented.

Lipid Digestion and Absorption

Because most of the body is an aqueous solution, lipids provide a challenge to digestion, absorption, and transport because of their **hydrophobic** nature. The first step of digestion of lipids is enhanced by bile acids secreted by the liver and stored in the gallbladder (Fig. 4-6). Bile acids are derivatives of cholesterol with polar components, making them **amphipathic.** This property allows them to solubilize fats and be carried through aqueous solutions. Thus, they are able to emulsify fatty molecules in the gut, providing enzymes with better access to them.

One such enzyme is **pancreatic lipase,** which catalyzes hydrolysis of triacylglycerols at their 1 and 3 positions (Fig. 4-7), forming 1,2-diacylglycerols and then 2-monoacylglycerols (monoglycerides). Monoacylglycerols and fatty acids are absorbed by intestinal epithelial cells. Within intestinal epithelial cells, triacylglycerols are resynthesized. **Phospholipase A$_2$** is secreted by the pancreas into the intestine. It hydrolyzes the ester linkage between the fatty acid and the hydroxyl on C2 of phospholipids, producing **lysophospholipids.** These lysophospholipids then aid digestion of other lipids by breaking up fat globules into small micelles.

Enterohepatic Cycle

Cholesterol can be readily synthesized and absorbed, but the only way it is metabolized and excreted is via conversion to **bile salts.** These are then secreted into the intestine and used to emulsify and digest fats, and they are most commonly reabsorbed. This process of the secretion, reabsorption, and return to the liver of bile acids is known as the enterohepatic cycle. Evolutionarily, this is important because there was very little dietary cholesterol available to our ancestors, but it provides a source of major morbidity and mortality, with hypercholesterolemia being a risk factor for atherosclerosis and CAD. Thus, the interruption of this cycle, which allows cholesterol products to be excreted into the GI tract without reabsorption, may help lower cholesterol. These agents include synthetic resins and soluble fibers.

Lipid Transport

Once absorbed by the intestinal cells, cholesterol may be esterified to fatty acids forming cholesteryl esters. This is catalyzed by **acyl-CoA:cholesterol acyltransferase** (ACAT). Fatty acids (which are poorly soluble and have detergent properties) are not bound to cholesterol and thus are kept sequestered from the cytosol by being bound by **intestinal fatty acid-binding protein** (I-FABP) or are transported in the blood bound to **albumin.** Other lipids are transported in the blood as part of **lipoproteins** (Fig. 4-8), complex particles whose structure includes a core consisting of a droplet of triacylglycerols and/or cholesteryl esters, as well as a surface monolayer of phospholipid, cholesterol, and specific proteins (apolipoproteins).

Lipoproteins differ in their contents of proteins and lipids. They are classified based on density.

- **Chylomicron:** largest; lowest in density due to high lipid: protein ratio; highest in triacylglycerols as percentage of weight
- **VLDL:** second highest in triacylglycerols as percentage of weight
- **Intermediate-density lipoprotein (IDL)**
- **LDL:** highest in cholesteryl esters as percentage of weight
- **HDL:** highest in density because of high protein:lipid ratio

After absorbing or synthesizing triacylglycerols, cholesteryl esters, phospholipids, free cholesterol, and apolipoproteins, the epithelial cells lining the intestine package these lipids into **chylomicrons.** The chylomicrons are then secreted and transported via the lymphatic system to the blood. **Apolipoprotein C-II** (apo C-II) on the chylomicron surface activates **lipoprotein lipase,** an enzyme attached to the luminal surface of small blood vessels. Lipoprotein lipase catalyzes hydrolytic cleavage of fatty acids from triacylglycerols of chylomicrons, and these fatty acids and monoacylglycerols are picked up by body cells for use as energy sources. As triacylglycerols are cleaved and removed through this process, the chylomicrons shrink, becoming **chylomicron remnants** with lipid cores having a relatively high concentration of cholesteryl esters. These chylomicron remnants are taken up by liver cells via receptor-mediated endocytosis involving

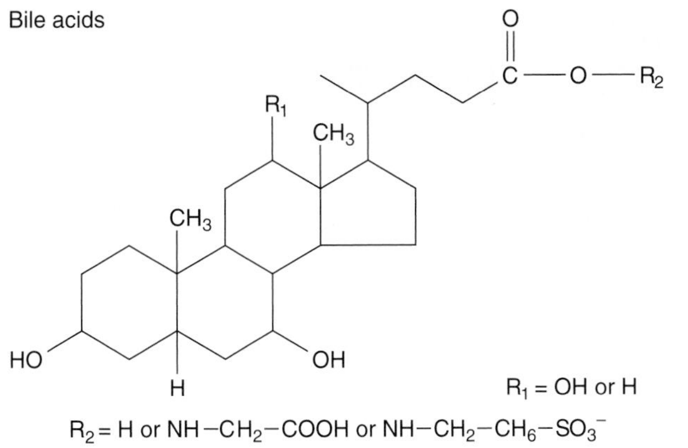

Bile acids

$R_1 = OH$ or H

$R_2 = H$ or $NH-CH_2-COOH$ or $NH-CH_2-CH_6-SO_3^-$

• **Figure 4-6.** Bile acids are amphipathic with both hydrophilic and hydrophobic regions.

recognition of **apo E** (apolipoprotein E) of the chylomicron remnant by receptors on the liver cells.

Liver cells produce and secrete VLDL into the blood. The core of this lipoprotein has a relatively high triacylglycerol content. One of the apolipoproteins of VLDL is B-100. Microsomal triglyceride transfer protein (MTP), in the lumen of the endoplasmic reticulum in the liver, has an essential role in VLDL assembly. MTP facilitates transfer of lipids to apo B-100 while apo B-100 is being translocated into the endoplasmic reticulum lumen during translation. VLDL assembly is dependent on availability of lipids and apo B-100. As VLDL particles are transported in the bloodstream, **lipoprotein lipase** catalyzes triacylglycerol removal by hydrolysis. With this removal, the percentage weight of cholesteryl esters increases. VLDLs are converted to IDLs, and eventually to LDLs. The lipid core of LDL is predominantly cholesteryl esters. Whereas VLDL contains five apolipoprotein types (apo B-100, apo C-I, apo C-II, apo C-III, and apo E), only one protein, apo B-100, is associated with the surface monolayer of LDL. Cell membranes contain an LDL receptor that binds LDL and leads to endocytosis and absorption of the LDL molecule.

HDL (the "good" cholesterol) is secreted as a small protein-rich particle by the liver (and intestine). One HDL apolipoprotein, apo A-I, activates **lecithin-cholesterol acyltransferase (LCAT),** which catalyzes synthesis of cholesteryl esters using fatty acids cleaved from the membrane lipid lecithin. The cholesterol is scavenged from cell surfaces and from other lipoproteins. HDL may transfer some cholesteryl esters to other lipoproteins. Some remain associated with HDL, which may be taken up by the liver and degraded. HDL thus transports cholesterol from tissues and other lipoproteins to the liver, which can excrete excess cholesterol as bile acids.

Clinical Correlation

A number of enzyme, receptor, and molecular deficiencies can result in syndromes that cause premature atherosclerosis. These include familial hypercholesterolemia, lipoprotein lipase deficiency, hypertriglyceridemia, and hyperlipoproteinemia. The pathophysiology of each of these conditions is interesting and depends on the pathways elucidated earlier. Patients with familial hypercholesterolemia, an autosomal dominant (AD) disease that occurs in 1 in 500 individuals, have a mutation in the LDL receptor gene. This leads to elevations in LDL and total cholesterol because LDL is not bound and endocytosed by cells.

Lipoprotein lipase deficiency (AR) results in diminished metabolism of the chylomicrons and their buildup in the plasma. In patients with type III hyperlipoproteinemia (familial dysbetalipoproteinemia), which is essentially AD, the uptake of IDL and chylomicron remnants is diminished or absent, leading to elevated plasma levels of these lipoproteins. Familial hypertriglyceridemia is also an AD disease in which patients have difficulty in catabolizing VLDL triglycerides. This can lead to elevated triglycerides over time.

Diagnosis and Treatment

All of these syndromes result in elevated lipoproteins and/or triglycerides. The two most common clinical presentations are xanthomas and premature **atherosclerosis.** Xanthomas are fatty deposits that are yellow and can erupt anywhere on the body, and certain cases of these syndromes show a clearer pattern of presentation than others. The premature atherosclerosis is most aggressive in familial hypercholesterolemia, often presenting in patients in their 20s and 30s as an MI. Still other patients, those with familial apo C-II deficiency, will present in childhood with pancreatitis. Patients with family histories of these outcomes should be screened with annual lipid profiles and physical exams, and they should be advised to avoid a high-fat, high-carbohydrate diet because patients with diabetes and obesity are more likely to experience the complications of this disease.

Although xanthomas can be surgically removed, removal of atherosclerotic plaques in the arteries throughout the body can be more difficult. CAD in these individuals can be treated with standard management. The prevention and treatment of these rare diseases can include the use of binding agents (e.g., cholestyramine) to reduce cholesterol and triglyceride absorption and distribution. In the syndromes in which there is primarily a cholesterol elevation, HMG-CoA reductase inhibitors, which block the synthesis of cholesterol at its rate-limiting step, can be used.

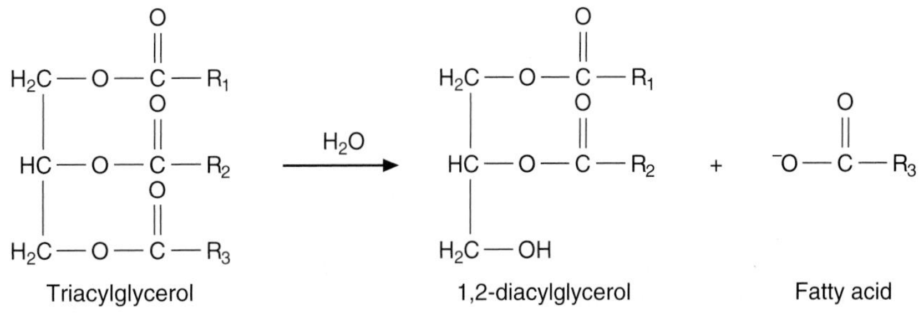

• **Figure 4-7.** Hydrolysis of triacylglycerol.   Triacylglycerol   1,2-diacylglycerol   Fatty acid

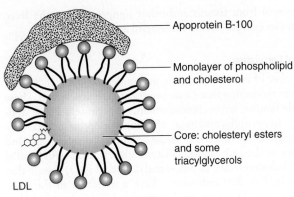

- Apoprotein B-100
- Monolayer of phospholipid and cholesterol
- Core: cholesteryl esters and some triacylglycerols

LDL

• **Figure 4-8.** The structure of LDLs.

CASE CONCLUSION

The ED physician, concerned about an acute MI, begins treatment for CP with an aspirin and a beta-blocker to control his BP, and CP is given morphine for his pain. His labs return with an elevated cardiac troponin I and myocardial muscle creatine kinase isoenzyme (CK-MB) elevation, which are both consistent with an acute MI. His triglycerides and LDLs are extremely elevated as well, leading most likely to a diagnosis of familial hypercholesterolemia. The ED physician consults cardiology to take CP for a cardiac catheterization.

THUMBNAIL: Cholesterol and Lipid Metabolism

Familial Hyperlipoproteinemias

Disorder	Defect	Lab Elevation	Presentation
Familial hypercholesterolemia	Absent LDL receptor	LDL	Xanthomas on tendons, atherosclerosis
Familial hypertriglyceridemia	?	VLDL	Eruptive xanthomas, atherosclerosis
Familial lipoprotein lipase deficiency	Lipoprotein lipase deficiency	Chylomicrons	Eruptive xanthomas, pancreatitis
Familial type III hyperlipoproteinemia	Abnormal VLDL Apo E	Chylomicrons, IDL	Palmar xanthomas, atherosclerosis
Familial apo C-II deficiency	Apo C-II deficiency	Chylomicrons, VLDL	Pancreatitis
Familial combined hyperlipidemia	?	LDL, VLDL	Xanthomas, atherosclerosis

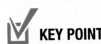 **KEY POINTS**

- Lipid digestion is begun by bile acids, which emulsify fatty molecules
- Then, enzymes such as pancreatic lipase catalyze hydrolysis of triacylglycerols
- Monoacylglycerols and fatty acids are absorbed by intestinal epithelial cells, and within intestinal epithelial cells, triacylglycerols are resynthesized
- Once absorbed by the intestinal cells, cholesterol may be esterified to fatty acids, forming cholesteryl esters catalyzed by ACAT

- Triacylglycerols, cholesteryl esters, phospholipids, and free cholesterol are packaged into chylomicrons in the GI tract epithelium for transport
- Chylomicrons have these fatty molecules removed by cells throughout the body until they become chylomicron remnants and are absorbed by the liver
- Cholesterol is further transported by VLDL, IDL, LDL, and HDL

QUESTIONS

1. The key step catalyzed by lipoprotein lipase is which of the following?

   A. Hydrolysis of triacylglycerols
   B. Hydrolysis primarily of monoacylglycerols
   C. Conversion of chylomicrons to HDLs
   D. Chylomicron conversion to triacylglycerols
   E. Binding to apo B-100

2. Which of the following patients is most likely to have atherosclerosis, xanthomas, and pancreatitis, but LDL and VLDL levels normal or only slightly elevated?

   A. 65-year-old man who is morbidly obese
   B. 42-year-old man with lipoprotein lipase deficiency
   C. 33-year-old woman with familial hypercholesterolemia
   D. 48-year-old man with familial hypertriglyceridemia
   E. 55-year-old man who smokes and has a family history of heart disease

CASE 4-8 Homocystinuria

HPI: EL is a 22-year-old woman who is concerned about her family history of blood clots. Her 19-year-old brother died last year of a stroke, and she had heard on TV that some blood-clotting diseases can run in families. EL has never had a stroke or blood clot. She is near-sighted but otherwise enjoys good health. She had a hard time in school, and throughout high school she was in a special education program. She states that her behavior is sometimes erratic, and that last summer she was admitted overnight to a psychiatric unit because of "psychosis." Further review of family history does not reveal any other family member with a history of thromboembolic events. EL has a sister who is 25 years old and who finished college. Both of her parents are healthy, in their late 50s, and of average stature.

PE: Height 5'11", weight 125 lbs. Tall, slender, young woman. HEENT exam is notable for poor visual acuity and high-arched palate. She has mild kyphoscoliosis, mild pectus excavatum chest deformity, and long, slender fingers. Cardiopulmonary exam is unremarkable.

Labs: CBC count shows platelets within normal limits; PT, INR, PTT within normal limits; factor V Leiden, methylenetetrahydrofolate reductase (MTHFR), and G20210A prothrombin molecular studies negative for any mutations; protein C and protein S studies normal; plasma amino acids show elevated methionine and homocysteine; plasma cystine and total homocysteine levels are markedly elevated.

THOUGHT QUESTIONS

- What is the diagnosis? How is the diagnosis made?
- What is the metabolic defect?
- What are the different strategies to correct the metabolic defect?
- Are there other disease states associated with elevated homocysteine levels?

BASIC SCIENCE REVIEW AND DISCUSSION

Homocystinuria is an AR inborn error of metabolism (IEM) characterized by the **accumulation of homocysteine, which may lead to ocular, musculoskeletal, CNS, and vascular manifestations.** Newborn screening for homocystinuria is possible, although not all state programs screen for this potentially treatable condition. Newborns appear normal, and early symptoms, if present, are vague. Visual problems may lead to diagnosis if the child is discovered on exam to have **dislocated lenses and myopia.** Displacement of the lens into the anterior chamber (ectopia lentis) is highly suggestive of homocystinuria and typically occurs by age 8 years. **Musculoskeletal manifestations** are similar to those of Marfan syndrome and include tall stature, thin body habitus, long, skinny fingers, pectus excavatum, and kyphoscoliosis. **Thromboembolic complications** occur in roughly 25% of patients by age 15 years if untreated. **Some degree of mental retardation** is usually seen, but some affected people have normal intelligence quotients (IQ range 10–138). When mental retardation is present, it is generally progressive if left untreated. Psychiatric disease such as personality disorder and psychosis can also result.

Metabolic Defect

Homocystinuria is due to cystathionine β-synthase (CBS) deficiency. **CBS** is an enzyme involved at the branching point between trans-sulfuration and remethylation in methionine degradation. Most of the homocysteine is converted to cystathionine and much less is remethylated back to methionine. However, in homocystinuria, the inactivity of CBS prevents homocysteine from trans-sulfuration to cystathionine and diverts it via remethylation to methionine. Consequently, there is elevated methionine and homocysteine, as well as low or absent cysteine. Diagnosis is confirmed by the detection of low levels of CBS on cultured fibroblasts. Once the diagnosis is established, a therapeutic trial with vitamin B6 (cofactor of CBS) should be performed. Fifty percent of patients respond to vitamin B6, some with full correction of the metabolic imbalance. Nutritional therapy with reduced amounts of methionine is necessary for all pyridoxine nonresponders and partial responders. Betaine, a methyl group donor that lowers homocysteine levels by remethylating homocysteine to methionine, is also helpful in these vitamin B6 nonresponsive patients.

Hyperhomocysteinemia and Vascular Disease Elevations of homocysteine can be a result of IEMs such as CBS deficiency but may also arise in common states like folate deficiency or B12 deficiency that impair remethylation. Folate and B12 are cofactors required in the one-carbon transfer reactions. There has been a well-established association between elevated homocysteine levels and vascular disease, in the coronary, carotid, and peripheral circulation. The mechanism by which this occurs is not fully understood, and whether interventions that decrease homocysteine levels can prevent the occurrence of these complications is not currently known.

CASE CONCLUSION

Homocystinuria is suspected, so a skin biopsy is performed for fibroblast culture, which shows no detectable CBS activity, confirming the diagnosis. EL then undergoes a trial of pyridoxine, showing marked metabolic improvement with normalization of homocysteine levels in plasma. Subjectively, EL says she feels better and has not had any more drastic mood changes. Because she has had a complete response to pyridoxine, there is no need for diet modifications.

⚙️ **THUMBNAIL:** Homocystinuria

Trans-sulfuration pathway showing key enzymes, cofactors, and rate-limiting steps

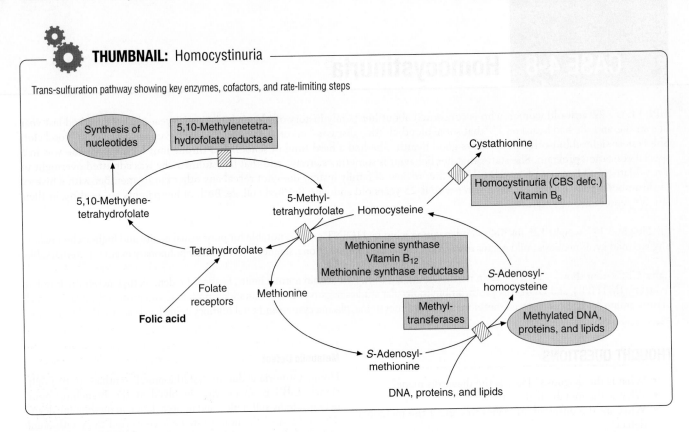

✓ **KEY POINTS**

- Features: ectopia lentis, tall and thin, mental retardation, thromboembolism
- Metabolic defect: elevated homocysteine, methionine, low cysteine level resulting from CBS deficiency
- Treatment: vitamin B6; diet and betaine for partial or nonresponders to vitamin B6 treatment

QUESTIONS

1. A 26-year-old man presents to the ED with severe chest pain. He is tall and slender, and he has dislocation of the lens and a pectus carinatum deformity. What is the molecular basis for the underlying disorder?

   A. Fibrillin gene mutation
   B. CBS deficiency
   C. Drug abuse
   D. MTHFR mutations
   E. None of the above

2. During a routine checkup, Mr. Smith, a 65-year-old patient, has an elevated level of homocysteine in plasma. Plasma elevations of homocysteine have been associated with which of the following?

   A. Dementia, coronary disease, neural tube defects
   B. Protein C deficiency, folic acid deficiency, vitamin B6 deficiency

   C. MTHFR mutations, CBS mutations, factor V Leiden mutations
   D. Dolichostenomelia, mental retardation, normal methionine
   E. Cleft lip and palate, neural tube defects, holoprosencephaly

3. A 4-year-old child with displacement of the lens and mild developmental delays is brought to your office. You suspect homocystinuria. Of the following, which would you not expect to find?

   A. Arachnodactyly
   B. Low CBS activity in cultured fibroblasts
   C. Elevated methionine and homocysteine in plasma
   D. Positive cyanide nitroprusside test
   E. Increased levels of phenylalanine in serum

CASE 4-9 Phenylketonuria

HPI: PF, a 7-day-old infant, is brought to her pediatrician by her parents after receiving a call from the State Lab Newborn Screening Division. Her heel-stick dried blood spot is suspicious for phenylketonuria (PKU). Her mother tells you that PF was born via normal spontaneous vaginal delivery (NSVD) at term after an uncomplicated pregnancy. Her birth weight was 3.5 kg, length 51 cm, and head circumference 50 cm, all near the fiftieth percentile. She was discharged from the hospital on her second day of life, along with her mother. PF is being breast-fed exclusively. Both parents are quick to assert that she seems perfectly normal, and that she is no different from her two older siblings at the same age. They are terribly worried though because they read that PKU could cause mental retardation.

PE: Detailed exam reveals a perfectly normal 1-week-old infant.

Labs: Blood work was ordered by the State Lab. Serum amino acid tests show marked hyperphenylalaninemia (phenylalanine >360 µmol/L), mild decrease in tyrosine.

THOUGHT QUESTIONS

- What is the outcome of untreated and treated PKU?
- What is the metabolic defect in PKU?
- What is the molecular basis of this disorder?

BASIC SCIENCE REVIEW AND DISCUSSION

Initially recognized in mentally retarded adults who had high concentrations of phenylpyruvic acid in the urine, PKU is a classic example of an **IEM** and has a successful history in terms of the prevention of mental retardation in affected individuals with PKU.

Natural History of Untreated Phenylketonuria

Children with PKU, if untreated, are severely mentally retarded and have hypopigmentation and neurologic symptoms. Neurologic symptoms include hypertonicity, irritability, hyperactivity, and, occasionally, seizures. The mental retardation and other neurologic manifestations in PKU are thought to result from the accumulation of excessive amounts of phenylalanine and its derivatives. High levels of phenylalanine are toxic to the brain in experimental models and in humans. The hypopigmentation of skin and hair occurs because of the competitive inhibition of tyrosine hydroxylase by high levels of phenylalanine.

Results of Patients Treated for Phenylketonuria

With accurate diagnosis and identification of PKU in the newborn period, and with initiation of a phenylalanine-restricted diet, children with PKU can develop normally. Phenylalanine is an essential amino acid, so it cannot be completely eliminated from the diet. Blood phenylalanine levels must be carefully monitored, particularly during the first 5 years of life, but continuation of the phenylalanine-restricted diet should be lifelong. Patients with PKU who go off the diet as teenagers or adults, although not mentally retarded, may develop neurologic symptoms such as irritability, agitated behavior, and difficulty in concentration. Women with PKU, if not under optimal metabolic control, are at risk of having mentally retarded offspring (maternal PKU syndrome).

Biochemistry and Molecular Basis

The enzyme responsible for the conversion of phenylalanine to tyrosine, phenylalanine hydroxylase (PAH), is deficient in PKU. This "enzymatic block" leads to the accumulation of phenylalanine and its metabolites (phenylpyruvic acid and phenylacetic acid, which are excreted in the urine), which are toxic to the brain. The levels in blood of tyrosine (the end product of PAH) are low, as anticipated. This decrease in tyrosine, in addition to the competitive inhibition of tyrosinase by the hyperphenylalaninemia, the enzyme that converts dopa to melanin (see the Thumbnail), is responsible for the hypopigmentation of untreated patients with PKU. There are many different mutations of the PAH gene, most of which are base substitutions found in exons 6 through 12. No single mutation seems to be predominant, and more than 70 have been identified. The frequency of PKU is about 1 in 10,000 newborns of western European descent and is lower in other populations.

CASE CONCLUSION

PF was immediately placed on a phenylalanine-restricted diet. She was bottle-fed with a special formula until age 1 year and then gradually advanced to low-protein foods and continued to take her special phenylalanine-free formula. For years, she was followed at the metabolic clinic in her region. She tested in the high end of normal in all of her periodic neuropsychologic tests. As a teenager, PF had difficulty with compliance with her diet and went through some rough times at school. Fortunately, with lots of support from her parents and staff, she has been back on her diet fully. She is now 25 years old and thinking about having children.

THUMBNAIL: Phenylketonuria

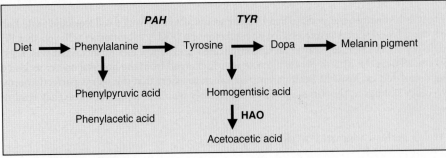

Phenylalanine, Tyrosine, Dopa Pathway

PAH = phenylalanine hydroxylase
TYR = tyrosinase
HAO = homogentisic acid oxidase

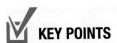

KEY POINTS

- A block in a metabolic pathway leads to accumulation of intermediaries and/or deficiency of the end product

- Several IEMs can be detected by newborn screening and successfully treated by dietary restriction, supplementation, or enzyme replacement

- Most IEMs are AR; most IEMs can be detected prenatally by either functional assays or DNA testing

QUESTIONS

1. PF is now 10 weeks pregnant. Her fetus is at risk of mental retardation if which of the following is true?

   A. Her fetus is homozygous for the PAH mutation.
   B. High levels of phenylalanine in maternal serum, independent of fetal PAH genotype
   C. Normal levels of tyrosine and normal levels of phenylalanine in maternal blood
   D. Low levels of phenylalanine, homozygous fetus for the PAH mutation
   E. The father is a carrier of the PAH mutation that is passed on to the fetus.

2. A couple who has a 5-year-old son with PKU is interested in a prenatal diagnosis. Their son has classic PKU, but only one mutant allele was identified on DNA testing. Prenatal diagnosis is possible by means of which of the following?

   A. Liver biopsy of the fetus
   B. Is not possible because only one mutation was identified in the child with PKU

   C. Amniocentesis measuring PAH activity from amniocytes
   D. Linkage of the mutant allele using restriction fragment length polymorphisms (RFLPs) by means of chorionic villus sampling (CVS) or amniocentesis
   E. DNA testing of the fetus for mutations of PAH using CVS

3. A 10-day-old male infant in the neonatal ICU (NICU) has jaundice, hepatomegaly, and sepsis caused by a gram-negative rod. On review of the family history, you learn that his older sister had a similar course as a newborn and later developed cirrhosis of the liver and cataracts. The most likely diagnosis is which of the following?

   A. Homocystinuria
   B. Maple syrup urine disease
   C. Galactosemia
   D. Tyrosinemia
   E. Biotinidase deficiency

HPI: HA is an 18-month-old male infant who is brought to the ED by his parents. They note that he has had symptoms of a viral illness for the past 3 days, but today his vomiting increased in frequency and he became uncooperative and combative. His mom says that he has behaved like this before when sick, but this is the most violent he has ever been. Upon further history, they note that he has had five to six prior episodes, and that during the last one, he was diagnosed with Reye syndrome at age 15 months.

PE: HA is febrile to 101.3°F, mildly tachycardic, and showing other signs of dehydration. On neurologic exam, you note that he is hyperreflexic, and has mild asterixis and a positive Babinski sign.

Labs: CBC count and LFTs return normal, except for an elevated ammonia level.

THOUGHT QUESTIONS

- What genetic diagnoses should the ED physician consider?
- What key findings help make this diagnosis?
- What are the key elements of the urea cycle?
- What are the common derangements of the urea cycle?

BASIC SCIENCE REVIEW AND DISCUSSION

The key finding in this patient's laboratory results is an elevated **ammonia** level. Interestingly, ammonia levels are not commonly ordered in routine work-ups of children, but they are ordered in this case because of the physical finding of **asterixis,** which is a flapping reflex of the hands when they are held out in front in a hyperextended position. Elevated ammonia levels are seen most commonly in the setting of liver failure, but this patient does not have liver function abnormalities. Elevated ammonia levels are also seen in the hyperammonemia syndromes, such as carbamoyl-phosphate synthetase (CPS) deficiency (type I hyperammonemia) or ornithine transcarbamoylase (OTC) deficiency (type II hyperammonemia), or other derangements of enzymes in the **urea cycle.** To better understand these deficiencies, we first need to understand the processes of the urea cycle.

The Urea Cycle

Twenty percent of nitrogenous waste can be excreted in the kidney, where **glutaminase** is responsible for converting excess glutamine from the liver to urine ammonium. However, about 80% of the excreted nitrogen is in the form of urea, which is also largely made in the liver, in a series of reactions that are distributed between the mitochondrial matrix and the cytosol. The series of reactions that form urea is known as the **urea cycle,** or the **Krebs-Henseleit cycle.**

Removal of Nitrogen from Amino Acids

The dominant reactions involved in removing amino acid nitrogen from the body are known as **transaminations.** This class of reactions funnels nitrogen from all free amino acids into a small number of compounds; then, either they are oxidatively deaminated, producing ammonia, or their amine groups are converted to urea by the urea cycle. The remaining carbon skeleton of these amino acids can then enter into carbohydrate metabolism either in gluconeogenesis or in the TCA cycle. Transaminations involve moving an α-amino group from a donor α-amino acid to the keto carbon of an acceptor α-keto acid. **Aminotransferases** catalyze these reactions and use pyridoxal phosphate as a cofactor.

Generation of Urea

The essential features of the urea cycle reactions and their metabolic regulation are as follows: Arginine from the diet or from protein breakdown is cleaved by the cytosolic enzyme **arginase,** generating urea and ornithine. In subsequent reactions of the urea cycle, a new urea residue is built on the ornithine, regenerating arginine and perpetuating the cycle (Fig. 4-11). Because the urea cycle is cyclic, the first step is often arbitrarily chosen to begin with ornithine arising in the cytosol. Ornithine is transported to the mitochondrial matrix, where **OTC** catalyzes its condensation with carbamoylphosphate, producing citrulline. The energy for the reaction is provided by the high-energy anhydride of carbamoylphosphate. The product, citrulline, is then transported to the cytosol, where the remaining reactions of the cycle take place.

The synthesis of citrulline requires a prior activation of carbon and nitrogen as carbamoylphosphate. The activation step requires two equivalents of ATP and the mitochondrial matrix enzyme **CPS-I.** There are two CPSs: a mitochondrial enzyme (CPS-I), which forms carbamoylphosphate destined for inclusion in the urea cycle, and a cytosolic CPS (CPS-II), which is involved in pyrimidine nucleotide biosynthesis. CPS-I is positively regulated by the allosteric effector N-acetylglutamate, while the cytosolic enzyme is acetylglutamate independent. In a two-step reaction, catalyzed by cytosolic **argininosuccinate synthetase,** citrulline and aspartate are condensed to form argininosuccinate. The reaction involves the addition of AMP (from ATP) to the amido carbonyl of citrulline, forming an activated intermediate on the enzyme surface (AMP citrulline), and the subsequent addition of aspartate to form argininosuccinate.

Arginine and fumarate are produced from argininosuccinate by the cytosolic enzyme **argininosuccinate lyase** (also called **argininosuccinase**). In the final step of the cycle, **arginase** cleaves urea from aspartate, regenerating cytosolic ornithine, which can be transported to the mitochondrial matrix for another round of urea synthesis. The fumarate, generated via the action of **argininosuccinate lyase,** is reconverted to aspartate for use in the **argininosuccinate synthetase** reaction. This occurs through the actions of cytosolic versions of the TCA cycle enzymes, **fumarase** (which yields malate) and **malate dehydrogenase** (which yields oxaloacetate).

Bioenergetics

Beginning and ending with ornithine, the reactions of the cycle consume three equivalents of ATP and four high-energy nucleotide phosphates. Urea is the only new compound generated by the

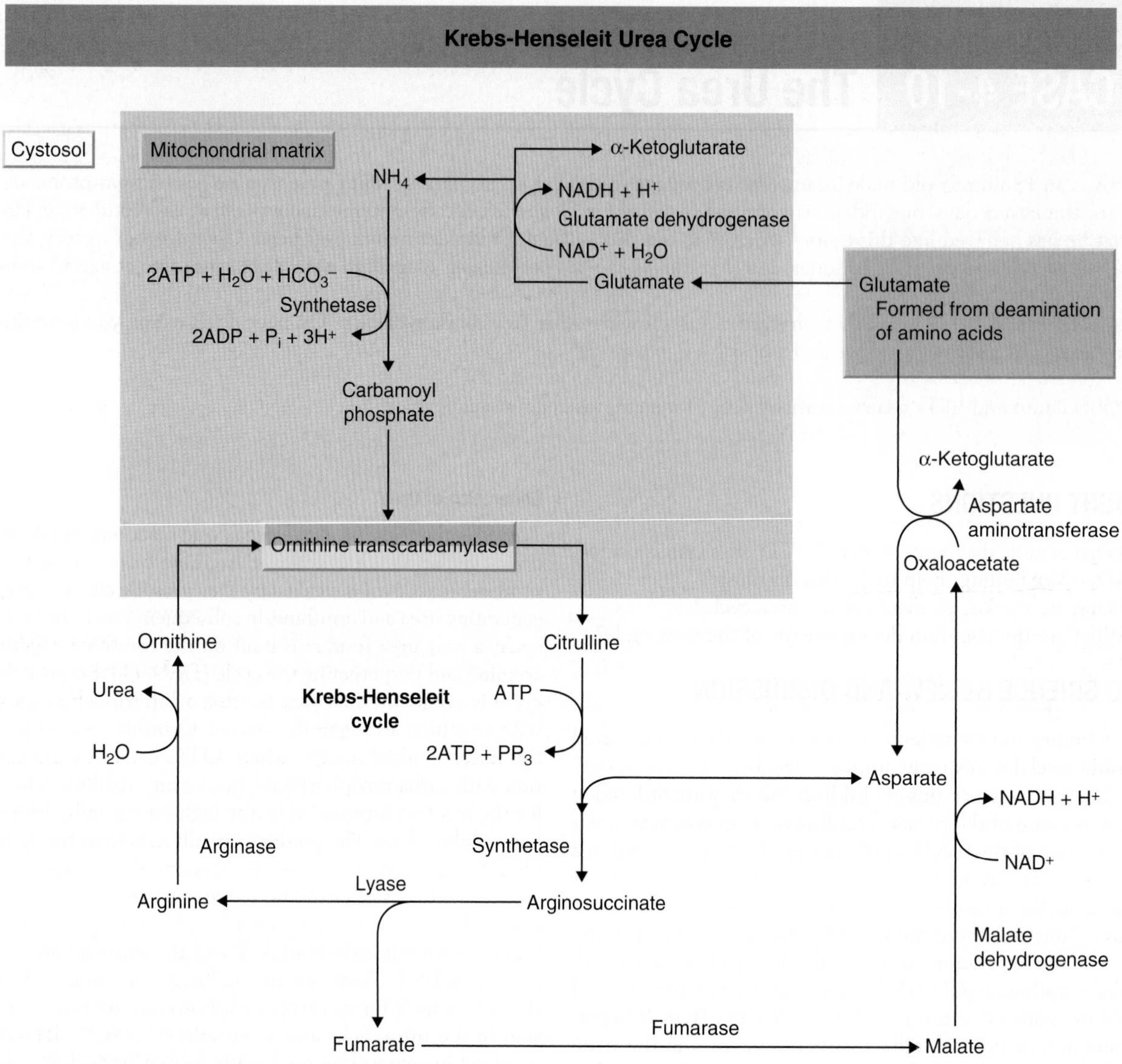

Krebs-Henseleit Urea Cycle

• **Figure 4-11.** The principle steps of the urea cycle. The rectangle encloses the reactions that occur in the mitochondrion. (Reproduced with permission from Greenstein B. Medical Biochemistry at a Glance. Oxford: Blackwell Science, 1996.)

cycle; all other intermediates and reactants are recycled. The energy consumed in the production of urea is more than recovered by the release of energy formed during the synthesis of the urea cycle intermediates. Ammonia released during the glutamate dehydrogenase reaction is coupled to the formation of NADH. In addition, when fumarate is converted back to aspartate, the malate dehydrogenase reaction used to convert malate to oxaloacetate generates a mole of NADH. These two moles of NADH, thus, are oxidized in the mitochondria, yielding six moles of ATP.

Regulation of the Urea Cycle

The urea cycle operates only to eliminate excess nitrogen. On high-protein diets, the carbon skeletons of the amino acids are oxidized for energy or stored as fat and glycogen, but the amino nitrogen must be excreted. To facilitate this process, enzymes of the urea cycle are controlled at the gene level. With long-term changes in the quantity of dietary protein, there can be up to a 20-fold increase in the production of urea cycle enzymes. Urea

cycle enzymes increase concomitantly with significant dietary protein increases. Under conditions of starvation, enzyme levels rise as proteins are degraded and amino acid carbon skeletons are used to provide energy, thus increasing the quantity of nitrogen that must be excreted. Short-term regulation of the cycle occurs principally at CPS-I, which is relatively inactive in the absence of its allosteric activator N-acetylglutamate. The steady-state concentration of N-acetylglutamate is set by the concentration of its components (acetyl-CoA and glutamate) and by arginine, which increases the activity of N-acetylglutamate synthetase.

Urea Cycle Defects

A complete lack of any one of the enzymes of the urea cycle will result in death shortly after birth. However, deficiencies in each of the enzymes of the urea cycle, including N-acetylglutamate synthase, have been identified. These disorders are referred to as urea cycle disorders (UCDs). A common thread to most UCDs is hyperammonemia leading to ammonia intoxication. Deficiencies in arginase do not lead to symptomatic hyperammonemia as severe or as commonly as in the other UCDs. Clinical symptoms are most severe when the UCD is at the level of CPS-I.

Symptoms of UCDs usually present shortly after birth and include ataxia, convulsions, lethargy, poor feeding, and eventually coma and death if not recognized and treated properly. In fact, the mortality rate is 100% for UCDs that are left undiagnosed. In general, the treatment of UCDs have as common elements the reduction of protein in the diet, removal of excess ammonia, and replacement of intermediates missing from the urea cycle. Administration of levulose reduces ammonia through its action of acidifying the colon. Bacteria metabolize levulose to acidic byproducts, which then promotes excretion of ammonia in the feces as ammonium ions, NH_4^+. Antibiotics can be administered to kill intestinal ammonia-producing bacteria. Dietary supplementation with arginine or citrulline can increase the rate of urea production in certain UCDs.

OTC deficiency is the most common of the UCDs. It is transmitted as an X-linked dominant disorder, with males affected more severely than females. It can present in infancy to early childhood. Episodes are usually instigated by periods of stress or a high-protein diet. Symptoms include vomiting, neurologic changes, ataxia, combativeness, and agitation. A hyperammonemic coma can evolve and, if untreated and undiagnosed, can lead to death. As far as development is concerned, these children will often be delayed and may have mild to moderate mental retardation. Specific diagnosis of OTC deficiency is made via laboratory findings during an acute exacerbation of symptoms finding hyperammonemia and elevated orotic acid secretion in the urine. This finding differentiates this disease from CPS deficiency, which may present identically. Prenatal diagnosis of OTC can be made via enzyme testing of a fetal liver biopsy specimen or via molecular genetic techniques on amniocytes or chorionic villi.

CASE CONCLUSION

HA has elevated urine orotic acid levels, making the diagnosis. He is acutely treated with levulose, sodium benzoate, IV hydration, and a nonprotein diet supplemented with simple amino acids. He recovers in the hospital after several days and is discharged home into the care of his parents with this new diagnosis and advice about management of this disease. The family is scheduled for follow-up in 1 week with the geneticist who saw them in the hospital.

THUMBNAIL: The Urea Cycle

Urea Cycle Disorder	Enzyme Deficiency	Symptoms/Comments
Type I hyperammonemia	CPS-I	1 to 3 days after birth, infant becomes lethargic, with vomiting, hypothermia, and hyperventilation; without measurement of serum ammonia levels and appropriate intervention, infant will die: treatment with arginine, which activates N-acetylglutamate synthetase
N-acetylglutamate synthetase	N-acetylglutamate synthetase	Severe hyperammonemia associated with deep coma, acidosis, recurrent diarrhea, ataxia, hypoglycemia, hyperornithinemia; treatment includes administration of carbamoylglutamate to activate CPS-I
Type II hyperammonemia	OTC	Most commonly occurring UCD; the only X-linked UCD; ammonia and amino acids elevated in serum; increased serum orotic acid due to mitochondrial carbamoylphosphate entering cytosol and being incorporated into pyrimidine nucleotides, which leads to excess production and consequently excess catabolic products; treat with high-carbohydrate, low-protein diet, ammonia detoxification with sodium phenylacetate or sodium benzoate
Classic citrullinemia	Argininosuccinate synthetase	Episodic hyperammonemia, vomiting, lethargy, ataxia, seizures, eventual coma; treat with arginine administration to enhance citrulline excretion, also with sodium benzoate for ammonia detoxification
Argininosuccinic aciduria	Argininosuccinate lyase (argininosuccinase)	Episodic symptoms similar to classic citrullinemia; elevated plasma and CSF argininosuccinate; treat with arginine and sodium benzoate
Hyperargininemia	Arginase	Rare UCD; progressive spastic quadriplegia and mental retardation; ammonia and arginine high in CSF and serum; arginine, lysine, and ornithine high in urine; treatment includes diet of essential amino acids excluding arginine, low-protein diet

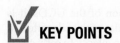 **KEY POINTS**

- Nitrogenous waste is primarily excreted by the kidney, although only about 20% of it is converted to ammonium in the kidney
- Eighty percent of nitrogenous waste is converted to urea primarily by the liver in the urea cycle
- Short-term regulation of the urea cycle occurs at CPS-I, which is activated by *N*-acetylglutamate

- *N*-acetylglutamate is increased by acetyl-CoA, glutamate, and arginine
- Long-term regulation of the urea cycle is primarily at the gene level that up-regulates with increases in dietary protein and starvation
- Without the normal functioning of the urea cycle, there is buildup of nitrogenous waste, which can cause the diseases discussed in the Thumbnail

QUESTIONS

1. The key regulatory step in the urea cycle is catalyzed by which of the following?

   A. CPS-I
   B. *N*-acetylglutamate synthetase
   C. OTC
   D. Argininosuccinate synthetase
   E. Arginase

2. The symptoms seen in patients with UCDs are primarily due to what?

   A. Excess serum urea
   B. Excess plasma orotic acid
   C. Hyperammonemia
   D. Hypoammonemia
   E. Decreased renal function

HPI: WE is a 59-year-old man who is brought to the ED in an acute state of alcohol intoxication. He is given IV hydration and put on a stretcher to "sleep it off." Several hours later he awakes, but his nurse finds him quite confused and calls the ED resident to examine him.

PE: He is noted to have a horizontal nystagmus and ataxia that is so severe, WE has difficulty standing. After a short time, he attempts to walk and is noticed to have a wide gait. The resident notices that WE is getting just IV hydration and orders a vitamin to be added to the hydration. He also orders neurology and psychiatry consults.

THOUGHT QUESTIONS

- What diagnoses are WE's history and exam most consistent with?
- What vitamin did the resident most likely add to the IV?
- What are the other important vitamin deficiencies and how do they present?

BASIC SCIENCE REVIEW AND DISCUSSION

WE's symptoms are most consistent with Wernicke-Korsakoff syndrome, where Wernicke disease describes the acute neurologic changes of the ocular nerves leading to nystagmus in this patient, as well as the ataxia, and Korsakoff psychosis describes symptoms of drowsiness, apathy, amnesia, and confusion. This syndrome is a result of thiamine (vitamin B1) deficiency. Reviewing vitamin deficiencies can be undertaken in each system separately or collectively as a series of vitamins. Here, we present them together.

Vitamins

Vitamins are **cofactors** and **coenzymes** used throughout the body in a multitude of reactions in synthesis and maintenance of homeostasis. The key importance of vitamins is that they must primarily be obtained from our diet; they either cannot be synthesized or are not synthesized at levels necessary to meet the body's demands. Deficiencies in these vitamins can lead to various diseases. Vitamins are usually broken down into the water-soluble (B and C) and the fat-soluble (D, E, A, and K) vitamins.

Vitamin B1—Thiamine Thiamine is converted to its active form, **TPP,** in the brain and liver by a specific enzyme, **thiamine diphosphotransferase.** TPP is necessary as a cofactor for the **pyruvate dehydrogenase** and **α-ketoglutarate dehydrogenase-**catalyzed reactions, as well as the **transketolase-**catalyzed reactions of the pentose phosphate pathway. A deficiency in thiamine intake leads to a severely reduced capacity of cells to generate energy as a result of its role in these reactions.

The earliest symptoms of thiamine deficiency include constipation, appetite suppression, nausea, mental depression, peripheral neuropathy, and fatigue. Chronic thiamine deficiency leads to more severe neurologic symptoms including ataxia, mental confusion, and loss of eye coordination (Wernicke-Korsakoff syndrome). Other clinical symptoms of prolonged thiamin deficiency are related to cardiovascular and musculature defects. Severe thiamine deficiency leads to **beriberi,** which can manifest as high cardiac output failure.

Vitamin B2—Riboflavin Riboflavin is the precursor for the coenzymes, **flavin mononucleotide (FMN)** and **flavin adenine dinucleotide (FAD).** The enzymes that require FMN or FAD as cofactors are termed **flavoproteins.** Several flavoproteins also contain metal ions and are termed **metalloflavoproteins.** Both classes of enzymes are involved in a wide range of redox reactions, for example, **succinate dehydrogenase** and **xanthine oxidase.** During the course of the enzymatic reactions involving the flavoproteins, the reduced forms of FMN and FAD are formed, $FMNH_2$ and $FADH_2$, respectively.

Riboflavin deficiencies are rare in the United States because of the presence of adequate amounts of the vitamin in eggs, milk, meat, and cereals. Riboflavin deficiency is often seen in chronic alcoholics because of their poor dietetic habits. Symptoms associated with riboflavin deficiency include glossitis, seborrhea, angular stomatitis, cheilosis, and photophobia. Riboflavin decomposes when exposed to visible light. This characteristic can lead to riboflavin deficiencies in newborns treated for hyperbilirubinemia by phototherapy.

Vitamin B3—Niacin Niacin is required for the synthesis of the active forms of vitamin B3, NAD^+ and **nicotinamide adenine dinucleotide phosphate** *(NADP⁺).* Both NAD⁺ and NADP⁺ function as cofactors for numerous dehydrogenases, for example, lactate dehydrogenase (LDH). Both nicotinic acid and nicotinamide can serve as the dietary source of vitamin B3. However, niacin is not a true vitamin in the strictest definition because it can be derived from the amino acid tryptophan. However, the ability to use tryptophan for niacin synthesis is inefficient (60 mg of tryptophan is required to synthesize 1 mg of niacin).

A diet deficient in niacin (as well as tryptophan) leads to glossitis of the tongue, dermatitis, weight loss, diarrhea, depression, and dementia. The severe symptoms, depression, dermatitis, and diarrhea, are associated with the condition known as **pellagra.** Several physiologic conditions and drug therapies can lead to niacin deficiency. In Hartnup disease, tryptophan absorption is impaired, and in malignant carcinoid syndrome, tryptophan metabolism is altered, resulting in excess serotonin synthesis. Isoniazid is the primary drug for the treatment of tuberculosis.

Interestingly, nicotinic acid (but not nicotinamide), when administered in pharmacologic doses of 2–4 g/day, lowers plasma cholesterol levels and has been shown to be a useful therapeutic for hypercholesterolemia. The major action of nicotinic acid in this capacity is a reduction in fatty acid mobilization from adipose tissue. Although nicotinic acid therapy lowers blood cholesterol levels, it also causes a depletion of glycogen stores and fat reserves in skeletal and cardiac muscle. Additionally, there is an elevation in blood glucose level and uric acid production. For these reasons, nicotinic acid therapy is not recommended for diabetics or persons who suffer from gout.

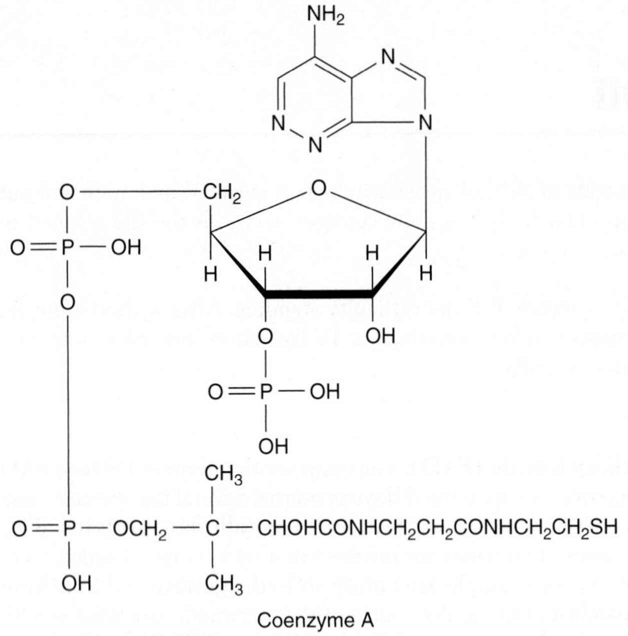

Coenzyme A

• **Figure 4-12.** The molecular structure of CoA.

Vitamin B5—Pantothenic Acid Pantothenic acid is formed from β-alanine and pantoic acid. Pantothenate is required for synthesis of **CoA** (Fig. 4-12) and is a component of the ACP domain of fatty acid synthase. Thus, pantothenate is required for the metabolism of carbohydrate via the TCA cycle and all fats and proteins. At least 70 enzymes have been identified as requiring CoA or ACP derivatives for their function.

Deficiency of pantothenic acid is extremely rare because of its widespread distribution in whole-grain cereals, legumes, and meat. Symptoms of pantothenate deficiency are difficult to assess because they are subtle and resemble those of other B vitamin deficiencies.

Vitamin B6—Pyridoxine Pyridoxal, pyridoxamine, and pyridoxine are collectively known as **vitamin B6.** All three compounds are efficiently converted to the biologically active form of vitamin B6, **pyridoxal phosphate** (PLP), catalyzed by the ATP-requiring enzyme **pyridoxal kinase.** PLP functions as a cofactor in enzymes involved in transamination reactions required for the synthesis and catabolism of the amino acids, as well as in glycogenolysis as a cofactor for **glycogen phosphorylase.** Deficiencies of vitamin B6 are rare and usually are related to an overall deficiency of all the B-complex vitamins. Isoniazid and penicillamine are drugs that complex with pyridoxal and PLP, resulting in a deficiency in this vitamin.

Vitamin B12—Cobalamin Vitamin B12 is composed of a complex tetrapyrrol ring structure (corrin ring) and a cobalt ion in the center. It is synthesized exclusively by microorganisms and is found in the liver of animals bound to protein as methylcobalamin or 5'-deoxyadenosylcobalamin. The vitamin must be hydrolyzed from protein in order to be active. Hydrolysis occurs in the stomach by gastric acids or in the intestines by trypsin digestion following consumption of animal meat. The vitamin is then bound by **intrinsic factor** (IF), a protein secreted by parietal cells of the stomach, and carried to the ileum where it is absorbed. Following absorption, the vitamin is transported to the liver in the blood bound to **transcobalamin II** (TCII).

Only two clinically significant reactions in the body require vitamin B12 as a cofactor. During the catabolism of fatty acids with an odd number of carbon atoms and the amino acids valine, isoleucine, and threonine, the resultant propionyl-CoA is converted to succinyl-CoA for oxidation in the TCA cycle. One of the enzymes in this pathway, **methylmalonyl-CoA mutase,** requires vitamin B12 as a cofactor in the conversion of methylmalonyl-CoA to succinyl-CoA. The 5'-deoxyadenosine derivative of cobalamin is required for this reaction. The second reaction requiring vitamin B12 catalyzes the conversion of homocysteine to methionine and is catalyzed by **methionine synthase.** This reaction results in the transfer of the methyl group from N^5-methyltetrahydrofolate to hydroxocobalamin, generating tetrahydrofolate (THF) and methylcobalamin during the process of the conversion.

The liver can store up to 6 years' worth of vitamin B12, so deficiencies in this vitamin are rare. Pernicious anemia is a megaloblastic anemia resulting from vitamin B12 deficiency that develops as a result of a lack of IF in the stomach leading to malabsorption of the vitamin. The anemia results from impaired DNA synthesis caused by a block in purine and thymidine biosynthesis. The block in nucleotide biosynthesis is a consequence of the effect of vitamin B12 on folate metabolism. When vitamin B12 is deficient, essentially all of the folate becomes trapped as the N^5-methyltetrahydrofolate derivative as a result of the loss of functional *methionine synthase*. This trapping prevents the synthesis of other THF derivatives required for the purine and thymidine nucleotide biosynthesis pathways.

Neurologic complications also are associated with vitamin B12 deficiency and result from a progressive demyelination of nerve cells. The demyelination is thought to result from the increase in methylmalonyl-CoA that results from vitamin B12 deficiency. Methylmalonyl-CoA is a competitive inhibitor of malonyl-CoA in fatty acid biosynthesis, as well as being able to substitute for malonyl-CoA in any fatty acid biosynthesis that may occur. Because the myelin sheath is in continual flux, the methylmalonyl-CoA–induced inhibition of fatty acid synthesis results in the eventual destruction of the sheath.

Folic Acid Folic acid is a conjugated molecule consisting of a pteridine ring structure linked to p-aminobenzoic acid **(PABA)** that forms pteroic acid. Folic acid itself is then generated through the conjugation of glutamic acid residues to pteroic acid. Folic acid is obtained primarily from yeasts and leafy vegetables, as well as animal liver. Animals cannot synthesize PABA and cannot attach glutamate residues to pteroic acid, so they require folate intake in the diet.

When stored in the liver or ingested, folic acid exists in a polyglutamate form. Intestinal mucosal cells remove some of the glutamate residues through the action of the lysosomal enzyme **conjugase.** The removal of glutamate residues makes folate less negatively charged (from the polyglutamic acids) and therefore more capable of passing through the basal laminal membrane of the epithelial cells of the intestine and into the bloodstream. Folic acid (Fig. 4-13) is reduced primarily within liver cells, where it is also stored, as THF through the action of **DHFR,** an NADPH-requiring enzyme. The function of THF derivatives is to carry and transfer various forms of one-carbon units during biosynthetic reactions. The one-carbon units are either methyl, methylene, methionyl, formyl, or formimino groups.

Folate deficiency results in complications nearly identical to those described for vitamin B12 deficiency. The most pronounced effect of folate deficiency on cellular processes is on

Folic acid

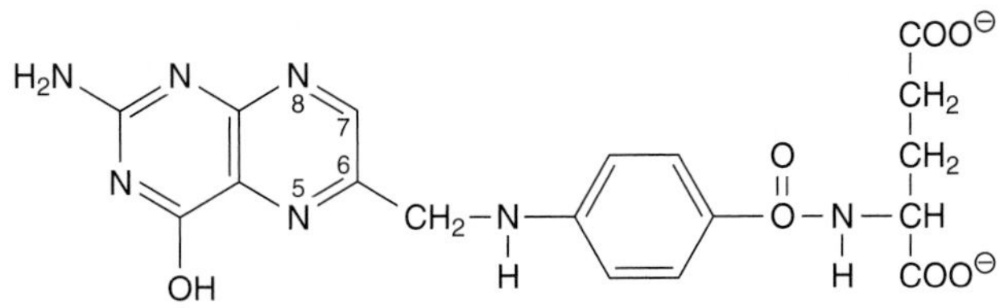

• **Figure 4-13.** In the molecular structure for folic acid, note that in DHF the double bond between 7 and 8 is gone, and these atoms are bound to hydrogen molecules. In THF, the same is true for 5 and 6 as well.

DNA synthesis. This is due to an impairment in dTMP synthesis, which leads to cell cycle arrest in the S phase of rapidly proliferating cells, in particular hematopoietic cells. The result is **megaloblastic anemia** similar to vitamin B12 deficiency. The inability to synthesize DNA during erythrocyte maturation leads to abnormally large erythrocytes, termed **macrocytic anemia.**

Folate deficiencies are rare because of the adequate presence of folate in food. Poor dietary habits can lead to folate deficiency. The predominant causes of folate deficiency in nonalcoholics include impaired absorption or metabolism or an increased demand for the vitamin. The predominant condition requiring an increase in the daily intake of folate is pregnancy. Folate deficiency has been associated with fetal anomalies, such as spina bifida, and its supplementation has been shown to decrease these defects. Certain drugs, such as anticonvulsants and oral contraceptives, can impair the absorption of folate. Anticonvulsants also increase the rate of folate metabolism.

Biotin Biotin is the cofactor required of enzymes that are involved in carboxylation reactions **(acetyl-CoA carboxylase and pyruvate carboxylase).** Biotin is found in numerous foods and is synthesized by intestinal bacteria, and, as such, deficiencies of the vitamin are rare. Deficiencies are generally seen only after long antibiotic therapies that deplete the intestinal fauna or after excessive consumption of raw eggs. The latter is due to the affinity of the egg-white protein, **avidin,** for biotin preventing intestinal absorption of the biotin.

Vitamin C—Ascorbic Acid Ascorbic acid is derived from glucose via the uronic acid pathway. The enzyme L-gulonolactone oxidase, which is responsible for the conversion of gulonolactone to ascorbic acid, is absent in primates, making ascorbic acid required in the diet. The active form of vitamin C is ascorbate acid itself. The main function of ascorbate is to act as a reducing agent in a number of different reactions. Vitamin C has the potential to reduce cytochromes *a* and *c* of the respiratory chain, as well as molecular oxygen. The most important reaction requiring ascorbate as a cofactor is the hydroxylation of proline residues in collagen. Vitamin C is, therefore, required for the maintenance of normal connective tissue and for wound healing because synthesis of connective tissue is the first event in wound tissue remodeling. Vitamin C also is necessary for bone remodeling because of the presence of collagen in the organic matrix of bones.

Deficiency in vitamin C leads to the disease **scurvy,** because of its role in the posttranslational modification of collagens. Scurvy is characterized by easily bruised skin, muscle fatigue, soft swollen gums, decreased wound healing and hemorrhaging, osteoporosis, and anemia. Vitamin C is readily absorbed, so the primary cause

of vitamin C deficiency is poor diet and/or an increased requirement. The primary physiologic state leading to an increased requirement for vitamin C is severe stress (or trauma). This is due to a rapid depletion in the adrenal stores of the vitamin. The reason for the decrease in adrenal vitamin C levels is unclear but may be due either to redistribution of the vitamin to areas that need it or to an overall increased utilization.

Vitamin A Vitamin A consists of three biologically active molecules, **retinol, retinal** (retinaldehyde), and **retinoic acid.** Each of these compounds is derived from the plant precursor molecule, **β-carotene** (a member of a family of molecules known as **carotenoids**). β-Carotene, which consists of two molecules of retinal linked at their aldehyde ends, is also referred to as the provitamin form of vitamin A.

Photoreception in the eye is the function of two specialized cell types located in the retina: the rod and the cone cells. Both rod and cone cells contain a photoreceptor pigment in their membranes. The photosensitive compound of most mammalian eyes is a protein called **opsin,** to which is covalently coupled an aldehyde of vitamin A. The opsin of rod cells is called **scotopsin.** The photoreceptor of rod cells is specifically called **rhodopsin,** or **visual purple.** This compound is a complex between scotopsin and the 11-*cis*-retinal (also called 11-*cis*-retinene) form of vitamin A.

Vitamin A is stored in the liver, and deficiency of the vitamin occurs only after prolonged lack of dietary intake. The earliest symptom of vitamin A deficiency is **night blindness.** Additional early symptoms include follicular hyperkeratosis, increased susceptibility to infection, and cancer and anemia equivalent to iron-deficient anemia. Prolonged lack of vitamin A leads to deterioration of the eye tissue through progressive keratinization of the cornea, a condition known as **xerophthalmia.** The increased risk of cancer in vitamin deficiency is thought to be the result of a depletion in β-carotene, which is a very effective antioxidant and is suspected to reduce the risk of cancers known to be initiated by the production of free radicals. Of particular interest is the potential benefit of increased β-carotene intake to reduce the risk of lung cancer in smokers. However, caution needs to be taken when increasing the intake of any of the lipid-soluble vitamins. Excess accumulation of vitamin A in the liver can lead to toxicity, which manifests as bone pain, hepatosplenomegaly, nausea, and diarrhea.

Vitamin D Vitamin D is a steroid hormone that functions to regulate specific gene expression following interaction with its intracellular receptor. The biologically active form of the hormone is 1,25-dihydroxyvitamin D_3 (1,25-$[OH]_2D_3$, also termed **calcitriol**). Calcitriol functions primarily to regulate calcium and phosphorous homeostasis.

Active calcitriol is derived from **ergosterol** (produced in plants) and from **7-dehydrocholesterol** (produced in the skin). **Ergocalciferol** (vitamin D2) is formed by UV irradiation of ergosterol. In the skin, 7-dehydrocholesterol is converted to **cholecalciferol** (vitamin D3) following UV irradiation. Vitamin D2 and D3 are processed to D_2-calcitriol and D_3-calcitriol, respectively, by the same enzymatic pathways in the body. Cholecalciferol is absorbed from the intestine and transported to the liver bound to a specific **vitamin D-binding protein.** In the liver, cholecalciferol is hydroxylated at the 25 position by a specific D_3-25-hydroxylase, generating 25-hydroxyvitamin D_3 (25-$[OH]D_3$), which is the major circulating form of vitamin D. Conversion of 25-hydroxyvitamin D_3 to its biologically active form, calcitriol, occurs through the activity of a specific D_3-1-hydroxylase present in the proximal convoluted tubules of the kidneys, as well as in bone and placenta. 25-Hydroxy-vitamin D_3 can also be hydroxylated at the 24 position by a specific D_3-24-hydroxylase in the kidneys, intestine, placenta, and cartilage.

Calcitriol functions in concert with **parathyroid hormone (PTH)** and **calcitonin** to regulate serum calcium and phosphorous levels. PTH is released in response to low serum calcium levels and induces the production of calcitriol. In contrast, reduced levels of PTH stimulate synthesis of the inactive 24,25-$(OH)_2D_3$. In the intestinal epithelium, calcitriol functions as a steroid hormone in inducing the expression of calbindinD_{28K}, a protein involved in intestinal calcium absorption. The increased absorption of calcium ions requires concomitant absorption of a negatively charged counter ion to maintain electrical neutrality. The predominant counter ion is P_i. When plasma calcium levels fall, the major sites of action of calcitriol and PTH are bone, where they stimulate bone resorption, and the kidneys, where they inhibit calcium excretion by stimulating reabsorption by the distal tubules.

The role of calcitonin in calcium homeostasis is to decrease elevated serum calcium levels by inhibiting bone resorption. As a result of the addition of vitamin D to milk, deficiencies in this vitamin are rare in this country. The main symptom of vitamin D deficiency in children is **rickets** and in adults is **osteomalacia.** Rickets is characterized by improper mineralization during the development of the bones, resulting in soft bones. Osteomalacia is characterized by demineralization of previously formed bone, leading to increased softness and susceptibility to fracture.

Vitamin E Vitamin E is a mixture of several related compounds known as **tocopherols.** The α-tocopherol molecule is the most potent of the tocopherols. Vitamin E is absorbed from the intestines packaged in chylomicrons. It is delivered to the tissues via chylomicron transport and then to the liver through chylomicron remnant uptake. The liver can export vitamin E in VLDLs. Because of its lipophilic nature, vitamin E accumulates in cellular membranes, fat deposits, and other circulating lipoproteins. The major site of vitamin E storage is in adipose tissue.

The major function of vitamin E is to act as a natural **antioxidant** by scavenging free radicals and molecular oxygen. In particular, vitamin E is important for preventing peroxidation of polyunsaturated membrane fatty acids. The vitamins E and C are interrelated in their antioxidant capabilities. Active α-tocopherol can be regenerated by interaction with vitamin C following scavenge of a peroxy-free radical. Alternatively, α-tocopherol can scavenge two peroxy-free radicals and then be conjugated to glucuronate for excretion in the bile.

No major disease states have been found to be associated with vitamin E deficiency, because of adequate levels in the average U.S. diet. The major symptom of vitamin E deficiency in humans is an increase in RBC fragility. Because vitamin E is absorbed from the intestines in chylomicrons, any fat malabsorption diseases can lead to deficiencies in vitamin E intake. Neurologic disorders have been associated with vitamin E deficiencies associated with fat malabsorptive disorders. Increased intake of vitamin E is recommended in premature infants who are fed formulas that are low in the vitamin as well as in persons consuming a diet high in polyunsaturated fatty acids. Polyunsaturated fatty acids tend to form free radicals on exposure to oxygen, which may lead to an increased risk of certain cancers.

Vitamin K The K vitamins exist naturally as K1 (phytylmenaquinone) in green vegetables, K2 (multiprenylmenaquinone) in intestinal bacteria, and K3 in synthetic menadione. The major function of the K vitamins is in the maintenance of normal levels of the blood-clotting proteins, factors II, VII, IX, X, and protein C and protein S, which are synthesized in the liver as inactive precursor proteins. Conversion from inactive to active clotting factor requires a posttranslational modification of specific glutamate (E) residues. This modification is a carboxylation reaction, and the enzyme responsible requires vitamin K as a cofactor. During the carboxylation reaction, a reduced hydroquinone form of vitamin K is converted to a 2,3-epoxide form. The regeneration of the hydroquinone form requires an uncharacterized reductase. This latter reaction is the site of action of the dicumarol-based anticoagulants, such as **warfarin.**

Naturally occurring vitamin K is absorbed from the intestines only in the presence of bile salts and other lipids through interaction with chylomicrons. Therefore, fat malabsorptive diseases can result in vitamin K deficiency. The synthetic vitamin K3 is water soluble and absorbed irrespective of the presence of intestinal lipids and bile. Because the vitamin K2 form is synthesized by intestinal bacteria, deficiency of the vitamin in adults is rare. However, long-term antibiotic treatment can lead to deficiency in adults. The intestine of newborn infants is sterile, so vitamin K deficiency in infants is possible if lacking from the early diet.

CASE CONCLUSION

The resident added 100 mg of thiamine to WE's IV infusion and he was admitted to the hospital, where he received daily IM injections of thiamine. He also received folate and vitamin B12 supplementation when it was noted that he had a macrocytic anemia. His acute symptoms slowly resolved over the ensuing 3 to 4 days, and concerned about these symptoms, he vowed never to take another drink.

THUMBNAIL: Vitamin Function

Vitamin Deficiencies

Vitamin Deficiency	Disease Caused
Vitamin B1 (thiamine)	Wernicke-Korsakoff syndrome; beriberi
Vitamin B2 (riboflavin)	Glossitis, stomatitis, cheilosis, photophobia
Vitamin B3 (niacin)	Pellagra (depression, dermatitis, diarrhea); also glossitis, weight loss, dementia
Vitamin B5 (pantothenic acid)	Rare, findings are subtle, similar to other B vitamin deficiencies
Vitamin B6 (pyridoxine)	Rare, findings are subtle, similar to other B vitamin deficiencies
Vitamin B12 (cobalamin)	Pernicious anemia, neurologic disease related to progressive demyelination
Folic acid	Macrocytic anemia, similar to B12
Biotin	Rare
Vitamin C (ascorbic acid)	Scurvy
Vitamin A	Night blindness, xerophthalmia
Vitamin D	Rickets, osteomalacia
Vitamin E	Hemolysis, neurologic disorders
Vitamin K	Coagulopathy, bleeding disorders

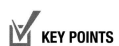

KEY POINTS

- Vitamins are **cofactors** and **coenzymes** used throughout the body in a multitude of reactions in synthesis and maintenance of homeostasis
- The key importance of vitamins is that they must primarily be obtained from our diet
- Some vitamins are synthesized by the body, but not at adequate levels
- Deficiencies in vitamins can lead to various diseases as shown in the Thumbnail

QUESTIONS

1. A 46-year-old man presents with progressive fatigue and weakness. He notices tingling in his lower extremities but attributes these symptoms to his being on his feet all the time as a manager of a local pizza restaurant. On neurologic exam, he actually has decreased position sense and vibration sense. His hematocrit is 28, with an elevated mean MCV of 114. His disease can most likely be attributed to a deficiency of which vitamin?

    A. Vitamin A
    B. Vitamin B12
    C. Vitamin C
    D. Vitamin D
    E. Vitamin E
    F. Vitamin K
    G. Biotin

2. Another employee at the same restaurant presents after he notices that a bruise he received 3 weeks ago is not resolving. He also has a burn from an oven from 6 weeks ago, which is still slowly healing. On exam, he has swollen gums, and a bone density measurement shows osteoporosis. His disease can most likely be attributed to a deficiency in which vitamin?

    A. Vitamin A
    B. Vitamin B12
    C. Vitamin C
    D. Vitamin D
    E. Vitamin E
    F. Vitamin K
    G. Biotin

PART V
Genetics

HPI: A 19-year-old man comes to your office with a complaint of "droopy eyelids." He notes a 2-year history of intermittent facial weakness and over the past 6 months has had increasing difficulty keeping his eyes open. He has been otherwise healthy and denies any past diseases. The patient's family history is significant for a grandmother with cardiac arrhythmias, who died suddenly at the age of 65 years. His father and an aunt both developed cataracts and mild hand weakness in their 40s. He also has a 16-year-old cousin with multiple illnesses, including neck and extremity weakness, chronic GI tract obstruction, and intellectual impairment.

PE: The patient is a thin-appearing man with limited facial expressions, thin hair, and a narrow face. On neurologic exam, he has bilateral eyelid ptosis, mildly slurred speech, mild generalized weakness, and difficulty rising from a seated position without assistance. The remainder of his exam is normal.

Labs: A creatine kinase level is mildly elevated at 250 U/L (normal <200 U/L). A muscle biopsy shows mild muscle fiber atrophy and other nonspecific myopathic changes. DNA analysis shows that the patient has approximately 200 CTG (cytosine-thymine-guanine) repeats present in a protein kinase gene on chromosome 19. (See case pedigree in Fig. 5-1.)

THOUGHT QUESTIONS

- What is the most likely diagnosis?
- What is the inheritance pattern of this disease?
- What is the significance of the DNA analysis?
- How would you counsel the patient regarding the risk to future children?

BASIC SCIENCE REVIEW AND DISCUSSION

Syndrome Description

Myotonic dystrophy is an **autosomal dominant (AD)** disorder and the most common adult-onset muscular dystrophy, with an incidence of 1 in 8000. The disease is slowly progressive and involves multiple organ systems, including skeletal, cardiac, GI, and respiratory systems. The onset of symptoms is usually after puberty with characteristic manifestations of **muscle weakness,** especially of the face and extremities, with progressive involvement of the proximal muscles. Smooth muscle involvement can lead to cardiac arrhythmias, decreased GI tract motility, and respiratory dysfunction. **Myotonia** is the inability to relax voluntary muscles after contraction. The most noticeable symptom may be an inability to relax the hand after a grip (grip myotonia), but symptoms are generally not severe enough to require treatment. Other associated symptoms of myotonic dystrophy include cataracts, testicular atrophy, and mental retardation.

Muscle biopsy reveals fiber atrophy; however, serum creatine kinase level is usually normal or only mildly elevated. A definitive diagnosis can be made by DNA analysis with either PCR or Southern blot analysis to determine the number of CTG trinucleotide repeats present in the myotonic dystrophy gene (*DMPK*), with CTG trinucleotide repeat expansions in excess of 35 repeats considered abnormal. There is no specific treatment for myotonic dystrophy. Ankle supports or leg braces can help with distal weakness, pacemakers can be used for cardiomyopathy, and cataracts can be surgically removed.

Autosomal Dominant Inheritance

The myotonic dystrophy gene is located on chromosome 19 and encodes for a protein kinase. It is inherited in an AD pattern and has several distinguishing characteristics. AD diseases affect an equal proportion of men and women. Because every carrier of the mutation is affected (complete penetrance), the pedigree shows no skipped generations. Finally, unlike X-linked or mitochondrial diseases, fathers can pass on the mutation to their sons. The most common pairing is between an affected heterozygote and a normal individual. Half of their offspring will be unaffected, whereas the other half will inherit the mutant allele and be symptomatic. Other common AD disorders include Huntington disease, neurofibromatosis type 1, familial hypercholesterolemia, and postaxial polydactyly (extra fingers or toes).

Anticipation and Repeat Expansion

The genetic cause of myotonic dystrophy is an expanded CTG trinucleotide repeat within a protein kinase gene on chromosome 19. An interesting phenomenon in familial myotonic dystrophy is that later generations afflicted with the mutation frequently have an earlier age at onset and more severe disease. This concept is termed *anticipation* and is caused by the increasing number of trinucleotide repeats found in the myotonic dystrophy gene in successive generations. Normal individuals have between 5 and 34 copies of the repeat, while premutation carriers have 35–49 repeats and are asymptomatic, but their children are at increased risk of inheriting a larger repeat size and being affected. Affected individuals have greater than 50 CTG repeats, and patients with severe disease can have hundreds or thousands of copies of the CTG repeat within the gene. Other disorders caused by such trinucleotide repeat expansions include Huntington disease (CAG), spinal and bulbar muscular atrophy (CAG), fragile X syndrome (CGG), and Friedreich ataxia (GAA).

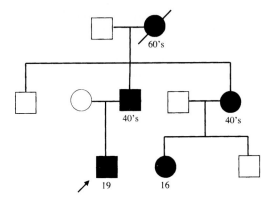

• Figure 5-1.

CASE CONCLUSION

The patient is started on annual cardiac exams with ECGs and counseled on his increased risk of eventual cardiac, pulmonary, and GI complications. The patient's cousin is also tested for trinucleotide expansions and is found to have more than 1000 copies of the CTG repeat.

THUMBNAIL: Autosomal Dominant Inheritance

Diseases Associated with Trinucleotide Repeat Expansions

Disease	Repeat	Description
Myotonic dystrophy	CTG	Facial/extremity weakness, cardiomyopathy, GI tract obstruction, respiratory tract muscle weakness, cataracts, testicular atrophy, and mental retardation
Fragile X syndrome	CGG	Mental retardation, macroorchidism in men, large ears, prominent jaw
Friedreich ataxia	GAA	Cerebellar dysfunction, limb ataxia, sensory defects, cardiomyopathy
Huntington disease	CAG	Loss of motor control (chorea), dementia
Spinal and bulbar muscular atrophy	CAG	Lower motor neuron disease, androgen insensitivity

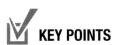 **KEY POINTS**

■ Myotonic dystrophy is an AD disorder.
■ AD disorders have the following characteristics:
  • Affects men and women equally
  • Does not skip generations
  • Fathers can transmit disease to sons

■ Anticipation defines the earlier onset and increasing severity of a disease from one generation to the next. In the presented case, this is caused by an expanding trinucleotide repeat in a gene on chromosome 19.

QUESTIONS

1. The patient meets a woman at a myotonic dystrophy support group who is also affected by the disease. They decide to marry but are very concerned about passing on the disorder to their offspring. If they eventually have two children, what is the chance that neither child will inherit the chromosomal abnormality?

   A. 50%
   B. 33.3%
   C. 25%
   D. 6.25%
   E. 0%

2. Myotonic dystrophy is inherited in an AD fashion. The AD trait can share similar characteristics with the pedigree of other inheritance patterns (e.g., AR and sex linked). Which of the following is true about the inheritance pattern of both AD and X-linked dominant disorders?

   A. Men and women are affected in equal proportions.
   B. Affected women have a 50% chance of passing the diseased allele to their children.
   C. Fathers cannot pass on the mutation to their sons.
   D. Skipped generations are commonly seen.
   E. Men have a 100% chance of passing on the mutation to their daughters.

3. A 35-year-old woman presents to your office with a complaint of abnormal, jerky facial and body movements. Over the past few years, her memory has deteriorated and she is becoming more depressed. The patient denies any significant family history but states that her father committed suicide when he was 40 years of age. Which of the following statements is true about the likely diagnosis?

   A. It is caused by a CTG trinucleotide repeat expansion.
   B. It is inherited in a sex-linked pattern.
   C. It is inherited in an AD pattern.
   D. Anticipation is not a factor in disease transmission.
   E. Dementia is not a common feature of this disease.

4. Molecular genetic techniques are becoming the standard methods for the diagnosis of many genetic disorders. Which technique is described by the following protocol: electrophoresis of DNA fragments through a gel, transfer to a membrane, hybridize with a labeled probe, and expose to x-ray film?

   A. PCR
   B. Western blot analysis
   C. Southern blot analysis
   D. Fluorescence in situ hybridization
   E. Northern blot analysis

HPI: FC is a 5-year-old boy with failure to thrive and chronic lung disease. Since age 11 months, he has suffered from malabsorption with increased fat content in the stools. In addition, he has recurrent, chronic bacterial lung infections often requiring hospitalization. Two weeks ago, he had an exacerbation of his cough and wheezing requiring hospitalization. Chest x-ray was consistent with bilateral lobar pneumonia. He was treated with systemic broad-spectrum antibiotics and intensive respiratory therapy. *Staphylococcus aureus* was isolated from his sputum. His medical history is significant for intestinal obstruction as a neonate. His parents are of Irish and German ancestry and are related only by marriage. He has an older sister who is healthy. No other family member is affected by a similar condition on either side of the family (Fig. 5-2). Although a tentative diagnosis has been raised in the past, the parents have come to you to try to establish a definitive diagnosis and for genetic counseling.

THOUGHT QUESTIONS

- What is the most likely diagnosis? How would you confirm it?
- What is the natural history and life expectancy of this disease?
- What treatment strategies are recommended for these patients?
- Which inheritance pattern does this pedigree suggest?

BASIC SCIENCE REVIEW AND DISCUSSION

Cystic Fibrosis

The association of symptoms presented is highly suggestive of cystic fibrosis (CF). The classic clinical triad consists of (*a*) chronic pulmonary obstruction and infections; (*b*) exocrine pancreatic insufficiency; and (*c*) elevations of both chloride and sodium concentration in sweat. It is the most common autosomal recessive (AR) disease in white populations, affecting about 1 in every 2500 to 3000 newborns.

In a patient with clinical suspicion of CF, a chloride sweat test result of more than 60 mmol/L confirms the diagnosis. Immunoreactive trypsin has been used as a screening test in newborns but requires a confirmatory test because of its poor specificity. DNA testing is helpful in confirming the diagnosis in atypical cases and is essential for prenatal diagnosis.

Natural History Sixty percent of patients with CF are diagnosed before 1 year of age and 90% by age 10 years. Eighty-five percent of patients have pancreatic insufficiency manifested by chronic malabsorption and failure to thrive. Almost all patients with CF have chronic lung disease resulting from recurrent infections, leading eventually to irreversible lung damage and strain on the right ventricle (cor pulmonale). Nearly all male individuals with CF are infertile because of the absence of the vas deferens. Chronic lung disease and its sequelae are the life-limiting factor for most patients with CF. Currently, survival for patients with CF in the United States is approximately 30 years.

Management strategies consist of improving nutritional status, preservation of lung function, preventing and treating complications, and ensuring psychosocial well-being. Exocrine pancreatic insufficiency can be effectively treated with enzyme replacement. Lung conservation is achieved by facilitating clearance of mucus and control of infection. Gene therapy is still investigational.

Inheritance The family tree shown is not characteristic of any particular inheritance pattern but is commonly seen in AR disorders. There are three features that suggest AR inheritance: it affects both men and women in equal proportions; it typically affects individuals in one generation of a single sibship; and it does not occur in prior or subsequent generations. Consanguinity is more frequently seen in families with AR traits than in the general population. Recessive traits require that the mutant allele is present in a double dose (homozygosity), although for most AR disorders, affected individuals have two allelic mutations at the same locus (compound heterozygote—e.g., $\triangle$F508/G542X, two of the most common mutations in CF).

Prenatal Diagnosis CF is one of a handful of diseases that are now commonly screened for via prenatal diagnosis. In the case of screening for AR disorders like CF, usually the mother is screened first. If her test returns negative results, then screening often stops there because the child would be at most a carrier. If her screen returns positive results, then the father is screened. If his screen returns negative results, again, the child can at most only be a carrier (assuming correct paternity). If the father has a positive result as well, then the fetus has a 25% chance of being affected, and invasive confirmatory testing is offered via either CVS or amniocentesis to obtain fetal cells. If the fetus is homozygous recessive, termination of the pregnancy may be an option for some couples because there is no effective treatment for this devastating condition. Because the prenatal diagnostic procedures are not without risk, patients need to weigh the decision regarding these options carefully after thorough counseling. In the case of CF screening, the parental screening can be further complicated given that not all of the mutations in the CF gene are identified, especially in non-Caucasian ethnicities, yielding a detection rate of less than 100%. Despite these limitations, CF screening is offered to any pregnant woman or couple considering pregnancy in the United States.

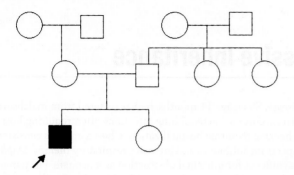

• **Figure 5-2.** Pedigree for Patient FC. Note that there are no other cases of CF in his family.

CASE CONCLUSION

FC undergoes DNA testing and is found to be homozygous for the F508 mutation. Commercially available DNA tests typically screen between 12 and 72 of the most common CF mutations, with a sensitivity of up to 97% for Ashkenazi Jews and more than 92% for northern Europeans, but as low as 60% in other populations. The cystic fibrosis transmembrane regulator (CFTR) genotype has a strong correlation with the phenotype in terms of age at disease onset, pancreatic insufficiency, and sweat chloride content. The correlation with pulmonary disease is less clear.

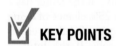

THUMBNAIL: Autosomal Recessive Inheritance

CF is the most common life-limiting AR disorder in Caucasians (1/3200 newborns)

Carrier frequency in Caucasians is approximately 1 in 30

Diagnosis: **Elevated chloride level in sweat glands; DNA analysis in cases of equivocal results**

Symptoms: **Exocrine pancreatic insufficiency, recurrent pulmonary infections**

Infertility in men, secondary to absence of vas deferens

Normal intelligence, decreased survival (mean, 30 years)

Genetics: **More than 1000 mutations have been identified; △F508 is the most common**

CFTR gene on chromosome 7q31; gene product CFTR protein

Mutations cause alterations in chloride transport and mucin secretion

Higher frequency of carriers than expected likely explained by *heterozygote advantage*

KEY POINTS

- AR disorders manifest only when the mutant allele is present in double dose
- Most AR diseases occur as a result of two different mutations at the same locus (compound heterozygotes)

- Parents of affected children are obligate carriers (heterozygotes) and are not affected
- Higher incidence of consanguinity in AR disorders

QUESTIONS

1. The underlying mechanism responsible for CF is which of the following?

   A. Defect in cholesterol synthesis
   B. Chloride channel abnormality
   C. Autoimmune response
   D. Calcium channel defect
   E. None of the above

2. A few years later, FC's older sister is considering pregnancy. Her husband is of northern European ancestry. Assuming a carrier frequency of 1 in 25 for northern Europeans, their chances of having an affected child with the same condition as her brother is what?

   A. 1 in 200
   B. 1 in 150
   C. 1 in 100
   D. 1 in 75
   E. 1 in 4

3. The couple in the question above decides to undergo carrier screening for 72 of the most common mutations of this disorder. The mother is found to be a carrier of one of the mutations screened. The husband screens negative for all of the 72 mutations tested. They decide to get pregnant. However, an ultrasound of the fetus revealed "echogenic bowel," the sonographic correlate of meconium ileus and concern for possible CF. How can this be explained?

A. Nonpaternity
B. Affected heterozygote
C. Father of fetus is carrier of mutation not identified by panel used
D. A and C are correct
E. A, B, and C are correct

CASE 5-3 X-Linked Dominant Inheritance

HPI: TR is a 10-year-old boy with moderate mental retardation and autistic-like behavior. His parents first noted that he was "kind of slow'" at 1 year of age, when he was not achieving his developmental milestones. He has an IQ of 68. On physical exam, he has nondysmorphic features, with average height and weight for his age. His initial newborn screening was normal. His parents are both healthy, of average intelligence, and nonconsanguineous. The family tree is shown in Figure 5-3, which as you can see shows an extensive family history of mental retardation. TR has come to see you for diagnostic evaluation at the request of his new pediatrician. As part of the work-up for his mental retardation, you ordered chromosome analysis, which showed a normal 46,XY karyotype.

THOUGHT QUESTIONS

- What type of inheritance pattern is suggested by the pedigree? Why?
- What is the molecular basis of fragile X syndrome?
- What is the phenotype of affected males and females with fragile X?

BASIC SCIENCE REVIEW AND DISCUSSION

The family tree depicted is somewhat atypical. It does not follow classic Mendelian inheritance. Fragile X syndrome was initially thought to be X-linked recessive, but two observations did not conform with this pattern: 30 to 50% of carrier females had some degree of mental retardation, a proportion much higher than anticipated by X-linked recessive, and the fact that normal males could pass a mutant allele to their daughters who were also normal but were at risk of having mentally retarded sons. This unusual pattern was not well understood until the molecular basis was revealed.

Unstable DNA Triplet Repeat Sequences

There are a number of disorders in which the mutation is an expansion of a triplet nucleotide repeat sequence that is unstable and can change in size on transmission from parent to offspring, sometimes called a **dynamic mutation.** Triplet repeat DNA sequences are present throughout the human genome, and unstable triplet repeats constitute dynamic mutations that account for at least seven disorders known to humans (see Thumbnail). In general, the longer the repeat, the more likely it is to expand further on transmission. Also, the longer the repeat,

the more severe the phenotype (in AD disorders). Premutations are expansions of triplet repeats beyond the normal range and are associated with a normal phenotype but can be unstable and expand to a full mutation associated with the disease phenotype on transmission from parent to offspring.

Fragile X syndrome is caused by an **unstable CGG repeat** in the 5′ untranslated region of the **FMR1** gene on the X chromosome. In the normal population, the size of the repeat varies from 6 to 50 and remains stable (i.e., does not expand) from one generation to the next. In fragile X syndrome, expansion from premutation to a full mutation only occurs when the premutation is transmitted by females. Expansions of 60 to 200 repeats are considered a premutation. The larger the size of the premutation, the greater the chance of it expanding into the full mutation range (>200). A mother carrying a premutation in the 60 to 69 repeat range has a chance of transmitting the premutation to a normal transmitting son, or it may expand to the full mutation range and she will have an affected son (8.5% risk). When the premutation is 90 or more repeats, the chance of expansion to full mutation is close to 100%.

Fragile X Phenotype Affected boys are mentally retarded in the moderate to severe range and often have autistic features. Speech tends to be halting and repetitive. Older boys and young adult men with the full mutation usually have discrete but recognizable physical features, including a high forehead, long face, prominent jaw, and large ears. After puberty, most boys develop macroorchidism. Females with the full mutation are mentally retarded about 30 to 50% of the time, usually in the mild to moderate range. Their physical features are not as clearly defined as those of their male counterparts.

CASE CONCLUSION

TR's parents decide to undergo DNA testing for fragile X syndrome. Southern blot analysis from TR shows an expansion of the CGG triplet repeat of 600 (full mutation). His mother is a premutation carrier with 98 repeats. His parents are counseled about the risk of recurrence in future pregnancies, and TR is enrolled at a special needs school that is better designed for his specific skill levels.

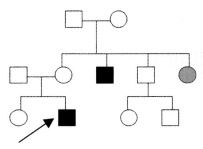

• **Figure 5-3.**

 THUMBNAIL: X-Linked Dominant Inheritance

Triplet Repeat Sequences

	Inheritance Pattern	Anticipation	Parental Sex Bias for Mutation Instability/Expansion	Repeat
Fragile X	X-linked dominant Partial penetrance in females	Yes	Maternal	CGG
Spinobulbar muscular atrophy	X-linked recessive	No	Predominantly paternal	CAG
Myotonic dystrophy	AD	Yes	No	CTG
Huntington disease	AD	Yes, but rare	Paternal	CAG
Spinocerebellar ataxia 1	AD	Yes	Unknown	CAG

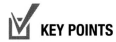 **KEY POINTS**

■ Regarding fragile X syndrome:

• Most common form of inherited mental retardation: 1 in 2000

• X-linked dominant inheritance: About one third to one half of females with the full mutation are mentally retarded

• Phenotype: Mild facial dysmorphisms and large testes after puberty; no obvious phenotype in affected females

QUESTIONS

1. What are the chances of TR's sister having a mentally retarded daughter with fragile X syndrome?

   A. 1 in 2
   B. 1 in 4
   C. 1 in 8
   D. 1 in 16
   E. She cannot have an affected daughter.

2. TR's maternal uncle is a carrier of a premutation containing 70 triplet repeats. What are the risks for his son and daughter of having mentally retarded offspring?

   A. They are not at risk because their father does not have fragile X.
   B. Both his son and his daughter are at risk of having mentally retarded children.

   C. His daughter is at risk of having mentally retarded sons.
   D. His daughter is at risk of having mentally retarded sons and daughters.
   E. Too high; they should adopt children instead.

3. Triplet repeat DNA expansions represent a newly recognized type of mutation. This type of mutation can explain which of the following concepts?

   A. Unusual pedigree patterns and anticipation
   B. Genetic heterogeneity and gene dose effect
   C. X-linked dominant inheritance and imprinting
   D. Founder effect and heterozygote advantage
   E. A and C are correct

HPI: A 26-year-old woman is brought by ambulance to the ED with a complaint of seizure, hemiparesis, and vision "blackout." She is well known to the ED staff and has been seen multiple times for similar stroke-like episodes that resolve over a period of days. Her husband states that these episodes have been occurring with increasing frequency for the past 3 years. He has also noticed personality changes since the strokes began, with increasing forgetfulness and irritability. The patient's medical history is significant for short stature, slight hearing deficit, diabetes mellitus, frequent migraine headaches and vomiting, and for becoming easily exhausted with mild exercise. She is an elementary school teacher but has been unable to work for the past year because of her constant fatigue. There is no family history of strokes, but the husband notes that her mother, an aunt, and an uncle frequently complain of low stamina and mild weakness. Interestingly, her aunt's children (cousins) also complain of these symptoms, but her uncle's children do not.

PE: The patient is somnolent, but arousable. HEENT exam reveals right-sided hemianopia and mild bilateral hearing deficit. On neurologic exam, she has mild muscle atrophy and decreased tone in all extremities. She is unable to move her right side against gravity and has proximal muscle weakness of the left side. The remainder of her exam is normal.

Labs: Serum lactic acid level is elevated at 6 mmol/L (normal <2 mmol/L). A brain MRI scan shows increased T2 signal in the posterior cerebrum that does not seem to correspond with the distribution of the major arteries. A Gomori trichome stain of a muscle biopsy reveals ragged red fibers, and Succinic dehydrogenase (SDH) stain reveals excessive mitochondrial accumulation.

THOUGHT QUESTIONS

- What condition is suggested by this clinical presentation?
- What is the likely inheritance pattern?
- Why is this disease presenting at a later age?
- What is the prognosis for this patient?

BASIC SCIENCE REVIEW AND DISCUSSION

Syndrome Description

The symptoms are consistent with a disease caused by mitochondrial DNA mutations. In this case, the patient was found to have **m**itochondrial myopathy, **e**ncephalopathy, **l**actic **a**cidosis, and *stroke-like* episodes syndrome (collectively called **MELAS**). Like most other mitochondrial disorders, this disease has a complex set of symptoms characteristically involving the CNS and muscle. These two organs have high-energy consumption and are very sensitive to any disruption to mitochondrial ATP production. Patients with MELAS may have a normal childhood, but in late childhood or early adulthood they will typically experience easy fatigability, exercise intolerance, stroke-like episodes with hemiplegia and vision changes, migraine-like headaches, seizures, and a progressive encephalopathy leading to dementia. Other associated symptoms include hearing loss, short stature, and diabetes.

The clinical diagnosis can be confirmed by serum lactic acidosis and a characteristic muscle biopsy showing a "ragged red" appearance from extensive mitochondrial proliferation. The biopsy sample can also be tested for decreased activity of mitochondrial respiratory chain enzymes, and mitochondrial DNA mutation analysis can be done on either a blood sample or a muscle biopsy sample. The prognosis is poor, and the disease frequently results in mental deterioration with eventual dementia. Currently there are no proven therapies, and treatment is generally supportive.

Mitochondrial Genetics

Each human cell contains hundreds (or more) of mitochondria in the cytoplasm. Each mitochondrion in turn has multiple copies of a circular double-stranded genome (mtDNA). In addition to the enzymes needed for oxidative phosphorylation, mitochondrial DNA also encodes for ribosomal and transfer RNAs that allow the mitochondria to produce proteins and to replicate independent of the nucleus. Although most genetic diseases are caused by mutations in the nuclear genome, an increasing number have been found to be due to mitochondrial defects. There are three different types of mitochondrial DNA mutations, which are used to classify the disorders. These include missense mutations, causing an amino acid substitution in the resulting protein (e.g., LHON). A second type of mtDNA mutation involves point mutations in a tRNA gene (e.g., MELAS), causing deficiencies in protein synthesis. The final class involves duplications and deletions (e.g., Kearns-Sayre disease) of the mitochondrial genome. There are three major differences between mitochondrial genetics and Mendelian genetics: maternal inheritance pattern, heteroplasmy/threshold effect, and replicative segregation.

Maternal Inheritance Pattern

Because mitochondria are found in the cytoplasm, the fertilized embryo receives most of its mitochondria from the egg and little from the relatively small sperm cytoplasm. In addition, the mtDNA of the sperm is actively degraded after fertilization. Therefore, mitochondrial mutations are inherited only from mother to offspring. Although a male can be affected by a mitochondrial disorder, he is unable to pass the mutation to his children. This inheritance pattern is seen only in mitochondrial diseases. It should be noted, however, that some mitochondrial disorders can be caused by mutations in nuclear DNA and are thus characterized by AR and AD inheritance patterns.

Heteroplasmy and Threshold Effect

Because a mitochondrion contains multiple copies of its genome, each mitochondrion (and therefore each cell) can contain a mixture of normal mtDNA and mutated mtDNA. The ability of a cell to be composed of several types of mtDNA is known as **heteroplasmy.** In most situations, the severity of the disease increases with an increasing proportion of mutant mtDNA to normal mtDNA. There is a threshold for the proportion of mutant mtDNA, below which mitochondrial function remains normal but above which function becomes impaired. Therefore, a patient will not become symptomatic until a minimal number of mutant mtDNA is reached. This threshold of mutant mtDNA numbers needed for cellular dysfunction is lower in tissue with a high ATP requirement. For example, the CNS and muscle are highly dependent on oxidative phosphorylation and so are two of the most severely affected organs.

Replicative Segregation

As mitochondria divide, the proportion of mutant to wild-type mtDNA changes. This phenomenon is known as **replicative segregation.** This process can occur either through chance or by a selective advantage of one mtDNA species over another. Over time, this process may cause the proportion of mutant mtDNA to increase past the threshold, leading to the unmasking of the disease phenotype. This may contribute to the delayed onset of the symptoms seen in the mitochondrial disorders.

CASE CONCLUSION

Mitochondrial DNA mutation analysis shows that the patient has an A-to-G substitution at nucleotide 3243 of the tRNA gene. This is the most common mutation seen in the MELAS syndrome and is found in 80% of affected individuals. After consultation with a geneticist, the patient and her husband decide to forgo having any children because of the high likelihood of passing the mutation on to any offspring. Her dementia worsens over the next few years, and she is finally placed in a nursing facility when her husband becomes unable to care for her.

THUMBNAIL: Mitochondrial Inheritance

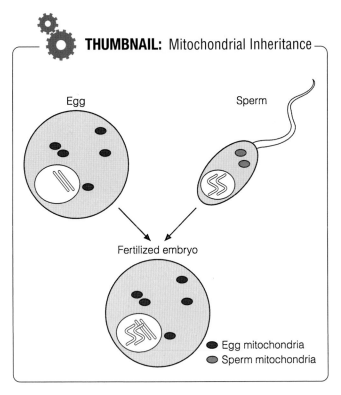

KEY POINTS

- MELAS is caused by a mitochondrial DNA mutation
- Key organs affected by MELAS include muscle (exercise intolerance, lactic acidosis) and the CNS (stroke-like episodes, seizures, encephalopathy)
- Laboratory diagnosis reveals serum lactic acidosis, muscle biopsy showing red ragged fibers, and DNA mutation analysis (3243A → G mutation most common)
- Mitochondrial genetics differ from Mendelian genetics in three aspects:
  - Maternal inheritance: Affected males cannot transmit a mitochondrial disorder that is due to mutations in mitochondrial DNA
  - Heteroplasmy: This is when multiple mtDNA species are found in a cell or tissue
  - Replicative segregation: As cells and mitochondria divide and proliferate, the proportion of mutant mtDNA to wild-type mtDNA can change

QUESTIONS

1. MELAS is transmitted via a mitochondrial inheritance pattern. It has similarities to both autosomal and sex-linked inheritance. Which of the following is true of both mitochondrial and X-linked recessive inheritance?

   A. Only females can transmit the gene to the next generation.
   B. Males are more likely than females to be affected (have symptoms).
   C. Females are more likely than males to be affected (have symptoms).

   D. No offspring of an affected male can be affected if his female partner has normal genotype.
   E. All offspring of an affected female can show symptoms of the disease, assuming the male has a normal genotype.

2. Assuming that the mitochondrial mutation was not de novo and all of the branches on a particular pedigree are blood related, what is the probability that a maternal aunt of an individual affected with MELAS will also have the mitochondrial mutation?

A. 100%
B. 75%
C. 50%
D. 25%
E. 0%

3. There are several differences between mtDNA and cell nuclear DNA. With the exception of the sex chromosomes, human nuclear DNA normally have two copies of each chromosome while hundreds (or thousands) of mitochondrial DNA may be present per cell. Which of the following terms describes the ability of a cell to have multiple different populations of mtDNA?

A. Threshold effect
B. Heteroplasmy
C. Homoplasmy
D. Pleiotropy
E. Imprinting

HPI: A 10-month-old girl is referred to you by her pediatrician for a growth on her back. The mother states that the mass was first noticed 3 months ago and has been growing slowly since then. She reports that the patient has fallen behind on her developmental milestones (she is still unable to crawl or sit without support) but denies any other significant medical problems. The only significant family history is the patient's 5-year-old brother, who has decreased vision in his right eye.

PE: The patient is an alert infant with normal weight and growth. HEENT exam reveals multiple scattered nodules on the left iris (Lisch nodules). She has numerous 5- to 10-mm hyperpigmented patches (café au lait macules) over her trunk and extremities, as well as freckling of the axillary and inguinal regions. A 4 × 5-cm firm, immobile mass is found left of the midline on her back. The remainder of her exam shows no abnormalities.

Labs: CT of the spine shows a large homogeneous enhancing mass at the level of T4–T5. An MRI of the brain shows no tumors.

THOUGHT QUESTIONS

- What is the most likely diagnosis?
- What is the inheritance pattern of this disease?
- Why might this patient have presented with a "negative" family history?
- What is the genetic basis of this disease?

BASIC SCIENCE REVIEW AND DISCUSSION

Syndrome Description

Neurofibromatosis type 1 (NF1) is an **AD** disorder affecting 1 in 3000 individuals. NF1 has a highly variable expression of symptoms, but features generally include **café au lait spots** (describing the hyperpigmented macules), **axillary/inguinal freckling, Lisch nodules** (benign growths on the iris), **neurofibromas** (benign proliferation of Schwann cells around peripheral nerves), **optic gliomas,** and **bone lesions** (scoliosis, vertebral dysplasia). Other symptoms may include learning disability, epilepsy, and hypertension. Because NF1 is an AD disease, it affects equal proportions of males and females, shows no skipped generations, and has male-to-male transmission.

Diagnosis is made clinically with imaging frequently finding optic gliomas, neurofibromas, and CNS hamartomas. Most patients do not require treatment, but disfiguring or painful peripheral neurofibromas can be removed surgically.

Variable Expression and Penetrance

The clinical presentation of NF1 can be highly variable, even between affected members of a family. Most patients have only mild cutaneous involvement—café au lait spots and few neurofibromas. However, those who are severely affected may have many if not all of the aforementioned symptoms, including hundreds or thousands of neurofibromas. The multiple potential manifestations of a disease phenotype is termed **variable expressivity.** Although the exact cause remains unclear in the case of NF1, variable expressivity in general can be attributed to environmental effects, interactions with other genes (modifier genes), or different types of mutations at a single disease gene locus (allelic heterogeneity).

Reduced penetrance is the concept that an individual with a disease genotype may not always manifest the disease phenotype, even though the individual is able to transmit the mutation to the next generation. The disease manifestation is not categorized based on severity but is seen as all or nothing. One example of this concept can be seen in retinoblastoma, in which one copy of the Rb1 tumor suppressor gene becomes nonfunctional due to a mutation. If the other copy of this gene also acquires a mutation during the lifetime of the individual, then the disease phenotype (malignant intraocular tumors) will be seen. This second mutation does not occur in 10% of patients, who remain disease-free throughout their lifetime. Thus, the penetrance of the Rb1 gene is said to be 90%.

Pleiotropy and Locus Heterogeneity

NF is caused by genetic mutations in the neurofibromin gene on chromosome 17. The gene product acts as a tumor suppressor, but in addition to benign and malignant growths, mutations in this gene can also cause a variety of other symptoms, including learning disabilities, hypertension, and bone defects. This is an example of **pleiotropy,** the ability of a gene to influence multiple phenotypes. Pleiotropy is involved in myriad other diseases, including **Marfan syndrome,** a connective tissue abnormality that leads to defects in the ocular, skeletal, and cardiovascular systems.

Although a gene can have several disease phenotypes, one disease phenotype can also be caused by mutations in multiple different genes. This is known as **locus heterogeneity** and can be seen in diseases such as autosomal dominant polycystic kidney disease (ADPKD). ADPKD can be caused by mutations in genes on either chromosome 16 **(PKD1)** or chromosome 4 **(PKD2).** These two genes produce membrane glycoproteins that interact with each other, and a defect in either will lead to a progressive accumulation of renal cysts, which are characteristic of this disease.

CASE CONCLUSION

The patient eventually undergoes an elective resection of the mass, which is determined by the pathologist to be a benign schwannoma, confirming the diagnosis of NF. The patient's father and brother are reexamined and several scattered café au lait spots are found on their trunks and backs. The brother is referred to an ophthalmologist who finds multiple Lisch nodules and an optic nerve glioma, the latter of which is the etiology of the decreased vision in his right eye.

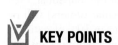

THUMBNAIL: Variable Penetrance

Key Principles of Medical Genetics

Genetic Principle	Definition	Examples
Variable expressivity	Variation in the severity/features of a disease among affected individuals	NF1, osteogenesis imperfecta
Allelic heterogeneity	Different mutations in the same gene that cause a single disease phenotype (although expression of phenotype may be variable)	CF
Penetrance	The proportion of individuals with a mutation who manifest the features of the associated disorder	Retinoblastoma
Pleiotropy	Ability of a gene to cause many phenotypes	NF1, Marfan syndrome
Locus heterogeneity	When mutations at different gene loci can cause the same disease phenotype	ADPKD

KEY POINTS

- NF1 is an AD disorder caused by a mutation in the neurofibromin tumor suppressor gene
- NF1 is characterized by café au lait spots, axillary/inguinal freckling, Lisch nodules, neurofibromas, optic gliomas, and bone lesions. Associated symptoms include hypertension, developmental delay, and malignancies.
- Potential reasons for a "negative" family history in a patient with a heritable disease include:

- New mutation
- Variable expressivity
- Reduced penetrance
- Wrong diagnosis
- False paternity

QUESTIONS

1. Osteogenesis imperfecta is a class of inherited diseases with varying severity, but all are characterized by abnormalities in the formation of the bone matrix, leading to an increased risk of fractures. It has been discovered that one possible cause for the highly variable symptoms is the location of the mutation in the gene. Mutations at the C-terminus of the procollagen gene results in more severe symptoms than those at the amino-terminal. This scenario is embodied by which genetic concept?

   A. Reduced penetrance
   B. Imprinting
   C. Pleiotropy
   D. Variable expression
   E. Anticipation

2. Multiple members of a single family are seen in your office with several presentations of a single disease. The mildest cases have only the dermatologic findings of hypopigmented "ash leaf spots," fibromas of the nail, and *shagreen patches* (leather-textured area of subepidermal fibrosis normally found on the back). The most severe cases have the additional symptoms of seizures, mental retardation, and facial angiofibromas (vascular tumors). What is the most likely diagnosis of this inheritable disease?

   A. Sturge-Weber syndrome
   B. NF2
   C. von Recklinghausen disease
   D. Marfan syndrome
   E. Tuberous sclerosis

3. Myotonic dystrophy is an AD disorder characterized by facial and extremity muscle weakness, cataracts, intellectual impairment, and abnormalities in the respiratory, GI, and cardiac systems. This disease is caused by a CTG trinucleotide expansion in a gene on chromosome 19. Recently, a family with myotonic dystrophy was found to have a mutation on chromosome 3 instead. The symptoms exhibited by members of this family are indistinguishable from those caused by the chromosome 19 mutation. Which of the following terms defines the ability of a disease to be caused by mutations at different gene loci in different families?

A. Pleiotropy
B. Allelic heterogeneity
C. Locus heterogeneity
D. Heteroplasmy
E. Reduced or incomplete penetrance

HPI: You are called from the well-baby nursery to evaluate JL, a full-term newborn who is having difficulty feeding and latching 1 day after delivery. He is the first child born to a 32-year-old mother after an uneventful pregnancy. The maternal serum prenatal screening revealed a risk for Down syndrome (DS) of 1 in 180, but his parents declined amniocentesis after genetic counseling and a normal obstetric US at 18 weeks. JL was delivered by uncomplicated vaginal delivery, at 40 and 3/7 weeks. He weighed 3.3 kg, was 51 cm long, and had a head circumference of 50 cm at birth. His Apgar scores were 7 and 9 at 1 and 5 minutes, respectively.

PE: JL has marked hypotonia and a poor Moro reflex. You also notice a flat facial profile, midfacial hypoplasia, and a special appearance of his eyes, particularly when he is crying. His tongue appears too big for the size of the mouth. His neck is short with redundant, loose skin posteriorly. He has clinodactyly of the fifth fingers and a wide sandal gap between his first and second toes. You also note a grade 3/6 pansystolic heart murmur.

THOUGHT QUESTIONS

- What is the most likely diagnosis?
- What are the clinical features of this disorder?
- Why is confirmation of the diagnosis so important?
- What is the etiology of this condition?

BASIC SCIENCE REVIEW AND DISCUSSION

Syndrome Description

DS is the most common cause of genetic mental retardation, with an incidence of 1 in 700 live births. In the newborn period, severe hypotonia and lethargy are the norm. A combination of associated minor anomalies, none of which is specific or pathognomonic, gives affected individuals a specific recognizable appearance. Craniofacial features include brachycephaly, flat facial profile, upslanted palpebral fissures, epicanthic folds, protruding tongue in a small mouth, small simple ears, and loose redundant neck skin. Skin and musculoskeletal findings can include a single palmar crease, small middle phalanx of the fifth digit (resulting in clinodactyly), hyperextensible joints, wide gap between first and second toes, and short stature. Cardiac malformations are present in 40% of cases and have a significant impact on infant mortality. Ventricular septal defects (VSDs), atrial septal defects (ASDs), common atrioventricular canal, and patent ductus arteriosus (PDA) are the most common heart defects. Other common major malformations include anal atresia and duodenal atresia. Hearing loss (both conductive and sensorineural) is common. Ocular anomalies (e.g., cataracts, strabismus, glaucoma, and major refractory errors) are also very common. Early recognition of hearing and visual impairment is essential because they may further worsen the mental retardation if untreated. Mental retardation is universal in DS, with an IQ range of 25 to 75. Children with DS are generally happy, have good social skills, and are very affectionate. Most adults with DS develop early onset Alzheimer disease. Life expectancy is approximately 50 years in the United States.

Chromosome Findings

Ninety-five percent of DS cases are a result of trisomy 21 (47,XX,+21 or 47,XY,+21 karyotype). The additional chromosome is of maternal origin 90% of the time, which arises as a result of **nondisjunction during maternal meiosis (75% meiosis I)**. There is a well-recognized maternal age effect and increased risk of **aneuploidy** (a chromosome number that is not an exact multiple of the haploid number). **Robertsonian translocations** account for 3% of DS cases, of which one third of the time, one of the parents is found to be a balanced Robertsonian translocation carrier. These couples are at a significant risk of recurrence, which varies depending of the type of translocation and who is the carrier parent (i.e., male or female, with males transmitting an unbalanced complement less frequently than do females). The rest of DS cases (2%) are due to mosaicism of trisomy 21. Individuals with mosaic trisomy 21 tend on average to have higher IQs than those with full trisomy. The phenotype of DS (and other trisomies) is the result of an increased dose of specific genes on the extra chromosome. Chromosome analysis is essential in suspected cases of DS to confirm the diagnosis, provide accurate recurrence risk counseling, and, to a lesser degree, provide some information about the prognosis (mosaic cases).

CASE CONCLUSION

After your assessment, you suspect that JL has DS. In a private setting, you meet with both of JL's parents and disclose your impressions and provide counseling. An echocardiogram showed a small VSD. Ophthalmology and hearing evaluations have been requested. Two days later, a fluorescent in situ hybridization (FISH) study using a fluorescent probe specific for chromosome 21 reveals an extra set in each of the 45 metaphases analyzed. Standard chromosome analysis reveals a 47,XY,+21 karyotype, confirming the diagnosis.

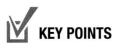 **THUMBNAIL:** Chromosome Structure

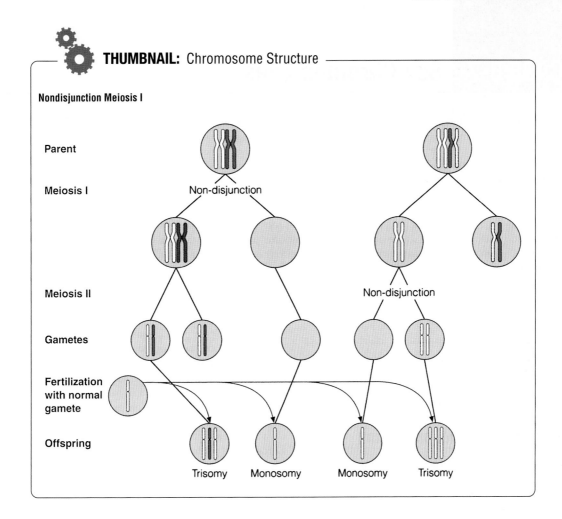

Nondisjunction Meiosis I

Parent

Meiosis I — Non-disjunction

Meiosis II — Non-disjunction

Gametes

Fertilization with normal gamete

Offspring — Trisomy — Monosomy — Monosomy — Trisomy

KEY POINTS

- Most common genetic cause of mental retardation, 1 in 700 live births
- DS: 95% trisomy 21, 3% Robertsonian translocation, 2% mosaic
- Most common trisomy: trisomy 16, but not compatible with life (all are spontaneous abortions)
- Maternal age effect: trisomy 21, trisomy 13, and trisomy 18
- Paternal age effect: increased incidence of spontaneous AD mutations (e.g., NF1, tuberous sclerosis complex, and achondroplasia)

QUESTIONS

1. After confirmation of the diagnosis, you inform JL's parents that the recurrence risk in the next pregnancy is what?

   A. Same as maternal age risk
   B. 1% greater than expected for maternal age risk
   C. 10 to 12%
   D. 100%
   E. Cannot provide adequate recurrence risk

2. Three years later, JL's parents are considering pregnancy and are interested in prenatal diagnosis. Upon discussion of the different modalities of invasive prenatal diagnosis, you explain which of the following?

   A. The incidence of trisomy 21 is the same with CVS and amniocentesis.
   B. The incidence of trisomy 21 is higher with CVS than with amniocentesis.

   C. Amniocentesis has a higher pregnancy-related loss rate than does CVS.
   D. Amniocentesis can be associated with confined placental mosaicism.
   E. A normal fetal US at 18 weeks rules out DS.

3. Children with DS are at increased risk for which of the following medical complications?

   A. Acute lymphoblastic leukemia
   B. Epilepsy
   C. Hypothyroidism
   D. Atlantoaxial subluxation
   E. All of the above

CASE 5-7 Sex Chromosomes

HPI: CA is a young female adolescent who has come to see you regarding her lack of sexual development. Unlike her two older sisters who initiated secondary sexual changes at ages 10 and 11, CA at age 14 still has not shown any signs of secondary sexual development. You learn that CA is a B+ student in the eighth grade who works an inordinate amount of hours to achieve her grades. CA's mother notes that she has always been a bit clumsy and has not shown much interest in sports, particularly those involving hand-eye coordination. Recently, it appears that she has been experiencing some low self-esteem because of her short stature and "not changing like the other girls have been."

PE: CA's height is at the fifth percentile and her weight is at the forty-fifth percentile for her age. Her facial appearance is unremarkable, but you do notice that her ears are a bit prominent and she has a low posterior hairline. There is mild posterior webbing of the neck. Cardiac exam including auscultation, BP readings of four extremities, and ECG is unremarkable. There is no evidence of secondary sexual development (Tanner stage I). Her chest is broad with widely spaced nipples. She has normal yet immature external genitalia. The rest of the exam is noncontributory.

THOUGHT QUESTIONS

- What is the most likely diagnosis?
- What are the clinical features of this disorder at different stages of life?
- What is the origin of the chromosomal defect?

BASIC SCIENCE REVIEW AND DISCUSSION

The most consistent feature in Turner syndrome is short stature and gonadal dysgenesis. Because the manifestations of ovarian failure are not evident in childhood, chromosome studies should be pursued in any girl with short stature and whose phenotype is not incompatible with Turner syndrome.

Syndrome Description

The majority of conceptuses with Turner syndrome will abort spontaneously. In the cases ascertained prenatally, fetal edema is commonly found, manifested as either increased nuchal translucency, nuchal edema, or generalized fetal edema (fetal hydrops). In the newborn period, congenital lymphedema with puffiness of the back of the neck, feet, and hands with hyperconvex nails as a result of the edema can be seen. Posterior webbing of the neck is common. The short stature is usually present from birth, although other manifestations can be present at any age. The thorax is broad with wide-spaced nipples. There can be subtle facial dysmorphisms—none of which is

characteristic or pathognomonic—such as low posterior hairline and short neck appearance. Cubitus valgus is very common. Cardiac malformations, including bicuspid aortic valve (30%) and coarctation of the aorta (10%), should be ruled out. The mean IQ is 90. Delays in motor skills, poor coordination, and visuospatial organization problems are common. Ovarian dysgenesis is present in more than 90%, manifesting as primary amenorrhea, but is *not* universal. A few girls with Turner syndrome will undergo secondary sexual development, and even fewer have been known to conceive spontaneously. The few that have spontaneous onset of menses will often experience early premature ovarian failure.

Chromosome Findings

The absence of a second sex chromosome is diagnostic of Turner syndrome. This absence may be a deletion of part or all of either an X or a Y chromosome. Nearly half of patients with Turner syndrome have monosomy X (45,X). Of these, 75% are due to the loss of either an X or a Y chromosome during paternal meiosis II. Other causes of Turner syndrome include mosaicism (e.g., 45,X/46,XX), isochromosome 46,X,i(Xp) in which there is loss of one chromosome arm and duplication of the other, ring chromosome 46,X,r(X) in which there is a break on each arm of the chromosome, leaving "sticky ends" that bind to form a ring, and chromosome deletions such as 46,X,del(Xp). You may see Turner syndrome written as 45,XO, which is incorrect nomenclature (there is no "O" chromosome).

CASE CONCLUSION

You obtain chromosome analysis that shows 45,X karyotype. FSH is markedly elevated at 89 mIU/mL. You discuss management in terms of using growth hormone therapy to enhance growth and starting estrogen replacement therapy to bring on secondary sexual changes and long-term prevention of osteoporosis. Lastly, you mention that conception, through in vitro fertilization (IVF) using donor eggs, is an option for her later in life.

THUMBNAIL: Sex Chromosomes

XXX females: No physical abnormalities; average IQ 10 to 20 points lower than that of controls; normal reproduction; approximately 80% due to maternal nondisjunction in meiosis I

XYY males: Normal appearance, taller than average; IQ 10 to 20 points lower than that of controls; tendency for emotional immaturity and impulsive behavior; can be associated with decreased fertility; result from nondisjunction in paternal meiosis II or postzygotic event

XXY (Klinefelter syndrome) males: Taller than average, breast development (gynecomastia), small testes, and infertility; IQ 10 to 20 points lower than that of controls; additional X chromosome either paternally or maternally derived

All trisomies (21, 18, 13, XXX, XXY) show a maternal age effect; the paternally derived trisomies have not been shown to have an advancing age effect (nondisjunction during meiosis II)

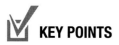 **KEY POINTS**

- Most common cause of primary amenorrhea
- Short stature, congenital lymphedema, ovarian dysgenesis, and mild decrease in IQ are hallmarks of Turner syndrome
- Growth hormone therapy, estrogen replacement therapy, and rule out (r/o) congenital heart disease are mainstays of management
- No advanced maternal age effect, usually sporadic (low recurrence risk)

QUESTIONS

1. A 10-year-old girl has hemophilia A. She is as severely affected as her 13-year-old brother. This could be explained by which of the following?

   A. Homozygous for this X-linked recessive disorder
   B. Skewed X inactivation
   C. 45,X karyotype female with hemophilia A
   D. X-autosome translocations
   E. All of the above

2. A newborn female with a prominent clitoris has been diagnosed with Turner syndrome. Her karyotype is 45,X/46,XY. Which of the following would you recommend?

   A. Immediate removal of the gonads
   B. Prophylactic removal of the gonads after puberty
   C. Bilateral oophorectomy if an ovarian tumor develops

   D. Routine management for Turner syndrome (same as for monosomy X)
   E. None of the above

3. The wide range of phenotypes for the various sex chromosome abnormalities can be explained at least in part by which of the following?

   A. Bias of ascertainment by studying only individuals who present with problems
   B. Imprinting effect due to parental origin of nondisjunction
   C. Data obtained prenatally may be different from data ascertained postnatally
   D. A and C are correct
   E. A and B are correct

CASE 5-8 Genomic Imprinting

HPI: EY is a 2-year-old boy who was referred to you by his pediatrician for seizures and developmental delay. You learn that as an infant, EY exhibited poor feeding, was hyperactive, and had trouble sleeping through the night. As he grew older, his developmental problems have become more pronounced, with significant delays in learning how to sit and walk. He is still unable to speak (at this age, children should have a vocabulary of 50 words and should be using two-word sentences). Six months ago, EY began having staring spells, which were eventually diagnosed as absence seizures. His parents are tired, frazzled, and very anxious for a diagnosis. Despite all that they have gone through, his parents added that EY is probably the happiest and most sociable of all their children.

PE: EY has a happy demeanor and laughs easily at trivial things in the office, but he does not speak during the entire exam. His skin is much fairer than that of either parent. He has a smaller than average head, deep-set eyes, and a wide mouth. His gait is wide and ataxic. The remainder of his exam shows no abnormalities.

THOUGHT QUESTIONS

- What is the most likely diagnosis?
- What is the inheritance pattern of this disease?
- What are some of the possible genetic defects causing this disease?
- What tests and/or studies would you order to confirm your diagnosis?

BASIC SCIENCE REVIEW AND DISCUSSION

Syndrome Description

Angelman and Prader-Willi syndromes are genetic disorders. These distinct diseases result from a deletion on the long arm of chromosome 15 (15q11-q13). **Angelman syndrome** occurs when this **deletion is maternal in origin** and **Prader-Willi syndrome** results when it is **paternal in origin.** Angelman syndrome consists of physical, neurologic, and developmental features, including severe mental retardation, global developmental delay, uncoordinated gait, seizures, hyperactivity, and disrupted sleep pattern. These patients often exhibit hypopigmented skin, mild physical dysmorphism (microcephaly, deep-set eyes, large mouth), and a characteristically happy disposition associated with excessive laughter. In contrast, the hallmarks of Prader-Willi syndrome include mild to moderate mental retardation, decreased muscle tone, hypothalamic insufficiency manifesting as hyperphagia and obesity, genital hypoplasia, incomplete or delayed puberty, and short stature.

Genomic Imprinting

Considering that the Angelman and Prader-Willi syndromes derive from deletions of the same chromosomal region, these syndromes have a surprisingly dissimilar constellation of symptoms. This difference in phenotype can be attributed to the concept of genomic imprinting. Genomic imprinting is the differential expression of genes depending on their chromosome of origin (either maternal or paternal). In other words, the expression of certain chromosomes—whether the genes will be turned "on" or "off"—depends on whether the chromosome is inherited from the mother or the father. This process is controlled by an imprinting center within the chromosome and is likely to be due to differences in DNA methylation (which involves adding methyl [CH_3] groups to nucleotides and thus inactivating the DNA). There are genes that are expressed only on the maternally derived chromosome, with the corresponding genes on the paternal chromosome remaining transcriptionally silent (and vice versa). Thus, deletion of part of a single chromosome will cause the loss of different sets of expressed genes, depending on whether the chromosome was from the mother or the father. This explains the differences between the Angelman and Prader-Willi syndromes: Angelman syndrome is caused by deletion of the 15q11-q13 region on the maternally derived chromosome and Prader-Willi is caused by deletion of the 15q11-q13 region on the paternally derived chromosome.

Genetic Defects

There are several causes for the Angelman and Prader-Willi syndromes, including mutations and uniparental disomy. Mutations are any changes in the DNA code, such as substitutions and deletions, that may eventually lead to a change in the protein end product. In many children with these syndromes, large deletions within the 15q11-q13 region have been found, as well as small microdeletions that are present either within the imprinting center or in other genes in the region. In other cases, children can be affected through uniparental disomy in which they inherit both copies of their chromosome 15 from one parent. If both copies are from the father, the child will have Angelman syndrome (consider this as the loss of the maternal chromosome), and if both copies are from the mother, the child will have Prader-Willi syndrome (consider this as the loss of the paternal chromosome).

CASE CONCLUSION

From EY's history and physical exam, you suspect Angelman syndrome. You perform a FISH analysis using a fluorescent probe specific for the 15q11-q13 region and find that only one of the probes lights up, demonstrating that there is a deletion in the 15q11-q13 region and confirming your diagnosis.

EY's parents are relieved to finally have a diagnosis after years of blaming themselves for their son's condition. His seizures have been brought under control with medications and his sleeping pattern has improved as he has grown older. Although EY is still unable to speak, he is beginning to learn sign language in a specialized school at age 5 years. With the help of physical therapy, he is also learning to feed himself and to become toilet trained.

THUMBNAIL: Genomic Imprinting

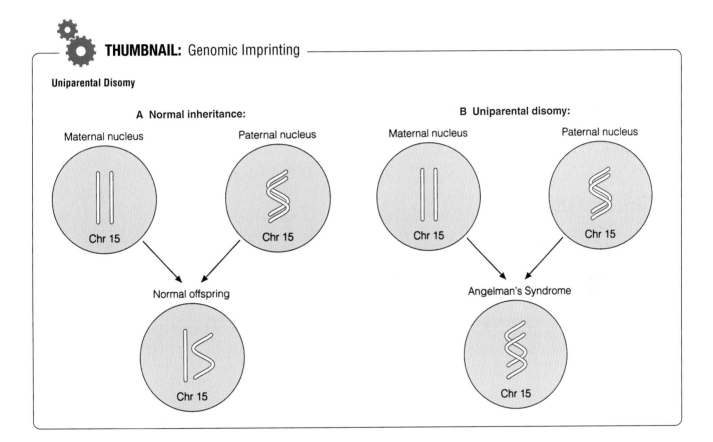

KEY POINTS

- Genetic defect on maternally derived chromosome 15 results in Angelman syndrome; defect on paternally derived chromosome 15 results in Prader-Willi syndrome
- The hallmarks of Angelman syndrome include (*a*) mental retardation, (*b*) uncoordinated gait, (*c*) seizures, (*d*) absent speech, and (*e*) an excessively happy demeanor
- The hallmarks of Prader-Willi syndrome include (*a*) mental retardation, (*b*) hyperphagia and obesity, (*c*) hypogonadism, and (*d*) short stature
- Genetic imprinting is the differential expression of genes depending on their parental origin
- Genetic defects can be due to large deletions, microdeletions, or uniparental disomy

QUESTIONS

1. Assume that EY is able to reproduce. Hypothetically, what are the chances that his children will have Angelman syndrome?

   A. 100%
   B. 66%
   C. 50%
   D. 25%
   E. 0%

2. Assume EY's mutation is heritable and is passed on for several generations to both male and female children. What inheritance pattern would the resulting pedigree (for Angelman syndrome) mimic?

   A. AR
   B. AD

   C. X-linked recessive
   D. Mitochondrial inheritance
   E. None of the above

3. The differences in Angelman and Prader-Willi syndromes are caused by differences in genetic imprinting defects. Which of the following disorders are also caused by defects in genetic imprinting?

   A. Duchenne muscular dystrophy
   B. Beckwith-Wiedemann syndrome
   C. NF
   D. CF
   E. Sickle cell anemia

CASE 5-9 | Cell Cycle

HPI: LA is a 2-year-old female brought in for a routine physical exam. Her family had been living in England for the last year, so she has not received care from you since she was 1 year old. The mother reports that LA has overall been healthy over the last year. LA has been eating well and developing appropriately in size, motor, and language skills. The primary concern she reports to you is that LA seems to be increasingly cross-eyed.

PE: Remarkable for moderate strabismus, an inequality of pupil size, a slight difference in iris colors, and mild proptosis of the left eye. The red reflex of the left eye is notably absent.

THOUGHT QUESTIONS

- What is retinoblastoma (Rb)? How is it acquired?
- What protein is responsible for this disease?
- Describe the normal cell cycle. What is the role of the Rb gene product?

BASIC SCIENCE REVIEW AND DISCUSSION

Rb is caused by a mutation in the tumor suppressor Rb gene, leading to a rare malignant tumor of the retina. It is found in approximately 1 in 20,000 births. Roughly 40% of cases are inherited, with an offspring obtaining a mutated allele through the germline, and the remaining 60% of cases occur sporadically. The signs of Rb include an absence of the red reflex, which typically is observed when light is directed at the retina. However, in the case of Rb, white is seen behind the pupils, which is also known as **leukocoria.** Other signs include strabismus or problems with eye movements, differences in pupil sizes, differences in iris colors, increased tearing, proptosis, nystagmus, and cataract formation. Most cases are diagnosed before the age of 5 years. The hereditary form is usually diagnosed earlier, with a mean age of 13 to 15 months, and the sporadic form is diagnosed at a mean age of 24 months. Treatment modalities include enucleation, external beam radiation, localized plaque radiation, photocoagulation, cryotherapy, and chemotherapy. The prognosis is overall good but generally depends on unilateral versus bilateral disease, extent of involvement, and age at diagnosis. One hundred years ago, the mortality rate from Rb was 100%. The death rate has since improved; in 1964, the mortality rate was 18%, and in 1990, it was less than 10%.

The Cell Cycle

To better understand the role of Rb, we will first review the general concepts of the cell cycle. The cell cycle is divided into four phases. **G1,** or gap 1, is the time when the cell prepares for DNA replication. Protein synthesis is significantly up-regulated at this time. In general, this is the portion of the cell cycle that varies from cell to cell, resulting in differences in doubling time between different cell types. On average, G1 lasts approximately 18 hours. **S phase** is the period when the cell undergoes **DNA replication,** and this typically lasts 20 hours. **G2,** or gap 2, is the period when the **cell prepares for cell division,** and this portion lasts roughly 3 hours. Lastly, **M phase,** or mitosis, is when the cell physically divides into two daughter cells and occurs over 1 hour. Cells that are not in the cell cycle are in **G0,** or quiescent. These cells may be temporarily out of the cell cycle, secondary to a negative stimulus such as lack of nutrients in the milieu or contact inhibition, which is a means of population control. Other cells are permanently out of the cell cycle because they have terminally differentiated—for example, neurons.

In general, three types of proteins interact with one another to orchestrate the progression through a cell cycle. **Cyclins** are proteins whose levels increase and decrease depending on the phase. There are different types of cyclins that are specific to each phase of the cell cycle or the transition of a phase. Cyclins serve a regulatory role to **cyclin-dependent kinases** (Cdks). The binding of a cyclin to its partner kinase allows the kinase to be activated. Cdks maintain a steady level throughout the cell cycle. Once bound to the appropriate cyclin, the kinase is able to *phosphorylate* downstream substrates, which include enzymes, structural proteins, and transcription factors. Cell cycle inhibitors also serve an integral role in the regulation of the cell cycle. These include tumor suppressors such as p53 and Rb and Cdk inhibitors like p27. Rb and p53 prevent cycle progression at the G1-S interface by interrupting transcription. p27 and other similar inhibitors, however, bind to active cyclin-Cdk complexes, inhibiting the kinase activity and the phosphorylation of downstream targets that are important for cell division.

Another important concept to understand is that multiple checkpoints exist within the cell cycle to prevent aberrant cell cycle progression. The first checkpoint is at the site of cell cycle entry from G0 to G1. This checkpoint ensures that the cell is ready for division with adequate resources available and an accommodating environment. The G1-S interface is the first checkpoint for DNA damage and is the point that p53 and Rb govern. Other DNA checkpoints occur within the S phase and between the S phase and G2. These checkpoints monitor the presence of Okazaki fragments during DNA replication, and a cell cannot proceed past the S phase until all the Okazaki fragments are gone. There is also a spindle checkpoint at the end of G2. It has been shown that cells that do not pass the checkpoints secondary to irreparable damage will undergo apoptosis.

Rb and p53 are guardians of the G1-S checkpoint. Rb has been shown to block cell cycle progression by binding to a transcription factor called **E2F** and thereby preventing the ability of E2F from binding promoters such as c-myc and c-fos. These proteins all regulate transcription of genes essential for proliferation. With one Rb allele absent, Rb can still be made from the unaffected allele, and Rb protein can still function to regulate the cell cycle. However, with two mutated Rb alleles, there is an absence of functioning Rb, and cells with errors in the DNA replication are able to pass through these checkpoints, complete the cell cycle, and propagate these errors.

CASE CONCLUSION

LA is diagnosed with Rb of the left eye. She is treated with localized plaque radiation therapy but because of a lack of substantial response, she ultimately had to undergo an enucleation of the left eye. A genetic work-up determined that she had the sporadic form of Rb and, therefore, the enucleation was curative.

THUMBNAIL: Cell Cycle

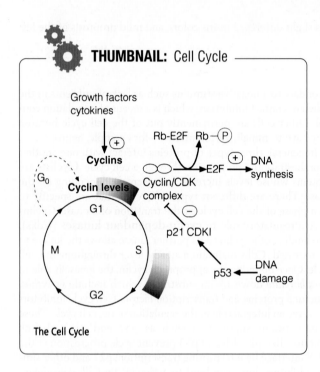

The Cell Cycle

KEY POINTS

- The cell cycle consists of four phases: G1, S, G2, and M
- Three types of proteins are important in the regulation of cell cycle progression: cyclins, Cdks, and inhibitors such as tumor suppressors or Cdk inhibitors
- Multiple checkpoints exist within the cell cycle to prevent the propagation of errors
- Rb is a rare malignant tumor of the retina resulting from a loss of function of the tumor suppressor Rb

QUESTIONS

1. Some chemotherapeutic agents affect cells that are cycling and are specific to certain phases of the cycle. Tumor cells typically have a quicker doubling time than healthy tissues, making tumor cells more sensitive to chemotherapeutic agents. Which phase of the cell cycle is most variable and responsible for the differences in doubling time between different cell types?

   A. G0
   B. G1
   C. S
   D. G2
   E. M

2. There are many points of regulation involved in cell population control. These are all important to prevent the propagation of errors and the formation of malignancies. Which of the following is a form of regulation?

   A. The presence of the Okazaki fragments, preventing progression through S phase
   B. A decrease in p53, leading to a block in the G1-S interface
   C. Rb dissociation from E2F, resulting in a conformation change in E2F and the inability of E2F from functioning as a transcription factor
   D. p27 binding to Cdks, leading to activation of these kinases
   E. Cyclins binding to Cdks directly dephosphorylating downstream protein targets

PART VI

Embryology

CASE 6-1 Embryonic Development

HPI: A 5-day-old baby girl is seen in the nursery by your team. She was found at birth to have bilateral congenital cataracts and low birth weight. She has also experienced poor feeding and failure to thrive. The mother is a recent immigrant and received no prenatal care. She states that during the second month of the pregnancy, she had an unusual pinpoint, nonpruritic rash lasting for several days, which was preceded by flu-like symptoms lasting about 1 week. The parents have two other children, now ages 3 and 5 years old, both of whom are healthy. They deny any significant family history of diseases.

PE: The infant appears lethargic and small. HEENT exam reveals mild microcephaly and bilateral cataracts. On cardiovascular exam, a grade 2/6 continuous machinery murmur is heard throughout the cardiac cycle. The remainder of her exam is normal.

Labs: Echocardiogram shows a PDA. CT scan of the head reveals intracerebral calcifications.

THOUGHT QUESTIONS

- What is the cause of the baby's defects?
- How is this disease transmitted?
- How is the timing of the mother's symptoms significant?
- What other infectious agents can cause birth defects?

BASIC SCIENCE REVIEW AND DISCUSSION

Syndrome Description

Rubella is an enveloped RNA virus that is part of the togavirus family. It causes a mild infection in adults characterized by flu-like symptoms for up to 1 week, followed by a fine, punctate, nonpruritic rash lasting for 3 to 4 days. Infection of the fetus before 16 weeks of gestation can cause a wide range of congenital defects, whereas infection after the fifth month rarely leads to any morbidity. The most common defects include **sensorineural deafness, cataracts, cardiovascular defects** such as PDA and pulmonary artery stenosis, CNS damage leading to mental retardation, and **fetal growth restriction.** The advent of the rubella vaccination led to a dramatic decrease in the number of rubella-associated neonatal defects, but it is not effective for every individual, and even when successful, the duration of the immunity is often variable.

Diagnosis can be made by the detection of rubella-specific IgM antibodies in the infant, isolation of the virus from nasopharyngeal or urine specimens, or the persistence of rubella-specific IgG in the infant beyond the time expected due to just the passive transfer of maternal antibodies (usually after 8–12 months of age). There is no specific treatment for congenital rubella syndrome. Heart and eye defects can sometimes be corrected with surgery, and children with vision, hearing, or cognitive deficits can benefit from specialized education programs.

Organogenesis

The period of **organogenesis** lasts from the third to the eighth week of gestation and is the time when most of the major organ systems are formed. For example, development of the embryonic eye begins on day 22 with the appearance of shallow grooves on either side of the forebrain. These grooves become the optic vesicle by the end of the fourth week and will induce the formation of the lens. By the end of the seventh week, the lens fibers are forming, as are the neural and pigment layers of the retina. During this critical period, the developing organs are very sensitive to both genetic and environmental insults. If a mother is infected with the rubella virus between the fourth and the seventh weeks of pregnancy, the resulting child will have a high risk of congenital cataracts. However, if infection is after the seventh week, the presence of a lens abnormality becomes rare. Similarly, cardiac malformations can occur with an infection before the first 12 weeks, and sensorineural deafness can occur if infection occurs before the first 16 weeks, but both defects are unusual with later infections.

Infectious Teratogens

Rubella is one of several infectious organisms (including toxoplasmosis, rubella, CMV, HSV, syphilis [ToRCHeS]) that can cause birth defects. Maternal infection with the protozoan *Toxoplasma gondii* can cause a flu-like infection in the mother, as well as ocular (chorioretinitis, optic nerve atrophy), systemic (hepatosplenomegaly, jaundice), and CNS (microcephaly, mental retardation) manifestations in affected infants. **CMV** is a DNA herpesvirus that can cause a variety of CNS (microcephaly, mental retardation, hearing loss) and systemic (low birth weight, hepatosplenomegaly) symptoms. **HSV type 2** (HSV-2) is most likely to be transmitted during the delivery of the infant through the birth canal and can cause a syndrome of meningoencephalitis, seizures, and skin lesions. Intrauterine infection can be manifested by prematurity, low birth weight, microcephaly, chorioretinitis, and skin lesions. **Congenital syphilis** occurs when the spirochete is transmitted to the fetus and can result in a 40% fetal mortality rate, as well as a multiorgan infection causing bone or teeth deformities, rhinitis, rash on the palms and soles, mental retardation, and vision and hearing defects. In addition, many other infectious organisms have been found to have teratogenic effects, including HIV, varicella zoster, hepatitis B, Parvovirus, and *Chlamydia trachomatis* (Fig. 6-1).

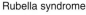

Rubella syndrome

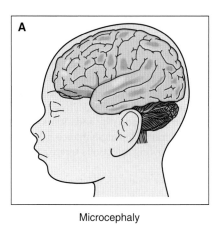

Microcephaly

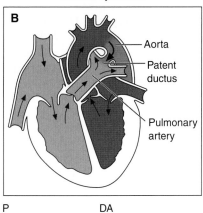

Aorta

Patent ductus

Pulmonary artery

P   DA

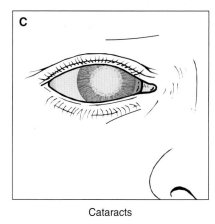

Cataracts

Figure 6-1. Teratogenic effects of rubella.

CASE CONCLUSION

The infant is found to have rubella IgM antibodies, confirming the diagnosis of congenital rubella syndrome. She undergoes surgery to repair her heart defects, and after an extensive search the parents are able to find an appropriate school for the visually and hearing impaired.

THUMBNAIL: Embryonic Development

Infectious Teratogens (ToRCHeS Organisms)

Teratogen	Symptoms
Toxoplasmosis (*T. gondii*)	Ocular (chorioretinitis) and CNS (mental retardation, hydrocephalus) malformations, hepatosplenomegaly
Rubella	Sensorineural deafness, cataracts, cardiac abnormalities (PDA), CNS defects (microcephaly), and growth retardation
CMV	Microcephaly, hepatosplenomegaly, and blindness
HSV	Most infections at birth, but fetal infection can cause prematurity, growth restriction, mental retardation, and chorioretinitis
Syphilis *(Treponema pallidum)*	Multiorgan involvement including defects in bone formation, rash, rhinitis, mental retardation, deafness, and vision loss

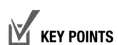 KEY POINTS

■ Rubella is an RNA virus that causes birth defects when fetal infection occurs before 16 weeks of gestation

■ Organogenesis lasts primarily from the third to the eighth week of gestation and is the period in which the fetus is most sensitive to teratogens

QUESTIONS

1. Infectious teratogens comprise a diverse class of organisms ranging from RNA viruses to DNA viruses to bacteria. Which of the following teratogenic syndromes is caused by a protozoan?

   A. Toxoplasmosis
   B. Rubella
   C. CMV
   D. HSV-2
   E. Syphilis

2. A newborn presents to your pediatric office with a history of poor feeding, failure to thrive, nasal discharge, and small blisters on the hands and feet. Which test would you order to definitively diagnose this infectious teratogen?

   A. Rubella IgG detection
   B. Rubella IgM detection
   C. HSV culture of blisters

   D. Urine culture for CMV
   E. Dark field microscopy

3. A 30-year-old pregnant woman at 15 weeks of gestation is brought to the ED by a friend for fever, lethargy, and excessive sleepiness. The woman is known to be HIV positive, but the rest of her medical history is unobtainable. Physical exam is significant for cervical lymphadenopathy and altered mental status. Head CT reveals multiple ring-enhancing lesions and edema. Which of the following infectious teratogens are you most worried about?

   A. Toxoplasmosis
   B. Rubella
   C. CMV
   D. HSV-2
   E. Syphilis

Teratogens

HPI: A 7-year-old boy is brought to your office by his parents because of difficulty at school. They state that he is unable to concentrate in class, has delays in his speech, and is quickly falling behind his classmates. In addition, his teachers have reported aggressive and impulsive behavior, as well as difficulty interacting with his peers. The patient was born premature with a low birth weight and has had a history of poor feeding and slow growth. The mother is a recovering alcoholic who has been sober for the past 5 years but admits to drinking heavily during the pregnancy. They deny any significant family history of any diseases.

PE: The parents are both of normal build, but the child appears small for his age. His height and weight are both measured to be below the tenth percentile. HEENT exam reveals mild microcephaly, a thin upper lip, flat mid-face, and short palpebral fissures. On cardiovascular exam, a grade 2/6 holosystolic murmur is heard at the left sternal border. The remainder of his exam shows no abnormalities.

Labs: Echocardiogram shows a small VSD.

THOUGHT QUESTIONS

- What is the most likely cause of the child's symptoms?
- How is your diagnosis made?
- What is the prognosis for the child?
- What are some other common chemical teratogens?

BASIC SCIENCE REVIEW AND DISCUSSION

Syndrome Description

Fetal alcohol syndrome (FAS) describes a set of irreversible signs and symptoms found in some children as a result of the maternal ingestion of alcohol during pregnancy. Although the phenotype of FAS can be highly variable, the most common clinical features include prenatal and postnatal **growth restriction, developmental disabilities, and distinctive facial dysmorphology** (microcephaly, short palpebral fissures, low nasal root, indistinct philtrum, and a thin upper lip). Other important findings include congenital heart defects, joint abnormalities, and structural defects in various other systems (renal, neurologic, ocular, genitourinary, hepatic, and immune). **Fetal alcohol spectrum disorder** (FASD) is a general term to describe the range of effects that can result from prenatal alcohol exposure, including the specific features that comprise a diagnosis of FAS. There is no safe level of alcohol use in pregnancy, but the incidence of FAS increases among women with a higher alcohol intake, especially during the first trimester. As children with FAS mature, the facial features become less recognizable, but their poor social/living skills may make independent living difficult as adults.

A diagnosis is made clinically by a history of maternal alcohol use in conjunction with the constellation of symptoms in the child. Although there is no specific treatment for FAS, it is important to evaluate the child for associated birth defects, some of which (e.g., cardiac) may be corrected surgically. Educational and community resources can be used to help support the family and help the child reach his or her fullest potential. Clinicians should recognize that this diagnosis might also be a sign of a continuing substance abuse problem in the family and the need for additional social support.

Early Embryogenesis and Organogenesis

After fertilization of the ovum by the sperm, the resulting **zygote** undergoes a series of cell divisions reaching the 16-cell **morula** stage by day 4. After the morula enters the uterine cavity, the blastocyst is formed when an influx of fluid separates the morula into the inner and outer cell masses, which will give rise to the embryo and the trophoblast, respectively. The blastocyst is implanted into the endometrium by the end of the first week. By the start of week 2, the **trophoblast** begins to differentiate into the inner cytotrophoblast and the outer syncytiotrophoblast, and together they will eventually give rise to the placenta. Meanwhile, the inner cell mass divides into the **bilaminar germ disc,** composed of the epiblast and the hypoblast. During the third week of development, the embryo is primarily preoccupied with the process of **gastrulation.** This is characterized by the formation of the primitive streak on the epiblast, followed by the invagination of epiblast cells to form the three germ layers of the embryo: the inner endoderm, the middle mesoderm, and the outer ectoderm. The **endodermal layer** eventually gives rise to the GI and respiratory systems. The **mesoderm** forms the cardiovascular, musculoskeletal, and genitourinary systems. The **ectoderm layer** will differentiate into the nervous system (neural crest, neural tube), skin, and many sensory organs (hair, eyes, nose, and ears). Alcohol has been shown to be toxic to the epiblast layer and therefore can have deleterious effects on multiple organ systems, although some organs (e.g., the brain and heart) seem to be especially sensitive. The period of organogenesis primarily lasts from the third week to the eighth week of gestation and is the time when most of the major organ systems are formed. Although fetal growth restriction can occur with alcohol use during any period in pregnancy, most major defects are the result of use during the first trimester (Fig. 6-2).

Classic Chemical Teratogens

Alcohol is just one of many chemicals linked to birth defects. Another classic example is **thalidomide,** which was used in the 1950s and 1960s for the treatment of nausea and insomnia. It was eventually discovered to cause major limb deformities, intestinal atresia, and cardiac defects. **Isotretinoin (Accutane)** is an

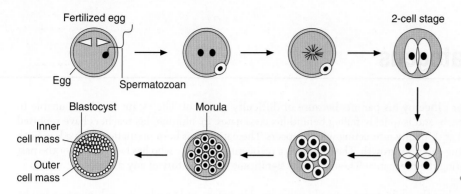

• **Figure 6-2.** Early events in fetal development.

analogue of vitamin A used to treat severe acne. However, this drug also produces a characteristic set of birth defects called isotretinoin/vitamin A embryopathy. The symptoms include abnormal ear development, mandibular hypoplasia, cleft palate, and neural tube and cardiac defects. **Diethylstilbestrol (DES)** is a synthetic estrogen that was used to prevent recurrent miscarriages in the 1940s through the 1960s. However, it was eventually found to cause early onset vaginal carcinomas and malformations of the genitourinary tract (T-shaped uterus, Müllerian fusion defects) in women exposed in utero.

CASE CONCLUSION

The diagnosis of FAS is made from the history of maternal alcohol use, characteristic facial features, and developmental abnormalities. The child was enrolled in the special education program at his elementary school, where he was able to receive greater attention and help with his language disabilities. Although he was found to have a low-normal IQ, the patient was unable to finish high school and eventually was placed in a group home for developmentally delayed adults because of his poor independent living skills.

THUMBNAIL: Teratogens

Chemical Teratogens

Teratogen	Symptoms
Alcohol	Craniofacial abnormalities, growth restriction, developmental delays, cardiovascular abnormalities (VSDs)
Thalidomide	Limb agenesis/deformities, intestinal atresia, cardiac abnormalities
Isotretinoin	Ear abnormalities, cleft palate, mandibular hypoplasia, neural tube and cardiac defects
DES	Genitourinary cancers and malformations

KEY POINTS

■ The stages of early embryo development include fertilization → cleavage and formation of morula → blastocyst → implantation → formation of bilaminar disc (epiblast and hypoblast) → gastrulation and formation of trilaminar germ disc

■ Inner cell mass → epiblast → ectoderm, mesoderm, endoderm → hypoblast → yolk sac

■ Outer cell mass → trophoblast → cytotrophoblast, syncytiotrophoblast → placenta

■ Ectoderm forms the nervous system, ears, nose, eyes, and skin

■ Mesoderm forms the musculoskeletal, cardiovascular, and genitourinary systems

■ Endoderm forms the GI and respiratory tracts

QUESTIONS

1. A 1-year-old girl is diagnosed with FAS and found to have the characteristic facial features and coordination difficulties, hearing loss, and a diffusely cloudy cornea. Which germinal layer(s) seem(s) to be affected?

   A. Mesoderm
   B. Endoderm
   C. Ectoderm
   D. Endoderm and ectoderm
   E. Endoderm and mesoderm

2. Most birth defects arise during the period of organogenesis between the third and eighth weeks of development. However, within that time span, each organ system is susceptible to environmental insults at specific times. For example, limb formation reaches a critical state around the fifth week of gestation when the limb buds appear. Which of the following teratogens would you be most worried about because of its effects on bone development?

   A. Isotretinoin
   B. Thalidomide
   C. Lithium
   D. Alcohol
   E. DES

3. Organogenesis cannot begin without the proper formation of the three germ layers (i.e., the ectoderm, mesoderm, and endoderm). Which of the following terms describes the events in the third week of development that establish these three layers?

   A. Cleavage
   B. Invagination
   C. Migration
   D. Compaction
   E. Gastrulation

CASE 6-3   Neural Tube Development

HPI: AC comes to your office for a second opinion after learning the results of her obstetric US. She is a healthy 28-year-old female currently at 19 weeks gestation. This is her first pregnancy, which was unplanned but desired. Her maternal serum prenatal screening at 16 weeks was abnormal, with an elevated maternal serum AFP (MSAFP) of 3.4 multiples of the median (MoM), which prompted further testing. Last week, she had a detailed US exam revealing a live single fetus appropriately grown for gestational age with a Chiari II malformation (Lemon-Banana sign, Fig. 6-3) and lumbosacral myelomeningocele (Fig. 6-4).

She reports no past significant illnesses. AC has being taking prenatal vitamins since her first visit at 12 weeks. She denies any tobacco, alcohol, or illicit drug use, past or current.

THOUGHT QUESTIONS

- What are the objectives of second trimester prenatal screening? When is it performed?
- What is the critical time period for neural tube closure?
- What are the known predisposing factors for neural tube defects (NTDs)?

BASIC SCIENCE REVIEW AND DISCUSSION

Maternal Serum Screening

Maternal serum screening in the second trimester of pregnancy is routinely offered to all pregnant women in the United States. It is a screening test for **Down syndrome** and **NTDs,** identifying a population at risk (screen positive) and a low-risk population. Additionally, a variety of other problems can also be identified, such as other chromosomal abnormalities and abdominal wall defects, but at lower detection rates (sensitivity). It is often referred to as the "quadruple screen" because four analytes are evaluated (AFP, unconjugated estriol, human chorionic gonadotropin [hCG], and inhibin A). Detection rates for Down syndrome (decreased AFP, decreased estriol, increased inhibin A, and increased hCG) are approximately 80%, and more than 90% of open NTDs (increased AFP) are detected among low-risk women, using a fixed cutoff of 5% false-positive results. The test is done between 15 and 20 weeks gestation and is most effective between **16 and 18 weeks.** Those women who screen positive are offered further testing.

Neural Tube Development

The **formation of the neural tube** begins between days 22 and 23 of gestation (fourth week) in the region of the fourth and sixth somites. Fusion of the neural folds occurs in cranial and caudal directions, probably at **multisite initiation.** The anterior neuropore (future brain) closes by day 25 and the posterior pore (future spinal cord) closes by day 27. Closure of the neural tube coincides with establishment of its vascular supply. Most NTDs develop as a result of defective closure at the fourth week of development (sixth week of gestation or from the last menstrual period [LMP]) (Fig. 6-5).

Etiology of Neural Tube Defects

NTDs are a classic example of **multifactorial inheritance (MFI),** emphasizing the interactions between environmental and genetic factors. Geographic and ethnic variations may reflect environmental and genetic factors affecting the occurrence of **NTDs.** Variations in the incidence of NTDs related to seasonal or temporal changes in the same region and among different areas in homogeneous populations support environmental contribution. Decreased levels of folic acid have been found among mothers who gave birth to babies with NTDs. Supplementation with periconceptional folic acid effectively reduces the incidence of recurrence of NTDs, as well as first occurrence, as shown by randomized controlled trials (RCTs). Doubling of the risk of NTDs has been associated with homozygosity for a common mutation in the gene for MTHFR, the C677T allelic variant, which encodes an enzyme with reduced activity. However, even if the association were causal, this MTHFR variant would account for only a small fraction of NTDs prevented by folic acid. The risk of NTDs seen with certain genotypes may vary depending on maternal factors, such as the blood levels of vitamin B12 or folate.

CASE CONCLUSION

AC and her partner decide to terminate this pregnancy after genetic counseling. Chromosome studies of the fetus reveal a normal 46,XY karyotype. An autopsy confirmed the presence of a large lumbosacral myelomeningocele. No additional major or minor anomalies were noted.

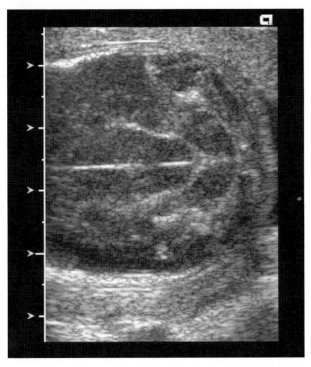

Figure 6-3. Lemon-banana sign. (Courtesy of Dr. Peter Callen, Department of Radiology, and Obstetrics, Gynecology and Reproductive Sciences, UCSF, San Francisco, CA.)

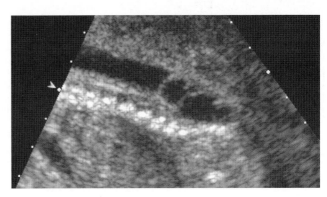

Figure 6-4. Lumbosacral myelomeningocele. (Courtesy of Dr. Peter Callen, Department of Radiology, and Obstetrics, Gynecology and Reproductive Sciences, UCSF, San Francisco, CA.)

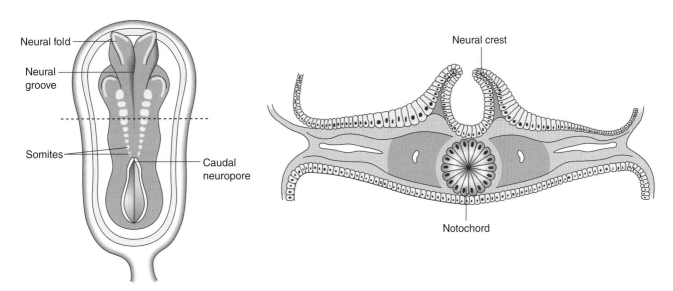

Figure 6-5. Neural tube development.

THUMBNAIL: Neural Tube Development

Spinal Cord and Brain Development

In embryology, the age of the embryo/fetus is given from the time of conception, whereas in clinical practice gestational age is derived from the LMP.

The neural tube gives rise to the CNS, consisting of the brain and spinal cord.

The neural crest gives rise to the peripheral nervous system (PNS) and the autonomic nervous system (ANS).

Formation of the neural tube (neurulation) begins at days 22 to 23 in the region of the fourth and sixth pairs of somites.

The cranial two thirds of the neural plate and tube down to the fourth pair of somites represents the brain, and the caudal one third of the neural plate and tube (below the fourth pair of somites) represents the future spinal cord.

The neural tube likely closes in a multisite fashion. Closure of the neural tube proceeds in the cranial and caudal directions until small areas at the ends remain open, the rostral and the caudal neuropores. By day 25 of development, the rostral neuropore closes, and by day 27, the caudal neuropore closes.

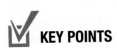 **KEY POINTS**

- NTDs are one of the most common major malformations; isolated NTDs, as well as other isolated single organ malformations, are explained by MFI

- Families with prior affected offspring with NTDs are at an increased risk of recurrence (10-fold over baseline); periconceptional use of folic acid can reduce the incidence and the recurrence of NTDs

- Drugs (valproic acid), hyperthermia, single-gene defects, and chromosomal abnormalities have been associated with NTDs; the recurrence risks in these cases are different from those for MFI and must be individualized

QUESTIONS

1. For this couple's next pregnancy, the greatest risk reduction for recurrence of NTDs is achieved by which of the following?

   A. FDA daily recommended allowance of folic acid (0.4 mg)
   B. High doses of folic acid periconceptionally (4 mg)
   C. Adoption; the risk of recurrence is too great
   D. Avoid alcohol consumption
   E. Avoid exposure to x-rays

2. Most NTDs are the result of which of the following?

   A. Teratogen exposure
   B. Vitamin deficiency
   C. Multifactorial etiology
   D. Single-gene defects
   E. Chromosomal abnormalities

3. A 20-year-old woman with seizure disorder on valproic acid has a positive pregnancy test 1 day after she missed her period. Regarding the teratogenic risk of the medication, how would you counsel her?

   A. The risk of NTDs is probably only slightly increased over background risk (1/1500) if she stops taking valproic acid now.
   B. The risk of NTDs secondary to valproic acid intake is not increased.
   C. Risk of NTDs is 10- to 20-fold over background (6%) with exposure during the first trimester.
   D. Continue taking valproic acid because the damage has already been done.
   E. A and C are correct.

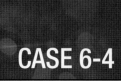

CASE 6-4 Branchial Arch Anomalies

HPI: A 15-year-old boy is referred to the cardiologist for HTN found during a routine physical exam. The patient notes no symptoms from the high BP but does complain of a long history of weakness and pain in both legs after mild exercise. He has been quite healthy and denies any significant family history of illness.

PE: BP 145/95 (arms) and 80/40 (legs); HR 85; RR 12

The child appears well developed and in no acute distress. On cardiovascular exam, a grade 3/6 systolic ejection murmur is heard at the suprasternal notch. Systolic murmurs can also be heard over the left and right sides of the chest, both laterally and posteriorly. Extremity exam reveals bounding carotid and radial pulses, and the lower extremity (femoral, popliteal, posterior tibial, and dorsalis pedis) pulses are weak. The remainder of the exam shows no abnormalities.

Labs: Chest x-ray shows a moderately enlarged heart with notching of the ribs. ECG reveals a left axis deviation, suggestive of left ventricular hypertrophy. Echocardiogram demonstrates a bicuspid aortic valve and decreased flow through the descending aorta.

THOUGHT QUESTIONS

- What is the diagnosis?
- What is the developmental process that forms the major arterial system?
- Which part of the embryologic system gives rise to this defect?
- How is this condition treated?

BASIC SCIENCE REVIEW AND DISCUSSION

Syndrome Description

Coarctation of the aorta is a congenital malformation that involves the abnormal **thickening of the aortic wall** that can cause narrowing of the lumen anywhere from the transverse arch to the origin of the iliac arteries (Fig. 6-6). An overwhelming majority (98%) occurs just distal to the ductus arteriosus. Coarctation can develop alone or in conjunction with other cardiac abnormalities, including bicuspid aortic valve, VSD, or transverse arch hypoplasia. The classic signs of coarctation are **unequal BPs and pulses** between the upper and lower extremities. Some children may also experience pain or weakness in the lower extremities with exercise. A systolic ejection murmur may indicate the presence of a bicuspid aortic valve, and flow murmurs along the lateral thoracic region are consistent with increased collateral circulation. Infants who are symptomatic generally have severe coarctation and can present with symptoms of heart failure, acidosis, and insufficient perfusion of the lower extremities.

Chest x-ray may show an enlarged cardiac silhouette due to ventricular hypertrophy, as well as rib notching from pressure erosion by enlarged collateral vessels. Left axis deviation and ventricular hypertrophy can also be seen on ECG. The diagnosis can be confirmed by an echocardiogram, which can visualize the segment of narrowed blood flow and detect other cardiac abnormalities. Treatment is by surgical correction of the defect through either excision of the area of coarctation or enlargement with a prosthetic patch. If untreated, most patients will experience chronic systemic HTN with associated complications of intracranial hemorrhage, CAD, and heart failure. In neonates with severe disease, heart failure and lower extremity cyanosis may be fatal if not treated immediately.

Pharyngeal (branchial) Arches The pharyngeal arches appear around the fourth to fifth weeks and are crucial in the development of the head and neck region. The arches are composed of **mesenchymal** and **neural crest cells** that are sandwiched between surface ectoderm (pharyngeal cleft) and a layer of endodermal epithelium (pharyngeal pouches). Each pharyngeal arch has its own artery (called **aortic arches**) and cranial nerve, which gives rise to distinctive skeletal and muscular components of the head and neck. The **first pharyngeal arch** gives rise to the mandible and maxilla and contributes to the formation of the bones of the middle ear (e.g., incus and malleus). The muscles of mastication (e.g., temporalis, masseter, and pterygoids) are also derived from the first arch and are innervated by the mandibular branch of the trigeminal nerve. The **second pharyngeal arch** produces the stapes and lesser horn of the hyoid bone, as well as the muscles of facial expression, the stapedius, stylohyoid, and posterior belly of the digastric. The innervation of these muscles is via the facial nerve. The **third pharyngeal arch** forms the greater horn of the hyoid bone. The musculature of this arch is the stylopharyngeus muscle that is innervated by the glossopharyngeal nerve. The **fourth and sixth arches** eventually fuse to give rise to the thyroid, cricoid, arytenoid, corniculate, and cuneiform cartilages. The fourth arch also develops into the cricothyroid, levator veli palatini, and pharyngeal constrictor muscles, and the sixth arch forms all of the intrinsic muscles of the larynx (except the cricothyroid). The muscles of the fourth arch are supplied by the superior laryngeal branch of the vagus, and the muscles of the sixth arch are innervated by the recurrent laryngeal branch.

Pharyngeal (branchial) Cleft Pharyngeal clefts are composed of **ectoderm tissue.** Of those present at 5 weeks gestation, only one makes a major developmental contribution. The **first cleft** gives rise to the external auditory meatus, and the other clefts form a temporary cervical sinus that disappears with the growth of the second arch.

Pharyngeal (branchial) Pouches The five pairs of pharyngeal pouches are composed of **endodermal** epithelium that develops into several important organs. The **first pouch** is involved in the creation of the middle ear, the eustachian tube, and the tympanic membrane. The **second pouch** forms the epithelial lining of the

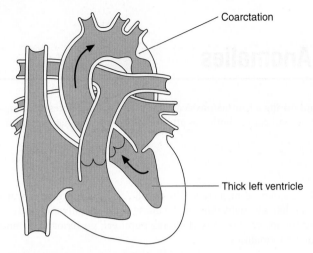

• **Figure 6-6.** Coarctation of the aorta.

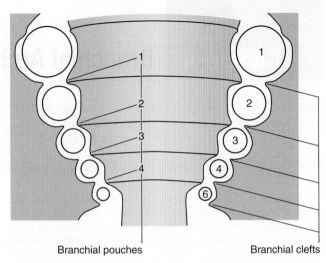

• **Figure 6-7.** Coronal section of the embryonic pharynx (arches are the circles numbered 1 through 6).

palatine tonsil. The dorsal wing of the **third pouch** develops into the inferior parathyroid gland, and the ventral wing differentiates into the thymus. The thymus eventually migrates medially and caudally while pulling the inferior parathyroid gland to its dorsal surface. The **fourth pouch** differentiates into the superior parathyroid gland, and the fifth pouch (usually considered part of the fourth pouch) gives rise to the ultimobranchial body of the thyroid. These cells develop into the parafollicular or C cells that secrete calcitonin.

Aortic Arches The aortic arches are derived from the aortic sac at the distal end of the truncus arteriosus and during development, each is paired with a pharyngeal arch. The **first aortic arch** has

mostly regressed by the end of the fourth week, with only a small portion remaining to form the maxillary artery. The **second arch** develops into the hyoid and stapedial arteries. The **third aortic arch** gives rise to the common carotid artery, the external carotid artery, and the beginning of the internal carotid artery. On the left side, the **fourth arch** forms the aortic arch, whereas on the right side, it differentiates into the proximal right subclavian artery. The **sixth aortic arch** is also known as the **pulmonary arch,** because the right side develops into the proximal right pulmonary artery and left side forms the ductus arteriosus. Coarctation of the aorta is caused by the abnormal development of the fourth aortic arch, which leads to thickening of the aortic wall and narrowing of the lumen (Fig. 6-7).

CASE CONCLUSION

The patient was found to have a bicuspid aortic valve and mild stenosis of the aorta just distal to the origin of the left subclavian artery. The area of the coarctation was excised and repaired by an end-to-end anastomosis of the transverse aorta and the descending aorta. After the operation, the patient was found to have markedly increased lower extremity pulsations and increased perfusion.

THUMBNAIL: Brachial Arch Anomalies

Head, Neck, and Arterial Development

Pharyngeal arch derivatives:

Pharyngeal Arch	Nerve	Skeleton	Muscles
First (mandibular)	CN V3	Mandible, maxilla, middle ear (incus, malleus)	Mastication (temporalis, masseter, medial/lateral pterygoids)
Second (hyoid)	CN VII	Stapes, hyoid (lesser horn)	Facial expression, stapedius
Third	CN IX	Hyoid (greater horn)	Stylopharyngeus
Fourth and sixth	CN X	Thyroid, cricoid, arytenoids, corniculate, cuneiform cartilages	Cricothyroid, levator veli palatini, constrictors (fourth); intrinsic muscles of larynx (sixth)

(Continued)

THUMBNAIL: Branchial Arch Anomalies *(Continued)*

Pharyngeal pouch derivatives:

Pharyngeal Pouch	Derivative
First	Middle ear, eustachian tube, tympanic membrane
Second	Epithelial lining of palatine tonsil
Third	Thymus (ventral wing), inferior parathyroid gland (dorsal wing)
Fourth	Superior parathyroid gland
Fifth	Ultimobranchial body (parafollicular cells of the thyroid)

Aortic arch derivatives:

Aortic Arch	Derivative
First	Maxillary artery
Second	Hyoid artery, stapedial artery
Third	Common carotid artery, proximal internal carotid artery
Fourth	Aortic arch (left), proximal right subclavian artery (right)
Sixth	Ductus arteriosus (left), proximal right pulmonary artery (right)

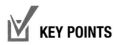

KEY POINTS

- The first pharyngeal cleft gives rise to the external auditory meatus

- The fifth pharyngeal and aortic arches do not make significant contributions to embryologic development

QUESTIONS

1. DiGeorge syndrome is a constellation of congenital defects that includes hypoplasia of the thymus and the inferior and superior parathyroid glands. Based on these symptoms, which of the following embryologic structures are involved?

   A. Second and third pharyngeal arches
   B. Third and fourth pharyngeal pouches
   C. First pharyngeal cleft
   D. Second and third aortic arches
   E. Fourth and fifth pharyngeal pouches

2. A neonate is diagnosed with hemifacial microsomia. This disorder comprises a number of craniofacial malformations, including small and flattened maxillary, temporal, and zygomatic bones. What type of tissue is involved in this abnormality?

   A. Ectoderm
   B. Endoderm
   C. Mesoderm
   D. Ectoderm and mesoderm
   E. Neural crest

3. The vocal cords are controlled by the intrinsic muscles of the larynx. Two patients are seen separately in your clinic for symptoms of hoarseness. Both patients have neck masses, but the lesions impinge on different nerves and affect different muscles. Which of the following statements is true about the embryology involved in these cases?

   A. The derivatives of the second and fourth pharyngeal arches are involved.
   B. One patient has dysfunction of the cricothyroid muscle, which is derived from the sixth arch and supplied by the recurrent laryngeal nerve.
   C. The levator palatini is the only intrinsic muscle of the larynx not supplied by the recurrent laryngeal nerve.
   D. Both masses affect the intrinsic muscles of the larynx, which are all derived from the sixth arch.
   E. One of the lesions affects the cricothyroid muscle that is innervated by the superior laryngeal nerve and derived from the fourth pharyngeal arch.

PART VII
Behavioral Science

HPI: Mr. and Mrs. B bring in their 2-week-old son to see you. Mrs. B says that the baby has been eating well and sleeping on and off for much of the day, but they notice that when he's turned abruptly he has a dramatic response and begins to wail. You reassure her and explain that this is a normal inborn reflex. She looks relieved and asks you what other inborn reflexes there are, how long they will last, and whether new ones will crop up.

THOUGHT QUESTIONS

- What is the reflex described above called?
- What other inborn reflexes are seen in a neonate? Describe each reflex, how it is elicited, and when it is extinguished.
- What physical milestones happen in the first year?
- What about social and language milestones?

BASIC SCIENCE REVIEW AND DISCUSSION

A number of reflexes are present at birth. These reflexes, called inborn reflexes, disappear as an infant develops normally (Table 7-1).

Early Development

In the first month the child is able to lift its head and develops a social smile. By 4 months he or she may be starting to babble, can reach for objects, and can sit with assistance. By 6 months the child can sit unassisted, and soon will roll over. Between 7 and 9 months the child develops stranger anxiety and separation anxiety. Both are normal responses, which demonstrate healthy attachment to parents and the ability to differentiate others.

By 1 year the child can crawl and has often taken his or her first steps. He or she can also drink from a cup, grasp things between thumb and forefinger (pincer grasp), and say his or her first word. By 18 months the child is furthering both fine and gross motor development and can climb up stairs, scribble, and use a spoon. Language also continues to develop, and the child can name common objects. Between 16 months and 2 years, the child practices moving away from the parent or caregiver and then coming back for reassurance and comfort. This practice is called rapprochement, which was described by Margaret Mahler, a developmental psychologist. In addition, between 18 months and 3 years core gender identity is established.

At age 2 the child can speak in two-word sentences, jump, and wash and dry his or her hands. By age 3 he or she can ride a tricycle, dress with supervision, speak in three- and four-word sentences, and recognize his or her whole name and some colors.

CASE CONCLUSION

You do a physical exam, which is unremarkable. You review the baby's eating patterns (normal, every 2–3 hours). The baby is eating well, urinating and moving his bowels, and gaining weight. You discuss the parents' concerns about changing and diaper ointments. It's a light day in your practice and, as new parents, Mr. and Mrs. B have many questions about what the next few years will hold for their newborn.

TABLE 7-1 Inborn Reflexes

Reflex	Description	Age of Disappearance
Moro	Sudden movement stimulates extension, abduction, then adduction of arms	4–6 months
Babinski	Scratching the lateral aspect of the sole (heel to toe) leads to dorsiflexion of the big toe and fanning of other toes	12–18 months
Grasp	Pressure on the palm causes infants to grasp	4 months
Suck/rooting	Oral or perioral stimulation will cause orientation toward the stimulus and sucking	4–6 months
Stepping	Hold the infant vertically, with pressure on feet; child will make stepping motions	2–3 months

THUMBNAIL: Behavioral Science—Developmental Milestones in the Early Years

Physical (average age attained):

1 month	Lift head
6 months	Sit unassisted
7 months	Roll over
10 months	Crawl
12–15 months	Walk
18 months	Walk up steps
24 months	Jump in place
36 months	Ride tricycle
48 months	Hop on one foot

Fine Motor (average age attained):

4 months	Grasp objects
9 months	Pincer grasp
14 months	Scribbles
18 months	Tower of 4 cubes
24 months	Imitates a vertical line
36 months	Copies an O
48 months	Copies a + (plus sign)

Social/Personal (average age attained):

1–2 months	Social smile in response to face or voice
7–9 months	Stranger anxiety–shows parental attachment and that the child can differentiate strangers
7–18 months (up to 3 years)	Separation anxiety (worry about being separated from parents or caregivers)
12 months	Drinks from a cup
18 months	Uses a spoon, removes a garment
24 months	Puts on clothing, washes and dries hands
36 months	Dresses with supervision, eats well with utensils
48 months	Dresses without supervision

Language (average age attained):

4–6 months	Babbles
12 months	Speaks first real word
18 months	Names some common objects
24 months	Two-word sentences
36 months	Says first and last name, some colors

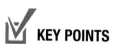

KEY POINTS

- Developmental milestones are usually grouped in terms of gross motor, fine motor, social, and language skills
- The age at which each milestone is reached is approximate, as each child develops differently

- It is important to understand the difference between separation anxiety and stranger anxiety.
  - Both start at about 7 months of age and indicate a secure attachment to the parents. Separation anxiety may last significantly longer. Both are normal developmental stages, and neither is pathologic.

QUESTIONS

1. You are a third-year medical student doing pediatrics and you go into the waiting room to call in a patient coming in for a routine checkup. From his chart you know that he has been developing normally. You watch the child in the waiting room go away from his mother to look at a toy, quickly return for a hug, and then go off to explore further, only to return again. What is this behavior called and at what age does it typically occur?

A. Separation anxiety—age 4 to 6 months
B. Rapprochement—age 16 to 36 months

C. Exploration—age 4 years
D. Insecure attachment—age 2 to 3 years
E. Stranger anxiety—age 7 to 9 months

2. You go into the waiting room of your pediatric practice to call in your next patient, a little girl who has been developing normally. You see her taking a couple of wobbly steps to a table, where she picks up a crayon and scribbles. In the waiting room there are three steps going up, and she cannot walk up them, but crawls her way up. Given this information, approximately how old do you think she is?

A. 6 months
B. 9 months
C. 13 months
D. 24 months
E. 36 months

3. A father brings his son in to see you for a routine checkup. He tells you that his son, who has been developing normally, has starting to speak in two-word sentences. Given his stage of development, which of the following would you also expect him to be able to do?

A. Copy a "+."
B. Ride a tricycle.
C. Wash and dry his hands.
D. Hop on one foot.
E. Dress without supervision.

4. You are doing a routine exam on an infant. You note that she smiles at you, grasps an object, but cannot sit independently or roll over. Given her likely age, which of the following reflexes is she most likely to have outgrown?

A. Moro
B. Stepping
C. Babinski
D. Grasp
E. Rooting

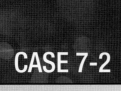

CASE 7-2 Depression in Pregnancy

HPI: AB is a 29-year-old married, nulliparous Caucasian female who is referred to your clinic during her third month of pregnancy. She complains about feeling anxious and tired, with occasional insomnia as well as some nausea and vomiting. Her husband has noticed that her mood has become more erratic and that she is "quick to fly off the handle" or burst into tears. She also reports diminished sex drive and expresses concerns about her body. She is afraid that she will become less attractive as the pregnancy proceeds. Her past medical history is unremarkable; she had a tonsillectomy at age 5 and a pregnancy termination at age 17. She takes no medications other than prenatal vitamins.

Her family history includes a mother who suffered from postpartum depression and a father with type 2 diabetes mellitus. She is the youngest of three children. She graduated from college and works full-time as an accountant. She has been married for 2 years. She and her husband live together in a rented apartment. She denies ever using illicit substances but before her pregnancy did drink two or three glasses of wine a couple of nights a week when socializing.

MSE: Appropriately dressed in business attire, good hygiene, eye contact, and rapport. Speech is soft but of normal tone. She shows no abnormal movements. Her affect is tearful during the interview as she discusses her hopes and fears for the pregnancy. She describes her mood as "up and down." Thought processes are logical and goal directed. She shows no indications of psychosis and no suicidal ideation (SI) or homicidal ideation (HI). Cognition, insight, and judgment are all intact.

THOUGHT QUESTIONS

- Is this young woman normal?
- Is pregnancy associated with increased rates of psychopathology?
- How should she be treated?

BASIC SCIENCE REVIEW AND DISCUSSION

The first trimester of pregnancy can be associated with a variety of physical and psychological concerns. The physical symptoms of early pregnancy include bloating, tiredness (or even insomnia), headaches, constipation, and morning sickness. Psychological symptoms include anxiety about the pregnancy itself, whether the baby will be alright, whether her husband will find her attractive, whether she will be a good mother, and whether she can balance her own needs and career with those of a young infant. A woman's sense of mothering is often influenced strongly by her own mother as her role model. It is important to inquire about levels of support from her husband, family, and friends. Also, ask about her future aspirations for her life. Some women may experience decreased libido during pregnancy. They may have concerns about harming the fetus during intercourse or physical discomfort. Sexual intercourse is not prohibited during pregnancy and some women may find they have increased sexual interest and satisfaction during this time. This may be due to engorgement of the sexual organs, which occurs in pregnancy.

Symptoms of depression are common in pregnancy; between 20 and 70% of pregnant women report some symptoms of depression (see Thumbnail). Nevertheless, rates of major depressive disorder in pregnancy, 10–16%, are similar to rates in nonpregnant women. A family history of postpartum depression increases the risk for depression in pregnancy as well as postpartum depression.

Treatment of such symptoms is generally supportive. Both the patient and her partner may benefit from psychoeducation and supportive psychotherapy. Since all psychoactive medications may cross the placenta, such medications are generally avoided unless the patient reaches diagnostic criteria for a major depressive disorder or any other *Diagnostic and Statistical Manual of Mental Disorders, 4th edition (DSM-IV)*, Axis 1 diagnosis.

Up to 85% of women experience some mood disturbance during the postpartum period. For most women, these symptoms are mild and self-limited. There is a reported increase in psychiatric admissions during the postpartum period. The majority of these conditions are mood disorders and are classified in *DSM-IV* as a subtype of depressive or bipolar disorders. Women with a history of bipolar disorder are particularly at increased risk for a relapse (between 20 and 50%) during this time. Care must be taken to rule out any medical conditions that may have psychiatric symptoms, such as hypothyroidism, Sheehan syndrome (pituitary infarction, usually the sequelae of postpartum hemorrhage, resulting in pituitary hypofunction), or delirium due to infection.

Pseudocyesis (false pregnancy) can occur in women who have an ardent desire to become pregnant and may be accompanied by many of the symptoms of real pregnancy.

CASE CONCLUSION

AB and her husband were relieved to learn that such symptoms could be normal during pregnancy. They were encouraged to attend antenatal classes offered at the hospital. During individual counseling sessions her fears and hopes for her pregnancy were explored fully and she was reassured. She was encouraged to follow the basic principles of sleep hygiene (i.e., regular exercise; avoidance of stimulating substances such as chocolate, caffeine, and alcohol; and relaxation exercises in the evening before bed). Six weeks later, she returned and was doing much better.

THUMBNAIL: Behavioral Science—Psychiatric Symptoms Associated with Pregnancy and the Postpartum Period

Condition	Epidemiology	Symptoms	Treatment/Prognosis
Depression during pregnancy	10–16%	Depressed mood, anxiety	Treatment includes psychotherapy and antidepressants if depression is severe Increased likelihood of postpartum depression
Baby blues	30–85% prevalence	Onset within 1 week postpartum; presents with labile mood, tearfulness, anxiety, and insomnia	Treatment includes support, reassurance, and education Symptoms tend to remit spontaneously by the 10th day
Postpartum depression	10–15% prevalence	Onset within the first 3 months, may be insidious, with depression, anxiety, and insomnia	Treatment includes antidepressants and psychotherapy Risk of recurrence is 50%
Postpartum psychosis	0.1–0.2% prevalence	Onset usually within the first month, with depressed mood or manic symptoms of euphoria, irritability, agitation, disorganized behavior, depersonalization, or delusions	Treatment includes antipsychotics with mood stabilizers if bipolar in presentation and antipsychotics and antidepressants if depressed If severe, may consider electroconvulsive therapy Risk of recurrence is 70%

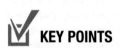 **KEY POINTS**

- Pregnancy is associated with a number of physical and emotional changes
- Between 20 and 70% of pregnant women report some symptoms of depression
- Ten to sixteen percent of patients meet diagnostic criteria for a major depression; this is similar to the rate of major depression in non-pregnant women
- A family history of postpartum depression or psychosis increases the risk for developing these disorders
- Treatment of psychiatric symptoms during pregnancy generally includes psychoeducation and supportive psychotherapy
- Psychoactive medications are avoided if possible during pregnancy but may be needed if symptoms are severe
- Up to 85% of women experience some mood disturbance during the postpartum period

QUESTIONS

1. A 16-year-old primigravid female presents at 14 weeks' gestation. Which of the following is associated with teenage pregnancy?

   A. It represents a small number of unmarried mothers.
   B. Low risk for obstetric complications.
   C. Depression and having divorced parents.
   D. About 50% of teenagers use contraception regularly.
   E. More than 70% of unmarried mothers are teenagers.

2. The patient from the preceding case is concerned about her risk of postpartum depression. Which of the following statements about postpartum depression is FALSE?

   A. The baby blues is a short-lived depressed mood experienced by up to 50% of women after delivery.
   B. Postpartum depression occurs in 5 to 10% of women.
   C. Postpartum psychosis develops in 1% of women.
   D. Postpartum disorders are influenced by a variety of psychosocial factors.

   E. Women with a family history of postpartum mood disorders may be at increased risk.

3. MB is a 39-year-old primigravida who had an 8-pound healthy baby boy by vaginal delivery 4 days previously. Her husband has brought her to the ER because he is concerned about her. Two days ago, she became restless and irritable, with a poor appetite. She then became very agitated and confused, and appeared to be hallucinating. Which of the following statements about postpartum psychosis is TRUE?

   A. Postpartum psychosis usually occurs in multigravida females.
   B. Family history is noncontributory.
   C. Approximately 50% recover fully.
   D. Approximately 50% have further episodes of psychosis.
   E. Approximately 10% of women commit infanticide.

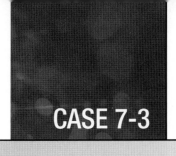

CASE 7-3 Psychopharmacology

HPI: TZ is a 26-year-old married woman who suffers from bipolar disorder and is well maintained on mood-stabilizing medications. At a routine follow-up appointment, she tells you that she and her husband are considering starting a family.

She was first diagnosed with bipolar affective disorder when she presented with a manic episode at age 19. She was originally stabilized on a combination of an antipsychotic haloperidol and lithium. After taking lithium for 2 years her mood stabilizer was changed to valproic acid, as she was complaining of intolerable side effects. She has been hospitalized twice for manic episodes and treated as an outpatient for depression. She has never abused substances and does not use tobacco products. She has never been suicidal. She has a family history of bipolar disorder and major depression. She graduated from college and works as a dental hygienist. She lives in a rented apartment with her husband of 2 years, who works as a mechanic. She is taking prenatal vitamins and valproic acid 750 mg PO twice daily.

PE: Results of a recent annual physical with chem 7, CBC, thyroid function test (TFT), and UA were all WNL. Recent valproic acid level was 80 μg/mL (reference range is 50–125 μg/mL).

MSE: She is well presented, her affect is of normal range, and her mood is euthymic. There is no evidence of psychosis and cognitive functions are intact.

THOUGHT QUESTIONS

- What are your concerns about medications should this patient become pregnant?
- What other psychiatric medications can cause problems during pregnancy and during breast-feeding?
- What are some of the adverse side effects of lithium? What are the potential toxic effects of lithium?

BASIC SCIENCE REVIEW AND DISCUSSION

Care must be taken when prescribing **any medications** during pregnancy and while breast-feeding, but particular caution should be taken with psychiatric medications. The dangers to the fetus must be balanced against the dangers of psychiatric illness, such as psychosis or depression. When a woman becomes pregnant her psychiatric medications and her mental state should be reviewed immediately, as the hormonal changes of pregnancy may cause changes in her psychiatric disorder and/or the metabolism of psychiatric medications.

Antipsychotic Agents

Antipsychotic agents should be avoided in the first trimester, if possible. Although there is no conclusive evidence that these agents are teratogenic, low-potency agents such as chlorpromazine may increase the risk of fetal malformations. Low-potency agents may also cause hypotension. In general, if they are needed, high-potency agents such as haloperidol should be used. Breast-feeding is not contraindicated in those taking phenothiazines. Antiparkinsonian agents should not be prescribed routinely to those who are pregnant. There have been case reports of feeding difficulties, hypertonicity, and dystonic and parkinsonian movements in infants exposed to antipsychotic agents.

Antidepressants

If possible, depressive symptoms in the first trimester should be treated with supportive measures and **psychoactive medications should be avoided,** but if severe depression develops, medications may be necessary; electroconvulsive therapy (ECT)

may also be considered. Limb deformities have been reported with tricyclics, but the studies of teratogenesis remain inconclusive. Some agents such as amitriptyline, trimipramine, and trazodone have been reported to be associated with poor outcomes in animal studies. There is concern about the neurologic development of the fetus with the use of tricyclic agents in the second and third trimesters, and a withdrawal syndrome has been reported in neonates. The long-term effects of exposure to tricyclic antidepressants in breast milk are unknown and thus they should be avoided, if possible. MAOIs are contraindicated in pregnancy, as there have been reports of growth retardation in animal studies and these agents may exacerbate pregnancy-induced HTN and affect placental perfusion. These agents are also contraindicated with the use of beta-mimetic agents in premature labor and opioids during labor itself. SSRIs are usually regarded as safe in pregnancy, but there is concern about possible behavioral teratogenicity. Fluoxetine may be associated with increased minor physical anomalies, but this finding remains controversial. There is less information about the safety of venlafaxine, nefazodone, and bupropion.

Mood Stabilizers

Lithium should be avoided in the first trimester because of possible teratogenesis, namely, Ebstein anomaly (hypoplasia of the right ventricle and abnormalities of the tricuspid valve), which may occur in 1 in 1000 exposed. Lithium may cause neonatal goiter and impair vaginal delivery, as well as result in neurologic and cardiovascular abnormalities in the neonate. Hence, it should be avoided in the first trimester and monitored closely during the rest of pregnancy because, if it must be used, the dramatic changes in fluid volume and renal function caused by pregnancy necessitate higher doses than that used in the nonpregnant state. After labor, rapid fluid loss may cause toxic effects, and lithium doses should be decreased 2 weeks before delivery and carefully monitored. The physician should look for evidence of toxic effects in the neonate. Lithium is secreted in breast milk, and neonatal renal function may lead to toxicity, with cyanosis, poor muscle tone, and cardiac abnormalities. It is therefore contraindicated during breast-feeding. Other agents, such as the anticonvulsants carbamazepine and valproic acid, have been reported to be associated with a ten-fold increased risk (1–5%) of NTDs such as spina bifida. There are reports of cleft palates in those exposed to these drugs in the first trimester; however, these agents may be safer than lithium in those who wish to breast-feed.

Benzodiazepines

Diazepam crosses the placenta and has been reported to have a two-fold increase in cleft lips and palate. The question of its teratogenesis remains unresolved; therefore, it should be avoided in

the first trimester. Occasional use in the second and third trimesters is not thought to have ill effects. Clonazepam may be used in the first trimester to control manic symptoms if antipsychotics cannot control symptoms. Impaired temperature regulation, apnea, low apgar scores, feeding difficulties, and hypotonicity have been reported in neonates exposed to benzodiazepines.

Miscellaneous

Neonates may show withdrawal effects if the mother has been dependent on alcohol or opiates. Alcohol itself is a known teratogen and causes FAS.

CASE CONCLUSION

TZ was encouraged to plan her pregnancy carefully in close coordinated care with her obstetrician. She returns to visit you when she finds out she is pregnant. After careful discussion with both the patient and her husband, you decide to taper and discontinue the valproic acid and maintain her on low doses of haloperidol. During the second trimester, you restart the valproic acid at a lower dose and monitor her carefully throughout her pregnancy. She delivers a healthy baby boy, her medications are increased to her usual doses, and she is further carefully monitored for her high risk of postpartum relapse.

THUMBNAIL: Behavioral Science—Pharmacology of Lithium

Uses	Control of acute mania and prophylaxis of recurrent bipolar, unipolar disorder and schizoaffective disorder; also used as an augmenting agent in schizophrenia
Pharmacokinetics	Rapidly absorbed by oral route, complete within 6–8 hours; peak plasma levels within 30 minutes to 2 hours; not protein bound; not metabolized; excreted unchanged by the kidney; **rates of clearance depend on renal function** and follow sodium reabsorption in the proximal tubules; increased sodium intake causes decreased reabsorption, and a sodium-restricted diet causes increased lithium reabsorption, leading to toxicity
Therapeutic action	Exact mechanism of action remains unknown but is thought to influence sodium and calcium transfer across membranes, affecting neurotransmitter release and receptor activity; also acts via inhibiting cAMP second messenger systems; stimulates Na- and Mg-dependent ATPase; increases uptake of tryptophan by serotoninergic neurons
Adverse effects	Early side effects: nausea, vomiting, and diarrhea, fine tremor, dry mouth, fatigue, drowsiness, nasal congestion, and metallic taste Long term: nephrogenic diabetes insipidus with polyuria and polydipsia due to distal tubule becoming resistant to alcohol dehydrogenase (ADH) in approximately 9–20% of users; hypothyroidism in approximately 5% of users; females more commonly affected than males Edema and weight gain; cardiac effects include T-wave flattening and arrhythmias; neurologic effects include choreoathetosis, ataxia, dysarthria, tardive dyskinesia, and memory impairment; acne and alopecia; increased risk of Ebstein anomaly in fetuses exposed in the first trimester of pregnancy; reported hypotonicity and cyanosis in infants
Drug interactions	Thiazides decrease lithium clearance by 30–50%; low-salt diets, pregnancy, and diarrhea/vomiting/dehydration may increase levels; NSAIDs also may increase levels; levels and risk of neurotoxicity may be increased by neuroleptics and carbamazepine Levels of lithium decreased by theophylline, caffeine, antacids, acetazolamide, and osmotic diuretics
Monitoring serum levels	Sampling should be drawn 12 hours after last dose to avoid peak levels; such peaks and troughs are avoided with slow-release preparations; in acute disorders, serum levels should range between 0.8 and 1.2 mEq/L, in maintenance, 0.6 to 0.8 mEq/L, and in older persons, keep at 0.5 mEq/L Toxic effects occur at levels >2 mmol/L and may include tremor, ataxia, slurred speech, confusion, convulsions, coma, and death

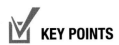 KEY POINTS

- Care must be taken when prescribing any medications during pregnancy and while breast-feeding
- Antipsychotic agents should be avoided in the first trimester, if possible
- If possible, treat depressive symptoms in the first trimester with supportive measures and avoid medications, but, if necessary, medications or ECT may be used
- Lithium should be avoided in the first trimester because of possible teratogenesis (e.g., Ebstein anomaly) and is contraindicated during breast-feeding
- Diazepam has been reported to cause cleft lips and palate, and should be avoided in the first trimester
- Neonates may show withdrawal effects if the mother has been dependent on alcohol or opiates
- Lithium is an effective mood stabilizer but requires monitoring to minimize adverse effects

QUESTIONS

1. Which of the following tests would you recommend to a patient taking lithium?

    A. Urea, electrolytes, creatinine, thyroxine, TSH, and EKG monthly

    B. Follow-up lithium levels weekly

    C. EKG every 6 months

    D. Urea, electrolytes, creatinine, thyroxine, TSH, EKG, and pregnancy tests at baseline, followed by lithium levels every 8 weeks, repeat chemistry, and TFTs twice a year and EKG annually

    E. Urea, electrolytes, creatinine, thyroxine, TSH, EKG, and pregnancy tests at baseline, followed by lithium levels every 12 weeks, repeat chemistry and TFTs three times a year, and EKG twice a year

2. When discussing the possible side effects of valproic acid with the above patient and her husband, which of the following do you warn her about?

    A. Nausea, vomiting, weight and hair loss

    B. Nausea, vomiting, weight gain, and hair growth

    C. Nausea, vomiting, weight gain, hair loss, agitation, neural tube defects in fetuses

    D. Nausea, vomiting, weight gain, hair loss, sedation, tremor, and neural tube defects in fetuses

    E. Nausea, vomiting, weight gain, hair loss, sedation, thyroid abnormalities, and neural tube defects in fetuses

3. In general, when prescribing medications to a patient, which of the following does not affect the distribution of a drug?

    A. Edema

    B. Pregnancy

    C. Hypoparathyroidism

    D. Obesity

    E. Age

4. Which of the following statements is correct?

    A. The therapeutic window is the ratio between the lethal dose and the clinically effective dose.

    B. The therapeutic index is the range of concentration of a drug in the serum in which the drug has a maximum clinical effect.

    C. Efficacy is a measure of a drug's maximum effect.

    D. Potency is a measure of a drug's ability to produce a desired effect.

    E. There are no drugs used in psychiatry that have a therapeutic window.

HPI: The W's have brought their 6-year-old son, FW, to see you because he is wetting his bed several nights a week and his pediatrician thinks that you may be able to help.

FW is the eldest of three boys and his parents describe him as a "happy, normal child." He started toilet training at about the age of 2 and achieved control of his bowels by the age of 3. He has never had complete control of his bladder functioning and has wet the bed at least once a week, but this has increased since the birth of this youngest brother 6 months ago. He is attending school and is doing well with no daytime wetting episodes. His pediatrician has seen him regularly since birth, and a thorough work-up was unremarkable (no evidence of structural problems, infection, or medical conditions that may be associated with bed-wetting [enuresis]). He achieved all the other developmental milestones without any delay. His appetite and sleep patterns are regular and he is very social but refuses to stay over at a friend's house because of his bed-wetting.

THOUGHT QUESTIONS

- You decide to use the bell-and-pad technique. What kind of conditioning is this an example of?
- What other learning-based techniques could you consider in this situation?
- What are other applications of behavioral techniques?

BASIC SCIENCE REVIEW AND DISCUSSION

Learning itself is the acquisition of behavior patterns and continues throughout the life cycle. Learning is divided into two major categories and includes classical conditioning and operant conditioning.

Classical Conditioning

Classical conditioning is based on the work of Ivan Pavlov. Here a conditioned stimulus is paired with an unconditioned stimulus to produce a desired response. The subject is passive and the response is typically emotional or autonomic. In Pavlov's classic experiment with dogs, he paired food (the unconditioned stimulus), which causes salivation (the unconditioned response), with bell ringing (the conditioned stimulus). After learning occurred, the bell alone stimulated the response of salivation (the conditioned response). There are two major phases in this type of learning. First is the **acquisition phase,** in which the conditioned response is learned. Second is the **extinction phase,** in which the conditioned response (salivation with the bell) fades when the conditioned stimulus is no longer followed by the unconditioned stimulus (food). Spontaneous recovery may occur when the conditioned response reappears. The link between the conditioned stimulus and conditioned response can also be recovered by repeating the pairing with the unconditioned stimulus. Stimulus generalization may also occur when a new stimulus similar to the conditioned stimulus (e.g., a buzzer instead of a bell) will provoke the conditioned response.

The bell-and-pad technique for the treatment of bed-wetting is also an example of classical conditioning. A fluid-sensitive pad is placed under the child's bedding; when urine wets the pad, a bell rings, the child wakes, and he is brought to the toilet to empty his bladder. Over time, the child learns to wake spontaneously to void his bladder.

Aversive conditioning has been used to treat unwanted behaviors (e.g., a sexual interest in children) with a noxious aversive stimulus, such as an electric shock or an agent that may cause vomiting. This type of learning also follows the preceding phases and patterns of extinction and spontaneous recovery.

Operant Conditioning

BF Skinner did much of the initial work on operant conditioning. The frequency of a spontaneous behavior can be determined by its following consequence (or reinforcement). Reinforcement affects the probability of a response being made. Therefore, a novel new behavior may be learned. Both positive and negative reinforcements can be used to increase desired behavior. **Positive reinforcements** are rewards that increase the rate at which the desired behavior occurs (e.g., buying a present if the child achieves bladder control). These rewards can be tangible, such as a present, or intangible, such as increased attention given to the child. **Negative reinforcements** are punishments that, when removed, increase the rate of the desired behavior.

There are several types of reinforcement scheduling (Table 7-2). **Punishment** is an aversive stimulus, which is aimed at reducing an unwanted behavior, but it may not work as well as extinction (e.g., ignoring unwanted behavior in a child). Punishment is also a negative reinforcer, as the adverse consequences of a response actually suppress a response. Escape conditioning is a particular type of reinforcement that is very resistant to extinction, as it provides complete escape from the unpleasant situation, such as the individual with agoraphobia running out of the supermarket.

Behaviors may also be shaped or modeled. In shaping, successive approximations to the desired behavior are reinforced/rewarded until the desired behavior is reached. In modeling, behaviors of role models are observed and then adopted and are an example of observational learning. With chaining techniques, more complex behaviors are broken into a sequence of steps, which are then learned. Behavior modification is important not only in working with children or mentally retarded patients but also in social skills training and managing wards with token economy systems.

All behavioral treatments involve the principles of learning theory, with an observation of behavior, concentration on symptoms, clear goals, directive treatment methods, and an empiric approach. They can be used successfully to eliminate unwanted behaviors, such as nicotine addiction. The Premack principle states that any frequently performed behavior can be used to positively reinforce a less frequent behavior.

TABLE 7-2 Schedules of Reinforcement

Schedule	Features
Continuous	Reinforcement/reward given after every time desired behavior occurs; least resistant to extinction, but although learned quickly it also disappears quickly without reinforcement
Variable ratio	Reinforcement given after an unpredictable and random number of responses and is highly resistant to extinction
Variable interval	Reinforcement given after an unpredictable and random amount of time; also highly resistant to extinction
Fixed ratio	Reinforcement given after a certain number of responses; produces a fast response rate
Fixed interval	Reinforcement given after a certain time; the rate of response increases as the agreed time approaches

CASE CONCLUSION

You decide to use a combination of the bell-and-pad method and star charts. You encourage the parents to toilet FW after each awakening and to remake the bed with the pad in place. Using star charts, dry nights are rewarded with a gold star, which in turn may be used to earn a specific reward. After several weeks, FW and his parents return to report excellent results. You tell them these techniques can be reused later if the bed-wetting begins again.

THUMBNAIL: Behavioral Science—Other Applications of Behavioral Techniques

Condition	Useful Behavioral Techniques
Phobias	Systematic desensitization and flooding are used to treat these irrational fears. With systematic desensitization, an individual is exposed in a graded hierarchical manner either to images of a stimulus or to the actual stimulus itself in combination with relaxation exercises, so as to decrease the fear response to the stimulus. During flooding, the paradoxical technique of entering the feared situation results in initially enhanced fear and arousal responses, which then decrease over time with the exposure and are extinguished.
Sexual deviancy	Aversion (as above) and covert sensitization (e.g., ridicule, arresting, and court appearances) are used.
Chronic schizophrenia	Token economy uses positive reinforcements or rewards for good behavior, which can be exchanged for desired objects later.
Mental retardation	Behavior modification and token economy can be useful.
Obsessional conditions	Response prevention is useful in the treatment of obsessional rituals with a motor component and includes thought stopping, in which a distracting stimulus, such as flicking a rubber band on the wrist, is used to "break" the cycle of rumination.
Sexual inadequacy	Masters and Johnson's techniques can help. Gradually, partners learned to relax and enjoy massage and nonsexual touching, which is gradually increased to achieve successful intercourse.
Marital difficulties	Contract therapy, wherein spouses agree to modify certain behaviors, may be helpful.
Depression and anxiety	Cognitive behavior techniques are used to replace distorted, negative thoughts with more positive, enhancing ones. This is used in combination with a graded schedule of homework activities designed to enhance the patient's sense of mastery and accomplishment.
Hypertension and headaches	Biofeedback is often successful.
Enuresis	Bell-and-pad technique, as discussed above.

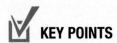 **KEY POINTS**

- Pavlov developed classical conditioning, in which a conditioned stimulus is associated with an unconditioned stimulus to produce a desired response
- Skinner initially described operant conditioning. The frequency of a spontaneous behavior can be determined by its consequence (or reinforcement). This reinforcement can be a reward or a punishment.
- There are several types of reinforcement scheduling, including continuous, variable ratio/interval, and fixed ratio/interval
- Behaviors may also be shaped or modeled

QUESTIONS

1. A child receives a course of immunizing injections from the nurse at his pediatrician's office. On a routine visit, he bursts into tears when he sees this nurse, even though he does not receive an injection. This behavior continues for several more visits before it subsides. This is an example of:

   A. Operant conditioning
   B. Classical conditioning
   C. Shaping
   D. Modeling
   E. The Premack principle

2. A patient is interested in exploring nonprescription techniques that may help her migraines. When discussing biofeedback techniques you tell her which of the following?

   A. It uses classical conditioning.
   B. It uses operant conditioning.
   C. It involves learning to lower blood pressure voluntarily.
   D. It does not need high levels of motivation to learn.
   E. It does not require much practice.

3. A mother smacks her toddler when he spits food on the floor, but this does not deter his spitting behaviors; in fact, he does it more often. What is happening in this situation?

   A. Aversive conditioning
   B. Classical conditioning
   C. Punishment
   D. Negative reinforcement
   E. Positive reinforcement

4. Which of the following techniques is correctly paired with the disorder it is used to treat?

   A. Aversive therapy—phobias
   B. Modeling—impaired social skills
   C. Token economy—generalized anxiety
   D. Flooding—encopresis
   E. Systematic desensitization—sexual inadequacy

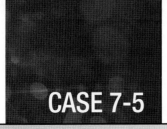

CASE 7-5 Defense Mechanisms

HPI: ED is a 40-year-old married businessman who was referred to you after he contacted the chairman's office seeking a "top-notch doc."

He says he has been experiencing some depressed mood since he has difficulties with his wife recently, but he does not endorse any other symptoms of major depression. He says she wants a divorce but he does not believe that she would leave him. On further exploration, he reveals that he has always had difficulties with people but that he attributes this to others being jealous of his success. He runs his own telecommunications firm and he tells you he will be number one in this field in the next 5 years. He says his wife is causing all the problems in their marriage because she does not understand all the sacrifices he has to make in order to be so successful. He thinks that all of their marital problems lie with her and says that he agreed to see you to stop her complaining. He has no previous psychiatric or medical history. He denied any family psychiatric history. He has been married for 8 years and has two sons. He admits to drinking socially 2–3 nights a week and has tried cocaine twice but denies abuse of other substances.

MSE: Significant for reported depressed mood; otherwise, there is no evidence of anxiety or psychosis. Cognitive functions are intact and he tells you that he is delighted to have had a "proper referral," as he was concerned that an ordinary doctor would not understand his situation.

THOUGHT QUESTIONS

- What personality disorder does this man have?
- What is a defense mechanism?
- Which defense mechanisms does this man display?

BASIC SCIENCE REVIEW AND DISCUSSION

This man is displaying the features of a narcissistic personality disorder. Personality disorders are defined as pervasive, maladaptive patterns of behavior that are deeply ingrained and recognizable from adolescence or even earlier. These patterns of behavior continue throughout adult life, causing difficulties for the patient and/or those around them. People with **narcissistic personality disorder** have a pervasive sense of grandiosity, need for admiration, and lack of empathy for others. They are preoccupied with fantasies of power, success, brilliance, love, or beauty. They believe that they are unique and can only be understood by those who are special or who have achieved high status. They require excessive admiration and attention. They can display a sense of entitlement, appearing arrogant or haughty. They may exploit others to achieve their own end and are often envious of others or believe that others are envious of them. Patients who have this type of personality disorder may actually threaten their physician and devalue his or her level of competence. These patients are at increased risk for developing major depression and substance abuse/dependence. They often present with marital problems and difficulties with interpersonal relationships in general.

Defense mechanisms are **unconscious** and habitual **processes that we use to protect the ego from conflicts between our basic desires and needs, our internalized controls, and the external environment.** They can sometimes be pathologic (see the Thumbnail). Defense mechanisms seen in narcissistic personality disorder include denial, distortion, and projection.

As with all personality disorders, these patterns of behavior are chronic in nature. Narcissistic symptoms may diminish with age and pessimism may develop. As these individuals do not perceive that they have a problem, they may only present in a crisis of marriage, family, or career with symptoms of depression, anxiety, or substance abuse.

In general, the treatment of personality disorders involves psychotherapy and pharmacotherapy aimed at correcting behaviors (e.g., aggression, impulsivity, anxiety, psychotic symptoms, and mood lability) and underlying neurobiologic mechanisms.

The different schools of psychotherapy are not mutually exclusive, complement each other, and generally fall into one of the following types:

1. **Dynamic psychotherapy:** The patient's symptoms are seen as expressions of the internal conflict between the patient's needs, emotions, and motivations (see Key Points).
2. **Behavioral therapy:** Treatment is focused on the external behaviors. The aim is to help the patient change or better control these behaviors. Types of learning include classical conditioning, operant conditioning, and cognitive behavioral and observational learning. Treatment techniques include aversive conditioning, positive reinforcement and extinction, systematic desensitization, and modeling.
3. **Cognitive therapy:** The distorted cognitive appraisals of external cues and underlying distorted beliefs are corrected or restructured and maladaptive behaviors are treated.

Psychoanalysis

Psychoanalysis is both a psychological theory of the mind and a therapeutic treatment. It is based on the work of Sigmund Freud. He described the topographic theory of the mind and the structural theory of the mind (Table 7-3).

The main strategy of psychoanalysis is to uncover these unconscious feelings and memories and to integrate them into the conscious mind. Several techniques are used and they include free association of words and thoughts, interpretation of the therapeutic relationship, dreams, and parapraxes (apparent errors in everyday life that symbolize underlying attitudes). For psychoanalysis to be suitable for a patient the problem must be understandable in psychological terms and the patient must be willing to understand these problems in psychological terms, must not be psychotic, must have enough ego strength to deal with the tensions caused by these inner conflicts, must have a stable life situation, and must be able to sustain a psychotherapeutic relationship. Psychoanalysis usually consists of three to five sessions a week for several years.

TABLE 7-3 Freud's Theories of the Mind

Topographical theory	1. The **unconscious** mind contains the repressed thoughts and feelings, and contains primary process thinking, which is associated with the primary drives; pleasure and wish fulfillment, and dreams, which represent the gratification of basic impulses and wish fulfillment. 2. The **preconscious** mind contains memories that can be accessed by the conscious mind. 3. The **conscious** mind does not have access to the unconscious mind and contains the thoughts and feelings that the individual is aware of.
Structural theory	The component parts of the mind operate mostly on an unconscious level. 1. The **id** represents the instinctual aggressive and sexual drives, is controlled by primary process thinking, and is not affected by external reality. 2. The **ego** is in direct contact with reality; it controls the drives of the id and adapts to the environment using reality testing to develop sustaining relationships. It also has cognitive and defensive functions. 3. The **superego** also controls the drives of the id, regulating moral values and functioning as the conscience.

CASE CONCLUSION

ED is not currently experiencing significant symptoms of depression or anxiety. You counsel him about the potential dangers of alcohol and substance abuse, and recommend a course of psychotherapy. He refuses to accept that he needs psychiatric treatment, because the problem is his wife, not him. He does not return for follow-up.

THUMBNAIL: Behavioral Science—Defense Mechanisms

Acting out	A direct expression of an unconscious impulse in order to avoid awareness of the accompanying affect (e.g., a patient throws furniture because his dinner tray arrives to his room late)
Altruism	Using a constructive service to others to provide vicarious satisfaction (e.g., an unhappy divorcee volunteers in a soup kitchen)
Denial	A conscious refusal to accept external reality (e.g., a patient who is newly diagnosed with cancer leaves the hospital against medical advice)
Distortion	Grossly reshaping external reality to accommodate internal needs (e.g., a substance abuser believes that amphetamine helps clear his/her thinking)
Displacement	The shifting of feelings onto a less cared for object (e.g., a disgruntled employee has a disagreement with his boss, then returns home and kicks his cat)
Dissociation	Temporary change of character or identity to avoid distress (e.g., a man who becomes bankrupt and develops amnesia)
Identification	Behavior patterns changed to emulate another (e.g., medical students wear white coats on the wards)
Intellectualization	Excessively using reason to avoid affective experiences (e.g., a physician who has a terminal illness constantly discusses the medical details with his/her colleagues)
Isolation	An idea is separated from its associated affect (e.g., an abused woman calmly plans to kill her husband)
Projection	Unacceptable feelings are attributed to others, may become delusional (e.g., a wife, who herself wants to have an affair, accuses her spouse of infidelity)
Projective identification	Unacceptable aspects of the personality are dissociated and projected onto another, who is then identified with (e.g., a person who wishes to have an affair projects this onto an admired close friend)
Rationalization	Reason is used to justify unacceptable emotions and feelings (e.g., an individual who has an indiscretion blames it on a single martini)

(Continued)

THUMBNAIL: Behavioral Science—Defense Mechanisms *(Continued)*

Reaction formation	An unacceptable impulse is transformed into its opposite (e.g., a televangelist who rails against illicit sex was caught on film with a prostitute)
Regression	Attempts to return to earlier behaviors to avoid anxiety (e.g., a child starts wetting the bed when his parents separate)
Repression	Refusal to accept into consciousness a feeling or instinct; it is the most basic defense mechanism (e.g., the wife of the traveling salesman says that she does not need intimacy)
Splitting	Positive and negative aspects of relationships are separately and alternatively conscious. Patients with this disorder think of others as either all good or all bad, with no medium ground. (e.g., a patient thinks that his physician is wonderful until one day the physician is late for an appointment and is then perceived as dreadful)
Sublimation	An unacceptable impulse is directed in a socially acceptable manner (e.g., a male with aggressive impulses becomes a surgeon)
Suppression	Ideas or feelings are consciously suppressed to minimize discomfort (e.g., a patient who has a life-threatening illness decides to worry about it for a limited time each day)
Turning against the self	Unacceptable aggression toward others is expressed indirectly toward the self (e.g., a teenager who dislikes her stepfather cuts herself superficially)

 KEY POINTS

- Defense mechanisms are unconscious and habitual processes that we use to protect the ego from conflicts between our basic desires and needs, our internalized controls, and the external environment. They can sometimes be pathologic.
- The main strategy of psychoanalysis is to uncover these unconscious feelings and memories and to integrate them into the conscious mind

- Personality disorders are defined as pervasive, maladaptive patterns of behavior that are deeply ingrained and recognizable from adolescence or even earlier
- Schools of psychotherapy include dynamic, behavioral, and cognitive
- Sigmund Freud described his topographic and structural theories of the mind. Topographic theory describes the unconscious, preconscious, and conscious mind. Structural theory describes the id, ego, and superego.

QUESTIONS

1. Which of the following is a mature defense mechanism?
   A. Repression
   B. Isolation
   C. Denial
   D. Acting out
   E. Suppression

2. Which of the following conditions is correctly paired with its associated defense mechanisms?
   A. Hysteria—displacement of affect
   B. Obsessional conditions—denial, projection, and identification
   C. Paranoia—turning on the self
   D. Phobias—displacement of affect
   E. Depression—isolation, reaction formation, and magical undoing

3. Which of the following examples is correctly paired with its associated defense mechanism?
   A. A woman who was sexually abused as a child develops multiple personalities as an adult: Splitting
   B. A man who is attracted to his sister-in-law begins to believe that his wife is having an affair: Reaction formation

   C. A woman who was physically abused as a child begins to physically abuse her own children: Identification
   D. A teenager whose parent has been diagnosed with cancer begins to neglect his schoolwork and becomes argumentative at home: Regression
   E. A man with bowel cancer tells you that he only worries about it for 20 minutes a day: Denial

4. Which of the following is correctly paired with its definition?
   A. Transference describes the therapist's attitude and response to the patient.
   B. Countertransference describes the shifting of a past person or object in the patient's life onto the therapist.
   C. Primary process thinking is unconscious and is based on the basic pleasure principle of the id; both logic and the sense of time are absent in this type of thinking.
   D. Secondary process thinking is also unconscious and unassociated with reality.
   E. Dream work is the process that examines only the manifest content of dreams.

CASE 7-6 Suicide Attempt

HPI: RC is a 29-year-old single Caucasian female who was brought in to the medical ER 5 days ago by her housemate, after she found her unconscious with an empty bottle of acetaminophen and vodka at her side. She was treated with gastric lavage and *N*-acetylcysteine, was monitored in the medical ICU, and then transferred to the medical floor with one-to-one observation. She is now stable. You are asked to evaluate her for transfer to psychiatry.

RC, a biology graduate student, has been depressed for the last month after the breakup of a relationship. She says that she has been feeling "horrible," is barely able to keep up with her duties as a teaching assistant in an undergraduate biology class, and has great difficulty focusing on her own studies. She has been waking up at 5 A.M., worrying about all of her unfinished work, unable to sleep. She has been feeling worthless and increasingly hopeless. She was seen in the psych ER last week and was referred for outpatient therapy and medication, saying that if she felt suicidal she would return to the ER. Over the past week things have not gone well. She slept through her appointment with the psychiatry outpatient services. The evening of the suicide attempt she finally went to her lab, only to find that her cells were overgrown and infected and that she would have to begin the complex experiment again. As she was walking home, she saw her ex-boyfriend across the quadrangle, walking hand in hand with someone else. She felt humiliated, worthless, and hopeless. She went home and took the acetaminophen and drank the vodka. She said that her housemate had been away for a few days and she thought no one would find her.

THOUGHT QUESTIONS

- How serious was this suicide attempt?
- Should she be transferred to psychiatry?
- What if she refuses hospitalization?

BASIC SCIENCE REVIEW AND DISCUSSION

This was a very serious **suicide attempt.** Acetaminophen overdoses are potentially lethal, may cause fulminant hepatic failure, and can be associated with significant hepatic damage. In addition, she thought her housemate was away and wouldn't find her, adding to her lethal intent. At this point there is no question that she requires hospitalization.

In general, in assessing safety and potential suicidality, one needs to ask directly about **plans** (hanging, overdose, crashing a car), **means** (pills, firearms, a vehicle), and **intent** to carry out suicide. It is also crucial to explore previous ideation and attempts, substance abuse history, and family history of completed suicide or attempts.

In this case, if she were to refuse hospitalization, even if she stated that she had "learned her lesson," she would still require hospital-level care and would meet criteria for involuntary hospitalization. She has an untreated major depression (depressed mood, impaired sleep with early morning awakening, decreased energy/motivation and concentration; see Case 8-1: Depression) and has just had an extremely serious suicide attempt. She is therefore a continuing danger to herself. In addition, although she had said in her initial evaluation that she would seek help if her suicidality worsened, she had not done so. The criteria for involuntary hospitalization (a.k.a. 5150) in most states include being a significant danger to oneself or others or being so gravely impaired that one cannot provide the basics of self-care.

Suicide

Although suicide can be the unfortunate outcome in a number of psychiatric disorders, it is most commonly seen in the context of **mood disorders.** The diagnosis of a current mood disorder is a risk factor for suicide; however, there are other risk factors.

Substance abuse alone or especially when it is comorbid with another psychiatric disorder is a significant risk factor for suicide.

Another psychiatric disorder with high prevalence rates of suicide attempts or completions is **schizophrenia.** Approximately 25 to 50% of schizophrenics attempt suicide, and about 10% die. Risk factors for suicide in schizophrenia include having made previous attempts, being male, being young, being hopeless (especially in the context of lost expectations, such as a college education and significant ambitions), having multiple relapses, being in a depressed mood, living alone, and using drugs.

In general, suicide attempts are more common in women than in men (by a factor of approximately 3:1), but completed suicide is more common in men than in women (by a factor of 4:1). There are an estimated 8 to 25 attempted suicides to 1 completion. Of all firearm suicides, 79% are committed by Caucasian men. During the year following an attempt, patients are at high risk for another attempt.

Other risk factors include age older than 60 years, current medical illness, comorbid substance abuse, and divorce. In 1999, suicide was the 11th leading cause of death in the United States. Suicide outnumbered homicides by 5 to 3. Suicide by firearms was the most common method for both men and women, accounting for 57% of all completed suicides. The highest rates of completed suicide, when categorized by gender and race, are in white men older than age 85, who had a rate of 59/100,000. (For more information, see the NIMH suicide research consortium and fact sheet: http://www.nimh.nih.gov/health/publications/suicide-in-the-us-statistics-and-prevention.shtml)

A mnemonic for remembering the risk factors for suicide is SADPERSONS:

- S–Sex male
- A–Age younger than 19 and older than 45 years
- D–Depression, clinical
- P–Previous attempts
- E–Ethanol and illicit substances
- R–Rational thinking absent (i.e., psychotic)
- O–Organized plan
- N–No spouse: single, divorced, or widowed
- S–Sickness/Stated future intent

CASE CONCLUSION

RC was admitted to psychiatry voluntarily after her discharge from the medical ICU. She was started on a course of antidepressants and began to have some individual psychotherapy to understand her suicide attempt. During the course of her 2-week hospitalization, she tolerated the medication well, was titrated up to a therapeutic dose, and met a therapist who she would continue to work with after discharge. At the time of discharge she was less dysphoric and more hopeful, and was able to describe alternate ways of coping should she become suicidal again.

THUMBNAIL: Behavioral Science—Medications in Overdose

Medications are potentially lethal. Of course, patients can overdose on any medication with varying potential lethality, depending on the amount ingested and the combination of medications and/or other drugs involved.

Medication in Overdose	Effects/Comments
Acetaminophen	Hepatic failure; overdoses are treated with activated charcoal +/− N-acetylcysteine (aka Mucomyst)
Aspirin	Metabolic acidosis and bleeding complications
Tricyclic antidepressants	Prolonged QT interval and AV block, may lead to ventricular tachycardia or torsade de pointes
SSRIs	Rarely lethal if taken alone, may be associated with drowsiness, tremor, nausea, vomiting, seizures, electrocardiogram changes, and decreased consciousness
NSAIDs	Disorientation, dizziness, lethargy, confusion, nausea, vomiting, abdominal pain, seizures, increased BUN and serum creatinine, tachycardia, and coma

KEY POINTS

- Suicide is between the 8th and the 11th leading cause of death in the United States
- In 2000 it accounted for 1.2% of all deaths; the three leading causes of death were heart disease (29.6%), cancer (23%), and stroke (7%)
- In young people (age 15–24 years), suicide was the third leading cause of death, following unintentional injuries and homicide
- The 2000 age-adjusted rate was 10.6/100,000, or 0.01% (age-adjusted rates are adjusted by population norms and allow for comparisons across time and among risk groups)
- The rate among elderly white men older than age 85 years was close to 60/100,000
- Women attempt suicide much more frequently than men (3:1), but men succeed more frequently (4:1)
- Approximately 50% of people who attempt suicide will have a second attempt, and 10% will succeed; the risk is greatest in the 3 months following the attempt
- Patients can be admitted involuntarily if they are deemed a danger to themselves or to others or are so gravely disabled that they cannot provide adequate self-care. The exact requirements vary from state to state. Usually either one or two licensed physicians must sign commitment papers that are valid for a finite time.
- Patients should always be asked about suicidal thoughts, intent, and possible plans; an assessment also needs to be made of the accessibility of the means

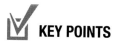

QUESTIONS

1. KH is a 30-year-old married female who presented to the ER after trying to poison herself with carbon monoxide in her car. She was found by her husband, who called for emergency services. Which of the following is true about people who attempt suicide?

   A. She says she is remorseful. She is unlikely to make another attempt.

   B. Approximately 75% of people who attempt suicide have another attempt.

   C. She is at serious risk for trying again, particularly in the next 3 months, and 80% of such attempts are subsequently successful.

   D. She is at serious risk for trying again, particularly in the next 3 months, and 10% of such attempts are subsequently successful.

   E. Approximately 5% of people who attempt suicide make another attempt.

2. LC is an 80-year-old, recently widowed African American male with chronic CHF, renal insufficiency, and osteoarthritis. He was in the military and has a gun collection. Which of the following characteristics does not increase his risk for suicide?

   A. Ethnicity—African American

   B. Age—80 years

   C. Chronic medical illnesses

   D. Access to a gun

   E. Male gender

3. JG is a 16-year-old boy who has taken an overdose of a medication from his parents' medicine cabinet. Which of the following is safest in overdose?

   A. Fluoxetine

   B. Ibuprofen

   C. Acetaminophen

   D. Aspirin

   E. Imipramine

4. BP is a 29-year-old schizophrenic who has recently been hospitalized after a suicide attempt. His parents want to know more about suicide. Which of the following statements about suicide is true?

   A. Seventy percent of schizophrenics attempt suicide.

   B. Ten percent of schizophrenics will die from suicide.

   C. The fact that he had completed 2 years at an Ivy League college decreases his risk of suicide.

   D. Men are at less risk of completed suicide than women.

   E. His current use of alcohol and marijuana does not affect his risk.

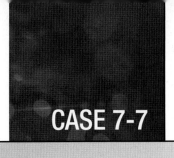

CASE 7-7 Abuse

HPI: PS is a 70-year-old retired postman with a history of schizophrenia who lives with his sister and her family. He has not been attending the outpatient clinic for his depot antipsychotic medication for a couple of months.

After the clinic staff called the sister several times, the patient came to the clinic. You decide to check his blood pressure; when you roll back his sleeve, you notice burn marks. You ask the patient to remove his shirt and you notice significant yellow and green bruises across his chest wall. You ask the patient what happened and he says that he must have fallen. He has a long history of schizophrenia, has been hospitalized several times, and was first diagnosed when he was 20 years old. However, he managed to maintain his job as a postman for approximately 40 years. He finished high school. He lives in his deceased parents' house with his sister, who is widowed, and her two children, who attend college locally. He never married and has no children. He has a small pension and says that his sister takes care of his finances. He does not drink alcohol or abuse substances. He has no forensic history.

MSE: He appears older than his stated age. His clothing is worn and he is badly shaven, but generally clean. Eye contact and rapport are fair. He appears a little anxious at times during the interview, though his affect is generally blunted. He describes his mood as "alright." Thought processes linear, with no evidence of psychosis. He denies suicidal or homicidal ideation. Cognitively, he scores 28/30 on the Mini Mental, missing two of three items on delayed recall. Insight and judgment fair.

PE: Vital signs are stable. He is a thin, frail male with superficial healing burn marks on both forearms and multiple fading bruises across the chest. No bony tenderness. The rest of his exam is WNL.

Labs/Studies: CBC and Chem 20 within normal limits. Chest X-ray reveals a dozen circular fractures of several ribs.

THOUGHT QUESTIONS

- What do you think has been happening to this man?
- What should you do? Should you file a report?

BASIC SCIENCE REVIEW AND DISCUSSION OF ABUSE AND NEGLECT

Abuse of elders and children is increasing across the United States. It has been reported that 4% of individuals older than 65 years of age may be abused. Sexual abuse of children is reported more nowadays than in the past. Up to 25% of females and 12% of males report sexual abuse. Between 5 and 20% of families have an abused member. Abuse of an elder may include physical abuse, sexual abuse, emotional abuse, financial abuse, and active and passive neglect.

First of all, this gentleman should be given a comprehensive physical evaluation, looking for signs of missed or other old injuries. Questions should be made in a nonjudgmental manner. Investigate the possibility of sexual abuse, which could involve bruising of the genitals or, in females, vaginal bleeding. Also look for evidence of malnutrition. Neglect is also a form of abuse, and can be both physical and psychological. In this particular case there may be concern that the patient's sister may misappropriate his funds.

The most common type of abuse in the elderly is financial abuse, followed by physical abuse and active neglect. Signs of physical abuse in an elderly person include signs of neglect and physical abuse. Look for signs of poor hygiene, self-care, and malnutrition. Other forms of neglect may include the withholding of needed equipment (such as a cane, hearing aids, dentures, eyeglasses, or even medication). Signs of physical abuse include evidence of old fractures, burns, and bruising, particularly on the arms, where the elder may have been grasped.

Signs of abuse or neglect in a child (see Thumbnail) also include poor personal care, such as diaper rash, malnutrition, bruises in areas not normally injured, old or healing fractures (including spiral fractures from rotating/twisting limbs), burns (including burns on the bottom or limb extremities from dipping the child in scalding water), and marks from whipping or beating the child with an instrument (e.g., a cane or belt). Mental and emotional abuse can be as harmful as physical abuse in children and may be more difficult to detect.

There is no increase in the rate of psychiatric disorders among parents who abuse their children. They may be isolated in a community without close friends and may seem unwilling to provide for the child's basic needs. They may make excessive demands of their children and fail to teach them how to correct their behavior. When asked about the child's injury, they do not provide an explanation or else they provide a conflicting one.

Mandatory reporting to Child Protective Services or Adult Protective Services of the local Department of Social Services is required by law throughout the United States. All doctors, nurses, hospital personnel, dentists, medical examiners, coroners, mental health professionals, researchers, social workers, teachers, school personnel, child care workers, and law enforcement officials must report suspected abuse of an individual. Some states require that all individuals report suspected cases of neglect and of physical and sexual abuse. Failure to report suspected abuse and malicious false reporting can lead to prosecution.

Forty-five states have physician-mandated reporting requirements for injuries sustained by knives, guns, or other weapons, crimes, or domestic violence. Physicians working in any state should check the state's regulations and requirements.

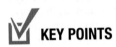

CASE CONCLUSION

PS was admitted to the hospital for his own safety. When told about the results of the chest x-rays, he confessed that his sister had hit and poked him with the end of a broomstick. She had also placed his forearms on the hot radiator because of his "bad table manners." His stay in the hospital was uneventful but significant for a 20-pound increase in weight. He did not wish his sister to be prosecuted, even though half of his pension money had been removed. A guardian was appointed and PS was placed in an independent living facility. A year later he was doing well.

THUMBNAIL: Behavioral Science—Sexual Abuse in Children

Physical signs	Signs of sexual abuse in a child include recurrent UTIs, bruising or injury to the genitals or anus, or presence of an STD.
Psychological signs	From a psychological perspective, the child may show signs of having inappropriate knowledge of sexual acts or may start sexual activities with their friends. There may be a change in behavior ranging from showing increased disruptive behavior to becoming more withdrawn and passive. Children's sleep may be disrupted, with nightmares, bed-wetting, the need for a night-light, or fear of sleeping alone.
Characteristics of the abuser	Most abusers are male and are known to the child. The abuser may abuse alcohol or illicit substances and may lack a suitable sexual partner or actually be a pedophile.
Characteristics of the victim	The majority of abused children are between 9 and 12 years of age, but some are younger. The children often report that they were afraid that the abuser would punish them or not care for them any longer if they reported the abuse. They may feel ashamed and guilty about the abuse.

KEY POINTS

- Four percent of individuals older than 65 years of age may be abused
- Twenty-five percent of females and twelve percent of males report sexual abuse; five to twenty percent of families have an abused member
- Twenty-five percent of murders occur among family members
- The most common type of abuse in the elderly is financial abuse
- There is no increase in the rate of psychiatric disorders among abusive parents
- The law requires mandatory reporting to Child Protective Services or Adult Protective Services of the local Department of Social Services

QUESTIONS

1. Which of the following characteristics are found in abusers of the elderly?

   A. They tend to be physically dependent on the victim.
   B. They usually have dementia.
   C. They are usually financially dependent on the victim.
   D. They often do not have a personal history of abuse.
   E. They are often the closest family member.

2. Which of the following are characteristics of physically abused children?

   A. Most were born full term.
   B. They are in good health.
   C. The majority are older than 5 years of age.
   D. They may be described as "slow."
   E. They usually report their injuries.

3. Which of the following statements is correct concerning the structures of family units in the United States today?

   A. Approximately 50% of families involve a single parent.
   B. Approximately 80% of children younger than 18 years of age have parents that both work outside the home.

   C. The number of children being born to married couples is declining.
   D. Approximately 55% of couples are childless.
   E. The majority of new marriages will divorce within 2 years.

4. TP is a 32-year-old married female who presented to the ER with a black eye. She told the ER physician that she had fallen in her home against the door of a kitchen cabinet. On exam you find evidence of red marks and recent bruises on her arms and legs. She tells you that she is 2 months pregnant. Which of the following is appropriate to tell her?

   A. She should leave home immediately.
   B. Dangers to the unborn child include low birth weight and premature birth.
   C. She does not need to report this to the police.
   D. Counseling should involve both partners together.
   E. Most female murder victims are killed by their partners.

HPI: You are called on to assess capacity of a 63-year-old single Caucasian female with schizophrenia who is refusing chemotherapy. JK has a 40-year history of paranoid schizophrenia and was diagnosed with colon cancer 3 weeks ago. She underwent a resection, and at that time was found to have stage IV adenocarcinoma with multiple metastases to the liver and carcinomatosis. On chest x-ray it appears that she has lung metastases as well. She is refusing chemotherapy. Her oncologist says that she is delusional and he questions her capacity to decide on a treatment. On exam you find her to be cooperative with the interview, sometimes digressing about her delusional material, but basically understanding that she has metastatic cancer and that her prognosis is poor with a less than 5% chance of 5-year survival.

On further exam of her psychiatric symptoms, she believes that when she was on a high school field trip to the museum, someone implanted an accessory uterus for use in experimentation and for control of her thoughts. Somehow this is connected to both the Hare Krishnas and the Kennedy assassinations. She believes that the Krishnas can implant thoughts in her mind, especially about politicians and TV newscasters. In discussing her treatment options, she explains that given her prognosis and the fact that she has had relatives die of this and other cancers, she feels that the morbidity from the chemotherapy outweighs the potential benefits. She has had numerous psychiatric hospitalizations and at present her medication is "optimized." She is not depressed or suicidal.

THOUGHT QUESTION

- Do you think she has the capacity to decide whether to accept chemotherapy?

BASIC SCIENCE REVIEW AND DISCUSSION

Competence vs. Capacity

It is important to understand that **competence** is a legal concept and can only be decided in the courts. **Capacity** is a clinical judgment about the patient's ability to make a decision. Capacity can be assessed by any physician, although psychiatrists are often called to make that assessment.

Decision-making capacity is based on four things. First, patients must be able to evidence a choice. They must understand that there is a choice to be made. Next, they must understand the relevant information. Often this involves being able to "explain back" what the doctor has said about the treatment or the procedure. Third, they should be able to understand the risks and benefits. Again, this can be evidenced by seeing if they can repeat or explain in their own words what was told to them. Finally, the highest level of capacity is to be able to manipulate the information and to explain the rationale behind the decision.

It is important to note that, depending on the risk of the treatment or procedure, physicians will expect different levels of capacity. For example, a low-risk procedure like drawing blood has no informed consent, and the patient basically just has to evidence a choice (i.e., letting the blood be drawn or refusing). When prescribing an antihypertensive with few side effects, physicians may document that they explained the risks of untreated hypertension and the potential side effects of the medication. Patients are rarely asked to sign consent about accepting a specific medication. Most often if patients are compliant and take the medication, they are evidencing a choice, and if they understand the purpose of taking the medication ("to treat my high blood pressure"), they are demonstrating that they understand the relevant information. When the stakes are greater (e.g., accepting an invasive procedure or potentially toxic treatment, or refusing a treatment that could be lifesaving), the expectations for the capacity of the patient are higher.

In terms of psychiatric symptoms, the greatest concern is that the symptoms are somehow influencing the person's decision. A severely depressed patient who believes there is no hope may refuse treatment because of his fatalistic outlook and severe depression. For example, a patient with a major depression may refuse to have a malignant melanoma removed because, "There is no hope; I will die anyway, and I deserve to die." With treatment and remission of the depression the patient would feel quite different, and probably would regret having let a potentially curable lesion evolve into a fatal one. Psychotic patients may have delusions that, for example, surgery is actually a plot to hurt them or a way for a governmental agency to implant a device. In this example the delusion is clearly influencing the patient's ability to think through the treatment decision.

Patients without capacity can have either healthcare proxies (if they have designated one) or court-appointed guardians make healthcare decisions. In some states a family member may make decisions on a patient's behalf if he or she lacks capacity, whereas in others only a court-appointed guardian or healthcare proxy can make decisions, unless the patient has clear documentation of his or her wishes. Although these concepts are used in all states, the details of the laws differ.

CASE CONCLUSION

You review the prognosis with the oncologist, who confirms the survival rates. Her prognosis is worse because of the distant metastases and the multiple intrahepatic and peritoneal lesions. The oncologist still believes that chemotherapy may improve the patient's quality of life. In your exam of this patient, although she is quite psychotic, her delusions do not appear to be related to or involve her illness. She understands that there is a choice to be made, can explain the risks and benefits of accepting the treatment, and can explain why she has decided not to accept treatment. You conclude that JK has capacity. Patients do not have to agree with their doctor's recommendations about treatment, quality of life, and so on, as long as they have the capacity to make their own decisions.

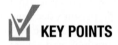

THUMBNAIL: Thumbnail: Behavioral Science—Decisions Involving Minors

Decision or Situation	Parental Consent Needed?
General healthcare for children younger than 18 years of age	Parental consent is required
Abortions	Parental consent required in approximately 50% of states
Prenatal care, treatment of STDs, or treatment of substance abuse	Generally does not require parental consent
Emergency treatment	Generally does not require parental consent; parents cannot refuse lifesaving medical treatment (Christian Scientists have been brought to court to ensure medical intervention for their children)
Emancipated minors (i.e., those who are self-supporting or are married)	Are treated as adults and do not require parental consent

KEY POINTS

- Competence is a legal standard
- Capacity is a clinical judgment about the patient's ability to make a decision that can be assessed by any physician
- Capacity is based on the ability to:
  - Evidence a choice
- Understand the relevant information
- Understand the risks and benefits of the treatment or procedure
- Manipulate the information and explain the rationale behind the decision

QUESTIONS

Questions 1 and 2 refer to the following case:

MS is an 88-year-old woman with dementia. At baseline she has severely impaired short- and long-term memory and cannot manage her activities of daily living, such as bathing, grooming, and toileting, without assistance. She has a receptive and expressive (fluent) aphasia and will talk "endlessly" without making much sense. She is admitted to the hospital for pneumonia.

1. Which of the following statements is true about her ability to make medical decisions?

   A. A physician cannot declare her incompetent to make decisions.
   B. If she refuses a procedure, her healthcare proxy cannot accept on her behalf.
   C. As long as she goes along with the treatment recommendations of her doctor, she does not have to demonstrate capacity.

   D. Although she had made a living will and discussed her preferences with her doctor prior to her dementia, her cousin's husband can decide that she needs to be resuscitated if she has a cardiac arrest, despite her wishes to the contrary.
   E. Only a psychiatrist can determine her decisional capacity.

2. MS wants to leave the emergency room before being admitted. She is very briefly evaluated and the inexperienced physician says, "She is an adult; she can decide to leave the hospital without treatment." She is allowed to leave and somehow manages to get home by showing her ID and giving $20 to a cab driver. The following day she becomes hypoxic, goes into respiratory arrest, and dies. In suing for malpractice, which of the following concepts is important?

   A. Demonstrating malicious intent
   B. Demonstrating that a crime was committed
   C. Demonstrating that there was a duty by the physician

D. Demonstrating that the physician was paid by the insurance company

E. Demonstrating that the hospital verified the physician's credentials

3. Which of the following clinical scenarios is absolutely true?

A. A patient with a stroke and hemiplegia does not have capacity.

B. A Jehovah's Witness who is cognitively intact cannot refuse a transfusion in an emergency.

C. A Christian Scientist who is cognitively intact may refuse surgery for appendicitis.

D. A patient with early-stage Alzheimer disease does not have capacity to accept a skin biopsy.

E. A Christian Scientist who is cognitively intact may refuse an emergency appendectomy for his or her child.

4. Which of the following patients probably has capacity?

A. A patient with a severe major depression who refuses treatment for a skin cancer because "it's all hopeless."

B. A 35-year-old patient with widely metastatic ovarian cancer who has had no response to four trials of chemotherapy and says "no more."

C. A patient with anorexia nervosa who is less than 60% of her ideal body weight, is bradycardic, and says she can gain on her own and doesn't need admission.

D. An 85-year-old man with moderate Alzheimer disease who requires 8 hours of home care daily, states that he wants to have a rhinoplasty, and can manage the postoperative care himself.

E. A schizophrenic who believed that chemotherapy was used as "mind control" by the CIA.

Eating Disorders

HPI: CF is a 15-year-old girl whose mother brings her in to see you, her family doctor, because she is concerned that her daughter has been losing too much weight. Her mother noticed a dramatic change in her daughter over the previous 3 months. Mrs. F says her daughter had always been a little "chubby" until about 1 year ago, when she gradually started to lose weight. Lately, she has been refusing to eat with the family, explaining that she would rather eat alone and prepare her own "healthy" food. She began exercising more with daily workouts of about 2 hours on top of her regular ballet training. When you ask CF about her weight loss she tells you that she needs to lose weight because the ballet teacher has been posting their weights on the wall and making comments about her size. She admits that she has been restricting her food intake but denies self-induced or laxative use. She has no psychiatric history and there is no significant family history. She is the middle of three girls. She is in her first year of high school and maintains an A average in her grades. Her mother discovered that she has been accessing a website called "Ana," which apparently is for anorexics, and she is concerned that her daughter may have anorexia.

PE: CF is 5'5" and weighs 100 lbs. Vitals signs are notable for a BP of 110/70 and a pulse of 50. She is a thin young woman with dry, yellow-colored skin and fine lanugo hair on both her face and back. She has bilateral parotid gland swelling. Neurologic exam is normal.

THOUGHT QUESTIONS

- What are the different types of eating disorders? What are the signs/symptoms of anorexia?
- What kind of treatments would you recommend?
- What are the principles of family and group therapy?

BASIC SCIENCE REVIEW AND DISCUSSION

There are two major types of eating disorders: anorexia nervosa and bulimia nervosa (see Thumbnail). Both are divided into two specific types. Anorexia subtypes include restricting and binge eating/purging types, whereas bulimia is divided into purging and nonpurging subtypes.

Anorexia Nervosa

To make a diagnosis of **anorexia,** several criteria must be met: a failure to maintain body weight at or above a minimally normal weight for age and height (85% below expected weight for size or a BMI = 17.5), a morbid fear of becoming fat, a distorted body image, and amenorrhea. Those individuals who restrict their food intake may develop the signs and symptoms of starvation, whereas those who vomit or abuse laxatives may show different symptoms. In the long term, patients are at increased risk of osteoporosis, impaired fertility, and perinatal mortality.

Many patients have increased rates of depression, obsessions, and compulsions. Those with the binging type are more likely to have substance abuse problems and other impulse-control problems than those with the restricting type.

The prevalence of anorexia is 1% or less of the general population. It affects males (10% of cases) and females, and seems to peak at both 14 and 18 years of age. Controversy exists as to whether this disorder is increasing in prevalence or whether it is simply being diagnosed more often. Higher rates are reported among certain groups, such as ballet dancers and gymnasts. First-degree relatives are at increased risk of developing the disorder, and monozygotic twins show increased concordance. Abnormalities in serotonin, cholecystokinin (CCK), and the hypothalamic-pituitary-gonadal axis have been suggested. Care should be taken to rule out any possible underlying medical illness, such as a tumor or AIDS. The prognosis is generally poor, with a high dropout rate from treatment and a mortality rate of 15%.

Bulimia

Individuals with **bulimia** tend to **binge-eat** and try to **compensate** for this by purging (with vomiting or laxatives), fasting, or exercising. During these binges, the patient consumes excessive amount of food in a short period of time. Typical binges may contain over 20,000 calories. This pattern of binging and compensating behaviors happens at least **twice a week for a 3-month period.** Notably, bulimic patients, although equally obsessed by their size/shape, tend to be in the normal weight range. They may also have depression, anxiety, and personality disorders (especially borderline). Approximately one third have substance abuse/dependence issues. They often have low self-esteem. The prevalence of bulimia is between approximately 1 and 3% of young women, with occasional binging reported in as many as 40% of college students. It occurs more rarely in males. Its peak age of onset is later than that for anorexia nervosa. Approximately one third of those with bulimia have a history of anorexia. The etiology is multifactorial as with anorexia, but abnormalities in serotonin have been more extensively studied in bulimia. The course may be episodic or chronic. The prognosis for individuals with bulimia is better than that for those with anorexia, but they continue to have high rates of relapse and impaired functioning.

Treatment for eating disorders includes attention to any comorbid conditions, such as depression, anxiety, or substance abuse. Treatment may also require hospitalization if these individuals are suicidal or medically compromised. A regular diet should be used in anorexics to achieve an ideal body weight (e.g., a BMI of 20 to 25). Depression in bulimic patients should not be treated with SSRIs, which may cause seizures. However, fluoxetine may help those with anorexia. Psychotherapies play an important role in the treatment of eating disorders and may involve individual, group, or family therapy. Individual therapy may be cognitive behavioral or interpersonal in type.

Family Systems Theory and Family Therapy

General systems theory is used particularly in family therapy and is based on the idea of concentric and overlapping systems with various subsystems formed by individuals. There are fundamental principles of a system and they include the following:

1. Homeostasis is maintained if possible.
2. Systems operate according to rules.

3. External problems may cause a crisis.
4. Crises may cause exploration of the problem.
5. This may lead to a reorganization and thus a new homeostasis.

The family therapist can have several roles: He or she can analyze the family system and provide feedback without involvement, get involved in conflicts, or act as an authority figure to change the system. Medical decisions can be made in the context of multidisciplinary groups, so doctors need to be aware about the dynamics of a group.

There are three main schools of family therapy:

1. **Behavioral-psychoeducational:** the aim is to identify the dysfunctional behaviors and improve them.
2. **Structural-strategic:** the aim is to identify the family structure and to fix faulty alliances.
3. **Intergenerational-experiential:** the focus is to identify transgenerational patterns using genograms and to improve communication.

Group Therapy

Group therapy provides the forum in which individuals can learn new and more appropriate behaviors, so the group functions as a microcosm of the individual's own world. Groups may be supportive (self-help) or psychodynamic. Analysis may be of the group as a whole or of individuals within the group. Groups can help members deal with the stressors of daily life. The therapist's responsibility is to provide support and to encourage an atmosphere in which change can occur.

Groups have several characteristics that may interfere with the group process. Groups may blame a particular individual (a "scapegoat") for difficulties that arise. Members may form alliances to protect their interests should a new leader arise. Members may also become dependent on the leader. Fight-or-flight responses may be provoked by perceived threats to the group.

Groups may generally influence behavior in several different ways through social facilitation (enhancement of task performance), social inhibition (inhibition of performance of a task as a result of the presence of others), social loafing (an individual's efforts are not evaluated, which leads to a lower work effort), identity functions, conformity, and minority influences. Some aspects of group activities may vary across different cultures (e.g., in some Asian communities, group participation enhances the individual's functioning).

An individual's sense of identity is affected by the groups (e.g., social/family) he or she belongs to in society. We may try to validate our own groups compared with others, which is called social identity theory. A member can feel less like an individual within a group when there is anonymity, high levels of cohesiveness, collective action, and an external focus of attention. Groups may be more effective at making decisions than are individuals. Cooperative, not competitive, atmospheres enhance such activities. Bad decisions can be made when there is polarization (may make too risky or overly conservative choices) or too much cohesion (no influence from groups within the group or from outsiders).

CASE CONCLUSION

After meeting with CF and her mother you decide to refer her to a psychiatrist who specializes in eating disorders. At this consultation, CF agrees to have individual psychotherapy and to participate in family therapy. A year later, CF has decided that she does not want to become a professional dancer after all and has reached a more normal weight for her size. The family therapy was very beneficial.

THUMBNAIL: Behavioral Science—Features of Eating Disorders

	Anorexia Nervosa	Bulimia Nervosa
Physical signs and symptoms	Emaciation, hypotension, hypothermia, bradycardia, may have yellowed skin due to hypercarotenemia, dry skin and lanugo hair, edema or petechiae (due to a bleeding diathesis). Amenorrhea is nearly universal, in postpubertal females. Vomiters may have erosions on the inside of their teeth, calluses on their fingers, and swollen salivary glands.	May have normal weight. The medical complications are similar to anorexia but occur less frequently and are often less severe. Binging may cause acute dilatation of the stomach. Vomiters may have enlarged parotid glands, elevated amylase levels, esophagitis, or esophageal tears. Electrolyte abnormalities are common, particularly low potassium, which may lead to renal impairment and cardiac arrhythmias. Seizures also may occur. Generally, TFTs are normal, but between 30 and 50% have menstrual abnormalities. Abuse of laxatives may lead to damage of the myenteric plexus.
Investigations/labs	Leukopenia, anemia, thrombocytopenia. Elevated BUN, cholesterol, cortisol, amylase, and liver function tests. Decreased levels of phosphate, magnesium, zinc; decreased levels of LH and FSH with low serum estrogen (females), low serum testosterone (males). T4 in low-normal range and T3 decreased. Vomiters may have a hypochloremic hypokalemic metabolic alkalosis, and those who abuse laxatives may have a metabolic acidosis. **Sinus bradycardia and arrhythmias, diffuse abnormalities on EKG. CAT scans of the brain may reveal reversible cortical atrophy.**	Low potassium, sodium, chloride, magnesium, phosphate, and calcium. Metabolic alkalosis in vomiters, and metabolic acidosis in laxative abusers. EKG as for anorexia. Leukopenia or lymphocytosis.

☑ KEY POINTS

- The prevalence of anorexia is 1% or less of the general population, with males accounting for approximately 10% of cases
- The mortality rate for anorexia is approximately 10%
- The prevalence of bulimia is between approximately 1 and 3 % of young women
- Both anorexics and bulimics tend to suffer from depression and substance abuse
- Group systems generally have rules, keep homeostasis, and have boundaries and feedback loops
- The three schools of family therapy include behavioral-psycho-educational, structural-strategic, and intergenerational-experiential approaches

QUESTIONS

1. CF tells you that she is not concerned that losing weight would affect her in the long term. Which of the following are considered to be more long-term complications of anorexia?

   A. Impaired fertility, osteoporosis, and seizure disorder
   B. Impaired fertility, osteoporosis, and renal stones
   C. Cardiac abnormalities, renal and cognitive impairments
   D. Cardiac abnormalities, renal and auditory impairments
   E. A mortality rate of greater than 50%

2. Which of the following is a characteristic physical finding in bulimia?

   A. Excess weight
   B. Calluses on the fingers
   C. Lanugo hair
   D. Hyperchloremic, hyponatremic alkalosis
   E. Alopecia

3. Which of the following models of family therapy is correctly paired with its own theory?

   A. Structural-strategic approaches: Behavior is caused by family developmental fixation.
   B. Behavioral-psychoeducational: Behavior is caused dysfunctional attempts to adapt.
   C. Intergenerational-experiential: Behavior is caused by family developmental fixation.
   D. Structural-strategic approaches: Behavior is shaped by current environmental events.
   E. Behavioral-psychoeducational: Behavior is caused by family developmental fixation.

4. Which of the following is considered a curative factor in group therapy?

   A. Scapegoating
   B. Triangulation
   C. Instillation of hope
   D. Humor
   E. Group-think

CASE 7-10 Obesity

HPI: LC is a 66-year-old man with HTN presenting to a new clinic for his regular care. He has exercised four times a week for 30 minutes for about a year but reports difficulty in maintaining a strict low-fat diet. He notes that he has struggled with his weight, and has tried several diet and exercise regimens without success. His highest weight was 280 pounds.

PMH: Non–Q-wave MI 10 years ago

Meds: Metoprolol, aspirin, atorvastatin

ROS: Snoring, chronic daytime fatigue, knee pain when walking for long periods. Denies having colicky abdominal pain, polyuria or polydipsia, depression, or anxiety.

PE: T 36.5°C; BP 130/90; HR 75; RR 20; Height 5′ 7″; Weight 240 lbs (weight 4 months ago was 245 lbs). He is obese with apparent truncal obesity and a waist-to-hip ratio of 1.6, and BMI of 34. His head, neck, lung, and cardiac exams are unremarkable. His abdomen is obese, soft, and nontender. His knees exhibit no apparent erythema or tenderness on exam. He has no peripheral edema or abnormal skin or hair texture.

Labs/Studies: Glucose 120; TG 205; total cholesterol (TC) 210; LDL 145; HDL 29; TSH 5.2. X-rays of both knees show mild narrowing of joint space without osteophytes, cysts, or subchondral bony sclerosis.

THOUGHT QUESTIONS

- How is obesity defined? What are the main characteristics of obesity?
- What are the main physiologic considerations and the medical consequences of obesity?
- Why are the psychological components of obesity?
- What treatment options are available for obesity?

BASIC SCIENCE REVIEW AND DISCUSSION

Body mass index (BMI = weight in kilograms divided by height in meters squared) is a measure of body fat based on height and weight. Using this calculation, overweight patients (BMI between 25 and 30) deserve clinical attention, since they meet the threshold weight associated with increased morbidity and mortality. Obese patients (BMI of 30 or above) are at especially increased risk (see Thumbnail). It is important to note, however, that BMI does not accurately predict risk for those who have increased lean body mass. In addition to overall weight, **central obesity,** a typically android pattern of obesity marked by increased intra-abdominal fat, is higher risk than **gluteal** or **subcutaneous obesity,** a typically gynecoid pattern. This is quantified by the **waist-to-hip ratio (WHR).** Truncal obesity is defined by a WHR of more than 0.9 for women and more than 1.0 for men.

From 1976 to 1998, the prevalence of obesity (BMI >30) in the United States has increased from 15 to 23%. Between 1991 and 1998, 50% of adults older than age 20 years were overweight. Women and the poor are particularly at risk. Childhood obesity has more than doubled since 1976.

Etiology

At the most basic level, obesity is caused by a consistent intake of calories in excess of one's metabolic requirements (i.e., calories in > calories out). Body weight is regulated homeostatically through endocrine and neural signals that influence either *energy expenditure* or *intake*. Seventy percent of our energy expenditure is from the **basal metabolic rate (BMR),** the energy required to run the basic bodily functions at rest. Another 20% of our energy expenditure comes from the metabolism and storage of food as well as adaptive thermogenesis. Only 5 to 10% comes from physical activity, that which we can modify in the form of exercise. Therefore, exercise alone is insufficient for weight loss; limiting food intake is the most important component of any weight reduction program.

Food intake is determined by appetite, which is influenced by several hormonal and metabolic signals (e.g., leptin, insulin, cortisol, cholecystokinin, serotonin, glucose, and ketone) as well as neural signals (e.g., those that come from the vagus nerve as a result of gut distension). **Leptin** is an important modulator of appetite, metabolism, and neuroendocrine function. It is released from adipocytes in the fed state and influences the hypothalamus by decreasing appetite, increasing energy expenditure, and influencing peripheral targets such as pancreatic beta cells. In those with typical obesity, leptin levels are found to be high, suggesting the presence of a "leptin-resistant" state. Along with psychological and cultural influences, all these factors are integrated in the hypothalamus and determine the subjective experience of hunger or satiety.

Although there are rare cases of well-defined familial obesity and secondary obesity from other medical conditions, the pathogenesis of common obesity is thought to be a result of a complex interplay of genetic and environmental influences on food intake and energy expenditure. Obesity commonly runs in families, although it may be difficult to separate the environmental influence from the genetic influence. Family and twin studies support the strong influence of genetics in obesity. Strong environmental influences include the availability of food, particularly those rich in fat and simple sugars, as well as increasingly sedentary lifestyles common in industrialized societies. For instance, the high-fat content of food readily available in poor neighborhoods contributes to the high prevalence of obesity in such communities. Cultural concepts of food and body image also contribute to the accepted patterns of food intake and adiposity. Childhood obesity has been linked to decreased physical activity and increased television watching.

Disease Associated with Obesity

The pathophysiologic consequences of obesity are manifold and increase mortality up to twelve times for morbidly obese individuals (>200% of ideal body weight). The cardiovascular diseases associated with obesity include **type II diabetes mellitus (DM), hypertension,** and **hyperlipidemia.** Together these are thought to contribute to the associated increased risk of developing **CAD, stroke,** and **CHF.** Other medical conditions include **male hypogonadism, polycystic ovarian syndrome, chronic hypoventilation, sleep apnea, cholelithiasis, osteoarthritis,** and **gout.**

Although these medical conditions are significant and dangerous, perhaps the most difficult and easily ignored consequences of obesity are the social and psychological challenges. Many individuals with obesity suffer from depression, anxiety, and poor self-esteem. Many cycles of failed dieting and exercising can lead to eating disorders, such as food obsession, compulsive eating, and patterns of bingeing and purging. Food addiction has been described in which food is used as self-medication to relieve depression or anxiety. People with obesity suffer from social ostracism and occupational discrimination, further compounding poor self-image. Often, these psychological effects are the greatest barriers to successful weight reduction and maintenance. For others, obesity has been accepted as a way of life, not just at the individual level but also at a larger, social and cultural level. Therefore, any physician attempting to evaluate and treat obesity needs to be sensitive to the complex and varied experiences and perspectives patients have about their weight and body image. However, a physician can offer objective information on the consequences associated with an individual's BMI and offer alternatives to current eating habits and sedentary lifestyles.

Diagnosis and Treatment of Obesity

To evaluate obesity, one must assess not only the objective indices of BMI and WHR but also the comorbid conditions that increase a person's risk of developing adverse clinical consequences. This includes measuring blood pressure, triglycerides, total cholesterol, LDL, HDL, and serum glucose. Obesity secondary to other medical conditions, such as Cushing syndrome, hypothyroidism, insulinoma, and tumors involving the hypothalamus, may be investigated if there is clinical suspicion from the history and physical exam. Familial obesity may be suspected in those with strong family histories, but with the exception of those with leptin deficiencies, further testing will unlikely result in changes in management. A patient's eating habits, stressors that lead to increased eating, level of physical activity, and, most importantly, motivation to lose weight, must be evaluated.

Treatment

Successful weight reduction and maintenance in obesity is difficult and, sadly, uncommon. The cornerstone of treatment is reduction in food intake to below that required to maintain current body weight. A 500-kcal/day deficit will result in a weight loss of 1 pound per week. There are several long-term community programs that focus on behavioral modification, such as helping an individual to maintain a low-fat, high-fiber diet; to change eating patterns; to identify and manage stressors that lead to overeating; and to provide long-term counseling and group support. Although exercise alone will not lead to significant weight reduction, it has been shown to improve long-term maintenance of reduced weight. There are several mildly efficacious drugs available for those with BMIs ≥30 or with BMIs ≥27 with concurrent obesity-related conditions. These include **sympathomimetic and serotonergic drugs** that decrease appetite and increase energy expenditure (e.g., phentermine, sibutramine, diethylpropion); these drugs are contraindicated in those with uncontrolled hypertension and other cardiac diseases. The other class of drugs includes the **lipase inhibitor** orlistat, which suppresses the conversion of triglycerides into free fatty acids in the gut lumen, preventing absorption. However, the most dramatic results come from surgical treatment of obesity. **Bariatric surgery** is available to those with morbid obesity (BMI >40) who have failed all other weight loss strategies. The procedures most commonly performed to maximize weight loss benefit and minimize adverse effects like short-gut syndrome are **Roux-en-Y gastric bypass** and **duodenal switch,** both of which can be done laparoscopically, thus minimizing postoperative morbidity associated with obesity.

CASE CONCLUSION

LC's BMI of 34 and central obesity place him at significant risk of adverse and perhaps life-threatening clinical consequences. You note that he already has several risk factors, including hypertension, hyperlipidemia, and CAD with a previous history of MI. He is also exhibiting other obesity-related conditions, such as osteoarthritis and sleep apnea. You also ruled out several associated conditions, such as type II DM and hypothyroidism. It is apparent that LC is highly motivated to lose weight but that, despite this, he is failing to limit his food intake, reflected by his minimal weight reduction in the last year and abnormal lipid profile despite medication. You therefore refer him to a community weight loss program, adjust his atorvastatin, offer NSAIDs for his mild arthritis pain, and suggest otolaryngology consultation for his sleep apnea.

THUMBNAIL: Behavioral Science—Obesity-Associated Medical Conditions

Condition	Description	Treatment
Hypertension	Increased peripheral resistance, cardiac output, sympathetic nervous tone, salt sensitivity, insulin-mediated salt retention	Diet, exercise, sodium restriction, beta-blockers, diuretics, ACE inhibitors
Hypercholesterolemia	Increased LDL, VLDL, and triglycerides. Decreased HDL, especially with abdominal obesity; leads to atherosclerosis and all subsequent clinical risks	Diet, statins, niacin, fibrates, resins
Sleep apnea, obesity, hypoventilation syndrome	Reduced chest wall compliance; increased intra-abdominal pressure, especially in supine position; increased minute ventilation due to increased metabolic rate; decreased total lung capacity; airway obstruction causing snoring and sleep apnea	Weight reduction, continuous positive airway pressure, surgical intervention with an ENT specialist
Type II DM	Hyperinsulinemia and insulin resistance; 80% of patients with type II DM are obese, especially associated with the presence of intra-abdominal fat	Metformin has efficacy in both weight reduction and glucose control
Polycystic ovary syndrome	Increased androgen production and peripheral conversion of androgen to estrogen, decreased sex hormone-binding globulin (SHBG) lead to anovulation, ovarian hyperandrogenism, oligomenorrhea, and fertility problems	Weight reduction, metformin, oral contraception
Male hypogonadism	Increased adipose tissue causes increased peripheral conversion of androgens to estrogens, reduced testosterone and SHBG leading to gynecomastia	Weight reduction
Cholelithiasis	Increased cholesterol levels promote the development of cholesterol gallstones, which could become symptomatic	Weight loss, low-cholesterol diets, cholecystectomy
Cancer	*In men:* higher mortality in colon, rectal, prostate cancer. *In women:* higher mortality in gallbladder, biliary, breast, endometrial, cervical, and ovarian cancer	Surgery, depending on cancer type
Osteoarthritis	Chronic added weight bearing causes gradual deterioration of weight-bearing joints (knees, hips)	Weight reduction, NSAIDs, joint replacement
Gout	Exacerbated by dietary excess and alcohol consumption	Allopurinol, colchicine

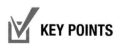 **KEY POINTS**

- Obesity is a multifactorial disease and results from the complex interplay of genetics and environment, causing a chronic intake of calories in excess of energy expended
- Obesity is associated with a number of different medical conditions (e.g., type II DM, hypertension, and hypercholesterolemia) as well as several-fold increases in overall morbidity and mortality

- Addressing issues of weight, body image, and obesity requires not only clinical knowledge of the problems but also cultural and emotional sensitivity to the patients that face this problem

QUESTIONS

1. BI is a 36-year-old woman with a height of 5 feet, 4 inches and weight of 170 pounds, giving her a BMI of 29. She also has hypertension and hyperlipidemia. What weight reduction strategy is included in the appropriate management of her obesity?

   A. Fasting
   B. Low-fat, high-fiber diet
   C. Strenuous exercise
   D. Laparoscopic duodenal switch
   E. Roux-en-Y gastric bypass

2. GL is an 11-year-old boy brought to his pediatrician for an annual physical exam. He is noted to be at the 98th percentile for weight. On further inquiry, you discover that the boy spends 8 hours a day watching TV or playing video games, participates in no sports or physical activity at school, and loves to drink soda and eat potato chips and candy bars. You note that the mother is also obese. Which is the *most* appropriate in the evaluation and treatment for this patient?

   A. Inquiring about family history of obesity with subsequent serum leptin testing
   B. Leptin replacement
   C. Family counseling on proper diet and exercise
   D. Sibutramine
   E. Roux-en-Y gastric bypass

3. LC (from the case presentation) returns 4 years later complaining of gradually worsening shortness of breath and dyspnea on exertion for 1 year. He came in because he was suddenly awakened from sleep the night before and was gasping for air, after which he got up and walked around to feel better. He notes having difficulty lying down flat because of difficulty breathing and now uses three pillows to sleep at night. He previously could walk 1 mile on flat ground to work but now cannot walk 1 block without getting short of breath. He also notes worsened knee pain, which limits his activity. In addition, he continues to have daytime fatigue. On exam, he is comfortable and in no respiratory distress, with a blood pressure of 165/89, pulse 83, RR 20, and an oxygen saturation of 97%. His BMI is now 41. His lungs are clear and he has normal heart sounds, but all other parts of his cardiac exam are difficult to assess due to his body habitus. He has bilateral pitting edema of both lower extremities. He has an EKG significant only for left ventricular hypertrophy. He has two negative tests for troponin I. Given this clinical picture, what is the *most* likely cause of his shortness of breath?

   A. Hypoventilation syndrome
   B. CAD
   C. Restrictive lung disease due to his large body habitus
   D. CHF with systolic dysfunction
   E. Acute MI

4. LC (from the above question) returns after having undergone all appropriate testing. He is shown to have a decreased ejection fraction of 40%. Having learned that his obesity may have something to do with his current medical condition, he would like you to help him lose weight. Which treatment is contraindicated for LC?

   A. Very low-calorie diet
   B. Orlistat
   C. Phentermine
   D. Moderate exercise three times a week
   E. Roux-en-Y gastric bypass

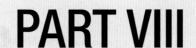

PART VIII

Neuroscience, Psychiatry, Psychopharmacology, and Psychopathology

HPI: MB is a 30-year-old mother of two who comes to your clinic complaining of depressed mood. She has noticed a gradual change in her mood over the past couple of months, but things have been particularly difficult for the past 2 weeks. She has difficulty sleeping, poor appetite, low energy, and low mood with tearful episodes. Her husband, who accompanies her, confirms these changes and says her libido has decreased and that things that she used to enjoy do not seem to lift her mood anymore. There have been no recent stressors, and MB has never had a problem like this before. She has never had an episode of mania or hypomania. No previous psychiatric history. No significant medical history apart from an allergy to bee stings.

In her family history, one maternal aunt has a history of recurrent depressions; otherwise, noncontributory. MB is the eldest of three daughters. Her parents are both well and live nearby. She graduated with a master's degree in art history and works as a curator in a local museum. Her husband is an accountant; they own their own home. They have two children, a son aged 4 and a daughter aged 2; both are healthy. She denies any illicit substance use, drinks alcohol rarely, and does not smoke. Lab tests were all normal.

MSE: A thin, well-dressed woman who appears her stated age; eye contact, limited; rapport, good. Affect dysphoric and tearful at times. Mood described as "down." Thought processes are logical and goal directed. Thought content includes expression of concern and guilt that she is not being a good mother or wife. She denies feelings of hopelessness or suicidal ideation. There is no evidence of psychosis. Her insight and judgment are good, and her cognitive functions are intact.

THOUGHT QUESTIONS

- Does this woman meet the criteria for major depressive disorder?
- What other mood disorders would you consider?
- How will you treat her?
- Which agents would you consider and why?

BASIC SCIENCE REVIEW AND DISCUSSION

Depressive symptoms are commonly reported by between 13 and 20% of the general population, but the lifetime prevalence for major depressive disorder is between 10 and 25% for females and between 5 and 12% for males. Patients who report symptoms of depression have higher rates of mortality, greater disability, and lower levels of social functioning. Approximately 15% of those suffering from major depression commit suicide. Major depression is reported to be higher among primary care patients than in the general population. Risk factors include female gender, younger age, early parental loss, disruptive childhood environment, lower socioeconomic status, family history of major depression, marital separation or divorce, chronic stress, residence in an urban area, and lack of a confidante.

Various medical disorders can cause depressive symptoms, including endocrine abnormalities (hypothyroidism, hyperparathyroidism, Addison disease, Cushing syndrome), CNS disorders such as Parkinson disease, multiple sclerosis, epilepsy, Huntington disease, cerebrovascular disease (particularly strokes with left anterior lesions), infections (HIV, brucellosis, infectious mononucleosis, hepatitis, postinfluenza), and various metabolic disorders (vitamin B12/folate and iron-deficient anemias, hypercalcemia, hypomagnesia). Various medications have also been implicated and include reserpine, L-dopa, steroids, barbiturates, NSAIDs, thiazides, digoxin, and prolonged use of amphetamines.

Major depression is the most common type of mood disorder and may occur as a single episode or recur throughout the life cycle. Major depressive episodes also occur in bipolar disorder (also called manic depression).

A mnemonic to easily remember the essential features of major depression is SIGECAPS:

- S—Sleep
- I—Interest
- G—Guilt
- E—Energy
- C—Concentration
- A—Appetite
- P—Psychomotor agitation or retardation
- S—Suicidality

Episodes of major depression may also have several specifiers, such as "chronic", with "catatonic features", with "melancholic features" (mood worse in the morning, early morning wakening, marked psychomotor agitation or slowing, and excessive or inappropriate guilt) or with "atypical features" (Table 8-1).

Psychopharmacology of Major Depression

There are four main classes of antidepressants. The choice of agent depends on an individual's symptoms, presentation, history of response to a particular type of agent (or a family history of response), and potential for adverse reactions to these agents. All antidepressants have a delayed therapeutic onset of action, although their effects on amine concentrations are relatively immediate. Antidepressant effects may be seen between 2 and 8 weeks after starting treatment. The main classes of antidepressants are outlined in Table 8-2.

TABLE 8-1 Other Mood Disorders to Consider When Taking the History and Mental State Examination

Disorder	Major Depression	Mild Depression	Mania	Hypomania
Major depressive disorder	+	±	−	−
Dysthymia	−	+	−	−
Cyclothymia	−	+	−	+
Bipolar I disorder	±	±	+	±
Bipolar II disorder	+	±	−	+

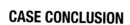

CASE CONCLUSION

MB indeed meets the criteria for major depressive disorder. After review of her history and discussion of the treatment options with the patient and her husband, she is started on a trial of sertraline, an SSRI that is titrated up to 50 mg per day without adverse reaction. You also arrange for her to receive weekly psychotherapy sessions. When she returns to your clinic 1 month later she reports feeling better; 6 months later her symptoms have completely resolved.

TABLE 8-2 Main Classes of Antidepressants

Monoamine reuptake inhibitors	1. **Tricyclics:** These are further subdivided into tertiary amines (amitriptyline and imipramine), secondary amines (desipramine and nortriptyline), and others (doxepin, clomipramine, protriptyline, and trimipramine). Tertiary and secondary amines have reuptake inhibition effects at both serotonin and norepinephrine neurons. All tricyclics affect 5-HT2 receptors as well as histamine, M muscarinic, and α_1- and α_2-adrenergic receptors. 2. **Heterocyclics:** Maprotiline (a tetracyclic) and amoxapine (a dibenzoxazepine). Tetracyclics cause reuptake inhibition of norepinephrine only but may have effects at D2 dopamine receptors. Amoxapine causes reuptake inhibition of both serotonin and norepinephrine. 3. **Triazolopyridines:** Trazodone and nefazodone. These agents cause reuptake inhibition of serotonin. 4. **Propiophenones:** Bupropion. This agent causes reuptake inhibition of dopamine, serotonin, and norepinephrine.
MAOIs	These agents inhibit monoamine oxidase A. 1. **Hydrazine compounds:** Phenelzine and isocarboxazid 2. **Nonhydrazine compound:** Tranylcypromine
SSRIs	These include fluoxetine, sertraline, paroxetine, fluvoxamine, and citalopram. These agents cause reuptake inhibition of serotonin, but some may also affect dopamine.
SNRIs	Venlafaxine. This affects both norepinephrine and serotonin as well as having a small effect on the reuptake of dopamine.

THUMBNAIL: Behavioral Science—Abnormalities Reported in Depression

Neurotransmitters	**Serotonin:** Decreased plasma tryptophan, CSF, 5-HIAA (particularly in suicides), platelet 5-HT uptake and prolactin response to challenge tests with tryptophan and fenfluramine (this normalizes after treatment with antidepressants); increased 5-HT2 receptor binding in platelets and the limbic cortex **Noradrenaline:** Decreased growth hormone response to challenge tests with amphetamine and clonidine, cAMP turnover in platelets when stimulated by clonidine; increased platelet alpha2-receptor binding and beta-receptors in suicides **Acetylcholine:** Agonists exacerbate depressive symptoms **GABA:** Decreased plasma, CSF, and brain levels
Neuroendocrine	**Hypercortisolemia:** Seen in up to 40% of depressed outpatients and in up to 60% of depressed inpatients; hallmark of the stress response; failure of suppression in the dexamethasone suppression test in up to 60% of depressed patients (also seen in anorexia, schizophrenia, and alcohol dependence) **Thyroid dysfunction:** 5–10% of depressed patients reported to have hypothyroidism; blunted TSH responses with thyrotropin-releasing hormone (TRH) challenge tests **Growth hormone:** Blunted response to clonidine **Somatostatin:** Lower CSF levels reported **Prolactin:** Blunted response to serotonin agonists
Neuropathology/ neuroimaging	**MRI** studies have reported decreases in caudate nucleus size; subcortical frontal and basal ganglia cerebrovascular lesions reported in late-life depression **Positron emission tomography (PET) studies** reported decreased metabolism in the anterior brain, reduced blood flow, and decreased metabolism in the mesocortical and mesolimbic tracts; increased glucose metabolism reported in limbic region; asymmetry of phosphorus metabolism in basal ganglia and left frontal lobe
Neuropsychoimmunology	Decreased natural killer cells, T-cell replication, and IL-2; increased monocyte activity

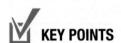 **KEY POINTS**

- Between 13 and 20% of the general population report depressive symptoms

- The lifetime prevalence for major depressive disorder is between 10 and 25% for females and between 5 and 12% for males

- Approximately 15% of those suffering from major depression commit suicide

- Risk factors include female gender, younger age, early parental loss, a disruptive childhood environment, lower socioeconomic status, family history of major depression, marital separation or divorce, chronic stress, residence in an urban area, and a lack of a confidante

- Medical disorders can cause depressive symptoms

- There are four main classes of antidepressants: monoamine reuptake inhibitors, monoamine oxidase inhibitors (MAOIs), SSRIs, and serotonin-norepinephrine reuptake inhibitors (SNRIs)

QUESTIONS

1. When discussing the side effects of SSRIs with the above patient and her husband, you mention the possibility of which of the following?

   A. Agranulocytosis
   B. Sexual dysfunction
   C. Dietary considerations
   D. Orthostatic hypotension
   E. Cardiac toxicity

2. Which of the following agents is incorrectly paired with other possible uses?

   A. SSRIs and OCD
   B. Tricyclics and enuresis
   C. MAOIs and narcolepsy
   D. SNRIs and bulimia
   E. Tricyclics and trichotillomania

3. A patient presents for treatment of depression. He is started on a tricyclic antidepressant medication. You counsel him that which of the following are all possible side effects?

   A. Arrhythmias, cholestatic jaundice, dry mouth, blurry vision
   B. Arrhythmias, cholestatic jaundice, priapism, constipation
   C. Dry mouth, arrhythmias, blurry vision, and constipation
   D. Dry mouth, priapism, constipation, and microcytic anemia
   E. Priapism, constipation, arrhythmias, and microcytic anemia

4. A patient presents with a depression with **atypical** features of hypersomnia and weight gain. You decide to give him a trial of an MAOI. Which of the following is a concern?

   A. Reversible binding to the enzyme MAO, hypertensive crisis with tyramine-containing foods and drinks
   B. Hypotensive crisis with tyramine-containing foods and drinks
   C. Little interaction with other CNS active agents, anticholinergic effects
   D. Little interaction with other CNS active agents, anticholinergic side effects, and postural hypotension
   E. Significant interaction with other CNS active agents, anticholinergic side effects, and postural hypotension

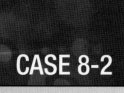

HPI: AD is a 32-year-old housewife. Her husband brought her to the ER because he is concerned that his wife is "going crazy."

AD has not been sleeping for the past few nights. Instead, she has been staying up night and day, cleaning the house from top to bottom. Her husband became especially concerned when he came home to find her emptying the woodshed of logs for the fire and cleaning it because she claimed it was "so dirty." She has no psychiatric history and no significant medical history. Her family history is significant for a male cousin who had been diagnosed as having bipolar disorder. She is the youngest of three daughters; her parents are well and live close by. She graduated from college and works as a primary school teacher. She has been married for 5 years and has no children. Her husband works as a software engineer. She denies illicit substance abuse and drinks one or two glasses of wine a week socially. She has no legal history.

PE: WNL

MSE: AD appears her stated age, wearing appropriate clothing with good hygiene. Eye contact is intense, staring. Speech is pressured and loud at times, particularly when she makes jokes. Very agitated at times. She keeps insisting that she has to go home to finish cleaning up and accuses you of trying to conspire against her with the headmaster of the school where she works. She describes her mood as "fantastic." Her affect is labile. Thought processes positive for flight of ideas and some loosening of associations. She denies suicidal or homicidal ideation. She further denies auditory or visual hallucinations, but does admit that she has "received a message" from the radio telling her to start preparing for her "next phase." Oriented to time, person, and place. She has no insight into her condition; judgment is impaired.

Labs: CBC, electrolytes, and thyroid function tests are normal. Urine toxicology (Utox) is negative.

THOUGHT QUESTIONS

- What is the most likely diagnosis?
- What are the characteristics of this type of disorder? What is the etiology?

BASIC SCIENCE REVIEW AND DISCUSSION

Bipolar disorder (aka manic depression) is characterized by episodes of depression and mania (Table 8-3). Only one episode of mania is needed to meet *Diagnostic and Statistical Manual of Mental Disorders, 4th edition* (*DSM-IV*) criteria. The episodes of depression in bipolar disorder have the same symptoms as in major depression but may differ in the following ways: The episodes of depression are less likely to have a specific triggering event, develop more gradually, usually do not last as long, and may be more atypical in presentation, with hypersomnia, increase in weight, and labile mood.

The *DSM-IV* criteria for mania include the following:

1. Abnormally **elevated or irritable mood for 1 week** (or less if hospitalized)
2. Three or more of these symptoms: grandiosity, decreased need for sleep, pressured speech, racing thoughts/flight of ideas, distractibility, increased goal-directed activity/psychomotor agitation, and involvement in potentially harmful activities, such as unsafe sex, gambling, or spending sprees

These episodes are not caused by substance abuse or a general medical condition and cause **marked impairment in functioning.**

Epidemiology

The lifetime risk of bipolar I disorder is between 1 and 1.5%, whereas that for bipolar II is 0.5%. Bipolar I affects both sexes equally, but women appear to have a higher incidence of rapid cycling and mixed states; bipolar II is more common in women than in men. It tends also to present earlier in men (late teens) with a manic episode, whereas women tend to experience depression first. There is another peak of onset for women aged 40. It may start in childhood and be misdiagnosed as ADD, but it can also occur with ADD. Studies have reported that a high percentage of adolescents with bipolar disorder also meet criteria for ADD. It can also start in later life in those with a history of previous depressions or in conjunction with neurologic conditions, such as stroke. Other risk factors reported include winter births and birth complications.

Etiology

The exact etiology of bipolar disorder is unknown. Genetics accounts for only 60% of cases, so other biologic and environmental factors must contribute to the development of this disorder. Increased rates have been reported in higher socioeconomic groups. It may share similar factors with schizophrenia or other psychotic disorders. These include deficiencies in Reelin (a brain protein important for information processing) or an elevation in the level of VMAT2 (a brain protein that regulates the transport of neurotransmitters) in the brainstem. However, brain imaging studies have reported differences in hippocampal structures, with a significant increase in volume on the left (compared with the right) in bipolar patients, whereas a decrease in volume was reported in patients with schizophrenia. Bipolar disorder may also share similar biologic mechanisms with epilepsy, including abnormalities in both of the neurotransmitters GABA and norepinephrine. This disorder may also be linked genetically to diabetes, as this condition has been reported to occur three times more commonly in those with bipolar disorder than in the general population.

TABLE 8-3 Subtypes of Bipolar Disorders

Bipolar I disorder involves at least one episode of **mania,** with or without a history of depression.

Bipolar II disorder is characterized by at least one episode of **hypomania** and at least one of **depression.** In hypomania, the symptoms are milder and last at least 4 days but do not cause much interference in functioning (and generally do not require hospitalization). Insight is lost in manic episodes but is retained in hypomania.

Mixed episodes occur when there is a **combination of both manic and depressed** symptoms.

Rapid cycling occurs when there are at least **four distinct episodes** of mood disturbance within 12 months. They happen in approximately 15% of patients with bipolar I and II disorders. Rapid cycling may be triggered by antidepressants. Those individuals with this disorder must be symptom-free for at least 2 months between episodes of mood disturbance.

Cyclothymic disorder is a chronic disorder lasting at least 2 years, with **milder episodes** of depression and elevation of mood that last more than 2 months. It may be chronic or may develop into a bipolar disorder.

Course and Prognosis

If untreated, manic episodes can last up to 6 months and depressed episodes can last up to 12 months. Manic episodes tend to occur in the summer and depressive episodes from autumn through late spring. As patients with bipolar disorder become older their episodes can become more frequent and more difficult to treat. A person with bipolar disorder tends to experience an average of 8 to 10 depressed or manic episodes in a lifetime. In most cases the number of depressed episodes is more than that of manic ones. Those who have early-onset bipolar disorder tend to have more complications (e.g., substance abuse, behavioral problems, and paranoid features) and a more severe form of the disorder. Between 15 and 20% of untreated bipolar patients may commit suicide, and it has been reported that up to 50% of bipolar patients may have attempted suicide at some stage during their illness. Periods of increased risk include depressed and mixed episodes. Studies have also reported that bipolar II patients may be at higher risk of suicide than those with either bipolar I disorder or depression.

Up to 60% of patients with bipolar disorder also have substance abuse problems during their illness. The most common substance abused is alcohol, followed by marijuana and cocaine. Males and those with mixed episodes appear to be at higher risk for developing substance abuse.

Other complications of this disorder may include high rates of divorce, legal problems due to impulsive manic behaviors, and high economic cost to the country. Direct costs include those due to patient care and suicide. Indirect costs include losses in productivity and costs to the justice system. Both have been reported to cost $45 billion.

CASE CONCLUSION

AD was admitted to the hospital and started on valproate and an atypical antipsychotic. Benzodiazepines were used as needed for anxiety, agitation, and insomnia. Her valproate was titrated with good effect (serum level of 85 μg/mL). A week later she was no longer manic, was sleeping normally, and was discharged to the care of her husband with close follow-up.

THUMBNAIL: Behavioral Science—Genetics of Mood Disorders

Data from twin, adoption, and family studies have provided support for the genetic contributions to bipolar disorder.

	Lifetime Risk in the General Population	Lifetime Risk in First-Degree Relatives	Twin Concordance
Bipolar disorder	1%	Bipolar 7.8% (1.5–17.9%) Unipolar 11.4% (0.5–22.4%)	MZ, 79% DZ, 19%
Unipolar depression	2–5%	Bipolar, 0.6% (0.3–2.1%) Unipolar, 9.1% (5.9–18.4%)	MZ, 58% DZ, 23%

MZ, monozygotic; *DZ,* dizygotic

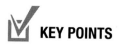

KEY POINTS

- In bipolar I disorder there is at least one episode of mania with or without a history of depression; bipolar II disorder is characterized by at least one episode of hypomania and at least one of depression
- The lifetime risk is between 1 and 1.5% for bipolar I and is 0.5% for bipolar II
- Bipolar I affects both sexes equally, bipolar II is more common in women; genetics accounts for only 60% of cases

- Women have a higher incidence of rapid cycling and mixed states
- Bipolar patients may experience 8 to 10 depressed or manic episodes in a lifetime
- Between 15 and 20% of untreated bipolar patients may commit suicide; up to 60% of patients with bipolar disorder also have substance abuse problems

QUESTIONS

1. When this patient's husband asks you about risk factors for developing bipolar disorder, you tell him that which of the following may be risk factors?

   A. Age >65 years
   B. Substance abuse
   C. A family history
   D. Female gender
   E. Male gender

2. He is concerned about any future children they might have. What other conditions have a higher incidence rate in the families of persons with bipolar disorder?

   A. Schizophrenia
   B. Eating disorders
   C. Kleptomania
   D. Depression
   E. Mental retardation

3. Which of the following statements concerning the genetics of psychiatric disease is correct?

   A. If twin concordance rates are higher ⌐ than in monozygotic twins, the⌐ implicated.
   B. Simple Mendelian modes of transm⌐ anisms of genetic transmission in psy⌐
   C. There is no evidence of trinucleotide re⌐ bipolar disorder.
   D. Linkage studies in bipolar disorder ha⌐ replicated.
   E. Chromosome 18 may be linked to bipolar disor⌐er.

4. Which of the following medical conditions may present with manic symptoms?

   A. Addison disease
   B. Hypothyroidism
   C. Cushing syndrome
   D. Turner syndrome
   E. Pancreatitis

HPI: You are going to co-lead a psychotherapy group for patients with anxiety disorders. Before the first group you review the descriptions of the group participants.

AG is a 30-year-old woman who works in the filing department of an accounting firm. She joined the group because of extreme shyness, an inability to participate in social activities for fear of people watching her and making a fool of herself.

RP is a 23-year-old man who has a new job in an advertising firm. He finds that when he has to make a presentation he becomes extremely anxious, tachycardic, and diaphoretic, with a dry mouth. He has been turning down projects or allowing his coworkers to get the accolades for his work, for fear of having to speak in public.

DB is a 20-year-old college student with a morbid fear of rats. He joined the group after realizing that his summer job in a prestigious laboratory included the responsibility of feeding and caring for the rats. He decided to address this fear rather than avoid the situation and find another summer job.

ET is a 47-year-old woman who describes a 20-year history of anxiety. "It's all of the time." It isn't related to any specific situation and it causes her a great deal of distress. Her sleep is often interrupted, she feels "wound up" and tense, is often irritable, and finds it hard to concentrate because of her anxiety.

THOUGHT QUESTIONS

- What disorders do these people have?
- What is known about their biology? Treatment?

BASIC SCIENCE REVIEW AND DISCUSSION

AG has social phobia, generalized type. RP has social phobia, specifically related to performance. DB has a specific phobia. ET has generalized anxiety disorder (GAD).

Social and Specific Phobias

A phobia is defined as an irrational fear that results in a compelling desire to avoid the phobic stimulus. This can be a specific object, activity, or situation. The person realizes that the fear is excessive or out of proportion to any danger.

Specific Phobia

A specific phobia relates to a persistent excessive fear of a specific thing (e.g., dogs, blood) or situation (e.g., flying, getting an injection, elevators). Exposure causes significant anxiety or distress, even a cued panic attack. The person realizes that the fear is excessive, and it causes significant distress or interferes with social or occupational functioning. Phobias are among the most common psychiatric disorders. Findings based on large community samples yielded lifetime prevalence estimates of approximately 11%. Most specific phobias are more common in women than in men. The mean age at onset differs, depending on the type of phobia. In childhood, phobias of animals, blood, storms, and water tend to begin, whereas phobias of heights tend to begin in the teens, and situational phobias (e.g., claustrophobia) have mean ages at onset in the late teens to mid-20s.

Blood–injection–injury phobias tend to cluster together, as do animal phobias, natural environment phobias, and situational phobias. Up to 30% of patients with an anxiety disorder have a comorbid specific phobia.

There is a higher risk of specific phobias in first-degree relatives of people with specific phobias than in controls (approximately 30% vs. 10%).

Social Phobia

In social phobia, the individual's central fear is that he or she will act in such a way as to humiliate or embarrass himself or herself in front of others. Socially phobic individuals fear and/or avoid a variety of situations in which they would be required to interact with or perform a task in front of other people. There are two subtypes of social phobias: generalized, in which the social fear encompasses most social situations, while the other is circumscribed to one or two specific activities (e.g. public speaking, eating in public). In social phobias the anxiety is stimulus-bound. When confronted with the phobic situation, the individual experiences profound anxiety accompanied by a variety of somatic symptoms, such as sweating, blushing, and dry mouth. Actual panic attacks may also occur in response to feared social situations.

Individuals who have only circumscribed social fears may function well overall and be relatively asymptomatic unless confronted with their phobic situation. When faced with this, they are often subject to intense anticipatory anxiety. Generalized social phobia can lead to chronic demoralization, social isolation, and disabling vocational and interpersonal impairment.

Epidemiology Social phobia may be slightly more prevalent in women. The median age of onset is in the mid-teens. The lifetime prevalence is between 3 and 13%. Interestingly, in a large epidemiologic study, despite significant functional impairment only a minority had sought professional help. Generalized social phobia usually has an earlier age of onset than more circumscribed social phobias, and affected patients are more often single and have more comorbidity with depression and alcoholism.

Genetics A strong familial risk for social phobia has been identified and is believed to be partly heritable and partly environmental. First-degree relatives of persons with generalized social phobia have an approximately ten-fold higher risk for generalized social phobia or avoidant personality disorder. Environmental factors also play a significant role. Prospectively, the personality trait of behavioral inhibition, assessed in toddlerhood, has been found to be a strong predictor of social anxiety in adolescence.

Neurochemistry and Neuroimaging The biology of social phobia has not been well documented. Despite the documented efficacy of serotonin reuptake inhibitors in treating social phobia, little is directly known about serotonergic involvement in the disorder. The neuroimaging of social phobia is also poorly elaborated, and studies are small and often not replicated. Provocation paradigms that evoke social anxiety symptoms during imaging suggest an increase in activity in areas involved in emotional processing, and possibly in the amygdala.

Course and Prognosis Social phobia has its mean age of onset in late adolescence and early adulthood, and the course is chronic, often lasting decades or longer. The onset of symptoms is usually insidious over months or years and without a clear-cut precipitant. Occasionally, the onset is triggered by a humiliating social experience. Predictors of good outcome in social phobia are onset after age 11, absence of psychiatric comorbidity, and higher educational status.

Generalized Anxiety Disorder

GAD is defined in the *Diagnostic and Statistical Manual of Mental Disorders, 4th edition* (text revision) (*DSM IV-TR*), as excessive anxiety or apprehension occurring more days than not, about a number of things, and lasting at least 6 months. There are three or more associated symptoms, such as feeling restless or keyed up, having difficulty concentrating, feeling easily fatigued or irritable, having muscle tension, and/or experiencing sleep disturbance (including difficulty falling or staying asleep). The anxiety must cause significant distress or impairment of functioning and should not be due to substance use, a medical problem, or another Axis I diagnosis (e.g., worry about dirt and contamination in someone with obsessive-compulsive disorder).

GAD is seen more frequently in women and often starts in the 20s. The lifetime prevalence is approximately 5%. The course may be chronic, with many people reporting years of symptoms before presentation for help. The literature on the course of GAD is sparse. Twin studies suggest that there does seem to be some heritable susceptibility to GAD, with a higher proportion of monozygotic twins being concordant.

There is some evidence that serotonin is involved in GAD. This is partially related to the data from pharmacologic intervention trials that demonstrate efficacy of $5\text{-}HT_{1A}$ partial agonists and $5\text{-}HT_2$ antagonists in the treatment of GAD symptoms. Challenge studies provoking symptoms in GAD patients have been consistent with this. A great deal of exploration is still needed to elaborate this system.

Treatment

Cognitive behavioral therapy (CBT) has been used in treatment of all anxiety disorders. The cognitive therapy is based on finding disordered cognitions (e.g., the expectation of failure or of anxiety), making it explicit, and then helping to find a way to replace it with a different cognition. The basic principle of the behavioral component to the therapy is that anything that triggers is avoided and thus becomes more frightening over time. If it is repeatedly confronted without leading to the anticipated bad or dangerous outcome, it becomes less frightening.

In social phobia, the cognitive work focuses on distorted expectations of negative social outcomes and hypercritical self-evaluations. The behavioral component is based on graded exposure (or systematic desensitization) to increasingly challenging situations to allow desensitization to occur. Groups are quite useful to practice exposure exercises and to help observe and correct other distorted self-assessments, which may lead to improved self-awareness as well. Specific phobias are treated with graded exposure as well. The patient must participate in creating a set of appropriate graded exposures and then practice them through imaging as well as "in the field." The treatment of GAD is less well defined but may respond to similar cognitive work in evaluating distorted expectations, using cognitive restructuring to reinterpret the physical symptoms of anxiety. Relaxation training also may be useful.

Pharmacology

GAD is often treated with buspirone, antidepressants (e.g., SSRIs or tricyclics), and/or benzodiazepines (BZDs). Generalized social phobia may also respond, in part, to antidepressants (e.g., SSRIs, tricyclics, or MAOIs and/or BZDs). In social phobia limited to performance situations, beta-blockers such as propranolol are often employed at low doses before the performance.

CASE CONCLUSION

You and your co-leader decide that the group will use a cognitive behavioral model. In the context of the group each participant will help the others find cognitive distortions and work out plans for graded exposures. In addition, AG, who had a generalized social phobia, started an SSRI; RP, who had a fear of public speaking, was given a prescription for propranolol, to use adjunctively with his graded exposure plan; DB, who had the specific phobia of rats, was not prescribed anything, although when he begins work he may have a short course of BZDs; and ET, who had GAD, had extra "homework" with relaxation exercises and was prescribed an SSRI.

THUMBNAIL: Thumbnail in Behavioral Science-Anti—Anxiety agents

Medication	Mechanism of Action	Metabolism	Side Effects
Buspirone	Serotonin (5-HT$_{1A}$) agonist; suppresses neuronal firing in the dorsal raphe	Primarily by oxidation to hydroxylated derivatives and an active metabolite	Dizziness, light-headedness, headache, little sedation, no tolerance or physical dependence
Benzodiazepines	Allosterically enhance GABA binding, causing increased influx of Cl$^-$ with GABA binding	Most are both demethylated and glucuronidated; lorazepam and oxazepam are only glucuronidated	Dizziness, ataxia, drowsiness, tolerance, physical dependence, confusion, amnesia; those with longer half-lives and active metabolites increase risk of falling among the elderly; withdrawal can lead to seizures
Barbiturates	Allosterically enhances GABA binding (different site than BZDs)	Hepatic, induces P450 enzymes	Tolerance (including cross-tolerance to all CNS depressants), withdrawal, life-threatening respiratory depression in overdose

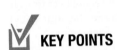 **KEY POINTS**

- *Specific Phobia*
  - Inappropriate persistent, excessive fear of a specific thing or situation.
  - Treatment includes CBT, systematic desensitization, sometimes BZDs.
- *Generalized Social Phobia*
  - Fear of humiliating oneself in a variety of social situations, with social avoidance
  - Treatment includes antidepressants and/or CBT

- *Limited Social Phobia*
  - Fear of humiliating oneself in a particular social situation (e.g., public speaking), with resultant dysfunction
  - Treatment includes beta-blockers, BZDs, and/or CBT
- *Generalized Anxiety Disorder*
  - Excessive anxiety occurring more days than not, about a number of things, lasting at least 6 months with associated physical symptoms
  - Treatment includes buspirone, antidepressants, BZDs, relaxation therapy, and/or CBT

QUESTIONS

Questions 1 and 2 relate to the following clinical scenario:

GZ is a 45-year-old woman who comes in to your office complaining of anxiety. She has restricted her activities, has taken a job where she can work from home, and sees only one long-standing friend and her siblings. She has a pervasive fear of humiliating herself and being ridiculed.

1. Which of the following is her likely diagnosis and what is the probable course?

   A. Social phobia—chronic, long-standing
   B. Social phobia—episodic, long-standing
   C. GAD—chronic, long-standing
   D. GAD—episodic, long-standing
   E. GAD—brief episodes followed by long remissions

2. What can be said about the treatment of this disorder?

   A. Propranolol is an efficacious medication.
   B. SSRIs are efficacious medications.
   C. CBT is not effective.
   D. Long-standing high-dose BZDs are the treatment of choice.
   E. Buspirone is the treatment of choice.

Questions 3 and 4 relate to the following scenario:

When JP is confronted with a social situation, especially a large party or a speaking engagement, he becomes extremely anxious and at times will have palpitations, diaphoresis, nausea, and tremulousness.

3. If he takes a lorazepam prior to the stressful event, he can circumvent these feelings. Which of the following is true about the pharmacology of lorazepam?

   A. It allosterically modulates the serotonin receptor.
   B. It allows an increase in the net efflux of calcium ions from the cell.
   C. It has multiple active metabolites and a half-life of 56 hours.
   D. It will not directly open the GABA receptor.
   E. It is an agonist at the 5-HT$_{1A}$ receptor.

4. His sister gives him some of her benzodiazepine prescription to take prior to her daughter's college graduation party. He is able to tolerate the experience with minimal anxiety. He decides that he wants to take this "all the time" and convinces his doctor to give him enough so he can take it four times a day. Which of the following is a likely adverse effect of this class of medication?

   A. Weight loss
   B. Weight gain
   C. Constipation
   D. Withdrawal seizures
   E. Headaches

HPI: RG is a recently married woman who comes to your office at the urging of her husband. She says that before their marriage she was always extremely neat and orderly, but since they are living together she is miserable because of his habits, and he is "going nuts" because of hers. She describes needing to have things "just so," with all of the CDs, books, and canned foods organized by size and color. She spends at least 2 hours each morning reorganizing these items. In addition, all the picture frames, shades, blinds, rugs, and incidentals (vases, decorative boxes, etc.) must be precisely in the correct place and orientation. This adds at least another hour to her day. She is always vigilant about dirt, allows no shoes or coats into the house, and washes her hands either 14 or 21 times a day, for 7 minutes each time. She worries that the dirt on the coats, bags, or shoes will somehow get into the house and make them sick. She works as an executive secretary and is extremely organized. Her boss, who is also "a bit compulsive," lets her keep the place "however she wants to."

Since her marriage, having her husband come in and move things, put his coat on the couch, inadvertently change the order of the CDs or books, or move things around the apartment makes her intolerably anxious, and she spends most of her evenings following him around "undoing his mess." He has tried to change his habits, but there is no way he can meet her "standards." Before her marriage she always thought of herself as "a little too neat," but now she realizes that her inability to "relax a bit" and allow some variability in her surroundings is excessive and might actually cost her her marriage.

THOUGHT QUESTIONS

- What is the likely etiology of her symptoms?
- What is known about the diagnosis, biology, and treatment of this illness?

BASIC SCIENCE REVIEW AND DISCUSSION

The essential features of **OCD** are obsessions and/or compulsions. In *Diagnostic and Statistical Manual of Mental Disorders, 4th edition* (text revision) (*DSM-IV*-TR), OCD is classified among the anxiety disorders because anxiety is often associated with obsessions. Resistance to compulsions causes anxiety or tension and is often immediately relieved by yielding to compulsions. Common presentations include obsessions about dirt and contamination, with rituals that include compulsive washing and avoidance of contaminated objects; pathologic counting and compulsive checking; obsessions but no compulsions; hoarding for fear of someday needing something discarded; and so on.

An obsession is an intrusive, unwanted mental event usually evoking anxiety or discomfort. Obsessions may be thoughts, ideas, images, or impulses and are often aggressive, sexual, or religious. Much obsessive thinking involves horrific ideas of an aggressive or sexual nature (e.g., rape, murder, child molestation). Obsessional fears often involve dirt or contamination, or harm coming to oneself or to others as a consequence of one's misdoings (e.g., failure to check the door and a killer getting into the house, or running over a pedestrian because of careless driving). Obsessional thinking may also involve persistent doubting. Patients variably try to resist these thoughts, causing significant anxiety or distress. Obsessions are usually accompanied by compulsions but may also occur as the main or only symptom. Approximately 10 to 25% of OCD patients are purely or predominantly obsessional.

Compulsions usually arise to try to control or decrease obsessional thoughts. For instance, excessive washing may arise to address obsessions about contamination, and repeated checking may arise because of persistent doubting. A compulsion usually reduces discomfort but is carried out in a rigid fashion. Compulsions include rituals involving washing, checking, repeating, avoiding, and being meticulous. The most common compulsion is washing, which represents about 25 to 50% of OCD cases. These individuals may spend many hours a day washing their hands, showering, or avoiding germs or bodily wastes. The second most common compulsion is checking. Checkers have pathologic doubt and compulsively check to see if they have run over someone with their car or left the ignition on. Not all compulsions are physically acted out. Mental compulsions include counting or mentally replaying conversations over and over. A rare and disabling form of OCD is called primary obsessional slowness. In this form of the illness it may take many hours to get dressed or get out of the house.

Obsessive-compulsive disorder should be distinguished from obsessive-compulsive personality disorder (see Thumbnail).

Epidemiology

OCD usually begins in adolescence or early adulthood. Almost one third of cases begin between ages 10 and 15 years, with 75% developing by age 30 years. The course is most often chronic. OCD was previously considered one of the rarest mental disorders. Current data suggest that OCD is actually fairly common, with a lifetime prevalence rate of 2.5%. The ratio of males to females is about 1:1, although in childhood-onset OCD, about 70% of patients are male.

Twin and family studies have found a greater degree of concordance for OCD among monozygotic twins compared with dizygotic twins, although there are no studies of OCD in adopted children or monozygotic twins raised apart. Studies of families and first-degree relatives of OCD patients show an increased incidence of anxiety disorders and obsessive-compulsive symptoms. OCD that begins before age 18 is associated with much higher rates of familial OCD. Family studies also suggest a genetic link between OCD and Tourette syndrome. No candidate serotonin-related genes have reliably emerged in familial studies.

Biologic Theories

There is a subset of patients whose symptoms result from a neurologic insult, including abnormal birth events, head injury and seizures, or association with the encephalitis epidemic of 1916–1918 (von Economo encephalitis). In addition, OCD may be associated with a number of subtle neurologic findings, including the presence of neurologic soft signs and abnormalities on electroencephalogram and auditory-evoked potentials.

Recent neuroimaging techniques suggest that orbitofrontal-limbic-basal ganglia circuits are involved in the pathophysiology of OCD. Interestingly, after effective treatment of OCD with serotonin reuptake blockers or with behavior therapy, functional imaging studies have shown a normalization of hyperactivity in areas such as the caudate, orbitofrontal lobes, and cingulate cortex. One hypothesis is that the basal ganglia act as a gating station, filtering input from the orbitofrontal and cingulate cortex and mediating motor patterns. Another theory is that OCD behaviors such as excessive washing or saving may be dysregulated manifestations of normal grooming or hoarding behaviors. The neurotransmitter serotonin has been implicated in the pathophysiology of the illness, particularly because of the therapeutic success of potent serotonin reuptake inhibitors.

Course and Prognosis

Approximately 5 to 10% of those afflicted have periods of remission or even sustained remissions; 5 to 10% may have a progressive, deteriorating course; 30% have a fluctuating course; and more than 50% have a continuous course. Before the use of current modalities, OCD had a poor prognosis. With the use of serotonin reuptake inhibitors and/or behavioral therapy, the prognosis is improved, although up to 30 to 60% may not have a significant clinical response, depending on how response is defined. Untreated, the disorder has a major impact on daily functioning, with some patients spending many waking hours consumed with their obsessions and rituals. This may lead to social isolation, marrying at an older age, and, in males, high celibacy rates. Depression and anxiety are common comorbid disorders with OCD.

Treatment

The principal pharmacologic agents used to treat OCD are the SSRIs, which include, for example, fluoxetine, fluvoxamine and sertraline, and the tricyclic antidepressant clomipramine. In general,

patients may require higher doses of SSRIs to treat OCD than to treat depression. If a patient fails to respond to an SSRI, an antipsychotic medication may serve as an augmenting strategy.

Either alone or in combination with pharmacotherapy, behavioral therapy has been shown to be effective in the treatment of OCD. Overall, 50 to 70% of patients are helped by behavioral therapy. About 20% refuse or cannot tolerate the anxiety that is induced, and another 25% fail to improve for other reasons. Behavioral therapy may have more long-term effects than pharmacology alone, with studies suggesting that up to 75% of people who respond to behavioral therapy continue to do well, although often not symptom-free, after the therapy has ended.

Behavioral therapy is based on the principle of exposure and response prevention. Briefly, the patient is asked to endure the anxiety that an obsession provokes while refraining from acting on the compulsion. For example, the patient with obsessions about contamination would choose a series of graded exposures (e.g., touching a doorknob, touching the floor, touching something in a bathroom) and not wash. By learning to tolerate the anxiety, it will eventually decrease on its own (i.e., habituation will occur) and the need to perform the ritual will eventually disappear. This principle is applied to many types of behavioral therapy and is referred to as **systematic desensitization.** For instance, in the treatment of phobias, patients are asked to create a hierarchy of anxiety-provoking experiences. Through imaging (i.e., imagining the experience) and through actually confronting the experience, the anxiety is tolerated and finally extinguished. This is done in a graduated manner, starting with the least threatening and gradually working up to the most anxiety-provoking exposure.

Occasionally, even with adequate pharmacotherapy and/or behavioral therapy, patients still experience intractable incapacitating symptoms. Obviously, the symptoms must be very severe, and the patient must have proven resistant to multiple psychological and somatic therapies over the course of many years. The success rate is about 50 to 70%. In general, the surgical procedures used (anterior capsulotomy, cingulotomy, and limbic leucotomy) aim to interrupt the connection between the cortex and the basal ganglia and related structures.

CASE CONCLUSION

RG decided to opt for a combination of pharmacotherapy and behavior therapy. She was treated with an SSRI and, with her therapist, devised a series of graded exposures first in the office and then at home. With the combination of these treatment modalities she was able to significantly decrease her time spent on her OCD symptoms and learned how to accept her husband (and his "mess"). Although in times of stress she had some recurrence of her symptoms, she was able to function well with only minimal disruption by her OCD.

THUMBNAIL: Behavioral Science—Obsessive-Compulsive Disorder vs. Obsessive-Compulsive Personality Disorder

Obsessive-Compulsive Disorder	Obsessive-Compulsive Personality Disorder
Obsessions	No obsessions
Compulsions	No compulsions
Ego dystonic (incompatible with the individual's self-concept)	Ego syntonic (compatible with the individual's self-concept)
Obsessions and compulsions are time-consuming and interfere with daily functioning	Personality style that is inflexible, perfectionistic, and detail oriented

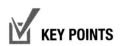 **KEY POINTS**

- **Obsessions:** Recurrent and persistent thoughts, impulses, or images cause marked anxiety or distress. They are not excessive worries about real-life problems. The person attempts to either ignore or suppress them, or to neutralize them with some other thoughts or actions.

- **Compulsions:** Repetitive behaviors or mental acts that the person feels driven to perform in response to an obsession, or according to rigid rules. The acts are aimed at preventing or reducing distress or neutralizing or preventing the obsessions and are clearly excessive.

- In the **diagnosis** of OCD, the obsessions or compulsions cause marked distress, are time-consuming (e.g., take more than 1 hour per day), or interfere significantly with the person's normal routine and social, occupational, or academic functioning.

- The orbitofrontal-limbic-basal ganglia circuits are implicated in OCD, and serotonin is thought to be the major neurotransmitter affected.

- The pharmacologic treatment of OCD is with SSRIs. Antipsychotics occasionally may be used as augmentation. Behavioral therapy is also effective. In rare cases of resistant, incapacitating OCD, psychosurgery is used.

QUESTIONS

1. PJ presented to the dermatologist for a cream for a rash on his hands. Upon exam his hands were red, irritated, and dry. He had no other manifestations on other parts of his body. In reviewing his habits, he admitted to washing his hands 50 or more times per day. His work in a hospital made him acutely aware of and concerned about germs and contamination. He is worried that if he does not continually wash, he will make his family or himself sick. He avoids touching most surfaces with his hands (e.g., doorknobs), and if he does he has to wash. Each time he washes he spends 10 minutes. If he is prevented from washing he becomes very anxious and upset. Which of the following would probably be the most beneficial treatment of his condition?

   A. Recommend that he not wash so frequently.
   B. Explain that he is causing the condition by his excessive washing.
   C. Educate him about universal precautions and when to wear latex gloves.
   D. Set up a structured program of exposure and response prevention.
   E. Encourage him to take a microbiology course to better understand which pathogens are harmful.

2. FD is a 22-year-old student who comes for an evaluation because of increased difficulty completing his work. He explains that when he reads he becomes overwhelmed with the idea that he has missed a paragraph or a page and thus reads everything six times. He has recently found it harder to get to class in the morning because he needs to check that the hot plate is off, the door is locked, his books are in a certain order, and his shoes are lined up in a particular way. He admits that he has an irrational fear that if things aren't perfect his dorm room will catch on fire or that something terrible will happen to his parents or brother. Which of the following neurotransmitter systems has been most consistently implicated in this disorder?

   A. Serotonin
   B. Norepinephrine
   C. Acetylcholine
   D. GABA
   E. Dopamine

Questions 3 and 4 relate to the following case:

SD is plagued with the notion that she has run over a child in her car or has inadvertently killed a baby. She stopped driving 5 years ago, but before that she would need to stop every block and get out to reassure herself that she had not hurt anyone. Whenever she saw a child in the street she would stare at him or her to convince herself that the child was well and unharmed. She has two grown children who are well, and she has never hurt anyone, child or adult, in her life. She has suffered from intrusive thoughts on and off throughout her adult life, but now, in her 40s, she spends hours every day plagued with these thoughts and horrific images of mutilated children or children crushed under the wheel of a car. This has been significantly interfering with her life and ability to function at work or socially over the past few years. She has had multiple psychiatric admissions because of her distress.

3. Which of the following is an appropriate treatment strategy?

   A. Decreasing her current SSRI medication (fluvoxamine)
   B. Adding lithium to her therapy
   C. Adding methylphenidate to her treatment
   D. High-dose clozapine therapy
   E. Adding behavioral therapy to her treatment

4. Assuming that she has failed multiple adequate treatment regimens and augmentation strategies, what is a possible treatment option for refractory OCD?

   A. Occipital lobe ablation
   B. Surgery on the cingulate cortex
   C. Frontal lobotomy
   D. High-dose desipramine therapy
   E. Augmentation of fluoxetine with an acetylcholinesterase inhibitor

HPI: EC is a 68-year-old woman who was brought to her doctor because of increasing confusion. Her family says that she was doing well living in an assisted-living apartment until yesterday, when she started to "act strangely." She called her daughters from her home and asked them about the family cat (who had died years ago) and when she was going to go home. She has no significant medical history. The assisted facility's nursing staff brought her to the ER for evaluation. Upon arrival in the ER, she fluctuated between being lucid and being agitated, disoriented, and confused.

PE: She is alert and oriented to person only. On exam, she has decreased breath sounds on the right. Her chest x-ray reveals a right middle lobe infiltrate. Her labs are all normal except for a WBC count of 15.

THOUGHT QUESTIONS

- What is wrong with this woman?
- What is the likely etiology of her cognitive problems?

BASIC SCIENCE REVIEW AND DISCUSSION

EC has pneumonia. Her change in mental status is probably due to **delirium.** Delirium is characterized by an acute, fluctuating change in mental status. Delirious patients exhibit reduced awareness of the environment, altered levels of consciousness, and reduced ability to focus attention. Delirium may be associated with perceptual disturbances in any modality (frequently tactile or visual) and with delusions, which are often disorganized and paranoid. The patient may be agitated, or psychomotorically retarded, may have a disturbance in the sleep-wake cycle, and may be emotionally labile. Symptom severity can fluctuate significantly.

Delirium is often undetected. As many as 70% of cases may go undiagnosed or untreated by physicians. Delirium generally presents in an acute or subacute manner (i.e., over hours or days), an important distinction that may help to distinguish it from **dementia,** which (except in the case of poststroke dementia) usually has an insidious gradual onset over months to years.

Epidemiology of Delirium

Risk factors for delirium include advancing age, dementia, drug/alcohol use, brain damage, chronic or severe physical illness, sensory impairment, and medications. Children may also be at greater risk. The prevalence of delirium in older persons living in the community is approximately 1%. In hospitalized inpatients the prevalence of delirium is approximately 10 to 25%. In hospitalized patients with dementia it may be up to 40%. In general, delirium is more frequent in post-coronary artery bypass graft (CABG) and in patients who have had hip surgery, in burn patients, and in people with low serum albumin (which can lead to increased free fractions of drugs). Of course, it is also frequently seen in people intoxicated with or withdrawing from various substances, most commonly alcohol or BZDs. Delirium can last from less than a week to more than a month. It is often more protracted in the elderly.

Delirium is associated with increased mortality rates during hospitalization and after discharge. It also is associated with increased hospital length of stay, increased healthcare expenditures, poor function, caregiver burden, persistent cognitive impairment, and increased costs for rehabilitation, institutionalization, and home care. In elderly patients, estimates of the risk of death during the incident hospitalization are 22 to 75%. Studies have also found a link between in-hospital delirium and functional decline, need for nursing home placement, increased length of stay, and so on. Thus, it is very important to recognize a delirium and treat the underlying cause.

Pathophysiology and Etiology

The pathophysiology of delirium is unclear. Dysfunction of the reticular activating system has been implicated, as has a reduction in CNS oxidative metabolism leading to neurotransmitter abnormalities and increased cerebral cytokines that impair neurotransmitter system function, neuronal signal transduction, and second messenger systems. In addition, older persons are at increased risk of delirium due to age-related changes in brain neurochemistry and pharmacodynamic and pharmacokinetic alterations in the metabolism and excretion of medications.

The etiologies of delirium are diverse. The following list provides a sample. The etiology of delirium is most often multifactorial but frequently involves medications.

- *Medications, drugs, pesticides, solvents*
  - Many medications are associated with delirium and psychotic symptoms, including NSAIDs, quinolones, and H2 blockers.
  - Many medications have anticholinergic side effects that can be cumulative. Medications that are not traditionally thought of as anticholinergic, such as cimetidine, meperidine, and prednisolone, do have some anticholinergic activity.
  - Drug-drug interactions (e.g., change of free fraction of drugs by protein-binding interactions or alterations in P450 metabolism) may cause a delirium.
- *Cardiovascular*—hypertensive encephalopathy, hypoperfusion
- *Intracranial bleeding*—especially with focal neurologic signs
- *Infections*—meningitis/encephalitis, sepsis, pneumonia, and in patients with dementia, even a UTI
- *Withdrawal* from various substances, including alcohol, BZDs, and barbiturates
  - Alcohol withdrawal is usually seen 24 to 96 hours after the last drink and is associated with autonomic hyperactivity (tachycardia, diaphoresis, HTN)
  - BZD withdrawal has similar signs and symptoms as alcohol withdrawal. The time required for symptoms of BZD withdrawal to develop depends on the half-life of the specific BZD.
  - Delirium tremens often has associated prominent visual or tactile hallucinations and seizures. The mortality of delirium tremens, if untreated, is about 20%.

- *Wernicke encephalopathy* (confusion, ataxia, lateral gaze paralysis)
  - Most commonly seen in alcoholics
  - Due to thiamine deficiency
  - If not immediately treated with IV thiamine it can progress to irreversible Korsakoff dementia (confusion, retrograde and anterograde amnesia). Remember that thiamine should always be given before glucose, so as to avoid precipitation of Wernicke encephalopathy.

- *Metabolic*—acid-base disturbances, electrolyte abnormalities, liver or kidney failure, hypoglycemia
- *Paraneoplastic syndromes* (sometimes called limbic encephalopathy) secondary to a number of neoplasms, including ovarian, small cell, thymoma, seminoma, testicular
- *Miscellaneous*—sleep deprivation, overstimulation in an ICU

CASE CONCLUSION

EC was diagnosed with delirium secondary to pneumonia. After a course of IV antibiotics her mental status improved. She was able to concentrate, was oriented to time and place, and had no more ruminations or confusion about the cat. She was able to return to her assisted-living situation with the same minimal level of care that she had before admission.

THUMBNAIL: Behavioral Science—Differentiating Delirium from Dementia

Delirium	Dementia
Impaired level of consciousness	Level of consciousness not impaired
Acute or subacute onset	Usually insidious onset over months to years
Marked fluctuation in symptoms	Symptoms more stable over time
Frequently reversible	Rarely reversible (~5%)
May have marked autonomic dysfunction	No autonomic dysfunction

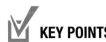

KEY POINTS

- *Risk factors:* Age (young children or elderly), dementia, drug/alcohol use, brain damage, chronic or severe physical illness, sensory impairment, and medications
- *Prevalence:* Hospitalized inpatients—10 to 25%; hospitalized patients with dementia—40%
- *Course:* Days to more than a month; more protracted in the elderly
- Delirium is associated with increased morbidity and mortality rates during hospitalization and after discharge
- Delirium is often underrecognized and often confused with dementia; remember that delirium, unlike dementia, typically has an acute onset

QUESTIONS

1. LS is a 75-year-old woman who was brought to her internist by her son. He notes that over the past week she has been more confused, at times hallucinating about a man coming into her apartment at night. On exam she is noted to be flushed, have a dry mouth, and to complain of constipation and blurry vision. She started a new medication within the past 2 weeks. Which of the following medications is most likely responsible for her symptoms?

A. Atenolol
B. Warfarin
C. Diphenhydramine
D. Diazepam
E. Ranitidine

2. A 56-year-old man is brought into the ER by the police after he was found staggering and incoherent in the train station. On exam he is ataxic, confused, and has lateral gaze paralysis. What treatment should be instituted immediately?

A. IV folic acid
B. IV thiamine
C. IV glucose
D. Oxygen
E. IV diazepam

3. A 45-year-old woman is admitted to the hospital for a broken leg. Two days after admission she becomes confused and begins to complain that groups of children are coming into her room and laughing at her. Later she tells you that she needs to pull her car out of the parking space and that you are blocking her way. She also is markedly tremulous, hypertensive, and tachycardic. What is the most likely etiology of her symptoms?

   A. New-onset schizophrenia
   B. Mania brought on by general anesthesia
   C. An adverse reaction to antibiotics
   D. Cocaine intoxication
   E. Alcohol withdrawal

4. An 83-year-old man has been admitted to the hospital for a UTI. On admission he is confused, disoriented, and disheveled. On exam, he is febrile and is intermittently irritable and falling asleep. He is treated for his infection with IV antibiotics and is rehydrated and discharged. At a follow-up visit 1 month later with his internist, he is able to sustain his attention and is able to groom himself but remains disorientated to time and the name of the street where his doctor is located; in addition, he cannot remember three words in 5 minutes. Otherwise, his neurologic exam is normal. In talking to the son, what is the most likely history? He was:

   A. Cognitively normal, working as a lawyer, and had a sudden onset of symptoms prior to hospitalization
   B. A retired lawyer, has impaired short-term memory, has been unable to pay his bills for the last year, but has been living independently; he experienced acute worsening of symptoms before hospitalization
   C. A retired lawyer and needed to move to a nursing home 4 years ago; there was no appreciable change in his cognition and behavior on admission
   D. A boxer who was knocked unconscious multiple times, with an acute worsening of cognitive symptoms before admission
   E. A man with a large middle cerebral artery stroke 1 year ago; he experienced acute worsening of his symptoms on admission

CASE 8-6 | Dementia

HPI: JD is a 79-year-old retired lawyer who is brought in by his wife for an evaluation of his memory. They note that he has been having difficulty with short-term memory, often forgetting what his wife told him hours before. He often asks her the same questions repeatedly, for instance, about social engagements or family concerns. He also describes that his desk and financial affairs, which were always immaculately organized, have become less so, to the point that last month he forgot to pay the electric bill and his broker had to call him three times to decide what to do with the money from a bond that was coming due. He was an avid bird watcher and notes that for the last 6 months he has been having problems naming the birds that he sees. He has no significant medical problems, his physical exam and laboratory work-up, including thyroid, vitamin levels, hepatic function, renal function, and blood counts, are all unremarkable.

THOUGHT QUESTIONS

- What is wrong with this gentleman?
- Given his normal physical, history, and lab results, what is the likely etiology of his problems?

BASIC SCIENCE REVIEW AND DISCUSSION

This gentleman meets criteria for dementia (see below) with deficits in short-term memory and difficulties with executive functioning and language. Given his history and work-up, he most likely has Alzheimer disease (AD).

Diagnosis and Epidemiology of Dementia

Dementia is defined as the presence of consistent deficits in short-term memory, coupled with a decline in another area of cognitive function—**aphasia** (impaired or absent comprehension or production of speech, writing, or signs), **apraxia** (difficulty in carrying out familiar purposeful movements not due to physical limitations [e.g., severe arthritis]), **agnosia** (impairment of ability to recognize or comprehend the meaning of various sensory stimuli), or disturbance of **executive function** (e.g., planning, organizing, sequencing, abstracting). Such cognitive deficits must cause marked impairment in social or occupational function and must represent a significant decline from a previous level of functioning. These deficits may not occur exclusively during the course of a delirium.

Dementia may be due to a medical condition (e.g., stroke, AD, Parkinson disease), the enduring effects of substance use (e.g., alcohol, toxins), or a combination of etiologies. The prevalence of moderate to severe dementia in different population groups is approximately 5% in the general population older than age 65 year; 20 to 40% in the general population older than age 85 years; 15 to 20% in outpatient general medical practices; and 50% in chronic care facilities.

The course of dementia varies according to the etiology, but most dementias are progressive. The following descriptions discuss general syndromes, although the actual presentation of diseases can vary enormously. Diseases that affect the cortical areas (such as Alzheimer or Pick disease) usually present with significant memory symptoms and difficulties in language, praxis, and executive functioning. Diseases that are primarily subcortical, such as Parkinson disease and Binswanger disease, often have prominent apathy, movement disorders, and less severe memory difficulties. Disorders affecting the frontal lobes, such as Pick disease, often have marked disinhibition, other personality changes, and slowed movement and thought. Dementias may be complicated by behavioral disturbances (e.g., wandering, hallucinations, paranoia, and aggression). These are more prevalent in the moderate and severe stages of disease. In the terminal stage patients may be contracted, immobile, incontinent, unable to swallow properly, unable to clear their secretions, and prone to pressure ulcers. Infections are usually the proximal cause of death (e.g., pneumonias, urosepsis, infected ulcers).

Etiology

The most common causes of dementia in individuals older than age 65 years are AD (which accounts for approximately 60%), vascular dementia (15%), and mixed vascular and Alzheimer dementia (15%). Other illnesses account for approximately 10%, including Pick disease, normal-pressure hydrocephalus, alcoholic dementia, infectious dementia such as HIV or neurosyphilis, prion diseases such as Creutzfeldt-Jakob disease (CJD), tumors, and Parkinson disease (see Thumbnail below). Some sources suggest that up to 5% of dementias evaluated in clinical settings may be attributable to reversible causes, such as metabolic abnormalities (e.g., hypothyroidism), nutritional deficiencies (e.g., vitamin B12 or folate deficiencies), or dementia syndrome due to depression. The dementia syndrome due to depression was previously referred to as pseudodementia.

The diagnosis of dementia is made by taking a careful history and using selected diagnostic tests. The clinical history should always be corroborated with a family member or other knowledgeable informant, as patients with memory disorders are often poor historians. The history and physical serve to evaluate various exposures, risk factors, potentially reversible etiologies, and neurologic findings (e.g., focal neurologic signs). A family history of dementia is particularly important in early-onset AD or other known genetically transmitted diseases, such as Huntington chorea.

Genetic Causes

Various etiologies of dementia are thought to have a genetic basis (e.g. Huntington disease). The genetics of AD is more complicated. There are known mutations on chromosomes 1, 14, and 21, which account for approximately 2% of all AD cases. These mutations are seen primarily in early-onset patients with strong family histories of AD, and they tend to be transmitted in an autosomal dominant pattern. The gene for Alzheimer precursor protein (APP) is coded on chromosome 21, and people with Down syndrome (trisomy 21) universally exhibit the microscopic pathology of AD as they age. The other two genes, on chromosome 1 and 14, code for presenilins, which are thought to be involved in APP processing.

Late-onset AD is also thought to have a genetic component. The precise genetic contributions have not been defined, but part of this is attributable to the effects of polymorphisms in the ApoE gene coded on chromosome 19. ApoE plays a role in redistribution of lipids associated with neurodegeneration, and promotes Aβ deposition into plaque (see possible etiologies below). The gene has three major alleles, ε2, ε3, and ε4, which code for the apo E2, E3, and E4 isoforms, respectively. The ε4 allele has been found in up to 50% of AD patients, versus 16% of controls, and the rare ε2 allele may be protective against illness development. A gene dosage effect exists, strengthening the association. Homozygosity for ε4 conferred an eight-fold increased risk over ε3/ε3 and a sixteen-fold increased risk over ε2/ε3.

Alzheimer Disease—Possible Etiologies

Overproduction or decreased clearance of Aβ (also called β-amyloid) is implicated as a central process in the pathophysiology of AD. Aβ is formed by processing of APP via the β- and γ-secretase enzymes. Aβ easily aggregates into β-pleated sheets, which aggregate to form insoluble extracellular amyloid plaque. All the known familial mutations (discussed earlier) are associated with an increase in Aβ production. APP can also be cleaved by the nonamyloidogenic α-secretase, which does not form toxic Aβ and releases soluble APP into circulation.

The other neuropathologic hallmark of AD is paired helical filaments of hyperphosphorylated τ (tau) seen in intracellular neurofibrillary tangles. τ is a CNS protein that is involved in microtubular assembly. Microtubules are vital to normal neurotransport, and the abnormal τ interferes with that process.

Many neurochemical deficits are observed in AD, but abnormalities in the cholinergic system are most consistently described. **Choline acetyltransferase activity is substantially reduced** in patients with AD, and this has been confirmed on autopsy of patients with at least a moderate stage of the illness, but not in patients with mild illness.

The diagnosis of AD is confirmed on autopsy. Macroscopically, the brains of early AD patients may appear grossly normal. As the disease progresses, widened sulci and increased ventricular size are seen. Atrophy in the temporal, parietal, and frontal lobes is often most prominent. The atrophy is due to neuronal loss, with up to 10% of the large neocortical neurons lost, primarily in the frontal and temporal lobes. Microscopically, the characteristic lesions of AD are **amyloid plaques and neurofibrillary tangles.** The early stages begin with relatively selective involvement of the entorhinal cortex and hippocampus. Later stages involve other areas of the limbic lobes and finally the neocortex. Plaque contains an amyloid core that is composed of β-pleated sheets of the peptide Aβ. The central core is surrounded by dystrophic neuritis, microglial cells, and reactive astrocytes. Neurofibrillary tangles are intracellular inclusion bodies, containing paired helical filaments composed of abnormally phosphorylated tau. Plaques and tangles are not unique to AD and are observed in other illnesses, but the presence of the two together in abnormally high density is pathognomonic for AD.

Alzheimer Disease—Management

The two strategies that are currently used in the management of the cognitive decline in AD are replacement and neuroprotection. Replacement strategies focus on the neurochemical deficits in AD (such as acetylcholine), whereas neuroprotective strategies aim to retard the progression of the illness by slowing further neuronal injury or loss.

The only class of drugs currently FDA approved for the treatment of AD are the acetylcholinesterase inhibitors (AChEIs). These medicines decrease the breakdown of acetylcholine in the synapse, increasing the effective amount of acetylcholine (ACh) available, and are generally associated with a clinical improvement of approximately 6 to 12 months' duration. After this, the patient continues to decline at a rate similar to that of untreated patients. The agents currently available are tacrine, donepezil, rivastigmine, and galantamine. The common side effects of this class of medications include nausea and diarrhea, although with gradual titration they are usually mild.

The most commonly used agent for neuroprotective effect is vitamin E, probably for its antioxidant properties. Vitamin E was shown in one double-blind randomized clinical trial to increase the time for moderate-stage patients to reach a poor outcome, suggesting a slowing of illness progression.

Other Dementias

Vascular dementia is the second most common cause of dementia after AD. The symptomatology depends on the areas of infarction. Vascular dementia may be distinguished from AD by its relatively sudden onset, its focal neurologic signs, its history of stroke, and the likely presence of multiple risk factors for cerebrovascular disease.

Binswanger disease, a vascular dementia, is characterized by microinfarctions of white matter with sparing of the cortex. It is a subcortical dementia with executive dysfunction, inattention, memory loss, slowed motor function, ataxia, incontinence, and loss of verbal fluency. Apathy, behavioral disturbance, and parkinsonian symptoms are also common findings.

Dementia with Lewy bodies (DLB) is a progressive dementia with parkinsonian symptoms and fluctuation in the level of attention and the severity of the cognitive deficits and visual hallucinations. Delusions and sensitivity to the side effects of neuroleptic medications are common. The exact prevalence is unknown, but it may be the third most prevalent dementia. Lewy bodies are eosinophilic intracytoplasmic structures and are composed of ubiquitin or alpha-synuclein. The presence of Lewy bodies in AD portends a more malignant course.

Frontotemporal dementia includes a heterogeneous group of sporadic and familial diseases that result in personality and behavioral changes, with variable degrees of language and cognitive impairment, including Pick disease, primary progressive aphasia, semantic dementia, and corticobasal degeneration. Frontotemporal dementias account for 5 to 20% of degenerative dementias. The age of onset ranges from 35 to 75 years. Pick disease is characterized by Pick cells, which appear swollen and stain pink with hematoxylin-eosin.

AIDS dementia complex (ADC) is seen in patients with advanced AIDS and is associated with high viral load. Before the introduction of HAARTs, ADC developed in 60% of patients. Now the incidence is less than 10% of AIDS patients. ADC is probably related to neuronal loss. The neuropathologic findings include diffuse inflammatory changes with microscopic foamy macrophages and multinucleated giant cells that invade subcortical white matter. ADC is characterized by cognitive decline and motor slowing; HIV is also associated with many CNS opportunistic infections.

Dementia due to Parkinson disease occurs in 20 to 30% of patients. The typical age of onset of Parkinson disease is 50 to 60 years. This dementia affects executive functioning and memory. Pathology reveals Lewy bodies in the cytoplasm of neurons in the substantia nigra. Classic symptoms of Parkinson disease include shuffling gait, "pill-rolling" tremor, decreased arm swing, and dysdiadochokinesia.

Dementia due to Huntington disease typically begins between the ages of 25 and 50 years. More trinucleotide repeats are correlated with earlier age of onset. Huntington disease is transmitted in an autosomal dominant pattern with complete penetrance and results from an unstable trinucleotide repeat sequence (CAG) on chromosome 4. Damage occurs through neuronal loss in the caudate nucleus and putamen by an unknown mechanism.

Huntington disease is characterized by psychiatric symptoms and cognitive impairment followed by the classic choreoathetoid movements. Psychopathology may include depression, psychosis, anxiety, and personality changes. Cognitive impairment is gradual and progressive. Initial symptoms may include mild memory deficits with subtle difficulty in executive functioning. Complex task performance worsens as the disease progresses, as do learning and verbal and visuospatial abilities.

Dementia due to CJD (aka "mad cow disease") occurs as a result of one of a group of rare but fatal neurodegenerative diseases. Transmissible spongiform encephalopathy results from CJD, Gerstmann-Straussler-Scheinker disease, fatal familial insomnia, bovine spongiform encephalopathy, and kuru. These diseases are caused by a *proteinaceous infectious particle*, or prion. Prions may incubate for decades before symptoms emerge. Transmission is through invasive body contact, such as corneal transplants, contaminated surgical instruments, cannibalism, or the ingestion of infected animal products. The infection produces a diffuse neurodegenerative process characterized by dementia, hypertonicity, and electroencephalographic changes. The progression is rapid, and death typically ensues within a year. Histopathology is diagnostic and shows neuronal loss, astrocyte proliferation, and a resultant spongiform appearance to the gray matter of the cortex, striatum, and thalamus. CJD is extremely rare.

CASE CONCLUSION

JD clearly has a dementia because he has difficulty with short-term memory, executive functioning, and mild difficulty with language. Given his negative work-up for other causes and his gradual and progressive course, his most likely diagnosis is AD. He was treated with a cholinesterase inhibitor and vitamin E, which had a modest effect in improving his cognitive functioning. He and his family were encouraged to discuss healthcare proxy and advanced directives with their internist, and were referred to the Alzheimer's Association for more information about financial planning and support groups available in the community.

THUMBNAIL: Behavioral Science—Possible Etiologies of Dementia

Degenerative dementias	AD Frontotemporal dementias (e.g., Pick disease) Parkinson disease Lewy body dementia Progressive supranuclear palsy
Cardiac/vascular/anoxia	Infarction Binswanger disease Hemodynamic insufficiency (e.g., hypoxia, hypoperfusion)
Tumor	Primary or metastatic (e.g., meningioma, metastatic breast or lung cancer)
Trauma	For example, dementia pugilistica, subdural hematoma
Metabolic/nutritional	Vitamin deficiencies (e.g., vitamin B12, folate) Endocrinopathies (e.g., hypothyroidism) Chronic metabolic disturbances (e.g., uremia)
Infection	AIDS Neurosyphilis Prion diseases (e.g., Creutzfeldt-Jakob, bovine spongiform encephalitis)
Drugs/toxins	Alcohol Heavy metals Irradiation Pseudodementia due to medications

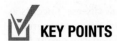
KEY POINTS

- *Neuropathologic and neurochemical hallmarks of AD*
  - Plaque—extracellular, made primarily of Aβ, seen very early in the disease in the hippocampus
  - Tangles—intracellular dystrophic neuritis with paired helical filaments of hyperphosphorylated τ protein
  - As the disease progresses, atrophy and ventricular enlargement are seen
  - In moderate-stage disease or more advanced disease, a loss of cholinergic neurons and a decrease in choline acetyltransferase are seen on autopsy

- *Genetics of AD*
  - Known mutations, usually associated with early-onset disease (<65 years) are on chromosomes 1, 14, and 21
  - The ApoE gene has polymorphisms (ε2, ε3, ε4), which seem to modify risk of developing AD
  - The ApoE ε4 gene confers the greatest risk, whereas the ε2 gene may be protective

QUESTIONS

Questions 1 and 2 relate to the following case:

WS is a 75-year-old woman who was brought in by her daughter for evaluation of her memory. She noted that her mother has been more forgetful over the past year but until recently had been paying her bills. Three months ago the daughter had gone to her house instead of meeting at a restaurant and was appalled at the stacks of papers, memberships, bills, and solicitations for contributions that were piled up on the desk. Since that time she has taken over financial management. She also noticed that her mother would repeat questions, forget conversations, and could no longer do the crossword puzzle.

1. Which of the following would be appropriate diagnostic tests?

   A. RPR, total body CT scan, TSH levels, vitamin K
   B. Vitamin C levels, RPR, MRI of the brain, TSH levels
   C. Vitamin B12 levels, RPR, MRI of the brain, TSH levels
   D. Total body CT scan, TSH levels, RPR, vitamin B12
   E. Ceruloplasmin, RPR, MRI of the brain

2. WS underwent all the appropriate testing above, as well as renal and hepatic function tests, a CBC, and a physical and neurologic exam, which were all unremarkable. Having ruled out other etiologies of dementia, she is presumed to have AD. Which of the following statements is most likely true?

   A. She has a mutation on chromosome 1.
   B. She has a mutation on chromosome 21.

   C. She has an ApoE ε4 allele.
   D. She has an ApoE ε2 allele.
   E. She has trinucleotide repeats on chromosome 4.

3. An 85-year-old woman died of pneumonia. Her sons requested an autopsy because they wanted a definitive diagnosis of her 8-year history of memory loss. At the time of her death she was incontinent, needed assistance in all of her activities of daily living, and often did not recognize her sons. Which of the following neuropathologic findings would confirm a diagnosis of AD?

   A. Alpha-synuclein containing intracellular inclusion bodies
   B. Astrogliosis, neuronal loss, and spongiform change
   C. Ischemic periventricular leukoencephalopathy
   D. Increased choline acetyltransferase
   E. Intracellular paired helical filaments of hyperphosphorylated τ protein

4. An 83-year-old man has had a stroke. His symptoms include irritability, impulsivity with poor executive functioning, and a marked change in his personality. Which area of the brain does the stroke most likely affect?

   A. Frontal
   B. Temporal
   C. Occipital
   D. Parietal
   E. Brainstem

HPI: KR is a 22-year-old female college junior who is brought in to the student health service by her roommates because they found her superficially cutting her arms with a razor blade when they came home from a dinner. She told them that she was "fine," but they insisted on bringing her into urgent care. Upon questioning you find that she felt "lonely and empty" when her roommates went out together to a dinner and that cutting herself made her feel more "real." She denies current suicidal ideation, although she admits to feeling suicidal in the past, with two overdoses at the time relationships were nearing an end. She took a leave of absence from college after the second suicide attempt. She returned to school 7 months ago. She admits that her relationships with friends and boyfriends are usually volatile, sometimes extremely close, sometimes with angry fights. She explains that it has been difficult because she has terrible troubles with self-image, can "never figure out who [she is]," and has had multiple problems with binge alcohol use, impulsive promiscuous sex, and binge eating and vomiting. She denies current bulimic behaviors. She has engaged in these self-mutilatory "cutting" behaviors since age 14. She was only in therapy once, briefly, after the second attempt.

THOUGHT QUESTIONS

- What is the likely diagnosis of this woman?
- Does she meet criteria for a personality disorder?

BASIC SCIENCE REVIEW AND DISCUSSION

This woman meets criteria for **borderline personality disorder (BPD).** *Diagnostic and Statistical Manual of Mental Disorders, 4th edition* (text revision) (*DSM-IV*-TR), defines BPD as a pervasive pattern, beginning in early adulthood, of instability of interpersonal relationships, self-image, and affect, associated with marked impulsivity. It must be present in a variety of contexts and may include frantic efforts to avoid real or imagined abandonment, unstable self-image, reckless impulsivity (e.g., sex, substance abuse, binging), mood instability, recurrent suicidal or self-mutilatory behavior, chronic feelings of emptiness, inappropriate intense anger, marked swings in interpersonal relationships that swing from idealizing to devaluing, and transient stress-related paranoia or severe dissociation.

Personality disorders, classified by the DSM-IV as Axis II disorders, represent pervasive maladaptive pattern of behaviors that begin in early adulthood and affect functioning. People with personality disorders do not necessarily see these symptoms/behaviors as an illness, or as alien to themselves, and therefore often do not seek treatment.

In general, there are three clusters of personality disorders as defined by the *DSM-IV*. **Cluster A, the "odd" cluster,** is comprised of paranoid, schizoid, and schizotypal personality disorders. This cluster is characterized by disturbance of interpersonal relatedness and cognitive function. **Cluster B, the "dramatic" cluster,** consists of histrionic, narcissistic, borderline, and antisocial personality disorders. It is characterized by disturbance of affective stability and impulsivity, with dramatic emotional expressiveness. **Cluster C, the "anxious" cluster,** is avoidant, dependent, and obsessive-compulsive personality disorders. It is characterized by the constriction of assertiveness and sociability in the service of avoiding anxiety.

Borderline Personality Disorder

The cluster B disorders are associated with the greatest morbidity and mortality. There are various theories about the pathogenesis of personality disorders and various theories by which to understand them. Psychoanalytic theory (especially Otto Kernberg) describes borderline personality structure as characterized by ego weakness (lack of impulse control, lack of anxiety tolerance, blurred self-other boundaries, occasional distorted reality testing), problematic object relations (seeing the same "object" as all good or all bad), immature defense mechanisms (e.g., splitting), and a fragmentary self-concept. These are seen at various immature phases of normal development, but in a personality disorder they persist. The psychobiologic approach sees personality disorders as an interaction of temperament (which has a strong genetic component) with character (which is formed more by family and other environmental influences). Family life and other environmental influences help form character, which allows the person, with his or her own unique temperament, to interact with the world. Thus, a person who is quite impulsive and novelty seeking could either be self-directed and cooperative and become a successful entrepreneur or be goal-less, undisciplined, and uncooperative and end up with a personality disorder. Studies show that maturation increases self-directedness and cooperation, leading to a decline in impulsivity and "acting out" with age.

Impulsive Aggression

A common component of many of the cluster B personality disorders is impulsive aggression. It is important to understand that impulsive aggression, whether self- or other-directed, is associated with decreased serotonergic activity, as reflected in reduced CSF 5-hydroxy indoleacetic acid (5-HIAA), and reduced prefrontal metabolic activity in response to serotonergic agents. The prefrontal cortex is implicated in aggression, as was seen by the famous case of Phineas Gage, who was a calm, capable, and efficient person who became irascible and impulsive following injury to the orbital frontal cortex (in a freak accident on a railroad construction site that left him with a tamping iron blown through his head).

Epidemiology/Course

BPD occurs in 2 to 3% of the general population. The male:female ratio is 1:3. It is five times more common in first-degree relatives than in the general population. The mortality is approximately 10%. The course often shows greatest instability and impulsivity in early adult years, often improving in the 30s and 40s. It is also associated with physical or sexual abuse in childhood. The morbidity of this disorder is high because of associated behaviors and disorders, such as impulsive promiscuity, reckless behaviors, substance use, depression, bulimia, other self-destructive or self-mutilatory behaviors, suicidality, and suicidal attempts.

Treatment

Medications may be useful in borderline or other personality disorders. In general, they are used to treat some of the comorbid axis I disorders. Some core symptoms of disorders may respond to medication. For instance, the impulsive aggression in borderline and antisocial personality may respond to SSRIs. In general, cognitive and behavioral approaches are often useful, as is group therapy. Since these are personality constructs, the support, reflection, and confrontation by other group members may be particularly useful. In BPD, various individual and group methods have been used to help patients find alternative ways to deal with feelings of emptiness, abandonment, depression, or anger rather than substance use or self-mutilation.

CASE CONCLUSION

KR meets criteria for BPD. She denies Axis I symptoms of major depression or an eating disorder. Because of her history of binging and vomiting, you check her electrolytes, which are within normal limits; she has no other stigmata of bulimia (e.g., parotid enlargement) and is of normal weight. Her cuts are superficial and do not require suturing. While she is in the ER, she is labeled as a "difficult patient," as she is somewhat seductive and idealizing of the medical student who examined her wrist and hostile and devaluing to the nurse and the ER resident. You note this behavior, evaluate her, and talk to her about her experiences and behaviors but decide not to admit her. She agrees to come in the following day to begin outpatient CBT.

THUMBNAIL: Behavioral Science—Review of Personality Disorders

Cluster	Disorder	Features	Epidemiology	Comments
Cluster A "Odd"	Paranoid	Suspiciousness over interpreting others' motivations or actions	0.5–2.5% of the population M > F	Experience of their paranoid symptoms as ego syntonic (part of who they are), thus rarely seek treatment
	Schizoid	Detached, restricted range of affect; disinterest in social relationships	0.5–7% of the population Possibly M > F Possible family association with schizophrenia	Experience of their symptoms as ego syntonic
	Schizotypal	Discomfort with and reduced capacity for close relationships, cognitive and perceptual aberrations, behavioral eccentricities	General population: approximately 3% Possibly M > F Increased in families of schizophrenics, and increased risk of schizophrenia in families with schizotypal personality disorder	Correlates of CNS dysfunction in schizophrenia seen in schizotypal personality disorder, including tests of visual and auditory attention and smooth pursuit eye movement
Cluster B "Dramatic"	Histrionic	Excessive emotionality; attention seeking; sometimes seductive, shallow, theatrical, speech may be vague or impressionistic	2–3% of the general population, much higher in psychological and medical samples Diagnosed in F > M	May have a higher rate of somatic complaints, depression, and substance abuse
	Narcissistic	Grandiosity; need for admiration; lack of empathy; interpersonally exploitative, envious, arrogant	M > F	Associated with devaluing parenting; sense of worth contingent upon accomplishment Increased risk of depression, rage, or paranoia with injury to self-image
	Borderline	Instability of interpersonal relationships, self-image, and affect; associated with marked impulsivity	General population: 2–3% M:F = 1:3	Associated with physical or sexual abuse; associated with substance use, suicide (approximately 9%), depression, eating disorders
	Antisocial	Disregard for and violation of rights of others; lying, illegal behavior, impulsivity, aggressive, remorseless	Rate in prison: 20–50%; general population: 3% of men, 1% of women Possible genetic predisposition	Childhood: physical or sexual abuse or neglect, empathy and warmth discouraged or punished Associated with substance abuse, depression

(Continued)

THUMBNAIL: Behavioral Science—Review of Personality Disorders *(Continued)*

Cluster	Disorder	Features	Epidemiology	Comments
Cluster C "Anxious"	Avoidant	Social inhibition, feeling inadequate, hypersensitive to criticism; avoiding people or occupational pursuits because of feeling inadequate	0.5–1% of the population M:F = 1:1	Intense desire for acceptance; overlap with social phobia
	Dependent	Need to be taken care of, clingy, fear of separation, need for constant reassurance, helpless	2–3% of the population; seen frequently in psychology medical settings because seeking help and support Possibly F > M	Intense need for relationships and social approval; treatment to help assertiveness; associated with depression and anxiety disorders
	Obsessive-compulsive	Preoccupation with orderliness, perfectionism, inflexibility, control	1% in the general population M > F Not significantly associated with OCD	View their symptoms as positive; no intrusive obsessions or ego dystonic compulsions; may be self-critical and lack social closeness and therefore may have increased depression

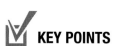 **KEY POINTS**

- The cluster A disorders may have the strongest genetic components, and schizotypal personality disorder may have the greatest genetic relationship to an Axis I disorder (schizophrenia)
- The cluster B disorders are associated with the greatest morbidity and mortality, especially borderline and antisocial personality disorders
- Some personality disorders are significantly associated with childhood trauma or neglect (e.g., borderline and antisocial)

- Borderline and histrionic personality disorder are diagnosed in more women than men
- Narcissistic, antisocial, and probably paranoid and obsessive-compulsive personality disorders are seen more frequently in men

QUESTIONS

1. DP is a 33-year-old man who is seen for an initial appointment for routine health maintenance. He comes in with a large folder in which his daily activities and diet are catalogued, along with his immunization history and record of all doctors' appointments that he has had since college. He reports that he has always been organized and it is one of the things he likes most about himself. He is self-employed as a computer programmer and cites the disorder and lack of rational structure in offices as the reason he works on his own. He admits that the environment in the office at his last job made him anxious. He has few relationships and he admits to being "a bit controlling." His most likely diagnosis is:

   A. Avoidant personality disorder
   B. Antisocial personality disorder
   C. Obsessive-compulsive personality disorder
   D. Schizoid personality disorder
   E. OCD

2. GR is a 39-year-old single female who comes in for a routine checkup because her astrologer told her that there was an excess of gamma waves and microwaves that she should be concerned about. She has few close social contacts or friends. She spends some time with a group of people with whom she discusses numerology and astrology. Her work history is somewhat checkered, because after working in a place for a while she usually has some conflict with the other staff or

management and feels singled out. She often feels that things are indirectly giving her messages (e.g., hearing a specific song while on a bus and knowing that it is a sign she should look for a job in the neighborhood of the next stop). She has no significant medical history, complaints, or physical or lab findings. Which of the following is probably true?

   A. She is no more likely to have a family member with schizophrenia than the general population.
   B. She may have abnormalities in smooth pursuit eye tracking.
   C. She has more than a 50% chance of developing schizophrenia.
   D. She probably sees her beliefs as being odd and not compatible with her self-image.
   E. This disorder is seen predominantly in women.

3. ZC is a 56-year-old businessman who comes in for treatment of depression after being downsized from his company. Before seeing you [he tells] you that he was referred by the chairman of another [department] and plays golf with a vice president of the hospital [and] confirms your academic rank and membership [and that] of a local philanthropic organization. In your evaluation you find that he has been downsized because his division did not weather the recession and that it was probably due to some poor management decisions on his part. He is furious and is convinced that it is their fault and that they will call him back. He seems to lack empathy and in many of

his stories comes across as being arrogant and exploitative. Which of the following is probably true?

A. This disorder is seen in women more frequently than in men.
B. This man probably has histrionic personality disorder.
C. This man probably has no difficulty accepting feedback.
D. This man probably has no difficulty in sustaining long-term intimate relationships.
E. His feelings of insecurity may be masked by arrogance.

4. NF is a 45-year-old man who has been running a prostitution and drug ring from his suburban home, where his wife and two young children also live. As a younger man he abused substances, was expelled from high school for selling home-work answers and marijuana, and tried to put the responsibility on his friend, who was actually uninvolved. He also had stolen various things as a child, and although he wasn't caught, he "borrowed" cars frequently and actually crashed two or three of them. He also frequently got into physical fights and at times had hit his wife. He laughs when he tells you about some of his exploits and how various people got hurt in the process. His wife apparently thought he was doing direct marketing and called the police when she found a crate of semiautomatic weapons in the basement. Which of the following is true?

A. This disorder is seen in 90% of prison inmates.
B. This disorder is seen in 3% of men.
C. This disorder has no association with childhood abuse or neglect.
D. This disorder is more common in women than in men.
E. This disorder has diagnostic EEG findings.

Schizophrenia: Biology and Pharmacology

HPI: JL is a 19-year-old single, white male college junior who you saw yesterday in the student health service and diagnosed with a first episode of schizophrenia, with auditory hallucination, paranoid delusions, and ideas of reference. You decided to hospitalize him, which made him feel much safer, and told him you would start him on medications in the morning. You are the attending physician on the psychiatry service, and during morning rounds you sit down with the medical students to review certain things about the etiologic theories of schizophrenia and pharmacologic options.

You review these theories and then go to the nursing report, in which the night nurse describes the patient's status overnight. She tells you that JL has been quite agitated and the resident on call had to prescribe multiple doses of haloperidol overnight. When you and the team go to see him, his neck is stiff and turned to one side. He says he is not sure how this happened but he is quite uncomfortable. He is also having difficulty moving his eyes. His vital signs are normal, as is the rest of his physical exam.

THOUGHT QUESTIONS

- What neurotransmitter abnormalities are thought to be associated with schizophrenia?
- What has happened to this young man and how is it treated?
- What kinds of medications are used for schizophrenia? What differentiates antipsychotics?

BASIC SCIENCE REVIEW AND DISCUSSION

Neurotransmitter Abnormalities in Schizophrenia

A number of hypotheses related to major neurotransmitter systems have been set forth to explain the symptoms of schizophrenia. The three major theories relate to dopamine, serotonin, and glutamate.

The Dopamine Hypothesis of Schizophrenia Schizophrenics have too much dopamine, especially in the striatum and limbic system, and this is responsible for the positive symptoms of schizophrenia. Many of these symptoms are mimicked by giving large doses of amphetamines, which cause dopamine release. Traditional antipsychotics act by blocking dopamine receptors, particularly the D2 receptor, in the brain. This model is overly simplistic, as negative symptoms seem to be associated with a hypodopaminergic state in the prefrontal cortex.

The Serotonin Hypothesis Because lysergic acid diethylamide (LSD), a serotonin (5-HT) postsynaptic agonist, causes hallucinations, some researchers have suggested that there is a relationship between serotonin and schizophrenia. Serotonin is implicated in many behaviors, including cognition, pain sensitivity, mood, impulsivity, aggression, and sexual drive. Alterations in serotonergic functioning affect multiple neurotransmitter systems (including dopamine, glutamate, GABA, and norepinephrine). There is now considerable evidence that the atypical antipsychotic drugs, such as clozapine, olanzapine, quetiapine, risperidone, sertindole, and ziprasidone, are more effective than the older medications (especially for negative symptoms), and they are all antagonists of the 5-HT_{2A} receptor. In fact, although most of them have some activity as D2 antagonists, they are much more potent at the 5-HT_{2A} receptor.

The Glutamate Hypothesis The glutamate hypothesis proposes a hypofunctional glutamate system in schizophrenia. The origins of the glutamate hypothesis of schizophrenia can be traced to the observations that the dissociative anesthetic ketamine, which is similar to phencyclidine (PCP), produced psychotic symptoms in a subgroup of surgical patients. This continues to be under investigation.

Neurotransmitters in Schizophrenia, Anatomic Location, and Metabolic Pathways

Dopamine is a catecholamine. Dopamine cell bodies are found in the substantia nigra (SN) and in the ventral tegmental area (VTA). The VTA sends its axons to the prefrontal cortex (implicated in attention and working memory) and the nucleus accumbens (associated with motivation). The SN projects to the striatum (associated with motor function) (Fig. 8-1).

Serotonin is an indolamine. Serotonin cell bodies are primarily found in the raphe nuclei. Most areas of the brain receive at least some serotonergic innervation (Fig. 8-2).

Glutamate is an excitatory amino acid neurotransmitter. Glutamate is the major excitatory neurotransmitter in the CNS and the glutamate receptors play a vital role in the mediation of excitatory synaptic transmission. It is synthesized either from α-ketoglutarate via an aminotransferase or from glutamine via glutaminase.

Antipsychotic Medications and Their Side Effects

This patient is having a dystonic reaction to haloperidol. **Dystonic reactions** are either spasmodic or sustained involuntary contractions of muscles in the face, neck, trunk, or extremities. Treatment with anticholinergic agents such as benztropine (Cogentin) or diphenhydramine (Benadryl) is extremely effective, and the symptoms resolve within minutes. The reaction is more common in young male patients and with high-potency drugs such as haloperidol. The usual etiology is nigrostriatal dopamine D2 receptor blockade leading to an increase in striatal cholinergic output

There are two broad classes of antipsychotic medications. One is the *typical*, or conventional, antipsychotic; the other is the *atypical*, or "second-generation," antipsychotic. **Typical antipsychotics** have their primary site of action at the D2 dopamine receptor. Examples include haloperidol, chlorpromazine, and perphenazine. They are usually classified by their potency, which reflects both the dosage used to have an effect and their side effect profile. In general, the high-potency medications (e.g., haloperidol) are less sedating and less anticholinergic but cause

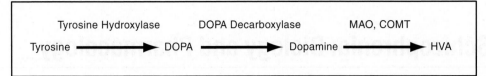

• Figure 8-1. Dopamine—metabolic pathway.

more extrapyramidal (Parkinsonian) symptoms. The low-potency medications (e.g., chlorpromazine) are more sedating and anticholinergic but cause fewer extrapyramidal symptoms.

Atypical antipsychotics usually have antagonistic actions at a number of receptors, including 5-HT$_{2A}$, dopamine D4, and some D2. As a rule they are better tolerated, cause fewer extrapyramidal side effects, and are less likely to cause a dystonic reaction. They still may be associated with sedation, weight gain, and orthostasis. Examples of medications in this class include risperidone, olanzapine, and clozapine.

Another common side effect of the typical antipsychotics and of risperidone is an increase in prolactin levels, caused by the dopamine blockade, which can result in galactorrhea, breast enlargement, amenorrhea, and sexual dysfunction. Many medications can also cause conduction abnormalities or QT prolongation.

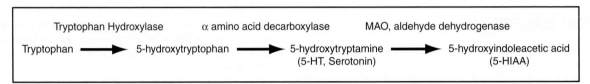

• Figure 8-2. Serotonin—metabolic pathway.

CASE CONCLUSION

JL was started on an atypical antipsychotic and tolerated it well. Over the next week he had a decrease in the auditory hallucinations and paranoia and felt "calmer." He was able to be discharged to outpatient follow-up.

THUMBNAIL: Psychiatry—Review of Antipsychotic Medications and Their Side Effects

Typical or Conventional Antipsychotics

Potency	Example	Side Effects
High	Haloperidol (Haldol), thiothixene (Navane)	Akathisia (an internal sense of restlessness), extrapyramidal (Parkinsonian) symptoms (EPS)
Mid	Perphenazine (Trilafon)	Mildly sedating, some anticholinergic effects, less EPS than with high-potency medications
Low	Thioridazine (Mellaril), chlorpromazine (Thorazine)	More sedating, significant anticholinergic effects (dry mouth, constipation, urinary retention, blurred vision), orthostatic hypotension, lowered seizure threshold Thioridazine may cause irreversible pigmentation of the retina Chlorpromazine may cause corneal deposits and/or photosensitivity and blue-gray skin coloration

Atypical Antipsychotic Agents

Medication	Comments/Side Effects
Risperidone	EPS in higher doses, some sedation, orthostatic hypotension, tachycardia, anticholinergic effects
Olanzapine	Sedation, weight gain, orthostatic hypotension, tachycardia, anticholinergic effects
Quetiapine	Orthostatic hypotension, tachycardia, anticholinergic effects
Clozapine	Indicated for resistant symptoms, is more effective, may improve negative symptoms, results in less tardive dyskinesia (TD), NMS, and EPS but is sedating, lowers the seizure threshold, causes orthostatic hypotension, and requires weekly blood work to monitor for agranulocytosis

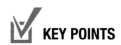

KEY POINTS

- The dopamine hypothesis is the classic hypothesis for the etiology of symptoms in schizophrenia.
  - Increased dopamine function in the limbic system is thought to be important in the etiology of the positive symptoms of schizophrenia.
  - Decreased dopamine function in the prefrontal cortex is thought to be important in the etiology of the negative symptoms of schizophrenia.

- Typical antipsychotics act as antagonists at the dopamine D2 receptor.
- Atypical antipsychotics have antagonistic actions at a number of receptors, including 5-HT$_{2A}$, dopamine D4, and some D2.
- In general, the atypical agents have a more benign side effect profile and are less likely to cause EPS, dystonia, and akathisia; clozapine is thought to confer minimal risk of TD.

QUESTIONS

Questions 1 and 2 relate to the following case:

TR is a 56-year-old female who has been maintained on the same conventional neuroleptic for the past 30 years. She comes into the ER with an exacerbation of her auditory hallucinations. She complains that there are too many side effects to her medications and admits to having stopped them 1 week before.

1. The medical student in the ER tells you that he's confused about the "typical antipsychotics" and asks which of the following is true:
   A. Their primary effect is through blockage of the muscarinic receptor.
   B. Haloperidol is a low-potency medication.
   C. Thioridazine is associated with sedation and orthostatic hypotension.
   D. Potent D2 receptor agonists are particularly effective medications.
   E. Akathisia refers to the parkinsonian rigidity associated with these medications.

2. Which of the following is true about the atypical antipsychotics?
   A. Perphenazine (Trilafon) is an example of an atypical antipsychotic.
   B. Clozapine is associated with agranulocytosis and lowered seizure threshold.
   C. Atypical agents have no effect on dopamine receptors.
   D. All atypical agents have marked agonist effects on the 5-HT receptor.
   E. Risperidone has its primary action at the nicotinic receptor.

3. BR has a 15-year history of antipsychotic use prescribed for chronic paranoid schizophrenia. He comes to your office for an initial visit and you notice that he is smacking his lips, his tongue occasionally protrudes from his mouth, and he seems to have some choreoathetoid movements in his hands. What is this syndrome called and what medication is most likely to have caused it?
   A. TD—chlorpromazine
   B. Akathisia—haloperidol
   C. Akathisia—olanzapine
   D. TD—clozapine
   E. EPS—clozapine

4. You are called to see a 38-year-old patient in the ER, who was brought in because he had a high fever and had become confused, rigid, and sweaty. You check his laboratory results and find that his WBC count and CPK are elevated. His other labs are pending, and his PE is otherwise unremarkable. He is on hydrochlorothiazide and perphenazine. What is the most likely etiology for his symptoms?
   A. Influenza A
   B. *Neisseria meningitidis meningitis*
   C. Neuroleptic malignant syndrome
   D. Malignant hyperthermia
   E. Enterovirus meningitis

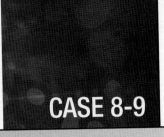

CASE 8-9 Alcoholism

HPI: WK is a 65-year-old man with a history of alcoholism who is brought in by ambulance to the ED after being found unconscious on a street corner, smelling of alcohol and vomit. He is somnolent but arousable to painful stimulus. His finger-stick blood sugar is 55. He is given oxygen, naloxone, thiamine, and vitamin B12, 1 amp of $D_{50}W$, and started on IV normal saline with 5% dextrose by the paramedics, to which he responds minimally.

PE: T 35.9°C; BP 110/65; HR 97; RR 16; SaO_2 92% room air.

He is lying in the bed, difficult to arouse. Glasgow Coma Scale (GCS) is 10. Head is atraumatic and anicteric. He has multiple spider angiomatas and telangiectasia on his chest. Lung and cardiac exam are normal. Abdomen is large and distended with a positive fluid wave, migrating dullness to percussion, and his liver is palpable 5 cm below the costal margin. Stool is brown and heme-positive. He has bilateral symmetric wasting of upper and lower extremities, palmar erythema, diffuse ecchymoses, and 2+ pitting edema to the sacrum. Pupils are equal, with his right eye slightly deviated inwardly, 1+ deep tendon reflexes bilaterally.

Labs: WBC 6200/mL; Hgb 10 (13.5−17.5); Hct 30% (41−53%); Plt 95,000 (150,000−400,000); MCV 100 (80−100); Na 132 (136−145); K 3.5 (3.5−5.0); glucose 115 (70−110); total bilirubin 1.7 (0.1−1.0); direct bilirubin 0.6 (0.0−0.3); AST 90 (8−20); ALT 45 (8−20); Alkphos 132 (20−70); Alb 2.5 g/dL; total protein 5.5 g/dL; PT/PTT/INR 30 s/43 s/3.2; UA −3+ ketones, lipase 205; ABG −7.35/50/95/20 ($pH/CO_2/O_2/HCO_3$).

Studies: Abdominal CT shows marked ascites and nodular cirrhotic liver; no evidence of acute pancreatitis. Head CT shows diffuse cortical atrophy with no other parenchymal abnormalities.

THOUGHT QUESTIONS

- What are the definitions of *alcohol abuse, tolerance,* and *dependency?*
- What are the clinical manifestations of alcohol intoxication? Withdrawal?
- What are the acute and chronic medical and cognitive complications of alcoholism?
- How are alcohol intoxication, withdrawal, and alcohol-related medical diseases managed acutely and chronically?

BASIC SCIENCE REVIEW AND DISCUSSION

Alcoholism is a common condition affecting 7% of adults, with a lifetime prevalence of 14%. While alcohol may be benign within the context of safe and responsible drinking, when taken to excess in unsafe conditions, a person may acutely fall victim to its secondary hazards, including falls, car accidents, sexual assault, and other violence. Alcohol is a pervasive element in crime, violence, and poverty, and its greatest effect may take place silently in an individual of any socioeconomic class or background.

Mechanism of Action

Ethanol is a CNS depressant and acts by enhancing the activity of the inhibitory **GABA$_A$ receptor** and inhibiting the excitatory **NMDA receptor.** Its immediate effects include sedation, disinhibition, impaired judgment and motor coordination, and, in severe cases, "blackout" (or a temporary amnesia of all events surrounding the period of alcohol ingestion). A person who drinks an excessive amount over a short period of time (e.g., in hazing rituals) may induce enough CNS depression to cause respiratory depression, a common cause of alcohol-induced death. Otherwise,

acute physiologic effects include some nutritional and metabolic derangements. A drink is approximately one 12-ounce can of beer, one 4-ounce glass of wine, or one shot (1.5 ounces) of liquor. One drink produces a blood alcohol level of about 30 mg/dL. "Legal intoxication" is reached at blood alcohol levels of 80 mg/dL and above (about two to three drinks, depending on a person's weight). Ethanol is metabolized to acetaldehyde by the liver primarily via the **ADH pathway** and does so at a constant rate of approximately 30 mg/dL/hr, approximately one drink per hour.

Epidemiology

Risk factors for alcoholism include male gender, low socioeconomic status, unemployment, depression, anxiety, narcotic abuse, antisocial personality disorder, family history or dysfunction, and peer pressure. Often psychological conditions, such as depression and anxiety, precede the substance abuse, which develops as a result of a person's attempt to self-medicate. Those susceptible to addiction may develop a habit of alcohol consumption, which can induce **tolerance.** First, a **metabolic tolerance** develops as hepatic clearance accelerates. Next, a **cellular tolerance** develops as alcohol induces neurochemical changes that make neurons dependent on alcohol for normal functioning. Finally, a person adapts to chronic intake by modifying behavior (**behavioral tolerance**). *Alcoholism* describes the interface between the physiologic event of *tolerance* and the internal and external ramifications of *behavior.* Two terms subdivide the syndrome of alcoholism, **alcohol abuse** and **dependence,** both of which predict recurrent problems with drinking and shortened lifespan (Table 8-4).

There are several classic signs of chronic alcoholism (Box 8-1). An established clinical screening method is the CAGE method (Box 8-2).

TABLE 8-4 *DSM-IV* Criteria for Alcohol Abuse vs. Alcohol Dependence

Alcohol Abuse	Alcohol Dependence
Continued drinking despite repetitive problems, at least one out of four of the following: *Mnemonic: "When alcohol takes **HOLD** of you."* **H**azardous situations—*e.g., driving under the influence* **O**bligations unfulfilled—social/occupational debilitation **L**egal problems—crime, violence **D**ifficulties with interpersonal relationships	Presence of three out of seven of the following within a 12-month period: *Mnemonic: "**WE** are unable **TO CUT** our drinking."* **W**ithdrawal symptoms **E**xcessive drinking (progressively increasing amounts) *Tolerance* **O**ccupational/social abandonment (in order to drink) **C**ontinued use despite occupational/social consequence **U**ncontrolled use—person unable to control drinking **T**ime increasingly occupied by drinking

Over time, physiologic and psychological dependence to alcohol can develop. Any decrease in alcohol intake can unmask the compensatory overactivity of the nervous system to alcohol and induce symptoms of withdrawal. Mild withdrawal symptoms include **tremors, agitation, mild anxiety, GI upset, headache, insomnia,** and **palpitations** 6 hours after the last drink. More severe withdrawal symptoms starting 1 to 4 days after the last drink include generalized tonic-clonic **seizures** within 48 hours, alcoholic **hallucinosis** (usually visual) within 12 to 24 hours, and **delirium tremens** 48 hours after the last drink. Delirium tremens is an uncommon but life-threatening condition without intervention. It includes unorientable delirium, hallucination, agitation, diaphoresis, and **autonomic instability** with increases in all four vital signs. **Benzodiazepines** (e.g., chlordiazepoxide, lorazepam) are GABA receptor agonists and are used to suppress withdrawal symptoms. **Thiamine** is also given to prevent Wernicke-Korsakoff syndrome, described later.

Otherwise, patients who present with acute intoxication and evidence of chronic alcoholism need to be stabilized and offered a long-term plan for rehabilitation. After discharge, those who express a desire to quit can undergo detoxification (monitoring and support for withdrawal symptoms) for several days. This can be followed by long-term rehabilitation; this includes organizations that support behavior modification, like Alcoholics Anonymous. Private therapy and residential rehabilitation programs are also effective. Pharmacotherapy to supplement the rehabilitation regimen includes **naltrexone** and **acamprosate,** which reduce cravings for alcohol and reduce relapse rates.

BOX 8-1 Classic Signs of Chronic Alcoholism (from Head to Toe)

Alcohol odor in breath

Scleral icterus/jaundice

Ophthalmoplegia (Wernicke)

Spider angiomata/telangiectasia

Firm, distended abdomen (ascites)

Caput medusa (portocaval shunt)

Large liver span (steatohepatitis)

Small liver span (cirrhotic liver)

Palmar erythema

Asterixis (encephalopathy)

Peripheral neuropathy/ataxia

Mental status changes (dementia)

↑ AST, ↑ ALT (AST:ALT = 2:1)

↑ Total and direct bilirubin

↓ Albumin/protein, ↑ PT/PTT

BOX 8-2 CAGE Screening

Have you ever tried to **C**ut down?

Have you ever been **A**nnoyed by people telling you to stop drinking?

Have you ever felt **G**uilty about drinking?

Have you ever needed an **E**ye opener?

≥ 2 *positive answers makes alcoholism likely*

CASE CONCLUSION

WK is stabilized with electrolyte repletion and lorazepam for withdrawal prophylaxis. He is also given a multivitamin and vitamin K injection for his coagulopathy. He is admitted to the hospital and is diagnosed with having had an episode of acute alcohol intoxication with combined respiratory and metabolic acidosis from respiratory depression and alcoholic ketoacidosis, respectively. During his stay it is established that he has cirrhotic liver disease that is causing ascites. This hepatic insufficiency is thought to be responsible for his hypoproteinemia and edema, hyperbilirubinemia, and coagulopathy from insufficient coagulation factor production. Poor nutrition, liver insufficiency, and occult GI bleeding may be responsible for his anemia, leukopenia, and thrombocytopenia. His moderately elevated lipase suggests that he has chronic pancreatitis. Paracentesis is performed to relieve him of some of the abdominal pressure from his ascites. He is given supportive therapy and discharged to a medical detoxification program, after which he enters a residential rehabilitation program. He is currently taking naltrexone and has been abstinent for 2 months.

THUMBNAIL: Behavioral Science—Common Medical Complications of Chronic Alcohol Abuse

	Acute Conditions	Chronic Conditions
Neurologic	Acute alcohol intoxication Alcoholic withdrawal syndromes Tremors—"shakes" Seizures Alcoholic hallucinosis Delirium tremens Hemorrhagic stroke Subdural/epidural hematoma	Alcohol tolerance/dependency Peripheral neuropathy (B12 deficiency) Organic brain syndromes Alcoholic dementia Korsakoff syndrome Wernicke encephalopathy
Respiratory	Respiratory depression/hypoxia Aspiration pneumonia	Pulmonary edema (from CHF) Bronchitis/COPD (from smoking)
Cardiovascular	Peripheral vasodilation → syncope	Cardiomyopathy CHF Gastroesophageal varices
Gastrointestinal	GI hemorrhage Mallory-Weiss tear Ruptured gastric varices Coagulopathy Acute pancreatitis	Occult GI bleeding Chronic pancreatitis PUD Oropharyngeal, esophageal, hepatic cancer
Hepatic	Acute hepatic failure with concurrent acetaminophen ingestion, hepatitis Disulfiram reaction (Antabuse) Metronidazole, cefotetan, INH, griseofulvin	Chronic liver failure, ascites Hepatic encephalopathy Hyperbilirubinemia, coagulopathy Hypoalbuminemia, hypoproteinemia Hypercholesterolemia/triglyceridemia
Renal	—	Hepatorenal syndrome
Metabolic	Alcoholic ketoacidosis Hypoglycemia, hypokalemia, hypomagnesemia	Malnutrition Vitamin B12/folate deficiency Thiamine (vitamin B1) deficiency Vitamin K deficiency (coagulopathy)
Endocrine Genitourinary	—	Gynecomastia, impotence, testicular atrophy, infertility, menstrual irregularities
Hematologic	Anemia from acute hemorrhage	Pancytopenia
Dermatologic	Cigarette burns Traumatic bruising, lacerations	Ecchymoses (platelet dysfunction) Palmar erythema, spider angiomata, telangiectasia, jaundice
Musculoskeletal	Traumatic fractures, rhabdomyolysis	Osteopenia Peripheral atrophy, myopathy
Infectious	Aspiration pneumonia	Klebsiella or Legionella pneumonia Gram-negative sepsis
Psychiatric	Suicide or homicidal ideation Sexual assault Violence	Alcohol abuse/dependency Multidrug abuse/dependency Depression/anxiety disorder

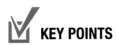

KEY POINTS

- Alcoholism is a common problem with significant effects on lifetime morbidity and mortality, affecting every system in the body
- The behavioral pathology of alcoholism stems from the development of alcohol tolerance and dependence due to metabolic, cellular, and behavioral adaptation; such dependence may subsequently result in social and occupational dysfunction with disease progression
- Alcohol withdrawal results from the unmasking of the compensatory overactivity of the CNS to chronic alcohol intake. Delirium tremens is a potentially life-threatening form of alcohol withdrawal that typically presents 48 hours after the last drink. Symptoms include delirium, hallucination, agitation, and autonomic instability. BZDs suppress this overactivity and are used to treat alcohol withdrawal.

QUESTIONS

1. TN is a 37-year-old man with a long history of alcoholism who is brought by ambulance to the ED severely agitated but oriented and cooperative. He is diaphoretic with vital signs stable at T 38.0°C; HR 98; BP 139/85; RR 24; SaO$_2$ 100%. He develops severe stuttering speech, a tongue wag, and generalized tremors, pronounced by intentional movement. He soon undergoes a generalized tonic-clonic seizure. Once he stops seizing, he is given longer-acting diazepam and is admitted to the hospital. He reports having had his last drink about 24 hours ago. What is his *most* likely diagnosis?

   A. Withdrawal tremors and seizure
   B. Delirium tremens
   C. Alcoholic hallucinosis
   D. Wernicke encephalopathy
   E. Korsakoff syndrome

2. NH is a 52-year-old woman with a long history of alcoholism who presents complaining of fatigue and palpitations. She notes having passed foul-smelling, black stool in the last 2 days. Her recent history is significant for three episodes of vomiting and dry retching after an alcoholic binge. Generally, she appears well, with an HR of 96 and BP of 125/87. Her exam is significant for general pallor, diffuse epigastric tenderness, and heme-positive stool. Laboratory findings are significant for Hct of 32%, Plt 150,000/μL, and MCV of 85 fL. What is the *most* likely cause of her anemia?

   A. Folate and vitamin B12 deficiency causing a megaloblastic anemia
   B. Anemia of chronic disease from chronic alcoholism

   C. Iron deficiency anemia
   D. Occult bleeding from Mallory-Weiss esophageal tear
   E. Ruptured gastroesophageal varices

3. A 19-year-old boy is brought by ambulance after being found collapsed in his college dorm room by his roommate, "blue and not breathing on his own." On the field, he is found to have an O$_2$ saturation of 75% and is quickly intubated, which resolves his cyanosis, bringing his saturation to 100%. He has a heart rate of 55 and a blood pressure of 95/55, for which he is given fluids. He has a GCS of 3, glucose of 85. He smells of alcohol and shows no signs of trauma. His pupils are equal and reactive, and the rest of his exam is normal. What is his *most* likely diagnosis?

   A. Acute heroin overdose
   B. Acute alcohol toxicity
   C. Acute cocaine overdose
   D. Insulin overdose
   E. Acute BZD overdose

4. HM is a 72-year-old man with a long history of alcoholism who is brought in by ambulance after having collapsed in his chair at home. He is eventually diagnosed with a hemorrhagic stroke. What is the *most* likely cause of this stroke?

   A. Thiamine deficiency
   B. Hypoglycemia
   C. Korsakoff syndrome
   D. Hepatic encephalopathy
   E. Vitamin K deficiency

CASE 8-10 Opioid Drug Abuse and Dependence

HPI: LW is a 37-year-old man who is brought by ambulance to the ER after having been found unconscious and unresponsive in his apartment by his sister. When emergency medical services arrived, he was found to have a heart rate of 60, respiratory rate of 8, and an oxygen saturation of 89%. He had "pinpoint" pupils, unresponsive to light bilaterally. He was immediately intubated and given naloxone, thiamine, and vitamin B12, to which he immediately responded with an oxygen saturation of 98% and GCS of 12. The sister knew of no known ingestions he could have taken and had no suspicion of suicidality. His sister says LW has no significant medical history except for mild insomnia for which he takes a "sleeping pill." He is a registered nurse in the ward and has no known habits, including cigarettes, alcohol, or drugs.

PE: T 36.0°C; BP 112/75; HR 65; RR 22; SaO_2 98% on oxygen.

He is lying in bed, somnolent but arousable. Pupils are equally small and minimally reactive to light. His head and neck exams were otherwise normal. He had a normal cardiac and abdominal exam. No track marks on his extremities or trunk.

Labs/Studies: Urine toxicology is positive for opioids. Head CT is WNL.

THOUGHT QUESTIONS

- What opioids are frequently used as drugs of abuse? How do they work?
- What are the definitions of *opioid abuse* and *dependence*? How does dependence develop?
- What are the clinical manifestations of opioid intoxication, overdose, and withdrawal?
- What are the complications associated with opioid addiction?
- How are opioid intoxication, withdrawal, and dependence managed acutely and chronically?

BASIC SCIENCE AND REVIEW

Opioids are derived from the poppy plant *Papaver somniferum* and have been used for centuries as a sedative and analgesic. Today they are used for the same purposes medically, but also illicitly as drugs of abuse. A 1997 study reported a 1% lifetime prevalence of heroin use, about 800,000 opioid-dependent persons in the United States, with rates higher in males than in females. All opioids produce similar effects of euphoria, sedation, and analgesia and can produce psychological and physical dependence over time (Table 8-5).

Mechanism of Action

Opioids bind different opioid receptors, whose endogenous ligands include **endorphins** and **enkephalins.** These include μ-, δ-, and κ-receptors, which are inhibitory G protein-coupled receptors. The **μ-receptor** mediates analgesia, euphoria, reinforcement, constipation, hormone level modification, and respiration. This receptor is mostly responsible for the effects of reward, tolerance, dependence, and withdrawal. The κ-receptor mediates some of the preceding effects as well as mood. These drugs can be injected intravenously, which produces the most potent effect, as opioids are quickly metabolized by the liver and have a high first-pass metabolism if taken orally. With increasing purity of heroin, intranasal use is increasing. In addition, street heroin includes **adulterants,** nonopioid additives like powdered milk, sugar, caffeine, and even strychnine, which may produce unexpected effects to the injector.

The *Diagnostic and Statistical Manual of Mental Disorders, 4th edition (DSM-IV)*, criteria for opioid abuse and dependence are the same as those for alcohol. Tolerance and dependence are thought to develop through similar neurochemical modifications of receptors and signaling pathways that opioids affect. Up-regulation of components of this pathway, such as adenylyl cyclase and protein kinase A, is thus implicated in the production of the withdrawal syndrome.

The primary effects of opioids are **sedation, analgesia,** and **euphoria.** Secondary effects include nausea, vomiting, and *decrease in GI motility*, producing **constipation** and **anorexia.** It decreases secretion of LH, causing **reductions in testosterone and sex drive** as well as **amenorrhea.** A particularly dangerous effect of opioids is **respiratory depression,** with a reduction in brainstem response to CO_2 tension. Opioids can also cause peripheral vascular dilation and orthostatic hypotension. However, the greater part of the morbidity and mortality of opioids is attributed to the risks of injection drug use, the criminal activity required to maintain the habit, and the generally poor social circumstances and functioning of some addicts. Injection drug use increases the risk of contracting hepatitis B or C, HIV, and bacterial endocarditis, each of which have their own short- and long-term complications.

Diagnosis

To recognize the stigmata of opioid dependence, signs and symptoms include constricted pupils that are poorly reactive to light (**pinpoint pupils**) and **needle marks** on the skin. In acute overdose, respiratory depression, bradycardia, and general unresponsiveness may subsequently produce anoxic brain injury, cardiorespiratory arrest, and death. Withdrawal produces opposite symptoms, such as diarrhea, mydriasis as well as coughing, lacrimation, and rhinorrhea (*think secretions of CN VII*), sweating and piloerection, as well as increases in all vital signs, especially temperature, blood pressure, and respiratory rate.

Treatment

Treatment of opiate overdose includes support for respiratory compromise and reversal of opioid effects with an **opioid antagonist** like **naloxone** or the longer-acting **naltrexone.** These antagonists

TABLE 8-5 Opioid Drugs and Their Effects on Opioid Receptors

Agonists		Mixed Agonist/Antagonists	Antagonists
Morphine Codeine Heroin Oxycodone Hydrocodone Meperidine	Propoxyphene Fentanyl *(most potent)* Methadone *(long acting)* LAAM *(longer acting)*	Buprenorphine Pentazocine	Naloxone Naltrexone

may precipitate withdrawal symptoms, however. Withdrawal symptoms, alternatively, are treated with an opioid such as **methadone**. Otherwise, **clonidine** may be useful for inhibiting autonomic hyperactivity with supplemental **BZDs** to decrease agitation. In general, altered mental status can be empirically treated with glucose, naloxone, thiamine, and vitamin B12. Other treatments may be considered, depending on their response to these empiric treatments and suspicion of other ingestions (e.g., flumazenil is an antidote for BZD intoxication).

Once stabilized, the patient requires support of withdrawal symptoms for several days (**detoxification**). This is followed by long-term rehabilitation and pharmacologic support of opioid dependence with the long-acting opioid agonist **methadone** or the even longer-acting **levomethadyl acetate (LAAM)**, administered through methadone maintenance programs. Counseling and psychotherapy can be provided in group settings or privately through residential programs and clinics, which may include therapy for concurrent psychiatric illness. Alternatively, opiate-dependent persons may choose to achieve complete abstinence from opiates by undergoing treatment with opiate antagonists (e.g., naloxone, naltrexone), although this has limited efficacy. Those with chronic pain syndromes are encouraged to take nonopioid analgesics and limit their opiate intake with the advice that their pain can be minimized but not eliminated.

CASE CONCLUSION

LW is monitored for the next 24 hours for overdose intoxication and withdrawal symptoms. After 3 hours, he demonstrated symptoms of opioid withdrawal and was thus given IV methadone. During this time, he admits to having used opiate analgesics (oral morphine and fentanyl he stole from the wards) for the last few years to relieve his stress and insomnia. He is now dependent on them for sleep. He agrees to undergo detoxification and subsequent long-term rehabilitation with methadone treatment. Several months later, he continues to attend group counseling and is on methadone maintenance.

THUMBNAIL: Opiate Drug Abuse and Dependence

Epidemiology	1% lifetime prevalence of heroin use; men > women
Molecular biology	Agonists to μ-, δ-, κ-opioid receptors; μ-receptor acts to produce tolerance and dependence
Physical exam	Track marks, constricted unresponsive pupils, tender liver edge (hepatitis)
Drug intoxication	Sedation, analgesia, euphoria, constipation, ↓ LH → ↓ testosterone/sex drive, amenorrhea
Drug overdose	Respiratory depression/arrest, orthostatic hypotension, hypoxic brain injury, death
Drug withdrawal	Diarrhea, mydriasis, coughing, lacrimation, rhinorrhea, sweating, piloerection ("goose bumps"), yawning, and increases in all vitals signs (temperature, blood pressure, respiratory rate)
Drug complications	Hepatitis B/C, HIV, bacterial endocarditis, cardiac valve disease, stroke, behavioral issues, skin cellulitis, abscesses, necrotizing fasciitis (skin infection with systemic spread and sepsis)
Treatment	*Overdose:* Intubation, oxygen, naloxone, naltrexone *Withdrawal:* Methadone, clonidine, BZDs *Rehabilitation:* Methadone or LAAM (if refractory), counseling

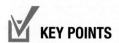

KEY POINTS

- Opioids primarily cause sedation, analgesia, and euphoria; secondary effects include constipation, nausea, and vomiting. Classic signs/symptoms of intoxication include pinpoint pupils and track marks. Overdose causes respiratory depression.

- Opioids exert their effects through opioid receptors and produce tolerance and dependence with continual use

- Most of the morbidity and mortality of opioids come from the risks associated with injection drug use, criminal behavior, and generally poor social circumstances and functioning

- Opiate addiction occurs not only in the stereotypical homeless heroin addict but in many individuals; therefore, it is important to screen for opiate use in all patients.

QUESTIONS

1. BR is a 42-year-old homeless man who presents to the clinic complaining of 2 days of runny nose, cough, night sweats, and shortness of breath. He has also had 1 day of watery, non-bloody diarrhea. His vitals are T 38.4°C; BP 150/90; HR 104; RR 28; and SaO$_2$ 100%. On exam, he appears agitated and diaphoretic. He has a III/VI mid-systolic murmur at the right lower sternal border and a diffusely tender periumbilical abdomen without rebound or guarding. He has multiple track marks on his skin and has decreased skin turgor from apparent dehydration. What is the *likely* diagnosis?

   A. Acute gastroenteritis
   B. Bacterial endocarditis
   C. Upper respiratory tract infection
   D. Heroin withdrawal
   E. All of the above

2. TS is a 39-year-old woman who presents with severe lower back pain to the ER. She has a history of multiple back surgeries for chronic back pain without successful relief of the pain and is chronically taking meperidine for pain. She is currently screaming in agony, demanding pain medication. What strategy is *most likely* to exacerbate her dependence on narcotic medication?

   A. Complete history of back pain, surgeries, pain management, and physicians from which she received pain medication.
   B. Complete physical of her back with attention to new findings complete with a neurologic exam.
   C. Review quickly her medical record and contact her primary care physician.
   D. Administer IV morphine for her severe pain immediately
   E. Give her a combination of ibuprofen and acetaminophen for pain immediately.
   F. Advise her to return to her primary care physician for review of her pain symptoms and the appropriate pain regimen.

3. UN is a 57-year-old man. He presents with a painful skin infection on his right leg and states that he has been "feeling very, very sick" for the last 2 days. He has had this skin infection for 4 days, has recently felt "sick," and cannot elaborate except to say that this was unlike his normal withdrawal symptoms. He last injected heroin 6 hours ago. He has a temperature of 39.1°C, HR of 105, BP of 96/52, RR of 28, and SaO$_2$ of 99%. He appears ill and in mild distress. He has a 7-cm poorly circumscribed area of erythema and swelling on his right thigh that is extremely tender. It also has a questionable central area of fluctuance. His lungs are clear and his heart is regular, with no murmurs. What is the *most* important diagnosis to evaluate?

   A. Necrotizing fasciitis
   B. Cellulitis
   C. Abscess
   D. Opioid withdrawal
   E. Bacterial endocarditis

4. AL is a 40-year-old man who is brought by ambulance to the ER after being found collapsed on a park bench. He is breathing at a rate of 8 breaths per minute with an O$_2$ saturation of 85% on room air. He has no odor of alcohol on his breath and a Breathalyzer test shows an alcohol level of zero. He has multiple track marks and pinpoint pupils. He is given IV normal saline, naloxone, thiamine, vitamin B12, and glucose with no response. He is given three more doses of naloxone with still no response. He is given flumazenil with improvement in his level of consciousness. What is the *most* likely etiology of his depressed level of consciousness?

   A. Hypoglycemia
   B. Heroin overdose
   C. Alcohol intoxication
   D. Hyponatremia
   E. BZD overdose

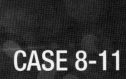

CASE 8-11 Altered Mental Status and Drug Intoxication

HPI: MG is a 17-year-old girl who was brought in by ambulance to the ER after her mother found her passed out and unresponsive on the bathroom floor after an evening out with her friends. Her mother wasn't sure where she had gone but suspected that she had gone to a party or dance club. MG did not smell of alcohol or vomit. She is otherwise healthy and has no significant medical or psychiatric history. When the emergency medical services team arrived, she had a GCS of 9, with equally dilated and responsive pupils bilaterally. Blood glucose was 75. She was given naloxone, thiamine, and vitamin B12 and started on normal saline IV infusion with 5% dextrose, with minimal improvement in her mental status.

PE: T 36°C; BP 98/65; HR 105; RR 32; SaO_2 100% on room air.

   She is lying on the gurney and is tachypneic. She had no apparent head trauma and no meningismus. Her jugular venous pulsation (JVP) is flat and she is tachycardic, with occasional irregular beats. Her lungs are clear and her abdomen is benign. She now has a GCS of 10, localizing painful stimulus (5), responding to pain with a garbled "no" (3), and opens her eyes to painful stimulus (2). Her deep tendon reflexes (DTRs) are diminished but symmetric and with a negative Babinski sign. She has diminished skin turgor diffusely and 2+ radial pulses.

Labs/Studies: CBC is normal. Labs otherwise notable for Na 125, BUN 40, Cr 0.7, and low serum osmolarity. UA is normal; Utox is negative; alcohol/acetaminophen/aspirin levels are zero. ABG is 7.37/36/100/20. EKG shows a sinus tachycardia with occasional premature atrial contractions. CSF findings are normal, cultures pending. Head CT is normal.

THOUGHT QUESTIONS

- What are the common drugs of abuse?
- What are the manifestations of intoxication and withdrawal for each drug?
- How does the body adapt to chronic drug exposure?
- What is the physiologic basis of reward, reinforcement, tolerance, and dependence?

BASIC SCIENCE REVIEW AND DISCUSSION

The common drugs of abuse can be divided into three main categories: (*a*) **stimulants,** (*b*) **sedatives,** and (*c*) **hallucinogens,** although any single drug may have effects that fall into at least two categories.

Stimulants

Stimulants include sympathomimetic drugs like **cocaine, amphetamines, PCP,** and **ketamine.** These drugs stimulate excitatory neurochemical pathway components (e.g., NMDA receptor) in the central and peripheral nervous systems. For instance, cocaine acts by inhibiting the reuptake of the excitatory neurotransmitters **norepinephrine, dopamine,** and **serotonin.** Peripherally, this results in vasoconstriction, hypertension, tachycardia, dry mouth, and mydriasis due to its **sympathomimetic effects.** Centrally, cocaine use produces subjective feelings of euphoria, alertness, increased confidence, and grandiosity. It may also produce anxiety and paranoid delusions. Other stimulant drugs will produce similar effects along with their own signature variations. PCP intoxication is distinguished by the associated hypersalivation and vertical nystagmus not present in intoxication due to other stimulants. These effects in overdose can produce severe vascular complications such as MI and cerebral hemorrhage, or other neurologic complications such as seizure or coma. **Generally, symptoms of withdrawal from chronic use of any drug will produce effects opposite to those that the drug produces.** Therefore, withdrawal from stimulants produces fatigue, hypersomnia, and depression.

Sedatives

Sedatives produce central and peripheral autonomic depression. Common sedative drugs of abuse include **cannabis, BZDs, barbiturates, ethanol, opiates** (e.g., heroin, narcotic analgesics), and a newer drug popular at clubs, **gamma-hydroxybutyrate (GHB).** Such drugs enhance the inhibitory **$GABA_A$ receptor** and inhibit the excitatory NMDA receptor, or target other receptors that mediate sedative effects (e.g., cannabinoid and opioid receptors). Centrally, these drugs produce subjective feelings of sedation, cognitive depression, and dyscoordination (e.g., ataxia, dysarthria). Autonomic manifestations include the **parasympathomimetic effects** of pupillary miosis and relative bradycardia and hypotension. In severe overdose, central CNS depression produces *respiratory depression* due to decreased central responsiveness to the CO_2 content in the blood. Clinically, these intoxications can be distinguished by their differing pharmacokinetics and dynamics (i.e., duration of action, severity of effect) and even the order in which neurologic functions are depressed. For instance, GHB can produce severe coma with a GCS of 3 (the lowest possible) without producing respiratory depression. The withdrawal symptoms of sedatives include restlessness, anxiety, insomnia, and autonomic instability, including tachycardia and hypertension. Severe withdrawal can produce seizures and **delirium tremens,** a life-threatening withdrawal syndrome consisting of tremors, delirium, and severe autonomic instability. Often these symptoms require re-intoxication with the offending drug (often as self-medication by the user) or with an analog (e.g., BZDs).

Hallucinogens

Hallucinogens, such as **LSD,** and 3,4-methylenedioxymethamphetamine **(MDMA, ecstasy),** are marked by their ability to produce vivid and bizarre visual, auditory, and tactile hallucinations. They can also produce unusual sensory perceptions, or **synesthesias,** such as colors producing the perception of different sounds. They have mild autonomic effects and tend to be sympathomimetic. With LSD, the main adverse effects result from the patient's inability to handle the state of altered perception.

Impaired decision making can cause a person to engage in risky and at times life-threatening behavior. For instance, ecstasy, a popular club drug, produces a relatively benign syndrome of euphoria, enhanced mood, and perception of increased energy, often leading to continuous dancing and exertion for several hours. However, this can subsequently produce the more dangerous conditions of dehydration, hyponatremia (due to replacement of fluid loss with pure water), hyperthermia, rhabdomyolysis (from muscle breakdown), and renal failure.

Legal Drugs

Lastly, included in the list of drugs of abuse are legal drugs, which can produce the same phenomena of tolerance and of psychological and physical dependence. These drugs include **caffeine, alcohol, and tobacco.** In addition to physical dependence, the latter two produce significant long-term medical complications. In fact, some of the most prevalent causes of morbidity and mortality in the United States are associated with chronic alcohol ingestion or tobacco use.

The unifying characteristic of all these drugs is that they produce some form of **euphoria,** a very rewarding stimulus. It is hypothesized that the experience of **reward** is mediated by the release of **dopamine** from the presynaptic terminals of the **VTA** via the **median forebrain bundle** to the **nucleus accumbens, amygdala,** and **medial frontal cortex** of the **mesocorticolimbic dopamine system,** otherwise known as the reward center of the brain. The rewarding stimulus produces a compulsion or **craving** to repeat the drug use, that which is called **psychological dependence.** With repetitive use, neurons adapt by altering receptor and ion channel function and expression, signal transduction, gene expression, and synaptic connectivity. For instance, chronic ethanol exposure down-regulates the expression of NMDA receptors. These changes are thought to mediate the development of **tolerance,** wherein a user requires progressively higher doses of a drug to produce the same level of intoxication. These adaptive changes are also responsible for the development of **physical dependence,** wherein real pathophysiologic responses occur if the drug is withdrawn. All drugs of abuse, by definition, produce psychological dependence, but only a subset produce real physical dependence. The latter require not only behavioral modification therapy but also medical management to lessen the severity of the withdrawal syndrome, which at times can be life-threatening.

Cessation and rehabilitation are difficult tasks to accomplish. The barriers that a user must overcome are manifold and include intense craving, withdrawal, environmental stimuli that promote use, social pressures, life stresses, and lack of resources to help in quitting. Once a person is thinking about quitting (i.e., **contemplation** phase), it becomes crucial to follow up with immediate referral to counseling and perhaps medical support for withdrawal symptoms. Pharmacologic agents are increasingly being used as adjunctive therapy in the treatment of addictions. For nicotine addiction, nicotine replacement and treatment with bupropion (an antidepressant) or clonidine have been used with good efficacy. Pharmacologic therapies for other drugs are listed later.

CASE CONCLUSION

The patient probably took the popular club drug ecstasy, which is not usually available in the urine toxicology screening. She probably developed a hyponatremia from prolonged exertion, followed by fluid loss and simultaneous free-water intake. During her fluid resuscitation with normal saline, her vital signs are monitored and stabilized. Her fluids and electrolytes are corrected. She is referred to drug counseling and is sent home, having suffered no long-term sequelae.

THUMBNAIL: Behavioral Science—Substances of Abuse and Common Symptoms

Narcotic	Routes/Mechanism	Effects	Withdrawal Signs
Sedatives[a]			
Benzodiazepines Clonazepam Diazepam	Oral, physical dependence[b] **GABA agonist** Rx: **Flumazenil**	Cognitive difficulty, ataxia, pinpoint pupils, *lateral gaze nystagmus*, respiratory depression	Insomnia, restlessness, nightmares, *less severe than symptoms for barbiturates*
Barbiturates	Oral, physical dependence **GABA agonist**	Similar to alcohol and BZDs with *worse outcomes*	Insomnia, seizures, *delirium tremens*, hallucinations
Cannabis (THC) Marijuana, hashish	Smoked, oral **Cannabinoid agonist (CB$_1$, CB$_2$)**	Altered perception, "*amotivational syndrome,*" conjunctival injection, increased appetite, dry mouth	No significant withdrawal syndromes; some insomnia and restlessness in heavy users
GHB	Oral, liquid form, physical dependence Unknown MOA	Similar to alcohol, seizures, ***coma** followed by respiratory depression*, death	Insomnia, tremor, ↑ HR/BP, diaphoresis, *mild delirium tremens*
Stimulants (Sympathomimetics)			
Cocaine Free-base cocaine, crack	Intranasal, IV, oral, smoked **Blocks reuptake of NE, DA, and 5-HT** Short effect duration	*Hypervigilance*, paranoid delusions, chest pain, ↑ T/HR/BP, arrhythmias, mydriasis, dry mouth, death	Fatigue, nightmares, insomnia/hypersomnia, increased appetite, psychomotor retardation, agitation

(Continued)

THUMBNAIL: Behavioral Science—Substances of Abuse and Common Symptoms *(Continued)*

Narcotic	Routes/Mechanism	Effects	Withdrawal Signs
Amphetamines and **methamphetamine** *Speed, meth, ice, crystal, crack*	Oral, IV, intranasal, smoked **Increased NE, DA, 5-HT release** Long effect duration	*Enhanced concentration and physical performance*, grandiosity, anorexia, paranoid psychosis, ↑ T/HR/BP, hemorrhagic stroke, seizure, death	Intense fatigue, agitation, anergia, hypersomnia, prolonged mental depression, suicidal ideation
PCP *Angel dust*	Oral, IV, inhalation **NMDA receptor modulator, ↓ reuptake, and ↑ production DA, NE**	Hypervigilance, ataxia, ↑ HR/BP, myoclonus, analgesia, psychosis, *hypersalivation, vertical nystagmus*, coma, death	No significant stereotyped withdrawal syndrome
Ketamine *Special K*	Oral, intranasal, smoked Physical dependence **PCP derivative, similar mechanisms**	*"Dissociative anesthesia," immobility, nightmares*, mood elevation, sedation, amnesia, ↑ HR/BP	Flashbacks with visual disturbances weeks after exposure; associated with risky sexual behavior
Hallucinogens **LSD** *Acid*	Sublingual, smoked, intranasal, injected **Acts on 5-HT, DA receptors**	*Bizarre hallucinations*, altered perception and mood, anxiety, nausea, vomiting, diarrhea ↑ HR/BP, mydriasis	No significant withdrawal symptoms; rare, persistent psychosis; *flashbacks*
MDMA *Ecstasy XTC, E, X (popular at raves)*	Oral (intranasal) Increases 5-HT release and decreases 5-HT reuptake	Increased confidence, *empathy*, ↑ HR/BP, *hyperthermia, dehydration, rhabdomyolysis, renal failure*	No significant withdrawal symptoms; associated with risky sexual behavior

[a]Alcohol and opiates are not included in this table but should fall under the category of sedatives.
[b]All addictive drugs, by definition, produce psychological dependence and tolerance with repetitive use. Only some drugs produce physical dependence, which are marked by adverse physiologic effects if withdrawn. Those drugs that produce physical dependence are noted as such; otherwise, they only produce tolerance and psychological dependence.
BZD, benzodiazepine; DA, dopamine; 5-HT, serotonin; GABA, gamma-aminobutyric acid; GHB, gamma-hydroxybutyrate; LSD, lysergic acid diethylamide; MDMA, 3,4 methylenedioxymethamphetamine (ecstasy); MOA, mechanism of action; NE, norepinephrine; NMDA, N-methyl-D-aspartate; PDE, phosphodiesterase; PCP, phencyclidine; Ψ, psychological; THC, Δ-9-tetrahydrocannabinol (marijuana).

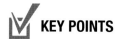

KEY POINTS

- Substances of abuse fall under three main categories: sedatives, stimulants, and hallucinogens; this simplification can aid with the diagnosis of a patient presenting with acute intoxication

- The effects of drugs are varied and may even be benign in isolation; however, intoxication may pose secondary dangers to the user due to impaired judgment, altered perception, and perhaps the unsafe social contexts within which the drug is used

- Reward and reinforcement of repetitive use are mediated by dopamine release in the mesocorticolimbic dopamine system; this produces psychological dependence

- Tolerance, physical dependence, and withdrawal syndromes are produced by the neurochemical adaptations that develop from chronic exposure to a drug

QUESTIONS

1. AT is a 16-year-old young man who is brought in by ambulance after being found by his mother "acting like he is on drugs." According to his mother, he was fighting with his 13-year-old brother and threatening to hit him for no apparent reason. He subsequently punched in the dry wall. When asked why he wanted to hit his brother, he said that his brother "wanted to steal his car and run off with his girlfriend." In the ED his vital signs were the following: T 38.5°C; HR 105; BP 148/89; RR 22; SaO₂ 98% on room air. He is found pacing the exam room with slight ataxic gait, answering appropriately but is at times tangential in his response. His pupils are equally dilated and minimally responsive to light; his extraocular movements are intact with a vertical nystagmus; his mucosal membranes are moist. He has diffusely exaggerated deep tendon reflexes. Which drug did he *most likely* take?

A. PCP
B. Cocaine
C. MDMA
D. Amphetamines
E. Methamphetamines

2. MA is a 35-year-old man who arrives in the ED agitated and tremulous. He is unable to give a history due to his altered mental status. His vital signs are as foll... 5°C; BP 150/100; HR 105; RR 24. He has no stig... holism and his physical exam is otherwise norm... valuation, he develops a generalized tonic-clonic... later given 4 mg of lorazepam, a BZD, to w... onds quickly with decreased agitation, tremulou... nal-izing vital signs. Which of the following co... ely cause of his presentation?

A. Alcohol withdrawal
B. BZD withdrawal
C. Barbiturate withdrawal
D. Methamphetamine overdose
E. All of the above

3. SJ is a 28-year-old woman who is brought in by ambulance after collapsing in the middle of a dance club. According to the bartender, she was noted to have three drinks that evening over the 3 hours she was in the club. A man who may have already left the bar bought one of those drinks for her. On the field she was unresponsive, with a GCS of 3, with the following vital signs: T 38.0°C; BP 135/85; HR 95; RR 20; SaO$_2$ 98% on room air. The rest of her physical exam and laboratory studies are normal. What is her *most* likely diagnosis?

A. BZD overdose
B. Alcohol intoxication
C. Barbiturate overdose
D. GHB overdose
E. Ketamine overdose

4. IL is a 21-year-old woman complaining of a recent episode of acute-onset 8/10 nonradiating, dull, substernal chest pain while at rest lasting for 30 minutes. She had one previous episode of such pain last night before going to bed. She denies having shortness of breath, nausea, vomiting, or diaphoresis. She was previously healthy and only taking an oral contraceptive (a low-dose estrogen-progesterone combination). Her vital signs are T 37.7°C; BP 147/82; HR 105; RR 24; SaO$_2$ 100% on room air. She is in mild distress, and her exam is otherwise normal. She currently has a normal EKG. What is the *most* important thing to ask her to help uncover the etiology of her chest pain?

A. Prior history of asthma
B. History of cocaine use
C. History of hypertension
D. Dosage of her oral contraceptive
E. Family history of early MI

HPI: CL is a 7-year-old boy who has been brought to the clinic by his parents, who are concerned that he might be "a little slow." His parents say that their son is a happy little boy who started school 2 years ago. His teacher reports that he has severe difficulties with reading, attention, and even memory. She recalls several episodes where he became very frustrated at his inability to understand the written word.

He is the youngest of five children and he had a normal birth. He achieved his developmental milestones, although some may have been a "little behind the others." He was slow to master language. He did not attend preschool, as his mother preferred to have him at home, but he had a year of kindergarten. He never appeared to have problems with hearing or vision. He had the usual childhood illnesses of chicken pox and the mumps. His parents describe him as a happy kid who enjoys playing with his toys. He still occasionally wets the bed.

FHx: There is no significant family history. His father is 50 years old, his mother is 49; both appear to be in good health. Their oldest son is 19 and attends junior college. None of their other children had any difficulties.

PE: WNL except for low-set ears. Neurologic exam is normal.

THOUGHT QUESTIONS

- How does mental retardation differ from learning disorders?
- What do you think is wrong with this child?

BASIC SCIENCE REVIEW AND DISCUSSION

Mental retardation is defined as significantly below-average intellectual functioning that begins before the age of 18 years and is associated with impairments in adaptive functioning. It is coded on Axis II. With mental retardation, IQ is approximately 70 or below (approximately two standard deviations). The IQ can be measured using standardized tests such as the Stanford-Binet or the Wechsler Intelligence Scales for Children. The severity of mental retardation is divided into four categories in the *Diagnostic and Statistical Manual of Mental Disorders, 4th edition (DSM-IV)*, based on IQ.

1. Mild mental retardation: IQ between 50–55 and 70
2. Moderate mental retardation: IQ between 35–40 and 50–55
3. Severe mental retardation: IQ 20–25 and 35–40
4. Profound mental retardation: IQ below 20 or 25

Patients with mental retardation also have deficits in more than two of the following skill areas: communication, self-care, home living, social/interpersonal skills, use of community resources, self-direction, academic skills, leisure, work, health, and safety.

Epidemiology

Mental retardation is found in approximately 1% of the population. This translates to 2.5 million people living in the United States. It is more common in boys than in girls; this may be due to higher rates of congenital abnormalities, x-linked conditions, prematurity, and stillbirths among boys.

Mild mental retardation accounts for approximately 85% of those with the disorder. These children may not be diagnosed until 5 to 10 years of age, and with special education techniques they can achieve academic levels of approximately a sixth grade level. With suitable supports these individuals can live in the community. Some can manage more independent living situations, but others need supervised settings.

Moderate mental retardation accounts for approximately 10% of those with the disorder. These individuals have communication skills and with vocational training and supervision can attend to some self-care. Educationally, they may reach a second grade level. They may be able work in sheltered workshops and live in supervised settings in the community.

Approximately 3 to 4% of those with mental retardation fall into the **severe** category. They can talk but cannot read adequately. They can manage to live in group homes or with their families unless they need specialized care. **Profound mental retardation** is found in approximately 1 to 2% of individuals with this disorder. Most of these individuals have an underlying neurologic disorder. They need constant supervision and help. Some may be able to perform simple tasks if training is successful.

Etiology of Mental Retardation

Those individuals who reside in long-stay facilities have higher rates of behavioral disturbances. Of those who are severely impaired approximately 32% have Down syndrome; genetic causes or associated malformations, perinatal injury, infections, and inborn errors of metabolism account for smaller percentages (see Thumbnail below).

A specific cause of mental retardation can be identified in approximately two thirds of cases. The more severe the impairment, the more likely it is that a cause will be identified. Individuals with mild mental retardation have an identifiable cause in approximately 30% of cases. More than 500 genetic disorders are associated with mental retardation (see Thumbnail below), and chromosomal disorders are responsible for 10% of all cases of mental retardation. Chromosomal abnormalities occur in 1 in 200 births and in 50% of first trimester miscarriages.

Fetal Alcohol Syndrome

FAS is the most common recognizable cause of mental retardation and is thought to occur in between 1 in 300 and 1 in 1000 newborns. The children have shallow philtrums without vertical ridges and short palpebral fissures. They also have growth retardation, particularly head circumference. The average IQ is approximately 65. These individuals often have problems with impulsivity, attention, psychiatric problems, and substance abuse. This may occur with in utero exposure to more than two units of alcohol a day during pregnancy. Milder variants of the disorder may be referred to as fetal alcohol effects.

Other nongenetic causes of mental retardation include the following:

1. **Toxic/nutrition:** Placental insufficiencies, malnutrition (includes neglect), lead encephalopathy, infantile hypoglycemia, teratogens such as medications (anticonvulsants), drugs (cocaine), FAS, and exposure to radiation
2. **Infection:** Toxoplasmosis, *Listeria*, rubella, CMV, syphilis, and herpes simplex in the mother; meningitis and encephalitis in the child
3. **Trauma:** Perinatal trauma, accidental and nonaccidental injury, including asphyxia

Prenatal factors account for the majority of individuals with severe mental retardation but less than half of those with mild retardation. Perinatal factors likely cause less than 10% of all cases of mental retardation, being more associated with cerebral palsy. Postnatal insults lead to approximately 5 to 10% of the cases of mental retardation.

Neurologic disorders are often associated with mental retardation. Seizure disorders are found in 15 to 30% of individuals with mental retardation; sensory impairments, in 10 to 20%; and motor abnormalities, in 20 to 30%. Mental retardation is found in approximately 50% of those with cerebral palsy.

Chromosomal abnormalities may be diagnosed by prenatal testing, such as amniocentesis, CVS, maternal serum alpha-fetoprotein, or ultrasound. Genetic counseling is offered to high-risk populations. Individuals with mental retardation should live as independently as possible, avoiding institutionalization and pursuing education and vocational training.

Learning Disorders

Difficulties in attaining intellectual skills at the same rate as others are known as **learning disorders** and were previously referred to as academic skills disorders. Learning disorders are diagnosed when the discrepancies between standardized tests in math, reading, or writing are more than two standard deviations behind those expected for age, schooling, and IQ. Learning disorders may also be referred to as learning disabled. Other disorders that affect academic performance include language and motor skills disorders. Difficulties can arise from inputting information (visual and auditory perception), integration of this input (sequencing and organizing), remembering of this information (short-term and long-term memory), and output (language). There are three types of learning disorders: **disorders of written expression, reading, and mathematics.**

Prevalence

Between 5 and 10% of the population have learning disorders, 4% of schoolchildren have a reading disorder, and 1% have a mathematics disorder. Boys have a higher prevalence of learning disorders than girls. Approximately 40% of children with learning disorders drop out of school.

Comorbid psychiatric disorders include conduct disorder, oppositional defiant disorder, major depression, dysthymia, attention-deficit/hyperactivity disorder (ADHD), and borderline personality disorder. These disorders may also lead to social problems, as they cause difficulties in peer group activities. These young people may also have problems with social skills. Between 20 and 25% of individuals with learning disorders have ADHD, and between 70 and 80% of those with ADHD have a learning disorder. Approximately 60% of those with Tourette syndrome have a learning disorder. Learning disorders may be caused by a variety of prenatal, perinatal, or postnatal insults. Studies have revealed a family pattern in between 40 and 50% of children, and monozygotic twins are more likely than dizygotic twins to have academic problems.

The differential diagnosis must include poor performance due to a lack of opportunity, poor teaching or cultural factors, impaired vision or hearing, mental retardation, and developmental disorder. These conditions may also coexist with a learning disorder.

Treatment of these disorders may include psychological, educational, and social skills training. These disorders are not cured but the individuals with these disorders and their families can be helped. Remedial methods are used to help those with reading disorders, which may include difficulties in decoding or comprehension, or a combination of both.

CASE CONCLUSION

You arrange for CL to have IQ testing. It reveals a nonverbal IQ in the normal range and a verbal IQ in the low-normal range, with some problems with vocabulary and language. Other testing found no difficulties with math but significant problems with reading skills in both recognition and comprehension. You persuade the parents to enroll him in extra individual reading classes three times a week; a year later he is doing well.

THUMBNAIL: Behavioral Science—Genetics Causes of Low IQ and Mental Retardation

Prenatal Causes	Examples
Genetic disorders: 32% of cases	
(1) Trisomies	Trisomy 21–22 (Down syndrome)
	Trisomy 17–18 (Edward syndrome)
	Trisomy 13–15 (Patau syndrome)
(2) Microdeletions	Cri du chat
	Wolf syndrome
	Prader-Willi syndrome
	Angelman syndrome
	Williams syndrome
(3) Multifactorial	Fragile X syndrome
	Familial mental retardation
	Tuberous sclerosis
	Metabolic disorders (PKU, Hunters, Lesch-Nyhan syndrome, galactosemia, Tay-Sachs, Niemann-Picks, etc.)
	Congenital hypothyroidism
Malformations of unknown cause: 8% of cases	
(1) CNS malformations	De Lange syndrome
	Sotos syndrome
	Neural tube defects
	Holoprosencephaly
(2) Multiple malformations	
Prenatal external causes: 12% of cases	
(1) Maternal infections	Toxoplasmosis, rubella, CMV, *Listeria,* syphilis, and HIV
(2) Toxins	FAS (discussed earlier)
(3) Placental insufficiency and toxemia	Prematurity
	Intrauterine growth retardation
(4) Miscellaneous	Radiation
	Traumatic injury
Perinatal causes: 11% of cases	
(1) Infection	HSV-2
	Meningitis
(2) Obstetric complications	Hypoxia
	Trauma
(3) Miscellaneous	Hyperbilirubinemia
Postnatal Causes: 8% of cases	
(1) Infection	Encephalitis
	Meningitis
(2) Toxic	Lead poisoning
(3) CNS disease and disorders	Trauma
	Tumors
	Cerebrovascular accidents
(4) Psychosocial problems	Poor nutrition, lack of stimulation, and abuse

✓ KEY POINTS

- Academic skills disorder may appear similar to mild mental retardation, visual or hearing impairments, or neurologic deficits
- Five to ten percent of the U.S. population have learning disorders
- Four percent of school children have a reading disorder, and one percent have a mathematics disorder; studies have reported that boys have a higher prevalence than girls
- Approximately 40% of children with learning disorders drop out of school
- Mental retardation affects approximately 1% of the population
- Approximately 85% have mild mental retardation, 10% have moderate retardation, and 3 to 4% have severe retardation

QUESTIONS

1. Which of the following statements concerning learning disorders is accurate?
   A. Between 30 and 40% of those diagnosed with reading disorder are males.
   B. Approximately 0.5% of schoolchildren have reading disorder.
   C. Approximately 5% of schoolchildren have mathematics disorder.
   D. It is rare to have a disorder of written expression without another learning disorder.
   E. They are not often found in association with general medical conditions.

2. A 32-year-old primigravida has just delivered a full-term baby girl. The midwife asks you to examine her more closely because she is concerned that the baby may have Down syndrome. Which of the following features would you expect to find in an infant with Down syndrome?
   A. Brushfield spots; high, arched palate; and floppy ears
   B. Brushfield spots; high, arched palate; and hypertonic muscles
   C. Prognathism, epicanthic folds, and protruding tongue
   D. Prognathism, single palmar crease, and blue eyes
   E. Epicanthic folds, protruding tongue, and single palmar crease

3. The parents of an 8-year-old boy with mild mental retardation bring him in for his annual physical. They are concerned about planning for his future. Which of the following could you tell them?
   A. The mortality rates are four times that of the general population for all individuals with mild mental retardation younger than age 20 years.
   B. The life expectancy is directly related to their IQ.
   C. Most individuals with mental retardation develop seizures.
   D. There is no increased risk of developing psychiatric disorders.
   E. They should plan for institutional care.

4. Which of the following features are associated with Rett disorder?
   A. Microcephaly, gait abnormalities, and increased purposeful hand movements
   B. Macrocephaly, gait abnormalities, and decreased purposeful hand movements
   C. Microcephaly, loss of previously acquired skills, and stereotyped movements
   D. Microcephaly, loss of previously acquired skills, equal sex distribution
   E. Microcephaly, loss of previously acquired skills, and increased male distribution

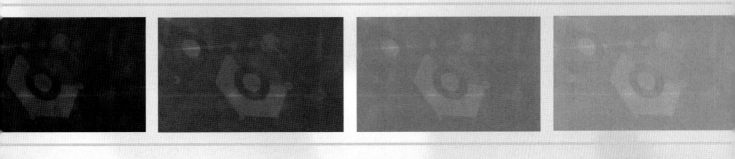

PART IX
Epidemiology, Biostatistics, and Health Policy

HPI: MM is a 56-year-old white male who presents for management of hypercholesterolemia to you, his primary care physician. You offer to start him on your favorite statin of choice and tell him that the mean reduction in total cholesterol is 15 points. MM then asks, "Does that mean that half the people who use the medication experience an even greater reduction in their cholesterol level?"

THOUGHT QUESTIONS

- What is the answer to MM's question?
- What are the three different measures of the center of a distribution?
- What are two ways that the dispersion of a distribution is measured?

BASIC SCIENCE REVIEW AND DISCUSSION

The measurement of most outcomes in a population of subjects will vary. Whether you are measuring height, weight, blood pressure, or the change in any of these, there is usually variation between subjects. The collection of data on one of these variables is known as a distribution. We are often interested in some central tendency of a distribution, or what subjects experienced, "on average." The three standard measures of the center of a distribution are the mean, median, and mode. The **mean** (also known as the arithmetic mean or average) is the weighted sum of all measurements in a distribution. For example, if there are N subjects, the mean is the sum of all of the measurements divided by N, denoted by:

$$\bar{X} = \Sigma x_i / N$$

where $\bar{X}$ is the symbol for the sample mean, Σ is the symbol for a sum, and x_i represents each of the measurements as i varies from 1 to N. The **median** of a sample is that value that falls directly in the middle of all of the measurements; that is, 50% of them are above the median and 50% are below. If there are an even number of measurements, then the median is the average of the middle two values. The **mode** is that value that occurs most commonly in a distribution.

Variation of Distributions

Although the mean and median give a feeling of the middle of a distribution, one also needs a measurement to describe the dispersion of the data. That is, while the data sets {49, 50, 51}

and {1, 50, 99} have the same mean, they are very different data. The **variance**, σ^2, or its square root the standard deviation, σ, is used to describe the dispersion of a distribution around its mean. If these values are higher, then the data are dispersed further away from the mean. In the most commonly assumed shape of a **distribution,** the normal distribution, the interval ranging from one standard deviation below the mean to one standard deviation above the mean, contains 68% of the data. If expanded to 1.96 standard deviations above and below the mean, 95% of the data is contained by the interval. A classic way to present data is the mean plus or minus 1.96 standard deviations, giving a 95% **confidence interval (CI).** If the analysis is part of a comparison of a study result to a null hypothesis, commonly 1 or 0, if the null hypothesis is not contained in the 95% CI, then it can be rejected.

Since the median measures the point at which 50% of the data are above it and 50% below, the dispersion measures used echo this technique; the most commonly used are the 25th and 75th centile points. This is where 25% of the data are below and above these points. Any centile mark can be used; 5th, 10th, 90th, and 95th are the most common after the 25th and 75th.

Types of Distributions

In a symmetric distribution (i.e., the distribution is a mirror image of itself when folded over on the mean), the mean and median are the same value. Symmetric distributions include the normal distribution, or bell-shaped curve, and uniform distributions where any value in the possible range has the same probability of occurring. Other distributions may not be symmetric and can be described as skewed to the right or to the left (Fig. 9-1), meaning that there are values that are farther away from the mean or median to the right or to the left, respectively. Another type of distribution seen commonly in medicine is the bimodal distribution (Fig. 9-2), where two disparate results are seen much more commonly than the others. Other common distributions include the Poisson, Bernoulli, and binomial, which are further described in the Thumbnail below.

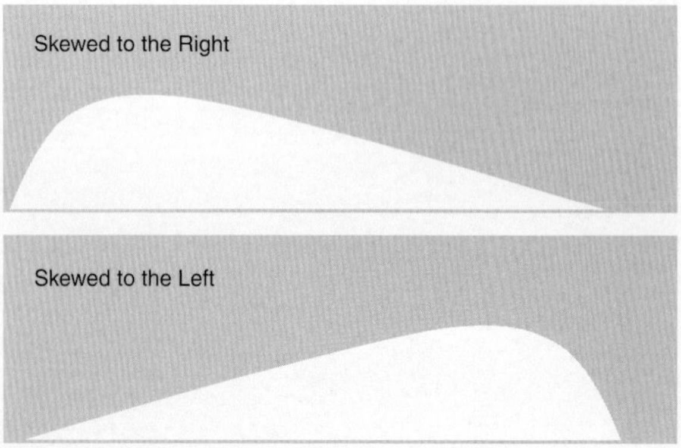

Skewed to the Right

Skewed to the Left

• **Figure 9-1.** Asymmetric distributions.

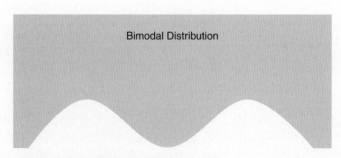

Bimodal Distribution

• **Figure 9-2.** Bimodal distribution.

CASE CONCLUSION

Given the preceding information, you discuss with MM that the mean decrement of 15 points means that the average person will lose 15 points off of their total cholesterol measurement. However, because the distribution is skewed to the left, toward 0, more than 50% will actually experience a less than 15-point drop, but a few people will experience a very large drop.

THUMBNAIL: Biostatistics—Common Distributions and Their Mean and Variance

Distribution	Parameter(s)	Formula	Mean $[E(X)] = \bar{X}$	Variance
Uniform Defined over an interval (a,b), where probability of outcomes is equal	a, b	$P(\bar{X} < c) = (c - a)/(b - a)$, where c is between a and b	$(a + b)/2$	$(b - a)^2/12$
Bernoulli Trial with binary outcomes 0 or 1	p	$P(\bar{X} = 1) = p$ $P(\bar{X} = 0) = 1 - p$	p	$p^*(1 - p)$
Binomial Number of occurrences x in a series of n Bernoulli trials	n, p	$P(\bar{X} = x) =$ $(nCy)^* p^y (1 - p)^{n-y}$	np	$np(1 - p)$
Poisson Number of occurrences x in a given time period t	$\lambda = x/t$	$P(\bar{X} = x/\lambda) = e^{-\lambda} \lambda^x/x!$	λ	λ

KEY POINTS

- The most common summary statistics utilized are the mean, or arithmetic average, and the median, which marks where 50% of the values are above and below
- The variance (and its square root–standard deviation) give information about the spread of a distribution around its mean
- When looking at a distribution around a median, more commonly, percentiles such as the 75th or 95th are used to communicate about the distribution
- The most common distribution assumed and used in biostatistics is the normal distribution (or bell-shaped curve)

QUESTIONS

1. Given the following collection of data {1,2,4,6,7,8,9}, which is correct?
   A. The mean is 5.0.
   B. The median is 5.0.
   C. The median is 5.5.
   D. The median is 6.0.
   E. The mean is 6.0.

2. Given the following collection of data {1,1,1,1,2,3,5,5, 6,6,7,7,9,9}, which of the following is correct?
   A. The mode is 1.
   B. The mean is 4.5.
   C. The median is 6.
   D. A and B are correct.
   E. A and C are correct.

3. Which of the following statements is true about a 95% confidence interval?
   A. There is a 95% chance that the true value is in the interval.
   B. Ninety-five percent of the time, the true value will fall in the interval.

   C. If you repeated the study 20 times, the true value would be in the interval at least once.
   D. If the interval does not contain the null hypothesis, you can be 95% certain that your result is the true value.
   E. If you repeat the study an infinite number of times, the results would fall in the interval 95% of the time.

4. You are told that your patient has a cholesterol result that is the mean of that in the population. Which of the following distributions would also mean that his result is necessarily greater than half of the population?
   A. Skewed to the left
   B. Skewed to the right
   C. Uniform
   D. Normal
   E. Bimodal

HPI: ST is a medical student who is working with you in an outpatient clinic. She comes to you with a research paper regarding an issue on a patient you saw together the previous day. The patient had high cholesterol and was asking to be treated with a drug that he saw in an advertisement. You had told the patient that there is no evidence to suggest that the drug is any better than the current medication he is on. The paper that ST brings to you found that in two groups of patients the mean value of total cholesterol points lowered was 12 for the new drug and 10 for the old drug in a study with a total of 40 patients. ST asks, "Doesn't this study show that the new drug is better than the old drug?"

THOUGHT QUESTIONS

- What is the answer to ST's question?
- What test is used to compare two means?
- What test is used to compare two proportions?
- What test can be used to compare more than two groups?
- When these tests are used, how do you know what kind of errors in the findings might be made?

BASIC SCIENCE REVIEW AND DISCUSSION

One of the fundamental purposes of biostatistics is to be able to compare the summary statistics of two or more groups and determine the likelihood that the two groups are different. In the preceding case, we are interested in whether the mean values of 10 and 12 are statistically different. A number of factors go into this. The most important is how different the numbers actually are. In this case, 12 and 10 are relatively close together in that the total difference is 2 and, proportionately, 12 is only 20% more than 10. Nearly as important is the size of the study. In a study with thousands of patients in each group, these findings are likely to be statistically different. In this study with 40 patients, they are less likely to be statistically different, but this needs to be examined.

It is equally important to ask, when considering a finding such as the preceding, not only whether the results are statistically significant but also whether the findings are clinically significant. Essentially, one must ask whether the difference suggested by the results is enough to make a difference in clinical outcome. In the preceding case, it is unclear whether two more points lowered by a cholesterol-lowering agent are likely to make a clinical difference.

Finally, when considering studies, it is important to think of the results not as absolute, but as possibly making one of two types of errors. Results can essentially fall into one of four categories, true positive, true negative, false positive, and false negative. The first two mean that the results indicated by the study are correct. A false-positive result is known as a **type I error.** This is what researchers attempt to avoid by having the null hypothesis be rejected only if it falls outside of a 95% confidence interval, or a $p < .05$ standard used in statistical tests. A false-negative result is known as a **type II error.** Unfortunately, the standards used to examine type II error are poorer. Many studies with negative results do not report the probability of a type II error. The probability of not making a type II error is known as power. As compared with the less than 5% chance of making a type I error, commonly the standard for making a type II error is less than 20%, or only 80% power. One of the reasons for this is that many times to ensure a negative finding it is not worth the cost of increasing the sample size to ensure greater power. For the purposes of clinicians, it is important to understand these issues and the statistical tests used to compare outcomes.

Comparison of Two Groups

The two common summary statistics that will be compared between two groups are the mean of some measurement and the proportion of the group that is positive for some characteristic. When comparing means, the test used is called the **student t test.** The t test takes the difference between two means, divides it by a pooled estimate of the variance, and compares the result against a table of values dependent on the degrees of freedom. When comparing two proportions, the **z test** is commonly used. This test statistic is normally distributed, so it resembles the t test with an infinite number of degrees of freedom.

The t Test An example of a situation in which the t test would be used is to compare the mean effect of an agent to lower cholesterol. Let us assume there are two agents, A and B, and we are comparing their effects in a small trial of 40 patients with the following results:

	A ($n = 18$)		B ($n = 22$)	
	Mean	SD	Mean	SD
Cholesterol difference	12	3	10	2

(where SD is standard deviation)

The formula for the t test is:

$$T = (X_A - X_B)/\{\sqrt{(s^2/n_A + s^2/n_B)}\} \ (s^2 = \text{pooled variance})$$

Where the pooled variance, $s^2 = \{(n_A - 1)(SD_A^2) + (n_B - 1)(SD_B^2)\}/(n_A + n_B - 2)$. So:

$$s^2 = \{(18 - 1)(3^2) + (22 - 1)(2^2)\}/(18 + 22 - 2)$$
$$= \{(17 \times 9) + (21 \times 4)\}/38$$
$$= 237/38 = 6.24$$

and the t test is:

$$t = (12 - 10)/\sqrt{(6.24/18 + 6.24/22)}$$
$$t = 2/\sqrt{(0.3467 + 0.2836)}$$
$$t = 2/\sqrt{(0.6303)} = 2/(0.79) = 2.53$$

We then examine the t test table for 38 degrees of freedom **(dof)** and find the following:

t test probability	0.5	0.2	0.1	0.05	0.02	0.01
	0.005	0.001				
38 **dof** t value	0.681	1.304	1.686	2.024	2.429	
	2.712	2.98	3.57			

So our value of 2.53 leads to a p value just under 0.02, or more than 98% certainty that the two means are different.

Interestingly, even with this relatively small sample size, these findings were statistically significantly different. Another way to examine these findings would be to see what proportion of patients experienced a certain outcome.

The z Test Now let us assume that instead of comparing the mean values in the two groups, we care about the proportion of patients whose cholesterol was decreased by 10 points or more. Examining the same group studied earlier, we find:

	A (n = 18)	B (n = 22)
Number > 10 points	14	10
Proportion (p)	0.78	0.45

Now, when comparing sample proportions, we need the proportions, sample size, and standard errors. Since these types of proportions are simply Bernoulli trials—that is, each subject either does or does not meet the criteria proposed—an estimate for the standard error can be used from the Bernoulli distribution. That is,

$$\text{Std error, } s = \sqrt{[p(1-p)/n]}$$

So the estimated standard errors for the preceding would be:

$$s_A = \sqrt{(0.78 * 0.22/18)} = \sqrt{(0.00953)} = 0.098$$
$$s_B = \sqrt{(0.45 * 0.55/22)} = \sqrt{(0.01125)} = 0.106$$

And the z test is: $z = (p_A - p_B)/\sqrt{(s_A^2 + s_B^2)}$

$z = (0.78 - 0.45)/\sqrt{(0.00953 + 0.01125)} = 0.33/0.144 = 2.29$

Since this is a z test, it is comparable to a t test with an infinite number of degrees of freedom and is based on the normal distribution.

z test Probability	0.5	0.2	0.1	0.05	0.02	0.01	0.005 0.001
z value	0.675	1.282	1.645	1.96	2.326	2.576	2.807 3.291

So, the results of the test are that it is almost 98% certain that the proportion of subjects in group A that had a 10-point or greater drop in diastolic blood pressure is greater than that in group B. This comparison is done using a two-tailed test, since there is no initial assumption regarding which group is assumed to have a higher proportion. Of note, instead of a z test, commonly the **chi-square test** is used to compare proportions. Interestingly, the z-distribution and chi-square distribution are related, in that as the sample size is large, the z-distribution squared is the chi-square distribution. One major advantage of the chi-square distribution is that it can be used not only to compare two proportions but also to analyze a study with multiple proportional results.

 CASE CONCLUSION

Going through the study with ST, you find that indeed there was a statistically significant difference in the two cholesterol-lowering agents. However, from a much larger clinical study you know that the difference of two points actually does not seem to make a long-term difference in rates of MI or stroke. Thus, you opt to wait for more evidence about the possibility that the drug will lower cholesterol more than this initial study showed or that this small difference will make a clinically significant difference in outcomes.

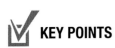 **THUMBNAIL:** Biostatistics—Types of Errors Made in Research

	True Results	
Study Results	Positive	Negative
Positive	True positive	False positive Type I error
Negative	False negative Type II error	True negative

KEY POINTS

- When comparing two means, commonly the student t test is used
- When comparing two proportions, either the z test or chi-square test may be used
- The chi-square test can also be used to compare more than two proportions
- It is important to consider whether findings are both statistically significant and clinically significant

TABLE 9-1 Results of Example Study for Question 4

Study Results	True Results	
	Positive	Negative
Positive	True positive 85	False positive 50
Negative	False negative 15	True negative 950

QUESTIONS

1. You read a paper in which the null hypothesis was not rejected with $p = 0.18$. A power analysis was done revealing 96% power. What is the probability that a type II error was made?

   A. 0
   B. 0.04
   C. 0.18
   D. 0.82
   E. 1

2. You are designing a study to investigate whether ethnicity is associated with type II DM. You have a cohort of 1000 patients of Asian, African American, Caucasian, and Latino ethnicity. Which of the following tests would be the best to compare the results of the study?

   A. Student t test
   B. Power analysis
   C. z test
   D. Chi-square test
   E. Bonferroni correction

3. Which of the following best describes a type I error?

   A. There is a positive result on a screening test, but the patient does not have the disease.
   B. There is a positive result on a screening test, and the patient does have the disease.
   C. There is a negative result on a screening test, and the patient does not have the disease.
   D. There is a negative result on a screening test, but the patient does have the disease.
   E. None of the above.

4. The following results from a screening study are available (Table 9-1). What is the rate of type I and type II errors, respectively?

   A. 0.15, 0.05
   B. 0.85, 0.05
   C. 0.95, 0.15
   D. 0.05, 0.85
   E. 0.05, 0.15

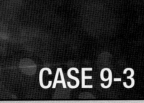

CASE 9-3 Screening Tests

HPI: AM is a 35-year-old G1P0 woman at 14 weeks' gestation. She comes for a routine prenatal visit. At the end of her visit she tells you that she saw a genetic counselor and despite his recommendation to obtain an amniocentesis she would prefer to avoid the risk of this procedure if possible. You validate her decision and ask if she would like to obtain a triple-marker screening test for Down syndrome, which has an 80% sensitivity in women age 35 and older. She is interested in this test because it involves only drawing blood and she will be quite happy to avoid the amniocentesis if the test is negative.

Her screening test returns the following week and is negative using a 1:190 cutoff. You tell her the happy news, and she asks, "Does this mean my baby does not have Down syndrome?"

THOUGHT QUESTIONS

- What is the answer to AM's question?
- What are the sensitivity and specificity of a screening test?
- What are positive and negative predictive values?
- What are likelihood ratios?

BASIC SCIENCE REVIEW AND DISCUSSION

Often in medicine there are two possible pathways to a diagnosis. One method, illustrated earlier by amniocentesis, involves a risky, often more expensive diagnostic test. The second often involves utilizing a much less risky, often cheaper screening test to identify the high-risk patients within a population in order to determine who should undergo the more invasive test. Which pathway to use is dependent on the importance of the diagnosis, the baseline risk of the patient, the risk of the diagnostic procedure, and the test characteristics of the screening test. The two classic test characteristics reported are usually the sensitivity and specificity, and these, in addition to the other attributes of the situation, are used to determine whether a patient will benefit from being screened.

Test Characteristics

Sensitivity is defined as the percentage of cases identified by a screening test. If among 100 cases, a screening test identifies 93 of them, then it has a 93% sensitivity. In a 2 × 2 table it is the number of true positives divided by the total number with disease

(Table 9-2). *Specificity* is the percentage of people without disease who are correctly identified as not having disease. For example, if in the same population above there were 100 people who were not cases, and 96 of them were identified as not being cases, then the test has 96% specificity. In a 2 × 2 table this would be the number of true negatives divided by the total number of individuals without disease (Table 9-2). Of importance is the relationship between sensitivity and specificity. Most screening tests return a value that is either above or below a threshold. Where the threshold is set determines the sensitivity and specificity. If the threshold of the test is set quite low, then the sensitivity will be high but the specificity low. Conversely, if the threshold is set quite high, then the sensitivity will be low but the specificity high. When the sensitivity versus 1 minus specificity are plotted for a series of possible threshold values for a test, it is called a receiver-operator curve (ROC). The ROC can be examined to look for an optimal point where the trade-off between sensitivity increase and specificity decrease is equalized (Fig. 9-3).

Predictive Value of Screening Tests

Although the trade-off between sensitivity and specificity is an important consideration, another is how useful the test is to differentiate individuals with a diagnosis from those without. One way to use the results of a screening test is to use its predictive value. The **positive predictive value** (PPV) is the proportion of screen-positive patients who actually have the diagnosis. These are

TABLE 9-2 Bacterial Organisms Sensitivity and Specificity in a 2 × 2 Table

		Disease	
		Present	**Absent**
Test Result	Positive	a = TP true positive	b = FP false positive
	Negative	c = FN false negative	d = TN true negative
	Sensitivity = a/(a+c) Specificity = d/(b+d)		

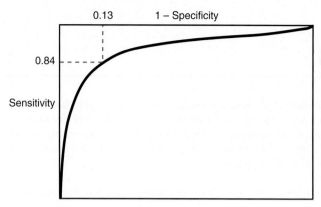

• **Figure 9-3.** The ROC diagram illustrates the trade-off between sensitivity and specificity. In the ROC above, the point chosen illustrates where the sensitivity is 84% and the specificity is 87%.

the true-positive patients divided by all those who test positive, or $a/(a + b)$ in a 2 × 2 table (Table 9-3). The **negative predictive value** (NPV) is the proportion of screen-negative patients who do not have the diagnosis. These are the true-negative patients divided by all who test negative, or $d/(c + d)$ in a 2 × 2 table (Table 9-3). In the example of the triple marker screen, because the test is positive for all women with a risk greater than or equal to 1:190, the PPV is poor, only about 1%. The NPV, on the other hand, is quite good, at 1:700 or better. This is because the baseline risk in the population is low.

Likelihood Ratios

The PPV and NPV of tests can also be calculated by using likelihood ratios (LR). A likelihood ratio is the probability of a particular test finding in a patient with disease divided by the probability of the same test finding in a patient without the disease. Thus, a likelihood ratio can be calculated for both positive and negative tests. A positive likelihood ratio, LR(+), is equal to the sensitivity divided by 1 − specificity, whereas the negative likelihood ratio, LR(+), is equal to 1 − sensitivity divided by the specificity. This is shown here:

$$LR(+) = \frac{\text{Prob(pos test given disease)}}{\text{Prob(pos test given no disease)}} = \frac{a/(a + c)}{b/(b + d)}$$
$$= \frac{\text{sensitivity}}{1 - \text{specificity}}$$

$$LR(-) = \frac{\text{Prob(neg test given disease)}}{\text{Prob(neg test given no disease)}} = \frac{c/(a + c)}{d/(b + d)}$$
$$= \frac{\text{specificity}}{1 - \text{sensitivity}}$$

Now that we know how to calculate likelihood ratios, we need one more concept in order to use them to calculate posttest probabilities. What we need is odds as opposed to probability. Odds is a ratio of probabilities, defined as the probability of an event occurring divided by the probability of the event not occurring.

$$\text{Odds} = p/(1 - p) \text{ and } p = \text{Odds}/(\text{Odds} + 1)$$

The likelihood ratio is actually multiplied by the pretest odds to calculate the posttest odds. So the pretest probability can be converted to odds using the first of the preceding equations, then multiplied by the likelihood ratio, and converted back to probability using the second equation. Of note, when the pretest probability is small, less than 1%, odds and probability are almost equal.

CASE CONCLUSION

You explain to AM that, despite a negative test, there is a small chance that her baby has Down syndrome, though using a LR(−) of 0.5, the probability is only half of what it was before having the test. Because she had not wanted an amniocentesis to begin with and now knows that her probability is lower, she decides to do without the diagnostic test. Her healthy 46XX baby girl is born five and a half months later.

TABLE 9-3 Calculating Predictive Value

		Disease	
		Present	Absent
Test Result	Positive	a = TP true positive	b = FP false positive
	Negative	c = FN false negative	d = TN true negative
	PPV = a/(a+b) NPV = d/(c+d)		

THUMBNAIL: Biostatistics—Example of How to Use a 2 × 2 Table

Let's assume we are given the following 2 × 2 table for Down syndrome screening:

		Disease	
		Present	Absent
Test Result	Positive	a = 10 true positive	b = 980 false positive
	Negative	c = 10 false negative	d = 9000 true negative

Sensitivity = $a/(a + c)$ = 10/(20) = 0.5
Specificity = $d/(b + d)$ = 9000/(9980) = 0.90
PPV = $a/(a + b)$ = 10/(990) = 0.01
NPV = $d/(c + d)$ = 9000/(9010) = 0.999
LR(+) = sens/(1 − spec) = 0.5/0.1 = 5
LR(−) = (1 − sens)/spec = 0.5/0.9 = 0.56

Example of using LR(+):
In this case, the pretest probability is 20/10,000 = 0.002
Odds = 0.002/(1 − 0.002) = 0.002
Posttest odds = 0.002 × (5) = 0.01
Posttest–rob. = 0.01/(1.01) = 0.01 = PPV

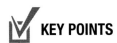

KEY POINTS

- Any screening test has a trade-off between sensitivity and specificity
- Because most screening tests are noninvasive, usually the goal is to get a maximum sensitivity
- The predictive value of a test tells you what the probability of disease is in someone with that test result
- The likelihood ratio can be used in a setting in which you do not have a 2 × 2 table to calculate the predictive value of the test

QUESTIONS

1. You are interested in developing a screening program to identify patients at high risk for a hematologic disease. The diagnostic test (bone marrow biopsy) for this disease is expensive, is painful, and has associated risks. There is no treatment at this time for the disease, but you feel it would be of some benefit to know whether you do have the disease earlier rather than later. If you are to be screening the general population, what test characteristics would you consider to be the best?

   A. 99% sensitivity and 10% specificity
   B. 98% sensitivity and 20% specificity
   C. 96% sensitivity and 40% specificity
   D. 90% sensitivity and 75% specificity
   E. 86% sensitivity and 99% specificity

2. A screening test is performed and there are 10 positive results. Of these, six are false positives. Of note, there are exactly 10 people with disease in the population screened. Which of the following is true?

   A. This test has a 40% sensitivity.
   B. This test has a 60% sensitivity.
   C. This test has a 100% sensitivity.
   D. This test has a 60% specificity.
   E. This test has a 40% specificity.

3. A screening test for diabetes is being evaluated. You know that 900 nondiabetics and 100 diabetics are being screened. There are 100 positive tests and of these, 90 have diabetes. Which of the following is true in this population?

   A. The NPV of the test is 0.9.
   B. The NPV of the test is 0.5.
   C. The PNV of the test is 0.1.
   D. The PPV of the test is 0.1.
   E. The PPV of the test is 0.9.

4. In the screening test in question 3, what is the LR(+)?

   A. 1
   B. 8
   C. 81
   D. 99
   E. 990

HPI: CP is a 24-year-old woman who presents to the hospital for the management of her first labor and delivery. During her labor, her fetus begins to show nonreassuring signs on the fetal heart tracing known as late decelerations, but the fetal heart rate variability is still excellent. Suddenly, the fetal heart rate drops down to the 80s (normal is between 120 and 160). The staff moves the patient to the operating room for an emergent cesarean delivery. This is accomplished with delivery of the fetus 14 minutes from the time the fetal heart rate decreased. Upon delivery, there was noted to be a complete placental abruption with extreme maternal blood loss and the development of a consumptive coagulopathy. CP is given blood products and is stabilized without need for hysterectomy. However, her baby has seizures on the first day of life several hours after delivery.

THOUGHT QUESTIONS

- Was this a case of malpractice?
- What factors might affect the probability of whether this will lead to a lawsuit?
- How can physicians decrease the chance that they will be sued?

MEDICAL-LEGAL REVIEW AND DISCUSSION

To determine whether the actions of a healthcare practitioner are consistent with malpractice, they need to be compared with existing national and local standards of practice. Medicine is not practiced in a vacuum, and what is considered standard practice can vary throughout the country (and certainly around the world). For instance, the procedure that is most commonly performed for an acute MI, angioplasty, stent placement, or CABG may vary between institutions and have regional trends. However, national standards also may be put forth by an accredited body, such as the American College of Surgeons, or research literature may be used to substantiate a particular clinical pathway.

In the preceding case, it is difficult to know from the description how long the fetal heart rate tracing showed the nonreassuring late decelerations. Even in light of these, fetal heart rate variability is more predictive of current fetal status, and that description did not necessarily merit action on the part of the obstetrician. Once the acute sign of fetal distress, the fetal bradycardia, occurred, the obstetrician and labor and delivery team acted quickly and were able to deliver the fetus in 14 minutes. The American College of Obstetricians and Gynecologists has used the standard of 30 minutes, and research suggests that the most serious fetal morbidity occurs once bradycardia is 15 minutes or longer. Given these two aspects of support for the care given, as well as the excellent care for CP intraoperatively and postoperatively for her coagulopathy, there is no evidence of malpractice in this case. However, whether a lawsuit will result in this setting is a different story.

Risk Factors for a Lawsuit

The principal risk factor for a lawsuit in medical practice is a bad patient outcome. If a physician makes errors in the care of a patient but the errors do not result in a bad patient outcome, the patient is unlikely to sue. Moreover, if the patient wants to sue, it is unlikely that such a suit would yield much, since there are little or no damages. Given this, what patients may define as a bad outcome can be quite varied, and often more pain and suffering or mental anguish than might have been experienced in another healthcare setting can be considered a bad outcome for

litigious patients. While having a bad outcome is an almost necessary risk factor for a lawsuit, it is not sufficient. Bad outcomes occur constantly in the healthcare setting. In fact, it is estimated that even among patients who do have bad outcomes and experience some degree of substandard care, 5% or fewer of these patients proceed to a lawsuit. Given these low numbers, what other factors might be predictive of lawsuits?

One clear factor that is predictive of whether a patient will sue is the type of relationship that the patient and the care provider enjoy. Thus, patients are more likely to sue physicians who they have only interacted with a short time than they are to sue those with whom they have longstanding relationships. Another factor is the nature of their relationship. If the physician has provided what the patient perceives as excellent care for a long time, then the patient is less likely to sue than if he or she perceives that the physician has made other mistakes or provided care different from what he or she would have liked in the past.

Another factor related to the relationship is that of the communication between the physician and the patient. Often physicians who are overworked and dealing with several ill patients simultaneously may be rushed in their communication with a patient and the patient's family. Furthermore, it is common that once a bad event or outcome occurs that the physician may avoid that patient either from feelings of guilt or simply because talking to patients about bad outcomes is difficult. It has been shown that physicians who simply spend more time with patients communicating about their disease, the plan of treatment, and the possible outcomes are sued less often. Similarly, physicians are also less likely to be sued if they seek to communicate with the patient and the family frequently after a bad outcome and explain what happened and what the plan of care is now.

It seems that certainly these two risk factors are the most important to a physician or a physician-in-training, as they are what can most easily be affected by physician behavior. However, other risk factors exist, such as patient demographics and socioeconomic status (wealthy > poor), region of the country (northeast > midwest), and the field of medicine (obstetrics > internal medicine) being practiced. However, a physician cannot affect these factors other than by moving or changing the field of medicine being practiced.

Evidence-Based Practice Opposed to Defensive Medicine

Because of concerns for lawsuits, many physicians practice defensive medicine. An example of this would be ordering a CT for every patient with a headache or at least for those who ask for one. It results in the waste of medical resources, causes unnecessary tests, and rarely results in better outcomes. In fact, because tests all have false-positive rates, it can lead to further risky diagnostic tests that may lead to complications.

A better way to practice that is also likely to avoid lawsuits, or at least avoid malpractice, is to practice evidence-based medicine. This seems obvious; however, with the number of medical journals and advances in medicine in the pharmaceutical, diagnostic technology, and procedural fronts, it can be difficult to keep abreast of all of the changes in medical practice once a physician completes training. Continuing medical education (CME) credits are required to maintain licensure, but one or two courses per year rarely update the clinical knowledge necessary to stay at the forefront of medical practice. Another way to maintain excellence is to attend weekly grand rounds and morbidity and mortality rounds at a university teaching hospital. Practicing in a group of physicians rather than in solo practice is another way to stay on top of changes in the practice of medicine. as is reading the current journals as much as possible. Usually, summaries of important journal articles and updates on clinical practice are published by medical societies. These are excellent substitutes for failing to read three or four journals per month and provide an idea of national standards.

CASE CONCLUSION

After CP's cesarean section, her physician meets with her family to describe what happened to her and her baby, and answers their numerous questions. In the following 5 days, CP's physician sees her every morning and evening while she recovers from her cesarean delivery and coagulopathy. He also checks in with the neonatologists frequently to determine how her baby is doing and communicates this information to CP. An MRI of CP's baby's brain shows no evidence of anoxic brain injury. CP is discharged home on postoperative day 5 and her baby is able to go home on day 10 of life. A week later, she sees her obstetrician in the clinic and they again discuss the events that led to her emergent cesarean delivery. A year later, she presents to her obstetrician's office again with a positive pregnancy test. She reports that her baby is slightly delayed, but making progress on all of his developmental milestones.

THUMBNAIL: Medical-Legal Issues—Decreasing Risk of Lawsuit

Risk Factor	Description
Relationship	Forming longstanding relationships with patients does decrease the risk of a lawsuit; however, this is impossible in an acute setting. A strong immediate relationship can be formed by acknowledging patient concerns, discussing tests and treatments before they are ordered, and breaking down some of the professional barriers that stand between a physician and patient in terms of power, paternalism, and information asymmetry.
Communication	It is important to communicate with patients regarding their diagnosis, tests, treatment, and prognosis in an unhurried fashion, allowing patients and their families to ask questions. It is also important to follow up with patients after bad events to make sure that they do not feel abandoned and to ensure that they are able to understand why a particular outcome has occurred.
Knowledge	More than in any other profession, updating medical knowledge by a practitioner is paramount in medicine. The available data change rapidly, and keeping up with national standards is difficult, but this above all else is the foundation for competent medical care.

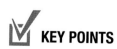

KEY POINTS

- Malpractice is providing healthcare in a way that does not meet local or national standards
- Many cases of malpractice go unnoticed because they do not necessarily lead to bad outcomes
- Even in cases of malpractice with bad outcomes, 5% or less actually lead to lawsuits
- Lawsuits occur less often when physicians have a good relationship with a patient; communicate thoroughly, allowing all questions to be answered; and do not avoid patients after bad events occur

QUESTIONS

1. You are a surgeon taking care of three patients in the ED. One has chronic back pain, one has abdominal pain suspicious for appendicitis, and one has a laceration of her hand requiring sutures. You are seeing your third patient who wants to discuss the possibility of scarring and is quite concerned; however, you are paged by the radiologist regarding the CT results on your abdominal pain patient. Which of the following is the likely best provision of care?

   A. Because you are currently with your third patient, continue your discussion with her and answer all of her questions.
   B. Tell your third patient, "I will be right back," and go see your first patient, who has been waiting the longest.
   C. Tell your third patient, "Let me go arrange a consultation with plastic surgery after I answer this page" and go to answer the page from radiology.
   D. Tell your third patient, "Don't worry; no one will notice this scar," and go to answer your page.
   E. Tell your third patient, "Don't worry; no one will notice this scar" and suture her hand.

2. You are an obstetrician providing care for a patient in labor. A nurse informs you that the fetal heart rate is experiencing a bradycardia, and on exam there is an umbilical cord prolapse. The patient is being moved to the operating room for an emergency cesarean section. Which of the following describes optimal documentation of this event?

   A. Immediately write down your impression of the situation and your plan of action.
   B. Go to the patient's bedside and facilitate the move to the operating room; after the cesarean, write a note documenting what occurred and when.
   C. Tell the nurse your plan of action, then postoperatively, time your note for when you told the nurse of the plan.
   D. Write a quick note, and then postoperatively, make changes to the note that reflect what actually occurred.
   E. There is no need to document what occurred because nursing will do the documentation.

3. A patient you are seeing for the first time has chronic back pain. He wishes to have an immediate MRI and a referral to a neurosurgeon. He tells you this is what his last doctor was going to do. Your best course of action is to:

   A. Order the MRI and make the referral.
   B. Tell the patient that because this is the first visit, you need to start the work-up of his back pain from the start.
   C. Give the patient ibuprofen and order an x-ray of the back.
   D. Ask the patient for the name and number of his prior physician and ask him to obtain his prior medical records, and reschedule him in 1 or 2 weeks.
   E. Order a CT and refer him to an orthopedic surgeon.

4. A physician is caring for a patient with atrial fibrillation and is prescribing medication to anticoagulate her blood. Which of the following actions is most likely to increase the risk of lawsuit?

   A. The physician prescribes twice the necessary dosage of medication, but there are no complications and a month later, the dosage is decreased.
   B. The physician prescribes the appropriate medication but the patient experiences a stroke despite the treatment. The physician sees the patient daily in the hospital.
   C. The physician prescribes the appropriate medication, but the patient experiences a stroke despite the treatment. The physician explains how medication does not always work.
   D. The physician prescribes the appropriate medication, but the patient experiences a stroke despite the treatment. The physician allows the hospital team to provide excellent care for the patient and plans to see the patient back in the office after discharge.
   E. The physician prescribes the appropriate medication, but the patient experiences a stroke despite the treatment. The physician updates the patient's family with daily changes in her status.

ANSWERS

PART I: MICROBIOLOGY

CASE 1-1

1. B. Vancomycin and linezolid will cover methicillin-sensitive staphylococci, but should be reserved for methicillin-resistant organisms. Penicillin and ampicillin are increasingly ineffective against *S. aureus*, as the introduction of penicillin in the early 1940s selected for penicillinase-producing strains. Approximately 85 to 90% of *S. aureus* strains in both the hospital and the community are now resistant to penicillin/ampicillin. The first-generation cephalosporins (e.g., cefazolin) will cover methicillin-sensitive strains of *S. aureus*. Of note, cefazolin has poor penetration into the CNS, and nafcillin should be used instead of the former in the case of staphylococcal meningitis.

2. C; 3. E. MRSA has carriage rates as high as 25 to 50%. Groups at higher risk for MRSA include injection drug users, persons with insulin-dependent diabetes, patients with dermatologic conditions, patients with long-term in-dwelling intravascular catheters, and healthcare workers.

4. D. *S. epidermidis* species tend to be much more antibiotic resistant than *S. aureus* species, with a methicillin resistance rate of approximately 80%.

CASE 1-2

1. D. Streptolysin O and streptolysin S both contribute to β-hemolysis. As streptolysin O is inactivated by oxidation (oxygen labile), it causes β-hemolysis only when the colonies grow under the surface of a blood agar plate. Because streptolysin S is oxygen stable, it is responsible for β-hemolysis when colonies grow on the surface of a blood agar plate.

2. C. Group A streptococcus is the only streptococcal species that is bacitracin susceptible, needs M protein for virulence, and has the species name of *S. pyogenes*. Group A streptococci are the most likely infectious agents to trigger poststreptococcal nonsuppurative infections, albeit such immunologic complications have rarely been seen following group C or group G infections. All streptococcal species are catalase negative, which distinguish them from the catalase-positive staphylococcal species.

CASE 1-3

1. B. Nutritionally variant streptococci (NVS) require pyridoxal or thiol group supplementation for growth. A streak of *S. aureus* on a sheep blood agar plate can provide these factors to the surrounding media so that the nutritionally variant streptococcus species will grow as satellite colonies around the *S. aureus* streak. Alternatively, 0.001% pyridoxal or 0.01% L-cysteine can be added to the agar media to promote growth of these *Streptococcus* species. Unsupplemented tryptic soy broth will not support the growth of NVS, and *S. pneumoniae* cannot provide these factors to the surrounding media to allow satellite growth of NVS colonies. Charcoal yeast extract agar plates are designed to allow culture of *Legionella* species.

2. D. In the setting of IE, emboli from the vegetative valvular lesion can lodge in the distal vasculature and immune complexes can form, leading to "stigmata" of endocarditis, such as:

Stigmata	Mechanism	Description
Roth spots	Immunologic	Retinal hemorrhage with a central area of clearing
Osler nodes	Immunologic	Erythematous painful nodes at the tips of digits
Janeway lesions	Vascular	Erythematous painless macules on the palms and soles
Splinter hemorrhages	Vascular	Petechiae underneath the nail bed

CASE 1-4

1. D. The following are CDC guidelines for the prevention of VRE. Situations in which the use of vancomycin is appropriate:

1. Treatment of serious infections due to β-lactam–resistant gram-positive organisms
2. Treatment of serious infections due to gram-positive organisms in patients with serious β-lactam allergies
3. Treatment of AAC when treatment with metronidazole has failed or if the AAC is potentially life threatening
4. Prophylaxis for endocarditis for certain procedures based on American Heart Association recommendations
5. Prophylaxis for certain surgical procedures involving implantation of prosthetic materials in hospitals with a high rate of MRSA or MRSE

Situations in which the use of vancomycin should be discouraged:

1. Routine surgical prophylaxis, unless the patient has a severe allergy to β-lactam antibiotics
2. Empiric treatment for febrile neutropenic patients, unless a gram-positive infection is suspected and the institution has a high rate of MRSA
3. Treatment of one positive blood culture for coagulase-negative *Staphylococcus* if other blood cultures drawn at the same time are negative (i.e., likely contamination)
4. Continued empiric use in patients whose cultures are negative for β-lactam–resistant gram-positive organisms
5. Prophylaxis for infection or colonization of in-dwelling central or peripheral intravascular catheters
6. Selective decontamination of the GI tract
7. Eradication of MRSA colonization
8. Primary treatment of AAC
9. Routine prophylaxis for infants with very low birth weight
10. Routine prophylaxis for patients on continuous ambulatory peritoneal dialysis or hemodialysis
11. Treatment of infection due to β-lactam–sensitive gram-positive microorganisms in patients with renal failure (for ease of dosing schedule)
12. Use of vancomycin solution for topical application or irrigation

Answers

2. **A.** VanA exhibits high-level resistance (MIC >128 μg/mL) to vancomycin and is resistant to teicoplanin (an investigational glycopeptide antibiotic). VanB exhibits moderate-level resistance (MIC 16–64 μg/mL) to vancomycin and is sensitive to teicoplanin. VanC, VanD, and VanE exhibit low-level resistance to vancomycin (MIC 8–16 μg/mL) and are sensitive to teicoplanin.

CASE 1-5

1. **B.** The most common location for diagnosed actinomycosis is the angle of the jaw.

2. **A.** *Listeria monocytogenes* is a nonfilamentous gram-positive rod that forms strongly catalase-positive, β-hemolytic colonies with a distinctive tumbling motility at 25°C in semisolid medium. This agent causes sepsis and meningitis in neonates and in immunosuppressed adults. The infection is acquired usually from unpasteurized milk or vegetables contaminated with animal feces. The treatment for *Listeria* infections is ampicillin plus or minus aminoglycosides. TMP-SMX can be used for penicillin-allergic patients.

CASE 1-6

1. **C.** Antibiotics that kill off normal flora but allow C. *difficile* to survive create ecological conditions for C. *difficile* overgrowth. Because metronidazole kills C. *difficile*, it is less likely than other antibiotics to give rise to the infection. Clindamycin (A) and cephalosporins (B, D, and E) kill a broad spectrum of bacteria but do not harm C. *difficile*; these antibiotics are associated with some of the highest rates of pseudomembranous colitis.

2. **B.** Toxic megacolon can be a lethal complication; this is why antimotility drugs are relatively contraindicated for C. *difficile* colitis. Gas gangrene (A) is due to C. *perfringens*. C. *difficile* does not cause the other listed conditions.

CASE 1-7

1. **C.** Rifampin will turn all of an individual's secretions, such as urine, sweat, tears, and stool, an orange color. Contact lenses can be permanently stained with this orange discoloration. This side effect is a source of great consternation to individuals who are not warned of its possibility.

2. **E.** *Moraxella catarrhalis*, formerly called *Branhamella catarrhalis*, is a gram-negative cocci that causes upper respiratory infections, including sinusitis, otitis media, and, occasionally, pneumonia.

CASE 1-8

1. **E.** B. *cereus* strains can produce two different toxins: a heat-stable toxin that can lead to an illness after 2 to 7 hours and a heat-labile toxin that causes disease manifestations 8 to 14 hours after ingestion. The syndrome of C. *perfringens* diarrhea usually occurs 8 to 14 hours after ingestion of the preformed toxin.

2. **D.** *Campylobacter jejuni* is a gram-negative rod that is S shaped or comma shaped on Gram stain.

CASE 1-9

1. **B.** The combination of an appropriate β-lactam antibiotic and an aminoglycoside is the most effective combination against *P. aeruginosa*. Penicillin does not have activity against *P. aeruginosa*. Both (C) and (E) are incorrect answers because combinations of two β-lactam antibiotics, even if they both have activity against *P. aeruginosa*, are antagonistic. Cefuroxime in (D) is a second-generation cephalosporin without activity against the organism.

2. **C.** Neutropenia in cancer patients is a risk factor for necrotizing enterocolitis. The syndrome can also occur in young infants and is often fatal.

CASE 1-10

1. **A.** Enteric pathogens, such as *Salmonella* and *Shigella*, are often distinguished from normal fecal flora by using plates such as MacConkey agar or Hektoen agar, which allow easy selection of lactose nonfermenters. The enterobacteraciae and *Salmonella* are glucose fermenters, oxidase negative, and nitrate reducing (B–D). *Salmonella* does produce hydrogen sulfide, which distinguishes it from *Shigella* and most enterobacteraciae.

2. **E.** *Salmonella typhimurium* is a nontyphoidal strain of *Salmonella* that causes gastroenteritis. Typhoid fever (D) is caused by *S. typhi* and *S. paratyphi*. Typhus (A–C) is a group of unrelated rickettsial diseases.

CASE 1-11

1. **B.** Only patients with active pulmonary or laryngeal TB are infectious. Patients with positive smears and cavitary disease have a higher organism load and are more infectious than patients who have positive cultures but no organisms found on direct sputum smears. Infections at other anatomic sites (A and E) do not make a patient infectious unless there is concomitant pulmonary TB. Positive skin tests (C) are a marker for past exposure, but do not necessarily indicate active disease; indeed, patients with overwhelming TB infection can have negative PPDs.

2. **B.** Pyrazinamide is one of the four first-line TB drugs. The other listed drugs are second line because of decreased or less proven efficacy, the necessity for parenteral administration (streptomycin), serious side effects (PAS and cycloserine), or cost and reservation for other uses (levofloxacin).

3. **C.** All the first-line drugs can cause hepatotoxicity, the major toxicity of TB therapy. INH can cause neuropathy (which can be prevented by co-administration of vitamin B6), ethambutol can cause optic neuritis, rifampin can cause serious drug-drug interactions (particularly with HIV protease inhibitors), and pyrazinamide causes hyperuricemia (although this is usually asymptomatic).

4. **C.** Active tuberculosis at any site (the presence of culturable organisms or evidence of progressive disease) mandates multidrug therapy. For patients with latent TB infection (A), treatment with a single drug will suffice to kill the small number of organisms. The calcified granulomas in patient B are a sign of old disease; he does not need new treatment unless he becomes symptomatic. The patients in (D) and (E) have had low-risk exposures and would not be treated unless there was evidence of a change in skin tests.

CASE 1-12

1. E. As with TB therapy, treatment of rapidly growing mycobacterial infections usually is very prolonged. Most skin and soft tissue infections require a combination of debridement and long courses of therapy; pulmonary infections may require even more than 6 months of appropriate chemotherapy for cure.

2. B. The various prophylactic regimens for MAC in HIV infection (usually initiated at CD4 counts = 50 cells/μl) include azithromycin 1200 mg orally every week, clarithromycin 500 mg orally twice a day, and rifabutin 300 mg orally every day.

CASE 1-13

1. E. β-Lactams (penicillins and cephalosporins) are often used to treat community-acquired pneumonia because they cover the most common causes (pneumococcus and gram-negative organisms such as *Moraxella* or *H. influenzae*). These drugs do not cover atypical agents and usually are given in combination with one of the other classes listed for atypical coverage, unless a firm etiologic diagnosis has been made. Ketolides are a new class of antibiotic that cover atypical organisms and have stronger pneumococcal coverage than do the macrolides.

2. D. *Legionella* is not known to be a colonizer; if it is found on culture, it should be treated. While *Mycoplasma* and *Chlamydia* cultures are rarely sent, these organisms can be found in asymptomatic subjects, so their mere presence does not require treatment. *Moraxella, Haemophilus,* and *Pneumococcus* can also be colonizers in asymptomatic patients. However, they should be treated in a patient with clinical signs of pneumonia and one of these organisms predominating in a sputum Gram stain and culture.

3. B. Mycoplasma are tiny free-living organisms that lack a cell wall. Because they have no cell wall, β-lactam antibiotics are ineffective against them. Bacteria (*Klebsiella, Moraxella,* and *Pneumococcus*) as well as yeast have cell walls. Because human cells do not have cell walls, the biosynthetic pathways for cell wall generation are important antibiotic targets.

4. B. Mycoplasma are extracellular parasites. The other agents all act intracellularly in human cells. Although the elementary bodies of chlamydia are extracellular, they are equivalent to spores; the reticular bodies, which are intracellular, are the form that carry out metabolism and reproduction.

CASE 1-14

1. C. All the treponemes cause skin disease, and most affect other organ systems as well. Pinta (which means "painted") affects only the skin (although the skin manifestations alone can be devastating and stigmatizing). Yaws and bejel can affect skin and bones. Syphilis affects skin and bones, but its dreaded manifestations are the cardiovascular, CNS, and ocular symptoms of tertiary syphilis.

2. D. Classic manifestations of tertiary syphilis include cardiovascular disease (aortic aneurysms), CNS disease (tabes dorsalis or general paresis), ocular disease, and the formation of lesions called gummas. Most skin manifestations are found at earlier stages; the chancre is the hallmark of primary syphilis, and the maculopapular rash and condylomata lata are found during the secondary stage.

3. D. Syphilis is one of the very few pathogens in which drug resistance has not become a clinical problem. It is still exquisitely sensitive to penicillin. The only reason not to use penicillin is if the patient has a severe allergy to the drug. Primary syphilis is a systemic infection and topical treatment is not possible. Neurosyphilis is still treated with penicillin, although the antibiotic is given via continuous IV to achieve higher CNS levels. Penicillin is the only drug approved for use in pregnant patients.

CASE 1-15

1. E. Resistance varies by the host and by the prior exposure of that host to antivirals. Approximate proportions of resistance in the U.S. population are as follows:

- 3% in normal hosts
- 5–7% in immunocompromised patients (such as organ transplant recipients and recipients of chronic corticosteroids)
- 15% in bone marrow transplant patients and in advanced HIV (due to extensive prior acyclovir exposure)

2. B. Asymptomatic viral shedding occurs 4.3% of the days tested in a year, accounting for 10% risk per year of transmission to an uninfected partner.

CASE 1-16

1. B. Foscarnet (and cidofovir) are second-line drugs against CMV, used to treat ganciclovir-resistant virus. Acyclovir, valacyclovir, and famciclovir are all active against HSV-1 and HSV-2, but not against CMV, which lacks the viral thymidine kinase required for their activation. Lamivudine is a reverse transcriptase inhibitor, used to treat HIV and HBV.

2. D. HIV patients are only at risk of CMV infection once they have reached a CD4 count below 50. These patients receive regular eye (the most common site of infection) exams to detect retinitis before vision is affected and irreversibly lost. CMV can also cause colitis in HIV patients, but they would be symptomatic with diarrhea; diagnosis requires endoscopic biopsy of the colon. Neutropenia (an absolute neutrophil count <500) is actually a contraindication to digital rectal exam because of the risk of bacteremia and subsequent sepsis. CMV can also cause CNS infection and rarely pneumonitis in HIV patients (pneumonitis is much more common in transplant patients), but asymptomatic patients are not screened.

CASE 1-17

1. B. Although there is some evidence of initiating antiretroviral therapy in the face of acute infection and such studies are currently in progress, most clinicians support acute HIV infection with symptomatic therapy alone at this point.

2. A. Retroviruses contain single-stranded, linear, positive-polarity RNA and a viral reverse transcriptase protein that "transcribes" the RNA genome into DNA upon viral entry into the host cell.

CASE 1-18

1. A. Mosquito repellant is thought to be the only effective measure against WNV infection. There is no evidence that handling dead, infected birds or other infected animals can lead to WNV infection.

2. D. Convincing epidemiologic evidence, especially from the 1999 New York outbreak, shows that older age is a risk factor for death from WNV infection, as is an increased incidence of chronic neurologic sequelae.

CASE 1-19

1. E. This patient has acute hepatitis, and the most likely cause is hepatitis A. Although sexual transmission is possible, the most likely source is food. Hepatitis B could potentially be transmitted from a sexual partner, a needlestick exposure from work (he should be vaccinated), or vertically (although vertical transmission would result in chronic hepatitis rather than acute disease in an adult). Ticks are not vectors for agents of acute viral hepatitis.

2. C. For nonimmune patients with potential future exposures to hepatitis A, preventive therapy is indicated. Rural Mexico would be a high prevalence area for hepatitis A, so she is at risk for acute infection. Vaccination is indicated in all travelers to endemic areas. Because it takes 2 to 4 weeks to develop protective antibodies from vaccination, immune globulin is indicated for patients in whom the potential exposure will occur in less than 1 month. Rimantadine is not effective against hepatitis A.

CASE 1-20

1. B. Anti-HBs shows protective immunity against the hepatitis virus. Production of this antibody is stimulated by past exposure to the virus or by administration of the recombinant HBV vaccine. Anti-HBc is a marker of past exposure to the virus, but in some cases current infection is still possible. HBeAg is a marker for high viral loads, and therefore high infectivity. Anti-HBe shows relatively low infectivity (although this test is rarely seen in practice). Finally, HBsAg is a marker for current infection.

2. D. Lamivudine is active against both HBV and HIV, as is tenofovir. Adefovir is also active against both viruses, but nephrotoxicity prevents adefovir from being used at the higher HIV dose. These drugs have activity against HBV because HBV replication includes a reverse transcriptase step. Other HIV drugs, including the rest of the nucleoside analogs like AZT and ddI, are not active against HBV.

CASE 1-21

1. E. Influenza can be distinguished from a generic upper respiratory infection (such as patient B) by the severe constitutional symptoms it causes. Despite the commonly used phrase "stomach flu," GI disturbances are minimal or absent in influenza. Patient A's diarrhea is likely due to another viral cause, or to bacteria or parasites. Patient C appears to have acute hepatitis, which could be caused by hepatitis A or B. The symptoms of patient D are worrisome for measles; he may not have been immunized against this disease.

2. D. Zanamivir and oseltamivir are both neuraminidase inhibitors. Hemagglutinin (B) is the other major surface protein of influenza virus, used for binding to target cells. No drugs currently target it. Protease and reverse transcriptase (C and A, respectively) are drug targets in HIV. Dihydrofolate reductase (E) is inhibited by sulfa drugs and is a target in bacteria and parasites.

3. D. Allergy to eggs is a contraindication to the vaccine because eggs are used to grow the virus for vaccine production. Because influenza virus is a killed virus, it is safe for AIDS patients (A) and pregnant women (C) to receive. Patients with severe pulmonary or cardiac disease (E) benefit the most from vaccination because they are the most likely to die from influenza, and vaccination programs should target them. Whereas the Pneumovax should not be repeated more than every 5 to 7 years (D), the influenza vaccination needs to be given every year to maximize protection against currently circulating virus.

4. C. Oseltamivir (and zanamivir) are neuraminidase inhibitors active against both influenza A and B. Amantadine (A) and rimantadine (E) are both only active against influenza A. Stavudine (B) is a nucleoside reverse transcriptase inhibitor active against HIV. Nelfinavir (D) is a protease inhibitor active against HIV.

CASE 1-22

1. B. Amphotericin B can lead to renal injury, ranging from mild renal tubular acidosis to severe renal toxicity with nephrocalcinosis. Hypokalemia and hypomagnesiumemia are frequent side effects from this medication, as are the more rare hepatotoxicity and bone marrow suppression.

2. D. *Mucor* and *Rhizopus* form nonseptate, true hyphae with broad irregular walls and branches that form at right angles (90°).

CASE 1-23

1. E. Flucytosine, which is given orally, is converted to 5-flurouracil, which is an antimetabolite that may result in bone marrow suppression. Drug levels of flucytosine may be monitored, as higher levels correlate with toxicity. The other answers are all potential side effects of amphotericin.

2. C. *Cryptococcus* does not secrete any toxins but rather relies on its capsule to evade host defenses through inhibition of phagocytosis and antibody production. Additionally, phenoloxidase uses the mycotoxic host catecholamines epinephrine in the process of melanogenesis, thus protecting the yeast.

CASE 1-24

1. E. Blood cultures growing yeast could theoretically be contaminants, but the physician is obligated to treat them. Yeast can colonize the other listed sites without causing disease, although yeast skin and UTIs are often diagnosed and treated. True yeast pneumonias are exceedingly rare; usually yeast in the sputum is a colonizer of the oropharynx.

2. A. Amphotericin B has both infusion-related toxicity (fever and chills) as well as cumulative nephrotoxicity, but doctors still frequently use the drug because they have the most clinical experience with it. Expensive lipid-based formulations have been developed to try and reduce these side effects. Topical antifungals (B, C, and D) all have minimal side effects. The new antifungal, caspofungin (E), also has minimal reported side effects.

3. E. Caspofungin, an echinocandin, blocks β-glycan synthesis required to make yeast cell walls. This is analogous to the *antibacterial* antibiotic penicillin (B). Polyenes, such as amphotericin and nystatin (A and D, respectively), and azoles, such as fluconazole (C), target ergosterol, a component of the yeast cell *membrane*.

CASE 1-25

1. E. In an immunocompetent patient, *Coccidioides* causes an acute pneumonia, which is self-limited, and most experts do not recommend treatment. A majority of people living in *Coccidioides*-endemic areas show skin test evidence of prior infection with the fungus. Of the listed drugs, levofloxacin is an antibacterial antibiotic, and terbinafine is usually reserved for onychomycosis; only fluconazole and amphotericin are routinely used for serious fungal infections.

2. B. Spherules filled with endospores are pathognomic for *Coccidioides*. Special medium can be used to induce *Coccidioides* grown in the lab to form spherules to confirm identification. A report of round encapsulated yeast would most often imply *Cryptococcus*. Acutely branching hyphae would suggest molds such as *Aspergillus* or *Pseudallescheria boydii*. (Although dimorphic fungi take the form of molds at room temperature, they usually appear as yeast in pathologic specimens from tissues at body temperature.) Do not confuse bacterial cocci, such as *Staphylococcus*, with *Coccidioides*. Finally, a morula is the hallmark of ehrlichiosis.

3. D. The most likely dimorphic fungus to be acquired in Arizona would be *Coccidioides*. *Histoplasma* is found in the midwest, *Blastomyces* in the southeast. *Penicillium marneffei* is another endemic dimorphic fungus that infects HIV patients in Southeast Asia. It is not found in the United States, except in patients who have traveled to that region in the past. *Sporothrix schenckii* is yet another dimorphic fungus, but is not restricted to a specific endemic area. It lives in the dirt and classically infects gardeners, particularly those stuck by rose thorns.

CASE 1-26

1. C. Glucose-6-phosphate dehydrogenase (G6PD) deficiency is the most common enzyme deficiency in humans, with an estimated 400 million people worldwide harboring this defect. Various drugs can trigger hemolytic anemia in a G6PD-deficient state, including primaquine. Hence, G6PD levels should always be checked prior to initiating primaquine therapy for the eradication of the intrahepatic stage of *P. vivax* and *P. ovale*.

2. E. Approximately 5% of native and imported malaria cases are the result of co-infection with *P. falciparum* and another *Plasmodia* species (i.e., *ovale*, *vivax*, or *malariae*), as the *Anopheles* mosquito can carry multiple malarial species concomitantly. It may be difficult to distinguish the different species on the patient's blood smear, however. Hence, the treatment of presumed *P. falciparum* almost always involves concomitant treatment for the intrahepatic stage of *P. vivax* and *P. ovale* (as seen in PF's case by the use of pyrimethamine in addition to the quinine).

PART II: IMMUNOLOGY

CASE 2-1

1. B. Transplant rejection is largely a T_h1 division cell-mediated immunity phenomenon promoting IgG production and cytotoxic activity. In acute rejection, there are presumably no preformed antibodies or prior T-lymphocyte sensitization. Therefore, the whole process of antigen presentation, T-helper cell activation, and subsequent activation of different cells starts from the time of the transplant. Recognition of "foreignness" by T-helper cells occurs through the direct and indirect pathways of sensitization, either by recognition of foreign HLA with foreign antigen on dendritic cells carried over by transplantation or by antigen processing and presentation by endogenous APCs of the recipient. These antigens (especially the allograft's surface MHC) activate T_h1 cells to release IL-2 and other cytokines that promote immune cell proliferation, B-cell IgG isotype switching, as well as CTL and macrophage activation toward cell killing and phagocytosis. CD40L is then up-regulated in T-helper cells, which bind CD40 on B cells, CTLs, and even dendritic cells to activate them further. TNF-α released from the site of inflammation promotes local edema by increasing vascular permeability and promoting cytotoxicity. Thus, (A), (C), (D), and (E) are incorrect.

2. D. Mycobacteria are eliminated by opsonization by IgG, phagocytosis, and oxidative degradation by macrophages. Without IFN-γ receptors, the IFN-γ cytokine cannot signal the activation of NADPH oxidase and iNOS to produce superoxide intermediates, crucial for the final elimination of phagocytized mycobacteria. IL-1 and TNF-α are responsible for acting on the hypothalamus to induce fever; thus, (A) is incorrect. TCR and BCR are the receptors responsible for specific antigen recognition; thus, (B) is incorrect. IFN-α and IFN-β are responsible for inducing "the antiviral state" among cells, which includes up-regulation of class I MHC to promote antigen presentation of intracellular pathogens, down-regulation of overall protein synthesis to prevent virus assembly, and increase of RNase synthesis to help degrade viral RNA. *Mycobacteria* become intracellular when phagocytized but remain outside of the cytosolic compartment and thus are not presented by class I MHC; genomic nucleic acids also consist of DNA, not RNA. Thus mycobacteria are not treated like viruses during the elimination process; (C) is incorrect. Finally, IL-4 is responsible for B-cell isotype switching to IgE, which is not involved in elimination of mycobacteria; (E) is incorrect.

CASE 2-2

1. E. The hematologic abnormalities found in SLE are caused by type II cytotoxic hypersensitivity reaction against red blood cells, white blood cells, and platelets, not by immune complex deposition. Immune complex-mediated tissue injury generally results from deposition of immune complexes in tissue, causing arthritis, glomerulonephritis, and vasculitis; (A) is incorrect. Antibodies against antigen at the dermo-epidermal region cause direct damage to the region, resulting in the erythematous and bullous lesions of the malar rash and discoid lupus; (B) is incorrect. Chronic lung interstitial inflammation may result in diffuse crackles of pulmonary fibrosis; (C) is incorrect. SLE is associated with immune injury due to a diffuse array of antibodies, and thus the spleen may become enlarged from follicular hyperplasia and increased plasma cell activity; thus, (D) is incorrect.

2. A. CTLA-4 antagonizes B7 on APCs, preventing the appropriate binding to CD28 on T-helper cells, thus blocking the needed second signal to allow proper activation of the immune response. This will theoretically prevent sensitization of donor T lymphocytes against the "foreign" antigen of host tissue, thus suppressing graft-versus-host disease among bone marrow transplant recipients. All of the others are incorrect mechanisms.

Answers

CASE 2-3

1. E. Nuchal rigidity as evidenced by the Kernig and Brudzinski signs is the least specific of all those listed. A positive Kernig sign is neck pain elicited by passive knee extension with hips flexed at 90 degrees. A positive Brudzinski sign is neck pain elicited by passive neck flexion. Both are signs of meningeal irritation from any cause of meningitis and do not necessarily reflect the presence of a complement deficiency. Answers (A) and (B) are incorrect, as people with complement deficiencies do have increased risk of pneumococcal and meningococcal infection. Those with terminal complement deficiencies are more likely to present with recurrent disseminated neisserial infection, including meningococcal and gonococcal septicemia and meningitis. Answers (C) and (D) are incorrect, as complement deficiency can present with arthritis and petechial rash, reflecting the presence of immune complex disease.

2. B. Given the fact that CD's serology showed IgM to meningococcus, one can assume that this is a first-time infection of this bacterium; therefore, there would be no IgG available for opsonization. This underscores the importance of innate immunity and the alternative and lectin pathways of the complement cascade in the defense against pathogens to which the body has never been exposed. The non–antibody-dependent mechanisms of pathogen recognition include recognition of molecular patterns widely expressed by microorganisms (e.g., LPS) and C3b binding. Thus, (A) and (C) are incorrect. Answers (C) and (D) are incorrect as they both describe parts of the complement cascade that can be activated via the alternative or lectin pathway, both antibody-independent pathways. Answer (E) is incorrect as IgM (all immunoglobulins except for IgE), can bind free-floating extracellular pathogens and form immune complexes that deposit in the joints and end vasculature of the dermis to produce arthritis and diffuse petechial rash, especially in dependent sites subject to higher pressure like the lower extremities. Last, answer (F) is incorrect, as the terminal cascade components are important for formation of the MAC, which is important in the complete elimination of neisserial infections, via their action in promoting bacterial leakage of immune mediators, cell lysis, and phagocytosis. (Think of a shark following the blood trail of wounded, bleeding prey until it localizes it and finally eats it.)

3. B. People with C5 deficiencies, as well as other terminal component (MAC) complement deficiencies, are subject to recurrent neisserial infections as well as immune complex disease. However, after the first infection, the subsequent infections are often marked by less severe disease with milder symptoms, such as low-grade fever, arthritis, rash, and, at times, nephritis (associated with hematuria). This reflects the development of adaptive immunity to *Neisseria* species and the availability of plasma cells producing specific IgG binding extracellular bacteria-forming immune complexes. Overwhelming infection and immune complex formation could surpass the body's ability to clear immune complexes, leading to their deposition in joints, vessels, and glomeruli. For those with MAC deficiencies, whereas the infection is better contained, there is still a defect in the final elimination of bacteria resulting in a more indolent course due to persistent infection. Answers (A) and (D) are incorrect, as both the complement cascade and NK cells represent parts of the innate immune system that are independent of prior exposure to pathogens. Answer (C) is incorrect, as it is unknown whether this mechanism exists. Answer (E) is incorrect, as these oxidative killing mechanisms exist in phagocytes and are unaffected by complement deficiencies.

CASE 2-4

1. E. BD's past medical history suggests an intact cell-mediated immune system responsible for the delayed-type hypersensitivity reaction of poison ivy contact dermatitis and the defense against fungal infections by *Candida albicans*, the main pathogen of thrush. This, in fact, does not necessarily represent the presence of immunodeficiency, as such a history suggests a *normal physiologic* response by T lymphocytes to poison ivy antigen and is the very immune mechanism that fights off fungal infections; (A) is incorrect. BD's disease is unrelated to mast cell- and IgE-mediated immediate hypersensitivity as suggested by (B). BD's disease is not an autoimmune disease, which represents *hyper*function of the immune system; it is, in fact, *hypo*function of the immune system; (C) is incorrect. Finally, as recurrent infection to mucosal membranes such as the respiratory tract may suggest poor defense against common mucosal pathogens, the lack of prior thrush suggests a more specific immunodeficiency in antibody production important in elimination of encapsulated bacteria like *H. influenzae*.

2. D. IgA is the main immunoglobulin of secretions and serves to protect all mucosal surfaces from infection and penetration by the many microbes that pass through the lumen. The congenital absence of IgA would make one susceptible to infections at these sites, which include the GI and respiratory tracts. Such infection would manifest as a recurrent gastritis and diarrhea. Unfortunately, this immunodeficiency cannot be treated with IV immunoglobulin replacement as can IgG deficiencies.

PART III: PHARMACOLOGY

CASE 3-1

1. B. Amiodarone reduces the clearance of digoxin by half, and the digoxin levels double approximately 1 to 2 weeks following the initiation of amiodarone therapy. Although hypokalemia increases the potential for any digoxin level to produce toxicity (pharmacodynamic effect), hypokalemia does not change the absorption, distribution, or metabolism/elimination of digoxin. With a digoxin $T\frac{1}{2}$ of 4 days, the digoxin concentration should decrease to 1.8 µg/L (3.6/2) after 4 days, and an additional 4 days (8 days total) would be required for the digoxin level to decline to about 0.9 µg/L (1.8/2). Digoxin is normally 20% metabolized and 80% renally eliminated. Even if the patient had half the normal renal function and the 80% was reduced in half, the remaining 40% would still be the majority of the route by which digoxin is cleared from the body. Benazepril does not change the pharmacokinetics of digoxin. It does have the potential to increase serum potassium.

2. G. Given the patient's, age, weight, sex, and serum Cr, his calculated CrCl rate is 20 mL/min:

$$\text{CrCl for males (mL/min)} = \frac{(140 - \text{age})(\text{weight})}{(72)(\text{Cr})}$$

$$= \frac{(140 - 80 \text{ yr})(72 \text{ kg})}{(72)(3 \text{ mg/dL})}$$

$$= 20 \text{ mL/min}$$

That would indicate that the recommended dose of cefepime is 0.5–1 g every 24 hours. Because the CrCl rate is in the middle of the recommended range, either dose would be reasonable. If only the serum Cr were used to approximate renal function, the serum Cr of 3 is three times higher than the usual value of 1 mg/dL, indicating a one-third normal value, or about 33 mL/min. Thus, only using the serum Cr to estimate a patient's renal function overestimates the actual value when patients weigh significantly less than 70 kg or are of advanced age.

CASE 3-2

1. B. This patient reports that he hasn't used this particular bottle of SL tablets for over a year. Because the SL tablets are volatile and lose potency when exposed to air, they must be used only for a maximum of 6 months after the original container is opened. Monitoring of the expiration date must be strict, and expired SL nitroglycerin should be replaced. This medication should be stored in a cool, dry place and should be closed tightly after each opening. In addition, the SL nitroglycerin must be protected from light and therefore be kept in the original amber bottle. Nitrate tolerance is not correct because tolerance occurs with continuous exposure to nitrates. Because short-acting nitrates have a rapid onset of action and short duration, it is unlikely to cause tolerance.

2. A. Isosorbide dinitrate tablets. Adding atenolol or verapamil for angina is not uncommon. However, this patient's BP and HR are within normal range. Adding nitroglycerin ointment is messy and is not the best alternative for an active lifestyle. SL isosorbide dinitrate has a slower onset of action but does not offer any advantage over SL nitroglycerin. Isosorbide dinitrate tablets are longer acting and can control symptoms throughout the day, especially for patients with active lifestyles. Isosorbide dinitrate should be given three times daily over a 10-hour period (e.g., at 7:00 a.m., 12:00 p.m., and 5:00 p.m.).

CASE 3-3

1. B. With long-term use of beta-blockers, there is an up-regulation of the beta-receptors. When beta-blockers are abruptly stopped after chronic use, these agents can cause rebound HTN. Exacerbation of angina, MI, arrhythmias, and death may occur. A gradual tapering of beta-blockers over 1 to 2 weeks may avoid the rebound. It is possible that the antihypertensive medications were not adequate; since he has not taken his medications for 5 days, this would be difficult to assess. Loratadine, asthma, or hyperglycemia are also unlikely to increase blood pressure.

2. C. The patient has COPD and renal impairment; thus, the beta-blocker selected should be β_1 selective and hepatically cleared. Atenolol is renally cleared. Nadolol is nonselective and renally excreted. Both propranolol and labetalol are nonselective. Metoprolol is the best choice because it is β_1 selective and hepatically eliminated.

CASE 3-4

1. C. Diltiazem. Quinidine can be used to maintain NSR after cardioversion of atrial fibrillation. Metoprolol is commonly used to control ventricular rate before conversion to NSR. However, this patient has two contraindications (COPD and diabetes) for beta-blocker use. Unlike diltiazem, amlodipine and nimodipine do not block AV nodal conduction; therefore, they would be ineffective at rate control.

2. D. Verapamil has been the calcium channel blocker most studied for migraine prophylaxis. In addition, verapamil is the calcium channel blocker associated with inducing both constipation and gingival hyperplasia. Nifedipine and diltiazem should not be used since studies have shown that their efficacy is questionable for migraine prophylaxis. Bepridil is used only for chronic stable angina. Amlodipine may be used for migraine prophylaxis, but it is not as likely to produce the side effects that this patient is experiencing.

CASE 3-5

1. B. Unlike other diuretics, furosemide at high infusion rates is associated with ototoxicity. Ototoxicity may occur will all loop diuretics, but the frequency is less with bumetanide and it has not been reported with torsemide. In addition, hypocalcemia is a side effect also experienced with loop diuretics and not with thiazide diuretics. In contrast, hydrochlorothiazide decreases urinary excretion of calcium, which may result in an elevation of serum calcium levels. Thus, thiazide diuretics may potentially reduce the risk of osteoporosis and be beneficial in postmenopausal women.

2. B. Diuretics that act on the distal tubule (thiazides and potassium-sparing diuretics) lose their effectiveness when CrCl decreases to less than 30–50 mL/min. The loop diuretics are more potent and retain their effectiveness at low CrCl (>5 mL/min).

CASE 3-6

1. E. One of the primary adverse effects of ACE inhibitors is hypotension. It may be manifested as dizziness, light-headedness, presyncope, or syncope. It occurs most commonly with the first dose. Patients at risk for developing hypotension are those with hyponatremia (serum sodium <130 mEq/L), recent increases in diuretic dose, and hypovolemia. Hypotension can be minimized by temporarily withholding or reducing the diuretic dose and/or starting an ACE inhibitor at lower doses.

2. B. ACE inhibitors such as captopril may cause angioedema. The incidence of angioedema is less than 1% and may occur any time during therapy. The swelling is usually confined to the face, lips, tongue, glottis, and larynx. Antihistamines may be used to relieve discomfort, but symptoms usually resolve without treatment. If the swelling obstructs the airway, then epinephrine should be administered immediately. Patients should not be rechallenged with an ACE inhibitor if they have a history of angioedema. The other adverse effects are not likely caused by captopril. The bradycardia is caused by metoprolol, flushing is caused by isosorbide dinitrate, and morphine may cause hallucinations, especially in the elderly.

CASE 3-7

1. A. Both ACE inhibitors and ARBs are contraindicated in patients with bilateral renal stenosis. Patients with bilateral renal stenosis have decreased blood flow to the glomerulus. When given ACE inhibitors or ARBs, the effects of angiotensin II are reduced, which leads to vasodilatation of the efferent arterioles. This will result in a decrease in pressure and glomerular filtration rate and a worsening of the renal function.

2. E. ACE inhibitors and ARBs may induce or potentiate renal impairment and elevate serum potassium, especially in patients who have underlying renal dysfunction or are taking concurrent medications that can increase serum potassium. Upon initiation of ACE inhibitors and ARBs, baseline serum Cr, BUN, and serum potassium should be obtained and then monitored periodically. BP also should be monitored regularly to evaluate efficacy and risk of hypotension.

CASE 3-8

1. D. Amiodarone may decrease warfarin metabolism within a week of coadministration, or the effects of the interaction may be delayed for several weeks. Patients who develop hyperthyroidism secondary to amiodarone may have an additional increased anticoagulant effect, because the turnover of clotting factors is more rapid. If amiodarone is discontinued, effects of the decreased warfarin metabolism may last 1 to 3 months.

2. A. The patient's INR is supratherapeutic. She is not having any major bleeding other than the slight nosebleed. Having a poor appetite may have decreased the amount of vitamin K that is absorbed. In addition, fevers also can increase the turnover of clotting factors. Because the patient has taken her morning dose of warfarin, her INR may continue to increase. Giving vitamin K orally at 2.5 mg would reverse the INR back toward the therapeutic range. Because it is given PO, effects are more predictable, compared with doses given subcutaneously. The IV route is not necessary in this patient because he is not bleeding. Also, there may be a small percentage of anaphylaxis with the IV route.

CASE 3-9

1. B. The sustained-release formulation of oxycodone would be inappropriate to administer via gastric tube since crushing the tablet would eliminate the sustained-release mechanism. The drug would then have to be administered more frequently to control pain, defeating the purpose of the long-acting formulation. IV opioids, liquid formulations, and immediate-release tablets that can be crushed are viable options.

2. E. Oxycodone/acetaminophen would be the most appropriate drug to start for this patient's acute postsurgical pain. The onset of action is rapid, and it can be titrated to effect. Morphine and meperidine have active metabolites that can accumulate in this patient with renal dysfunction, increasing the risk for seizures, sedation, and respiratory depression. The fentanyl patch is primarily indicated in chronic pain. The onset is slow, and the patches cannot be titrated up rapidly to cover acute pain, nor titrated down as the patient recovers and requires less opioid.

CASE 3-10

1. B. In patients with low albumin, their phenytoin levels should be "corrected" because phenytoin is a highly protein-bound drug. In this patient with an albumin of 2.8 g/dL, her phenytoin level of 5 μg/mL functions as a level of 7–8 μg/mL (still below the desired target), necessitating a dose adjustment. If a patient has the phenytoin level drawn a few hours after taking the dose, the level will appear falsely elevated. This patient's level

was drawn appropriately, and her compliance was verified. The therapeutic level of an antiepileptic is only as effective as the control of a patient's seizures. Although 10–20 μg/mL is generally the target for phenytoin, based on patient presentation the target may differ. In a patient such as this one, with no history of seizures, a target of at least 10 μg/mL is typically the goal. Her transaminases were normal and would not influence a decision to change her dosage at this time.

2. C. Valproic acid can be given IV while the patient is NPO and then she can be converted back to her oral regimen as soon as possible. Valproic acid has no interactions with propoxyphene or doxycycline. Valproic acid troughs (not peak levels) should be monitored to ensure minimal effective concentrations.

CASE 3-11

1. A. Benzodiazepines have long been used to treat social phobia, but RM is particularly afraid of the potential for physiologic and psychological dependence. Buspirone has not been found to be particularly effective for social phobia. Beta-blockers may be worth considering, particularly if his symptoms are more suggestive of stage fright, but issues around decreased exercise tolerance may discourage their use in a professional athlete such as RM. Because SSRIs are quite effective for this condition, sertraline and paroxetine are excellent options to consider, and because paroxetine appears to carry a greater propensity for weight gain, sertraline is the preferred treatment in this patient.

2. C. The abrupt discontinuation of long-term benzodiazepines may precipitate a serious withdrawal syndrome consisting of anxiety, restlessness, insomnia, agitation, sensory disturbances, and diaphoresis. Seizures may result from the abrupt discontinuation of benzodiazepines, although this is much more common with the more potent short- and intermediate-acting agents (e.g., alprazolam, triazolam). The onset of withdrawal symptoms is usually 2–3 days for short- and intermediate-acting agents and 5–6 days for longer-acting benzodiazepines (e.g., clonazepam).

CASE 3-12

1. B. Sexual dysfunction is generally believed to be a dose-dependent side effect with SSRIs and may be relieved or prevented with lower doses. Although RH may run the risk of relapse at a lower dose, many patients will achieve a therapeutic response at lower doses. If this approach is unsuccessful, bupropion is an excellent antidote and may also provide additional antidepressant effects (i.e., augmentation). Sildenafil has actually been found to reverse SSRI-induced sexual dysfunction but is an expensive alternative, with potential cardiovascular complications, that should only be considered after other measures fail.

2. C. Although a more complete history and physical exam is recommended to confirm the diagnosis (including vitals, CK, LFT, BUN/CR, and complete medication history), the constellation of symptoms that this patient is reporting is strongly suggestive of SSRI withdrawal syndrome. It is now widely recognized that the abrupt discontinuation of certain antidepressants (most notably paroxetine and venlafaxine) will precipitate the sudden onset of symptoms 48–72 hours after drug discontinuation.

Although this syndrome is ordinarily self-limiting, it can be quite uncomfortable for patients or incapacitating. Often, younger patients are reluctant to take psychotropic medications for a full course of therapy, and it is quite possible that she stopped the venlafaxine when she felt better or simply ran out of the medication. It may be necessary to remind her that antidepressants need to be continued for at least 4–9 months after remission is achieved. If the antidepressant is to be discontinued at a later date, it should be slowly tapered over a few weeks.

CASE 3-13

1. C. Risperidone. Although the incidence of adverse effects associated with hyperprolactinemia is rare with atypical antipsychotics, risperidone can increase prolactin levels in a dose-dependent manner. Blockade of the dopaminergic tone in the hypothalamus and 5-HT$_2$ antagonism by risperidone may explain this effect. Other adverse effects associated with persistent prolactin elevation include sexual dysfunction, female menstrual disorders, and reduced bone mineral density.

2. B. Diphenhydramine. Diphenhydramine would not be the optimal choice in this patient who is also taking haloperidol. Anticholinergic agents such as diphenhydramine have the potential to decrease the efficacy of antipsychotic agents due to their effects on the cholinergic-dopamine receptor balance. The other agents do not significantly interact with antipsychotic medications.

CASE 3-14

1. A. Methimazole has a longer T1/2 than PTU and can be dosed once daily; PTU requires three to four daily doses, which may affect compliance. PTU does not cause pretibial myxedema; rather, Graves hyperthyroidism leads to pretibial myxedema. Methimazole does not interact with amiodarone; however, amiodarone can affect thyroid function, leading to both hypothyroidism and hyperthyroidism. PTU therapy may result in spontaneous remission, but patients typically require therapy for many years (1–15 years).

2. B. Of the thioamides, PTU is less likely to cross the placenta compared with methimazole and is the preferred agent in pregnancy. PTU is also preferred over methimazole because it decreases the peripheral conversion of T$_4$ to T$_3$, whereas methimazole does so minimally. Both thioamides are used before surgery to decrease thyroid hormone stores and prevent intraoperative complications. PTU is routinely used during thyroid storm and not myxedema coma.

CASE 3-15

1. D. RC is currently experiencing hypoglycemic episodes in the mid-afternoon. This can be attributed to too much insulin lispro at lunchtime. It also would be a good idea to assess her food intake at each meal to see if she has consistent carbohydrate intake. While an A1C of 7.1% is close to goal, she is not in good glycemic control because she is experiencing hypoglycemia with her current insulin regimen.

2. E. Absorption of SC insulin can be affected by a number of factors. To achieve the most predictable pattern absorption of insulin, it is important to minimize factors that can affect the absorption. In general, factors that increase blood flow to the site

of injection will increase the insulin absorption rate. For example, patients should not take a shower immediately after injecting insulin because heat can cause the insulin to be absorbed more quickly. Lipohypertrophy can result when a person uses the same injection site repeatedly. Fat deposits can build up, which will cause a delay in insulin absorption.

CASE 3-16

1. B. AK has renal dysfunction and therefore metformin is contraindicated. Use of an alpha-glucosidase inhibitor would likely not achieve the target A1C, which requires a 1.5% lowering to attain the goal of less than 7%. He is not overweight (BMI is in normal range of 18.5–24.9). Therefore, a sulfonylurea would be an appropriate oral agent to select. It is important to select a sulfonylurea that is metabolized in inactive metabolites given his renal dysfunction. In renal dysfunction, metabolites can accumulate; thus, using a sulfonylurea with active metabolites would increase the risk of hypoglycemia. While not a choice in the answers, a thiazolidinedione would be a possibility. However, in a thin patient, in whom insulin resistance is likely playing a lesser role in hyperglycemia, a thiazolidinedione would not be the most appropriate choice. Thiazolidinediones also require frequent liver function monitoring (every month for the first year and periodically thereafter). Thiazolidinediones bind to the PPARγ (peroxisome proliferator activated receptor, gamma) nuclear receptors, which causes an upregulation of the glucose transporter, GLUT 4, resulting in enhanced insulin sensitivity.

2. A. The BP goal for a person with diabetes is less than 130/80 mm Hg. His BP is well controlled on the ACE inhibitor benazepril. His A1C is above goal at 7.8% (goal is less than 7%). The LDL-C goal for a person with diabetes is less than 100 mg/dL (HDL-C more than 45 mg/dL in men; TG less than 150 mg/dL); he is above goal with an LDL-C of 137 mg/dL. He should have a dilated retinal exam at least once yearly and a pneumococcal vaccination at least once. A one-time revaccination is recommended for people older than 64 years of age if they were previously vaccinated at younger than age 65 years and it was administered more than 5 years ago. Finally, a microalbuminuria test is recommended annually, which requires a patient to bring a urine sample to the laboratory for assessment of protein in the urine (and thus renal function).

CASE 3-17

1. E. Response to a change in therapy should be evaluated at 6 weeks. Upon achieving goals, response to therapy and patient adherence should be evaluated every 4–6 months.

2. F. Before initiating statin therapy, it is recommended to have baseline measurements of the lipoprotein profile and LFTs. If the LFTs are more than three times the ULN, statins should be avoided. If the LFTs are less than three times the ULN, statin therapy can be initiated, but the patient should be monitored closely. If LFTs become elevated, reversal of the transaminase elevation is common upon discontinuation of the statin. Some experts also recommend obtaining a baseline CK level. If the CK level is more than 10 times the ULN while on a statin, the statin should be discontinued. The combination of a statin with niacin or a fibrate should be used cautiously because of an increased risk of myopathy. Although most statins are taken at dinner or

bedtime, atorvastatin can be taken at any time of the day due to its longer T½ (~14 hours). Lovastatin should be taken with food because this increases its bioavailability.

CASE 3-18

1. A. The preferred treatment for EIB is pretreatment with a short-acting inhaled β_2-agonist (e.g., albuterol) just prior to exercise. Aerosolized albuterol induces bronchodilatation shortly after administration, and JC should be instructed to use his albuterol inhaler 5–15 minutes before engaging in physical activity. Oral β_2-agonists are not recommended due to the increased potential for systemic adverse effects (tremor, tachycardia) and slower onset of action. Similarly, nonselective β_2-agonists (epinephrine, metaproterenol) are not recommended due to the increased potential for excessive cardiac stimulation. Regular administration of short-acting inhaled β_2-agonists is not recommended in the management of intermittent asthma due to the increased risk of adverse effects without additional clinical benefit. Although daily administration of inhaled corticosteroids is effective in the management of EIB, given JC's mild intermittent asthma symptoms, the initiation of high-dose inhaled corticosteroid therapy is not appropriate at this time.

2. D. This patient has symptoms consistent with oral candidiasis (thrush), a fungal infection caused by *Candida albicans*. Thrush presents as discrete white plaques or small red spots on the oral (especially the tongue) and pharyngeal mucosa. The lesions are generally painless, but some patients experience "burning" pain or pain on swallowing. Other symptoms of thrush include nausea and taste alterations. Oral candidiasis is one of the most common side effects associated with inhaled corticosteroids. Local corticosteroid deposition on the oral and pharyngeal mucosa facilitates fungal colonization and overgrowth. Thrush is more likely to occur with high doses of inhaled corticosteroids. Appropriate preventative measures include the use of a spacer device and rinsing of the oral cavity with water after inhalation to decrease oral and pharyngeal corticosteroid deposition. All inhaled corticosteroid formulations cause thrush, and the substitution of an alternative corticosteroid without instituting the above measures is unlikely to help. Oral corticosteroids are associated with more severe systemic side effects and should not be used in the management of asthma unless absolutely necessary.

CASE 3-19

1. E. Antiplatelet and anticoagulant medications such as aspirin and warfarin would increase the risk of bleeding during surgery. Heparin and anticoagulant therapy will likely be required, however, immediately postoperatively because this surgery involves the lower extremity and will require prolonged immobilization. COC use should be discontinued at least 4 weeks prior to surgery to avoid increasing the risk of blood clots postsurgically. COC use should be reinitiated only after the patient is ambulating.

2. B. A mean delay of 10 months is observed after the discontinuation of Depo-Provera injections. All of the other formulations listed are associated with minimal delay in return to fertility (typically 1 month or less).

CASE 3-20

1. A. Famotidine, as well as some of the other antisecretory agents, can lead to headaches, dizziness, and other CNS side effects. This is particularly true in older patients or in those with compromised renal elimination.

2. C. Of the agents listed, only tetracycline has activity against *H. pylori* when used in combination with other antimicrobials. Although doxycycline belongs to the tetracycline family, it has not been shown to have activity against *H. pylori*. Miconazole is an antifungal agent and has no activity against *H. pylori*. Amoxicillin and not ampicillin has activity against *H. pylori*.

CASE 3-21

1. A. PPIs are most effective when given 30 minutes before a meal or breakfast (and not with food). This ensures that large amounts of inactive H+/K+-ATPase pumps are present. PPIs should not be coadministered with H$_2$ antagonists. PPIs work best if taken routinely to promote healing rather than on an as-needed basis.

2. E. Cardiac arrhythmias have been observed when cisapride has been used at greater than recommended doses or in those patients taking drugs that are CYP450 inhibitors. Cisapride can help to relieve constipation and nausea because it has prokinetic effects, facilitating the emptying of gastric contents. Cough and anemia also may resolve because cisapride will help to reduce the frequency of reflux episodes and allow time for healing of the esophageal erosions.

CASE 3-22

1. D. The patient has signs and symptoms consistent with cellulitis. Because the patient does not have any drug allergies and requires an oral outpatient regimen, cephalexin is the best choice. Cephalexin provides adequate empiric coverage against the most likely pathogens that cause cellulitis, *Streptococcus pyogenes* and *Staphylococcus aureus*.

2. D. Because the patient is exhibiting signs of an IgE-mediated reaction to nafcillin, the best choice is a non–β-lactam antibiotic with good gram-positive activity such as clindamycin. While rare, IgE-mediated reactions or type 1 reactions to penicillin are the most worrisome adverse effect. IgE-mediated reactions usually occur within 72 hours of starting penicillin and are characterized by laryngeal edema, wheezing, and urticaria. Anaphylaxis usually occurs within the first hour of administration. In this patient, it would be prudent to avoid the use of cephalosporins as well since the risk for cross-reactivity between penicillins and cephalosporins is 3–7%.

CASE 3-23

1. E. Because JK has experienced anaphylaxis to amoxicillin, prescription of any type of penicillin or cephalosporin should be avoided. Cross-reactivity between penicillins and cephalosporins is incomplete, but with a history of anaphylaxis to penicillins, cephalosporins should not be prescribed. Clindamycin would be an appropriate alternative to use to treat the cellulitis.

2. C. Cephalosporins do not have clinically significant drug interactions. However, drugs containing a methylthiotetrazole group such as cefotetan can cause disulfiram-like reactions when taken with ethanol. While MN is receiving cefotetan he will have to refrain from drinking alcohol.

CASE 3-24

1. A. Although pneumococcus remains the most common cause of acute otitis media, CT's otitis media is due to *H. influenzae*, a gram-negative coccobacilli. Although amoxicillin is active against *H. influenzae*, approximately 30% of *H. influenzae* strains in the United States are β-lactamase producing; thus, CT may be infected with a β-lactamase–producing strain. The addition of clavulanate to amoxicillin prevents the degradation of the amoxicillin β-lactam ring. Levofloxacin is not indicated due to early reports of tendonitis in young animals given quinolones. Similarly, tetracyclines are not indicated in children younger than 8 years of age because of their deposition in bone and teeth and propensity to cause teeth discoloration. Erythromycin does not have activity against *H. influenzae*, unlike clarithromycin and azithromycin.

CASE 3-25

1. B. Nongonococcal urethritis is primarily caused by *C. trachomatis*. Infections caused by *C. trachomatis* can be treated with tetracyclines, azithromycin, or macrolides. Doxycycline is contraindicated in pregnant women because of the effects on fetal teeth and bone growth. In the setting of pregnancy, erythromycin is the recommended regimen; however, preliminary data suggest that azithromycin is also safe and effective.

2. C. The tetracyclines interact with multivalent cations such as Ca^{+2}, Mg^{+2}, Fe^{+2}, or Al^{+3}. The major mechanism of these drug interactions is the formation of iron-drug complexes (chelation or binding of iron by the involved drug).

CASE 3-26

1. C. Ciprofloxacin is the best choice due to its good penetration into the prostate. Although TMP-SMX also has good penetration into the prostate, it should be avoided due to his allergy to sulfa medications. β-Lactams and nitrofurantoin are not used for prostatitis because they do not adequately penetrate into the prostate.

2. D. Trimethoprim is the best option since it can be taken by patients with sulfa allergies and has not been shown to increase QT_c interval. Gatifloxacin and moxifloxacin should be avoided in this situation due to her cardiac history and increased risk of QT_c prolongation with the quinolones. Also, due to the minimal excretion of moxifloxacin into the urine, it is not a preferred agent for UTIs. TMP-SMX should be avoided due to her history of anaphylaxis to sulfa medications.

CASE 3-27

1. H. Risk factors for ototoxicity include preexisting renal dysfunction, prolonged therapy, and concomitant receipt of other ototoxic drugs such as furosemide. Because KC is only 45 years old, age is not a risk factor. β-Lactam antibiotics and ACE inhibitors are not typically ototoxic and would not contribute to KC's ototoxicity.

2. C. Of the aminoglycosides, tobramycin has the best activity against *P. aeruginosa*. Streptomycin typically is reserved for infections due to mycobacterial TB. Amikacin is typically reserved for resistant gram-negative infections or infections due to atypical mycobacterial infections. Neomycin is an oral agent that is poorly absorbed in the GI tract and is used for GI decontamination only.

CASE 3-28

1. C. Treatment for catheter-related infections is often initiated empirically, with definitive therapy based on culture results and susceptibility. Dialysis catheters are usually permanently inserted lines, and patients on chronic hemodialysis are at higher risk for developing catheter-related infections secondary to staphylococcal species, particularly coagulase-negative staphylococci. Oral vancomycin is not appropriate because it does not achieve adequate blood levels to treat systemic infections.

2. F. Red man syndrome is an infusion-related reaction that is mediated by release of histamine and is not considered a hypersensitivity or allergic reaction. Thus, treatment with epinephrine is not warranted. In patients who experience red man syndrome, prolonging the duration of infusion or premedication with diphenhydramine will prevent further reactions.

CASE 3-29

1. B. Antibiotic-associated diarrhea due to *C. difficile* can occur with any antibiotic, but particularly with clindamycin. With the administration of antibiotics, normal GI flora is inhibited, which allows *C. difficile* to overgrow. Metronidazole is the treatment of choice for *C. difficile* infections. Although oral vancomycin also has activity against *C. difficile*, it is typically used as second-line treatment.

2. C. Alcohol ingestion should be avoided when taking metronidazole. The coadministration of alcohol with metronidazole can result in an uncomfortable disulfiram-like reaction in patients due to inhibition of aldehyde dehydrogenase, leading to an accumulation of acetaldehyde. A disulfiram reaction manifests as flushing, nausea, vomiting, throbbing headache, sweating, and HTN. The effect may last 30 minutes in mild cases to several hours in severe cases.

CASE 3-30

1. E. The dose of ganciclovir should be decreased due to his worsening renal function, which is a risk factor for increased bone marrow suppression. His neutropenia can be managed by administering filgrastim (granulocyte colony-stimulating factor) in an attempt to increase his WBC count. Cidofovir and foscarnet can both exacerbate SL's renal insufficiency and so would be contraindicated at this time.

2. F. Because foscarnet is an inorganic pyrophosphate analogue, foscarnet can cause electrolyte disturbances, particularly hypocalcemia, and hyperphosphatemia or hypophosphatemia. Thrombophlebitis with foscarnet can be severe, requiring a central line for administration. The main adverse effect of foscarnet is renal insufficiency, including acute tubular necrosis and interstitial nephritis.

Answers

CASE 3-31

1. H. Infusion-related toxicities secondary to amphotericin are common and may be prevented with premedication with diphenhydramine and acetaminophen. Meperidine is effective in halting rigors and muscle spasms. Thus, it is typically given in response to rigors and not as premedication. Sodium loading with normal saline may prevent some of the renal toxicities, particularly prerenal azotemia, associated with amphotericin and is administered prior to amphotericin.

2. B. GM is at risk for vulvovaginal candidiasis due to her poorly controlled insulin-dependent diabetes. Vulvovaginal candidiasis can be effectively treated with any of the topical azole antifungals, such as clotrimazole. Because this is not a systemic infection, amphotericin is not warranted. Ketoconazole, itraconazole, and voriconazole may be alternatives in patients with refractory disease. However, ketoconazole and itraconazole require an acidic environment for adequate oral absorption. PPIs, such as omeprazole, and H_2-receptor blockers can increase the gastric pH and thus inhibit absorption. If GM required systemic therapy for treatment of her vulvovaginal candidiasis, fluconazole would be the preferred agent because it is not dependent on gastric pH for absorption.

CASE 3-32

1. D. Dexrazoxane has been found to provide some protection against anthracycline-induced cardiotoxicity without compromising antitumor effectiveness. The mechanism of protection is thought to be related to intracellular iron chelation, which lessens formation of toxic oxygen-free radicals. It has been most studied with doxorubicin and is indicated for patients who have received cumulative doses of doxorubicin ≥300 mg/m² who would benefit from continued anthracycline therapy. The other agents listed do not clinically reduce cardiotoxicity from anthracyclines. Leucovorin has been used to rescue normal cells from high-dose methotrexate toxicity. Mesna binds toxic acrolein metabolites of ifosfamide and cyclophosphamide and reduces hemorrhagic cystitis. Amifostine is used to reduce renal toxicity from cisplatin. Although N-acetylcysteine has been postulated to reduce anthracycline-induced cardiotoxicity via sulfhydryl repletion and antioxidant effects, it has not been found to provide effective cardioprotection.

2. E. Bilirubin. Cholestasis may dramatically impair clearance of anthracyclines (including doxorubicin), and dose reductions are recommended for elevated bilirubin levels. Diabetes and asthma are unlikely to affect doxorubicin clearance or toxicity. Although the baseline platelet count is somewhat low in this patient, the myelosuppression from anthracyclines is primarily seen as leukopenia, and thrombocytopenia is rarely severe. Because anthracyclines are primarily eliminated in the bile, renal impairment (often present in patients with multiple myeloma) does not affect routine dosing.

CASE 3-33

1. D. Cisplatin has been associated with severe hypomagnesemia. Replacement with both PO and IV supplementation has been shown to be of benefit. Cisplatin is also the most emetogenic chemotherapy agent. Blocking serotonin receptors with **serotonin type III antagonists** (ondansetron, granisetron, or dolasetron) has led to complete prevention of nausea and vomiting in approximately 50% of patients. Dacarbazine is not known to cause pulmonary toxicity, but other alkylating agents (carmustine and busulfan) have been associated with delayed **pulmonary fibrosis.** Pulmonary effects usually present as shortness of breath, nonproductive cough, and hypoxia. Steroids are often used for symptomatic treatment.

2. E. Adequate hydration is absolutely necessary for the safe administration of high-dose cyclophosphamide. Often NS is used as hydration, since cyclophosphamide can be associated with the development of SIADH. The sodium will help minimize the incidence of hyponatremia. Mesna is often used with high-dose cyclophosphamide. As with ifosfamide, cyclophosphamide forms the acrolein metabolite that can be directly toxic to the bladder, leading to hemorrhagic cystitis. The incidence of hemorrhagic cystitis is much lower with cyclophosphamide than with ifosfamide, so usually only higher doses (>2000 mg) will require mesna, whereas all doses of ifosfamide should be given with mesna. High doses of cyclophosphamide can be very emetogenic. It causes both acute and delayed N/V. Acute chemotherapy-induced N/V (occurring within 24 hours of chemotherapy administration) is mediated by the stimulation of serotonin type III receptors, which then stimulate the vomiting center. Blocking the receptors with serotonin antagonists will help minimize acute N/V. On the other hand, delayed chemotherapy-induced N/V (N/V occurring more than 24 hours after chemotherapy administration) is not serotonin mediated, so the use of a serotonin antagonist is of minimal benefit. Only the use of steroids, such as dexamethasone, have been shown to offer significant benefit for delayed N/V.

CASE 3-34

1. E. All of the above conditions should be evaluated in patients receiving high-dose cytarabine. Although cytarabine is hepatically metabolized, one of the major active metabolites, Ara-U, is renally eliminated. Ara-U accumulation may lead to feedback inhibition of cytidine deaminase, which will lead to accumulation of ara-CTP, which is a neurotoxin. In the presence of renal impairment (which may be common in the elderly population), the accumulation of Ara-U may cause cerebellar toxicity. Often cerebellar toxicity is manifested as nystagmus, dysarthria, ataxia, and slurred speech. The cerebellar toxicity may be slowly reversible or it may be permanent in some cases. Cytarabine is extensively excreted through the lacrimal ducts, causing chemical conjunctivitis. The use of steroid eye drops during treatment and for at least 48 hours after the end of high-dose cytarabine may significantly minimize conjunctivitis. Rashes, characteristically starting on the soles and palms, are common with cytarabine administration. Diphenhydramine, topical steroids, and hydroxyzine are often used for pruritus associated with these rashes. Narcotic analgesics may be necessary for pain. Fevers are also a common side effect. In many situations, drug-induced fevers must be distinguished from fever due to infections.

2. B. Fluorouracil is a prodrug that is metabolized to F-dUMP and a triphosphate metabolite. F-dUMP binds and interferes with thymidylate synthase, whereas the triphosphate metabolite interferes with RNA function. Leucovorin is a reduced form of folic acid. Leucovorin provides folate cofactors that stabilize the binding of F-dUMP and thymidylate synthase, thus enhancing the cytotoxic effects of fluorouracil.

CASE 3-35

1. E. All of the above. Vinblastine is hepatically eliminated and must be dose adjusted for hepatic dysfunction. Because vinca alkaloids may cause neurotoxicity (including paralytic ileus), it is important to evaluate the patient's bowel status prior to administration. Of the vinca alkaloids, vinblastine is the most likely to cause severe myelosuppression (may be dose limiting), and baseline WBC counts should be obtained. Vinblastine is a vesicant. It can only be given as an IV infusion via a central line. It also may be given as a slow IV push if there is no central line and good peripheral access.

2. B. Administer via a central line. The risk of extravasation is too high if a vesicant is administered via peripheral venous access. If vesicants are to be administered as a continuous infusion, a central line is mandatory. Applying warm compresses to the affected area or administration of hyaluronidase are measures often used to treat extravasations should they occur.

CASE 3-36

1. C. It is recommended that all patients receiving paclitaxel receive pretreatment to reduce the risk and severity of hypersensitivity reactions. The preferred regimen includes a combination of a corticosteroid (such as dexamethasone), an antihistamine (diphenhydramine or equivalent), and an H_2 antagonist (such as cimetidine or ranitidine). Omeprazole and other PPIs will not block H_2-receptor sites and do not provide protection against hypersensitivity reactions.

2. E. It is recommended that all of the above laboratory parameters be evaluated prior to each course of docetaxel. Myelosuppression (especially neutropenia) is dose limiting with docetaxel, and patients with absolute neutrophil counts of less than 1500/mm³ should not receive this drug. Patients with baseline abnormalities in LFTs are at higher risk for severe side effects (including myelosuppression and death). Docetaxel should not be administered to patients with bilirubin levels above the ULN. Additionally, patients with AST or ALT levels greater than 1.5 times the ULN with concomitant alkaline phosphatase greater than 2.5 times the ULN should generally not receive docetaxel.

PART IV: BIOCHEMISTRY

CASE 4-1

1. E. Each molecule of glucose generates two NADH molecules during glycolysis, two more from the conversion of two molecules of pyruvate to acetyl-CoA, and six more (three each) from the oxidation of acetyl-CoA in the TCA cycle. Of note, the NADH molecules created during glycolysis in the cytosol each generate only two ATP molecules as compared with the three generated by the other NADH molecules in the mitochondria.

2. D. Pyruvate dehydrogenase is the enzyme that converts pyruvate to acetyl-CoA. Although its absence or diminished activity can be quite detrimental, it has little effect on erythrocytes, which primarily convert pyruvate to lactate with LDH. Hexokinase, aldolase, and phosphoglycerate kinase are each enzymes in glycolysis that can lead to hemolytic anemia. G6PD deficiency is the most common carbohydrate metabolism enzyme deficiency that can lead to hemolysis. It functions in the pentose phosphate or hexose-monophosphate shunt. This shunt is responsible for regenerating reduced glutathione, which protects the RBCs in the setting of oxidative stress. Thus, patients with G6PD deficiency have a normal hematocrit at baseline but will undergo a hemolytic anemia in the setting of exposure to various conditions, including viral or bacterial infections or treatment with drugs such as antimalarials, sulfonamides, and nitrofurantoin.

CASE 4-2

1. B. The glycogen storage diseases can be broken into several categories. One category encompasses those diseases leading to hepatic hypoglycemic pathophysiology. Of these, there are the varieties of type I, which have elevated levels of G6P and its metabolites, and types III (Cori), VI (Hers), and VIII in which G6P levels are usually diminished. In this case, because of the increased serum lactate level, there is a good chance that this is a variety of type I disease. However, with the normal level of G6Pase, it is not von Gierke disease. The second most common cause of type I disease is G6P microsomal translocase deficiency, which leaves the hepatic tissue without the ability to transport G6P into the endoplasmic reticulum and eventually convert to glucose and be transported out of the cell. The increased lactate essentially rules out Cori and Hers diseases. McArdle disease is one of diminished muscle capacity.

2. E.; 3. C. Another group of the glycogen storage diseases includes those that specifically affect the muscles. These include type V (McArdle) and several varieties of type VII. These diseases usually present between ages 10 and 30 years with painful cramps, muscle weakness, and myoglobinuria. They can be diagnosed by muscle biopsy and assessment of enzyme activity. In McArdle disease, which is an AR disorder mapped to chromosome 11, the inactive enzyme is muscle glycogen phosphorylase. The enzyme deficiencies in type VII include phosphofructokinase and phosphoglycerate mutase. Treatment of these diseases includes avoidance of vigorous activity and ingesting glucose before exercise. See Table A-1 for how these diseases commonly present.

TABLE A-1

Glycogen Storage Disease	Enzyme Deficiency	Presentation	Prognosis/Rx
Type IA—von Gierke	G6P	Hypoglycemia by age 12 mo	**Developmental delay;** renal failure (dietary Rx)
Type IB	G6P microsomal translocase	Hypoglycemia by age 12 mo	Similar to IA plus neutropenia, recurrent infections

(Continued)

TABLE A-1 *(Continued)*

Glycogen Storage Disease	Enzyme Deficiency	Presentation	Prognosis/Rx
Type II—Pompe	α-1,4-glucosidase	Weakness, cardiomegaly	Death by age 2 or 3 yrs
Type III—Cori	Debranching enzyme	Hepatomegaly, hypoglycemia	Dietary Rx
Type IV—Andersen	Branching enzyme	Hypotonia as infant, cirrhosis	Death by age 2 or 3 yrs
Type V—McArdle	Glycogen phosphorylase (muscle)	Cramps and pain after exercise	Avoid exercise, pre-feed
Type VI—Hers disease	Glycogen phosphorylase (liver)	Hepatomegaly, mild hypoglycemia	Dietary Rx
Type VII	Phosphofructokinase (muscle)	Cramps and pain after exercise	Avoid exercise, mild anemia, pre-feed
Type VIII	Phosphorylase kinase (liver)	Hepatomegaly, mild hypoglycemia	Dietary Rx

CASE 4-3

1. D. The α-glycerol phosphate shuttle produces $FADH_2$ in the mitochondria rather than NADH produced by the malate shuttle. Thus, there are two as compared with three ATP molecules produced per NADH molecule from the cytosol. The conversion of pyruvate to acetyl-CoA results in production of 1 NADH molecule, and a turn of the citric acid cycle produces 3 NADH, 1 GTP, and 1 $FADH_2$ molecule, all in the mitochondria, so the net result is 15 ATPs produced. When added to the four produced via the $FADH_2$ from the α-glycerol phosphate shuttle, this makes a total of 19.

2. A. Mitochondria and therefore mtDNA are only inherited maternally because the ovum is the sole source of mitochondria. Because LA is male, his children have no chance of being affected as long as their mother is not affected.

3. E. There are two NADH and two ATP molecules produced by glycolysis in the cytosol. There are also two pyruvate molecules formed, which rapidly pass into the mitochondria. As in question 1, each pyruvate molecule generates 15 ATPs. Because the two NADH molecules in the cytosol cannot enter the mitochondria without a shuttle, the net total ATP production is 32.

CASE 4-4

1. C. The carnitine diet supplementation can help provide carnitine as a substrate for CAT-I to transport fatty acids into the mitochondria. Because the very short fatty acid chains and the long-chain fatty acids can undergo some β-oxidation, yielding a fuel source of acetyl-CoA molecules, carnitine's effect is to increase the transport of the activated fatty acids across the mitochondrial membrane. The body behaves when carnitine deficient despite having elevated total levels because the carnitine molecules remain bound to CAT-II in the mitochondria. Carnitine does not influence the enzyme listed, and it cannot enter the TCA cycle at a later point.

2. A. Hardy-Weinberg equilibrium uses $p^2 + 2pq + q^2 = 1$. Because the homozygous recessive rate in that population was 0.81, the prevalence of the mutation K304E is 0.9. If $p = .9$, then $q = .1$, or 10%. Nine is the percentage of non-K304E mutations. Heterozygotes would number 2pq, or 18%. This leads the other homozygous population to be 1%, or .01.

3. B. Insulin and glucagon do much to maintain homeostasis. In general, glucagon leads to increased levels of fuel for tissues, and thus breakdown of fats and glycogen and increases in glucose levels. Insulin does the opposite, leading to storage of carbohydrates and fatty acids. So, of the four changes, only a decrease in CAT-I activity would lead to more storage. CAT-I and CAT-II are responsible for getting fatty acids into mitochondria so they can be oxidized. Fatty acyl-CoA synthetase activates fatty acids, so an increase would also lead to oxidation. Fatty acyl-CoA carboxylase is an enzyme in the fatty acid synthesis pathway, and thus would be increased by insulin. Protein catabolism would be stimulated by glucagon, not insulin.

CASE 4-5

1. E. If the 11β-hydroxylase enzyme is absent, the patient does experience CAH, but in this case because it is a male infant, there will not be any obvious phenotypic changes, and usually presentation is with failure to thrive. In CAH, cholesterol and pregnenolone levels are usually relatively normal. The immediate substrates of 11β-hydroxylase, 11-deoxycortisol, and 11-deoxycorticosterone would be elevated, as would androstenedione and often testosterone. However, in this male infant, without aromatase enzyme, estrone would not be elevated.

2. C. CAH is a constellation of absence of glucocorticoids, often mineralocorticoids, buildup of precursors and androgens, and the phenotypic response to these hormonal changes. 3β-Hydroxysteroid dehydrogenase deficiency is the third most common cause of CAH. If the C20,22-desmolase was missing, cholesterol would not be able to proceed down the common pathway, and none of the steroid hormones would be synthesized. If C17,20-desmolase was missing, the androgens would not be synthesized, but the other steroid hormones would undergo normal synthesis. If the 18-hydroxy enzymes were missing, aldosterone synthesis would not occur, but cortisol would still be synthesized.

CASE 4-6

1. A. Patients with SLOS have an enzymatic defect in the enzyme DHCR7, which takes 7-DHC into cholesterol. Thus, these patients have elevated levels of 7-DHC. A patient on enormously high quantities of HMG-CoA reductase inhibitors would have increased levels of HMG-CoA, the molecule that is reduced, and decreased levels of mevalonate, the product of this enzymatic reaction, as compared with normal patients. They would also have decreased levels of all of the molecules downstream (such as 7-DHC and cholesterol). Patients with SLOS are likely to have normal or high levels of these molecules because they have an enzymatic block in this pathway much further downstream.

2. C. HMG-CoA to mevalonate, the rate-limiting step of cholesterol synthesis, is catalyzed by HMG-CoA reductase. This is the key site of regulation and a target for cholesterol-lowering agents. The first two steps (A and B) are not important regulatory steps. Mevalonate to isopentenyl pyrophosphate actually takes several steps and requires three ATP molecules. 7-DHC to cholesterol is the step that does not occur in patients with SLOS.

CASE 4-7

1. A. Lipoprotein lipase primarily hydrolyzes triacylglycerols in either chylomicrons or VLDLs. This hydrolysis results in an increase in the percentage weight of these molecules, converting into VLDLs, LDLs, HDLs, and so on. Chylomicrons do get converted into VLDLs, but it is rare for HDL to be an end product. Apo B-100 facilitates the production of VLDLs.

2. B. All of these patients are at risk of developing cardiovascular disease, but only one fits the description in the question. The patient with lipoprotein lipase deficiency will have relatively normal or even low levels of LDL and VLDL because the enzyme normally helps produce these molecules, particularly from chylomicrons. The other two genetic-risk patients will have elevated LDLs and VLDLs. The other at-risk patients would be likely to have increased LDLs and VLDLs as well with the smoking and obesity histories and would not be at particular risk of having xanthomas.

CASE 4-8

1. A. There is significant overlap in the phenotype of **Marfan syndrome** and homocystinuria. Both disorders have similar musculoskeletal and ocular findings. Cardiac manifestations are one of the hallmarks of Marfan (mitral valve prolapse, aortic dilation) but are not part of homocystinuria. In addition, mental retardation and thromboembolic complications are *not* typical features of Marfan syndrome. The sudden onset of severe chest pain in a patient with the phenotype described suggests dissection of the aorta in a patient with Marfan syndrome. Marfan syndrome is caused by mutations in the **fibrillin-1 gene.** CBS deficiency is the enzymatic defect responsible for homocystinuria. Patients with homozygosity of MTHFR mutation variants may have mild elevations of homocysteine and are at an increased risk of vascular complications but do not have a distinct phenotype and are not at increased risk of aortic dilation/dissection.

2. A. Mild elevations of homocysteine have been associated with common medical problems, including vascular disease in the coronary, carotid, and peripheral circulations, increased risk of dementia, increased risk of NTDs, and possibly cleft lip and palate. The mechanism by which this occurs is not fully understood. Proposed mechanisms include oxidative injury to the vascular wall, vascular cell proliferation, and development of a prothrombotic state. The elevations of homocysteine may be the result of vitamin or cofactor deficiency in the homocysteine pathway, genetically determined (as in MTHFR homozygote variants), or a combination of genetic and environmental interactions. Protein C deficiency and factor V Leiden mutations are procoagulant conditions but are not associated with elevated homocysteine. Dolichostenomelia (tall, slender) and mental retardation are in keeping with homocystinuria, which has elevated, *not* normal, levels of methionine. Holoprosencephaly is genetically heterogeneous but is not associated with homocysteine elevations.

3. E. For those children with homocystinuria not identified through newborn screening, the diagnosis may be first suspected between 3 and 5 years of age when ocular manifestations become apparent. The mental retardation is progressive if untreated. Some musculoskeletal findings might be present but become more apparent with age. **Cyanide nitroprusside test** is used as a screening test in some **newborn screening** programs. The metabolic abnormality consists of elevations of homocysteine and methionine and low or absent cysteine. The diagnosis is confirmed by decreased or absent CBS activity. Hyperphenylalaninemia is the hallmark of PKU, the most common IEM associated with mental retardation, if left untreated.

CASE 4-9

1. B. Females with PKU who are not on a strict phenylalanine-restricted diet are at risk of having children who are mentally retarded, microcephalic, growth restricted, and have a high incidence of congenital heart defects. This phenotype is directly related to the levels of phenylalanine in the maternal blood and not related to the fetal genotype. It is essential that females with PKU remain in contact with a metabolic facility, are offered effective means of contraception, and receive optimal preconceptional treatment. With adequate dietary treatment, evidenced by phenylalanine and tyrosine levels within the normal range, the outcome in offspring of mothers with PKU should be the same as that of controls.

2. D. For nuclear families in which there is an affected individual with PKU and both parents are available, it is possible to offer linkage analysis and predict whether the fetus carries the defective haplotypes by either CVS or amniocentesis. Although it is possible to do a fetal liver biopsy and test for PAH activity, it is a procedure that carries significant risk to the fetus. PAH activity is not expressed in amniocytes. DNA testing is not possible because we know that mutation analysis failed to identify one mutation in the affected (homozygous) son.

3. C. Galactosemia is due to a deficiency of **galactose-1-uridyltransferase (GALT).** The neonatal presentation with liver failure and *E. coli* sepsis is classic. Infants who survive develop mental retardation, chronic liver failure, and cataracts. Females will develop ovarian failure. Treatment consists of removal of all galactose from the diet. **Tyrosinemia I** is characterized by liver dysfunction, liver failure, and cirrhosis but is not associated with cataracts. The defect is due to a deficiency in the distal pathway of tyrosine catabolism, leading to accumulation of succinylacetone, the hallmark of this disorder. **Homocystinuria** due to CBS deficiency is characterized by mental retardation, skeletal abnormalities, ectopia lentis, and a tendency for thromboembolism. **Biotinidase deficiency** can be successfully treated with large doses of biotin and will not lead to the serious neurologic symptoms (seizures, mental retardation, hearing loss, and hypotonia) seen in untreated patients. All of these disorders are AR IEMs that are currently screened in most newborn screening programs.

CASE 4-10

1. A. From the text in this case, we know that short-term regulation of the cycle occurs principally at CPS-I, which is relatively inactive in the absence of its allosteric activator *N*-acetylglutamate. The steady-state concentration of *N*-acetylglutamate is set by the concentration of its components acetyl-CoA and glutamate and by arginine, which is a positive allosteric effector of *N*-acetylglutamate synthetase. The other enzymes are from the urea cycle, but they are minimally involved in the regulation of the cycle.

2. C. IEMs can cause symptoms in two primary ways: not making enough of something or not breaking down or clearing a molecule. In patients with UCDs, what they have in common is the decreased ability to break down and excrete the nitrogenous waste from proteins and amino acids. This leads to a buildup of ammonia, which leads to the neurologic and mental status changes seen in patients with UCDs. These patients clear urea and orotic acid relatively quickly via renal excretion, so although orotic acid may be slightly elevated in OTC-deficient patients, it is not thought to be a cause of their symptoms. Urea is actually decreased, not elevated. There is no particular change in renal function in these patients.

CASE 4-11

1. B. This patient has both pernicious anemia and the neurologic symptoms that accompany vitamin B12 deficiency. These neurologic symptoms begin as paresthesias, progressing to an awkward unsteady gait and eventually stiffness of the limbs. These symptoms are related to demyelination of the nerves. If vitamin B12 supplementation is begun within a week or two of symptoms, there may be complete resolution of disease, although with a prolonged presence of symptoms, recovery may be only minimal. Folate (not listed) can also cause a macrocytic anemia. Thiamine (vitamin B1) deficiency, as in the case, can cause neurologic symptoms, but the presentation is different from this.

2. C. Deficiency in vitamin C leads to **scurvy** because of the role of the vitamin in the posttranslational modification of collagens. Scurvy is characterized by easily bruised skin, muscle fatigue, soft swollen gums, decreased wound healing and hemorrhaging, osteoporosis, and anemia. Vitamin C is readily absorbed, and thus the primary cause of vitamin C deficiency is poor diet and/or an increased requirement. Classically, scurvy was seen on long sea voyages where citrus fruit was not available. The osteoporosis in this case may have led to a diagnosis of vitamin D deficiency. However, rickets and osteomalacia do not present with decreased healing.

PART V: GENETICS

CASE 5-1

1. D. Because both parents are carriers, they have a 25% chance of having an unaffected child. The chance of having two unaffected children is 0.25 × 0.25, or 6.25%.

2. B. In both disorders, affected mothers have a 50% chance of transmitting the disease to their children. In X-linked dominant disorders, females are affected twice as commonly as males. One of the characteristic features of AD diseases is male-to-male transmission, which is not seen in X-linked disorders. Skipped generations are not seen in either AD or X-linked dominant pedigrees. In AD traits, affected males have a 50% chance of passing on the diseased allele to both their sons and their daughters.

3. C. This patient has Huntington disease, an AD disorder caused by expanding CAG trinucleotide repeats in the Huntington gene. Characteristic features of this disorder include involuntary twitching movements (chorea) and progressive loss of voluntary muscle control. Depression, dementia, and other psychiatric symptoms are common in patients with Huntington disease. Anticipation is known to occur in Huntington disease.

4. C. The above protocol describes the Southern blot technique and is used in the diagnosis of myotonic dystrophy. PCR involves the amplification of a specific DNA sequence. Western blot is a technique in which protein is run through a gel, transferred to a membrane, and then hybridized with labeled antibodies. This test is used for the diagnosis of diseases such as HIV and Lyme disease. FISH is a procedure in which fluorescence-labeled probes are hybridized with chromosomes and then visualized with a fluorescence microscope. Northern blot is similar to the Southern blot, except that RNA is run through the gel instead of DNA.

CASE 5-2

1. B. The gene product of the CF gene or CFTR protein is believed to participate in chloride transport and mucin secretion. The protein has a complex three-dimensional structure, with two transmembrane domains, which anchor it to the cell membrane, two nucleotide-binding folds, which bind ATP, and a regulatory domain, which has several phosphorylation sites.

2. B. In AR disorders, if each parent has one mutant allele, the chances of having an affected offspring is 1 in 4, a carrier is 1 in 2, and an unaffected noncarrier is 1 in 4, according to the Mendel law. However, in the case presented, the sister is not affected, so she can only be a carrier (2/3 chance) or not a carrier (1/3 chance). Because the husband has not been screened, we must use the known carrier frequency for that population (1/25). The chance that the mutant allele is passed on is 1 in 2 for each parent. So then the equation is: 2/3 * 1/2 * 1/25 * 1/2 = 1/150, or 1 in 150.

3. D. Nonpaternity may be as common as 15% in certain populations. Genetic testing may incidentally disclose nonpaternity in the work-up of a genetic disorder of an affected offspring. This issue must be addressed in the counseling before testing. Given that commercially available DNA panels screen only for the more common mutations (usually 32–72 for patients with CF), but there are more than 1000 known mutations, the possibility that an individual may carry a mutation not assessed by the DNA panel utilized must be discussed. This is particularly important among certain ethnic groups in which CF is rare and a large proportion of the mutations are unknown (e.g., Hispanics and Asians). In AR disorders, heterozygotes (carriers) are by definition not affected.

CASE 5-3

1. C. MR's sister has a 50% chance of having the full mutation and a 50% chance of having a normal allele (she cannot be a premutation carrier because it almost always expands when the mother has a premutation in the more than 90-repeat range). She has a 50% chance of transmitting the mutant allele to each of her daughters and a 50% chance of being mentally retarded (affected) if they inherited the mutation. So the risk is $\frac{1}{2} * \frac{1}{2} * \frac{1}{2} =$ 1 in 8 chance (the risk of having a mentally retarded son would be 1 in 4 because all males with the full mutation are mentally retarded).

2. D. MR's uncle is a premutation carrier, so neither he nor his children are affected. Because the mutant allele is on the X chromosome, he cannot pass the premutation to his son. All daughters of premutation carrier fathers will inherit the premutation unchanged (stable) or with mild expansion (but still in the premutation range) and hence be unaffected. The premutation daughter can then transmit and have an expansion of repeats to the next generation to 50% of sons and daughters. If the mutation expanded to the full mutation range (>200), all males will be affected and roughly one half of the females will inherit the full mutation with potential for mental retardation.

3. A. Unstable or dynamic mutations caused by triplet repeat sequences of DNA can expand over the course of generations, explaining complex inheritance patterns (such as for fragile X or myotonic dystrophy) that were largely unexplained until recently. Some AD disorders exhibit earlier disease onset in the offspring than the parents and increasing disease severity in subsequent generations. This phenomenon, known as *anticipation*, is well established in **myotonic dystrophy** and **Huntington disease,** which are both examples of AD unstable expansion triplet repeat DNA sequences. In myotonic dystrophy, an expansion of a CTG triplet repeat can account for the severe neonatal presentation of myotonic dystrophy, which occurs only when the mutation is inherited from the mother. In Huntington disease, an expansion of a CAG triplet repeat can account for the juvenile form of the disease when the mutation is passed on by the father. The cause of this sex bias in anticipation is unclear.

CASE 5-4

1. D. Males with a mitochondrial disorder that is due to mutations in mitochondrial DNA (as opposed to nuclear DNA) cannot pass on the mutation to offspring, whereas males with an X-linked recessive mutation can only produce either a normal son or a carrier female. Assuming that the female partner has a normal genotype, no offspring of a male with either a mitochondrial or an X-linked recessive disorder will be affected. In X-linked disorders, both the male and the female can pass the mutation on to the next generation. In mitochondrial inheritance, males and females are affected at an equal rate, but it is only the female who can transmit the mtDNA mutation. A mother with an X-linked recessive disorder will have affected sons but asymptomatic carrier daughters such as herself.

2. A. A female with a mitochondrial mutation will transmit the mutation to all of her children. Because we know that the affected individual's mother has the mutation, all of the maternal aunts must also have the mutation but may or may not be symptomatic due to heteroplasmy and replicative segregation.

3. B. Heteroplasmy defines the ability of a cell to have multiple species of mtDNA. The threshold effect describes the phenomenon of when symptoms are manifested only after a certain level of mutant mtDNA has been reached. Homoplasmy occurs when a cell has only one population of mtDNA. Pleiotropy is the ability of a gene to direct more than one phenotype. Imprinting is the concept that differences in phenotype occur depending on whether a genetic mutation is inherited from the mother or the father.

CASE 5-5

1. D. Variable expression is the concept that the severity of a genetic disease can be modified by the environment, allelic heterogeneity, or modifier genes. Reduced penetrance occurs when an individual has a disease gene, but not the disease phenotype. This is an all-or-nothing phenomenon. Imprinting is the variable phenotype of a genetic mutation depending on the parental origin of the disease gene. Pleiotropy defines the ability of a gene to influence multiple phenotypes. Anticipation refers to the earlier expression and increasing severity of a disease phenotype with successive generations.

2. E. This family has features characteristic of tuberous sclerosis. Tuberous sclerosis is an AD disease with highly variable expressivity, even among family members, and is the second most common neurocutaneous syndrome (the first being NF1). Manifestations of Sturge-Weber syndrome include congenital, unilateral capillary angiomas of the head and neck, as well as seizures. NF2 is also an AD disease characterized by eighth nerve tumors and is frequently associated with other intracranial or intraspinal tumors. von Recklinghausen is the German pathologist who first described the constellation of symptoms in NF and his name is now synonymous with NF1. Marfan syndrome is an AD disorder with a defect in the connective tissue protein **fibrillin.** Characteristic defects are seen in the ocular (detached lens), skeletal (long, slender limbs and fingers), and cardiovascular (mitral valve prolapse, aortic aneurysm) systems.

3. C. Locus heterogeneity is the ability of mutations in different genes to cause the same disease phenotype. Pleiotropy describes genes that can cause multiple phenotypes. Allelic heterogeneity is defined as the variation in disease phenotype depending on the type or location of mutations in a disease gene. Heteroplasmy is seen in mitochondrial genetics and is the presence of multiple species of DNA at a particular locus within a cell. When there are individuals in a population who have a disease genotype, but not the disease phenotype, the disease genotype is said to have reduced or incomplete penetrance.

CASE 5-6

1. B. For couples who have had one prior affected offspring with trisomy 21, the empiric recurrence risk is 1% greater than that expected for age-specific risk. This high incidence (particularly for younger couples) can be explained by trisomy 21 **gonadal mosaicism.** In 3% of DS, the extra chromosome 21 is fused with another acrocentric chromosome, known as a **Robertsonian translocation.** The parents of translocation DS children need to be karyotyped because one third of the time, one of the parents will be a **balanced translocation carrier.** These individuals are at a particularly high risk of recurrence of DS and for spontaneous abortion, which, depending on the translocation and the parent carrying it, can be as high as 100%.

2. B. Because a high proportion of trisomy 21 (30%) are spontaneously lost, earlier detection by **CVS** detects a proportion of cases that would not have been picked up by a later procedure (i.e., amniocentesis). This phenomenon is true for the other chromosomal aneuploidies as well. CVS is generally performed between 10 and 13 weeks' gestation. Its main advantage over amniocentesis is earlier diagnosis. The disadvantages of CVS over amniocentesis are a higher risk of pregnancy loss (0.5% higher) and **confined placental mosaicism.** Because chromosome mosaicism arises in somatic cells at a later stage in development, the abnormal cells may be confined to the placenta, the fetus, or both. Detection of mosaicism in placental tissue (CVS) is not absolutely indicative of abnormal karyotype in the fetus, the large majority of which are subsequently confirmed to be karyotypically normal. A second invasive procedure (usually amniocentesis) is necessary to provide reassurance to the parents after the detection of mosaicism through CVS.

3. E. Children with DS have a 1–2% chance of developing acute lymphoblastic leukemia (20-fold greater than the general population). Interestingly, **acquired** trisomy 21 is one of the most common chromosomal abnormalities seen in leukemia. A high incidence of seizure disorders (5–10%) is seen in children and adults with Alzheimer-like dementia who have DS. A high proportion of individuals with DS have thyroid dysfunction and hypothyroidism due to thyroid autoantibodies. Clinical recognition of hypothyroidism may be limited in DS, so routine screening is recommended. Atlantoaxial subluxation is a rare but serious complication of DS, associated with neurologic signs of spinal compression. It is likely related to the hyperextensibility of joints seen in DS and should be screened for starting in childhood.

CASE 5-7

1. E. Manifesting heterozygote females for X-linked recessive disorders have been well documented, albeit rare. Homozygosity (two mutant alleles [one on each X chromosome]) can occur when there is an affected father and the mother is a carrier female, or as a result of a new spontaneous mutation passed on by the mother (exceedingly rare). **Skewed X inactivation** is another explanation, although it is unlikely that the phenotype is as severe as an affected male. There are several cases of Turner syndrome girls with X-linked recessive conditions such as hemophilia A and DMD who expressed the trait as X-linked dominant. The X chromosome involved in an autosomal translocation remains preferentially active, in order for the autosomal component of the derivative chromosome to maintain activity. So if the **breakpoint of the translocation disrupts a gene** on the X chromosome that remains preferentially active, a female can be affected with an X-linked recessive disorder. This concept has been used in **gene mapping.**

2. B. Females with the Turner phenotype and signs of virilization should be screened for the presence of the Y chromosome. The karyotype may show various degrees of 45,X/46,XY mosaicism or the Y component may be detected by molecular methods such as FISH or PCR in cases of cryptic 45,X/46,XY mosaicism. These individuals with gonadal dysgenesis with a Y chromosome component are at increased risk of developing a malignant germline tumor (gonadoblastoma). The recommendation is for removal of the gonads after reaching puberty because the gonads generally do not undergo malignant changes before then and their presence may aid in sexual development.

3. D. Initial reports of individuals with sex chromosome abnormalities came from institutions for the mentally retarded or correction facilities for criminals. This selection bias contributed to descriptions of severe phenotypes, particularly for the XYY males and their "criminal Y chromosome," which have not held up in prospective studies of unselected populations. The phenotypes of prenatally ascertained cases (amniocentesis and CVS) are not always the same as those for postnatally ascertained cases. For example, 45,X/46,XY cases diagnosed by amniocentesis secondary to screening due to maternal age are usually (90%) normal males at birth who would not have been otherwise recognized as abnormal, whereas postnatally diagnosed 45,X/46,XY have phenotypic abnormalities (usually ambiguous genitalia) 100% of the time! (That's why the study was ordered.) Imprinting has not been shown to play a role in phenotypic variability of sex chromosome abnormalities.

CASE 5-8

1. E. There is a 50% chance that EY's children will receive the microdeletion. However, because his children would be receiving the mutation from their father, the affected children would have Prader-Willi syndrome and *not* Angelman syndrome.

2. E. In AD disorders, any affected parent can pass on the disorder. In AR disorders, two copies of a defective gene need to be inherited, one from each parent. In X-linked recessive disorders, only male offspring are affected while female offspring are carriers. Although the inheritance pattern of Angelman syndrome has similarities to mitochondrial inheritance, there is a key difference. In Angelman syndrome, a father can theoretically pass on the disease. For example, if an affected father gives the chromosome 15 deletion to his daughter, she will have Prader-Willi syndrome. If the daughter then gives it to the grandchild, the grandchild will once again have Angelman syndrome. This pattern would be impossible for mitochondrial inheritance.

3. B. Beckwith-Wiedemann syndrome results from the overexpression of a growth factor gene, which is normally expressed only on paternal chromosome 11 and imprinted (inactivated) on the maternal chromosome. This syndrome occurs when two copies of paternal chromosome 11 are inherited or if the imprinted maternal gene on chromosome 11 becomes activated. The symptoms of Beckwith-Wiedemann syndrome include large gestational size, large tongue, abdominal wall defects, and increased risk of Wilms tumor (a renal cancer). DMD is an X-linked disorder, NF1 is an AD disorder, and CF and sickle cell anemia are AR diseases.

CASE 5-9

1. B. G1 is known to vary most between cell types and accounts for the differences in doubling time between cell types. G0, or quiescence, refers to cells not in the cell cycle. Typically, the S phase lasts 20 hours, G2 lasts 3 hours, and the M phase lasts 1 hour for most cell types.

2. A. The presence of Okazaki fragments causes a block in the S phase, and progression through S does not occur until they are all cleared. An increase in p53 leads to a block in G1/S. Rb acts to block the cell cycle by binding to E2F, thereby preventing its action. p27 binds to cyclin-Cdk to prevent their activity. Cyclins bind to Cdk and the active cyclin-Cdk complexes phosphorylate downstream targets.

PART VI: EMBRYOLOGY

CASE 6-1

1. A. Only toxoplasmosis is caused by the protozoan *T. gondii*. Rubella is part of the togavirus family made up of enveloped RNA viruses. CMV and HSV are enveloped linear dsDNA viruses and are members of the herpesvirus family. Syphilis is caused by the spirochete *T. pallidum*.

2. E. The distinctive presentation of rhinitis, rash on the palms and soles, and poor feeding is consistent with congenital syphilis. This diagnosis is made definitively by dark field microscopy. As an older infant, other abnormalities will likely become apparent as well, including bone and/or joint pain, mental retardation, and vision and/or hearing loss. Rubella can be diagnosed by the detection of rubella-specific IgM antibodies in the infant, isolation of the virus from nasopharyngeal or urine specimens, or the persistence of rubella IgG after 8–12 months. HSV is made by culturing samples from vesicles, urine, or the nasopharynx. The diagnosis of CMV can be made by neonatal urine culture or serum antibody titer.

3. A. Although infection generally presents with flu-like symptoms in a healthy adult, the symptoms can be much more severe in an immunocompromised individual. This intracellular parasite can invade the CNS, and patients present with fever, mental status changes, lethargy, headache, seizures, and focal neurologic findings. CT scan is significant for multiple ring-enhancing lesions and cerebral edema. The source of the infection can be from the soil, undercooked meat, or cat feces, or it can be due to reactivation of oocytes in an immunocompromised host.

CASE 6-2

1. C. Only organs arising from the ectoderm (CNS, face, ears, eyes) seem to be affected in this patient. The mesoderm layer gives rise to the musculoskeletal, cardiovascular, and genitourinary systems, whereas the endoderm forms the GI and respiratory tracts.

2. B. The major birth defect associated with thalidomide is deformity of the long bones, resulting in amelia or meromelia (total or partial absence of the extremities). Isotretinoin causes abnormal ear development, cleft palate, and NTDs/heart defects. Lithium has been implicated in heart malformations (Ebstein anomaly), whereas alcohol causes FAS (growth restriction, facial dysmorphisms, mental retardation, and heart defects). DES is a synthetic estrogen that has been linked to genitourinary cancer and malformations in young women who were exposed in utero.

3. E. The formation of the embryonic germ layers occurs during gastrulation, starting with the appearance of the primitive streak on the epiblast and ending with the invagination of the epiblast cells to form the endoderm and mesoderm. Cleavage represents a series of cell divisions without an increase in overall size that characterizes early development of the embryo. Compaction is the process by which blastomeres form a compact ball of cells during the cleavage process.

CASE 6-3

1. B. Periconceptional (from before conception to at least 10–12 weeks of gestation) ingestion of high-dose folic acid (4 mg) has been shown to reduce the recurrence of NTDs in RCTs. First occurrence of NTDs is reduced by the periconceptional intake of 0.4 mg of folic acid. Women of reproductive age should be encouraged to take adequate amounts of folic acid, given that approximately half of pregnancies in the United States are unplanned. Consumption of large amounts of alcohol in pregnancy may lead to FAS, which is characterized by mild mental retardation and distinctive facial features, not to NTDs. Heavy doses of ionizing radiation, far greater than those from x-ray exposure, have been associated with microcephaly and ocular defects.

2. C. Like most other malformations involving a single organ (e.g., VSD and cleft lip), most NTDs show an MFI, implying an interaction of many genes with the environment. Other causes are rarer but well-established as causes of NTDs, such as **teratogens** (valproic acid), **vitamin deficiency** (coal-mine regions of Wales before dietary supplementation of folic acid), **single-gene defects** (Meckel syndrome: AR condition characterized by polydactyly, encephalocele, and polycystic kidneys), and **chromosomal abnormalities** (trisomy 13 and trisomy 18).

3. E. Valproic acid is a well-established teratogen, increasing the risk of NTDs 10- to 20-fold over background risk (6%) when administered during the first trimester of pregnancy. Most of the defects occur during the third and fourth week of development (5–6 weeks of LMP). Earlier exposures (1–2 weeks of development) either are associated with early pregnancy loss or are of no consequence to the fetus (**all-or-nothing phenomenon**). Other **anticonvulsants** are also associated with an increased risk of NTDs (carbamazepine) and minor congenital anomalies (phenytoin) but to a much smaller degree than valproic acid.

CASE 6-4

1. B. DiGeorge syndrome is caused by abnormal development of the third and fourth pharyngeal pouches that give rise to the thymus and the parathyroid glands. The second pharyngeal arch develops into the stapes and hyoid bones, as well as the muscles of facial expression. The third arch forms the remainder of the hyoid bone and the stylopharyngeus muscle. The first cleft develops into the external auditory meatus. The second aortic arch forms the hyoid and stapedial arteries, and the third aortic arch creates the common carotid, external carotid, and part of the internal carotid arteries. The fifth pharyngeal pouch differentiates into the ultimobranchial body that eventually becomes the parafollicular or C cells of the thyroid.

2. C. These bones are mostly formed by the first pharyngeal arch and are derived from embryologic mesodermal cells. The cells of the pharyngeal cleft are composed of ectoderm, and those of the pharyngeal pouch are of endodermal origin.

3. E. The cricothyroid muscle is derived from the fourth pharyngeal arch and is the only intrinsic muscle of the larynx not produced by the sixth arch. It is supplied by the superior laryngeal nerve, and all muscles of the sixth arch are innervated by the recurrent laryngeal nerve. Recurrent laryngeal nerve dysfunction (from trauma or mass lesion) is the most common cause of vocal cord paralysis and hoarseness.

PART VII: BEHAVIORAL SCIENCE

CASE 7-1

1. B. Rapprochement was defined by Margaret Mahler as the process by which the child practices moving away from the parent or caregiver, coming back for reassurance and comfort. Separation anxiety typically occurs at 7–9 months, as does stranger anxiety.

Answers

Exploration is not a stage, as it happens to everyone at all ages in differing forms. Attachment theorists, such as Mary Ainsworth, defined different types of attachment patterns in infants: secure, insecure, and unattached. The type of attachment defined how the infant interacted with the world, parents, and strangers.

2. C. Children usually take their first steps around their first birthday. Usually by 18 months they can walk up steps.

3. C. As this child is speaking in two-word sentences, his age should be 2; thus, he should be able to wash and dry his hands. Riding a tricycle is usually accomplished around age 3. Copying a +, hopping on one foot, and dressing without supervision are usually accomplished by age 4.

4. B. This child has a social smile (1–2 months) and can grasp (4 months) but cannot sit unassisted (6 months). The stepping reflex (in which if the infant is held vertically with pressure on the feet, she will make stepping motions) disappears at 2–3 months. All the others except Babinski are gone by 4–6 months. These include the Moro reflex (movement causing extension, abduction, and then adduction of the extremities), grasp reflex (pressure on the palm causes infants to grasp), and rooting reflex (oral or perioral stimulation causing orientation toward the stimulus and sucking). Babinski (scratching the lateral aspect of the sole [heel to toe] leads to dorsiflexion of the big toe and fanning of other toes) is consistently negative (flexor, downward) after 18 months.

CASE 7-2

1. C. Predisposing risk factors for teenage pregnancy include depression, poor planning for the future, academic difficulties, and divorced parents. Teenage pregnancy is a serious social problem in the United States, with approximately 600,000 births and 400,000 abortions annually. Teenagers are not consistent in their use of contraception; only about a third use contraception regularly. The average age of first intercourse in the United States is 16 years. By 19 years, 80% of men and 70% of women have experienced intercourse. Teenagers are at high risk for obstetric complications because of their physical immaturity and lack of prenatal care. Almost 50% of unmarried mothers are teenagers.

2. B. By the age of 30 years, between 60 and 70% of those individuals living in the United States are married and have children. Erik Erikson defined this period of psychosocial development as one of intimacy versus isolation. During this phase, there is pressure to develop intimate, stable relationships. If the individual lacks the capacity and ego strength to develop a mutually beneficial relationship, then emotional isolation may develop. During early adulthood (20–40 years) the individual's role in society is defined, independence is achieved, and physical development peaks. Daniel Levinson describes this transition phase as one in which a reappraisal of the individual's life occurs; this happens at approximately 30 years of age.

3. C. Postpartum psychosis occurs in between 0.1 and 0.2% of women after delivery. This is the most severe of all the postpartum psychiatric syndromes and usually develops 2–4 weeks after delivery. The postpartum blues occurs in between 30 and 85% of women after childbirth. Crying, irritability, depressed mood, anxiety, and insomnia characterize the condition. It generally appears within the first week and is a self-limiting condition that usually responds to reassurance, support, and some education about the condition. However, it has been estimated that 20% of women with the baby blues go on to develop major depression. In postpartum depression, ambivalent or negative feelings toward the infant are often reported, as are doubts about the mother's ability to care for her infant. When severe, suicidal ideation is frequently reported, but suicide rates appear to be relatively low. Increased risk may be associated with stressful life events during pregnancy or near delivery. Marital dissatisfaction or inadequate social supports may increase the likelihood of developing a postpartum depressive illness. Rates of 26% among teenagers have been reported. Factors suggested that might place women at increased risk of depression at this time include the fall in serum estrogen, progesterone, thyroid hormone, and cortisol and psychosocial issues surrounding the adjustment to having an infant. Treatment involves antidepressant medications and psychotherapy.

4. D. Approximately 50% of women have further episodes of psychosis. Postpartum psychosis occurs in 1.5 per 1000 deliveries. It is associated with primigravida females. Risk factors include a family history of psychiatric disorders and a history of bipolar or mood disorder in the mother. Psychological risk factors include the previous (or current) death of a child, poor social support, the quality of the relationships between the patient and her partner, his family, and her own mother. Most of these episodes are due to mood disorders. Very few are due to organic/medical causes. A prodromal period may begin 2 days after birth, with restlessness, insomnia, irritability, and changes in mood. This may be followed by confusion, overactivity, labile mood, and psychotic symptoms, including hallucinations and delusions (often focused on the baby). Approximately 5% of women with this disorder commit suicide and 4% commit infanticide. These women are at increased risk of developing further episodes of psychosis in the postpartum period or at any time.

CASE 7-3

1. D. Baseline exams prior to starting lithium treatment should include the following: urea, electrolytes, creatinine, urine tests, TFTs, weight, EKG, and pregnancy test if of child-bearing age. During treatment with lithium, levels should be drawn approximately every 8 weeks once the dose has been stabilized. Urea, electrolytes, creatinine, TFTs, and urine should be checked every 6–12 months. An EKG should be performed annually. Lithium treatment can cause a benign leukocytosis with an increase in neutrophils.

2. D. The side effects of valproic acid include nausea (25%), vomiting (5%), diarrhea, weight gain, hair loss (5–10%), sedation, ataxia, dysarthria, tremor (can be treated with beta-blockers if troublesome), elevated LFTs (5–10%), thrombocytopenia, and platelet dysfunction, which can increase bleeding times, and, more rarely, pancreatitis and fatal hepatotoxicity (0.85 per 100,000 patients). Use of valproic acid in the first trimester of pregnancy has been reported to cause neural tube defects in 1–2%. It is contraindicated in this situation (and while breastfeeding) and in those with hepatic disease.

3. C. Hypoparathyroidism does not influence the distribution of a drug. Edema can be caused by a variety of conditions, such as cardiac failure, cirrhosis, and nephrotic syndrome, all of which can both increase distribution and decrease clearance. Pregnancy causes an increase in blood volume, increasing distribution. Obesity increases the distribution of lipophilic agents and increases distribution and the half-life of such agents. Weight is of consideration when planning dosages of medications. Increasing age is associated with an altered volume of distribution, as lean body mass decreases and fat increases, which affects the volume of distribution.

4. C. Efficacy of a drug is a measure of the maximum effect a drug can produce. Potency is a measure of the amount of a drug required to produce a particular effect. Therapeutic indexes are used to measure the safety of drugs. (**The therapeutic index** is the ratio between a lethal dose and a clinically effective dose.) SSRIs usually have a high therapeutic index, and tricyclics have a lower one. A **therapeutic window** is the range in which a drug has a maximum clinical effect. Above and below this range, decreased clinical effects may occur. The tricyclic nortriptyline has a therapeutic window.

CASE 7-4

1. B. This is an example of classical conditioning. The nurse is the conditioned stimulus, which has become associated with an unconditioned stimulus, the injection, and the ensuing discomfort provoking the conditioned response of crying. After a period of time when the conditioned stimulus has not been paired with the unconditioned stimulus, extinction of the conditioned response occurs.

2. B. Biofeedback is a technique that is based on operant conditioning. Patients are trained to control peripheral skin temperature using galvanic measurements and have reported decreased migraine attacks. Biofeedback techniques are also used to help control hypertension, tension headaches, asthma, and generalized anxiety. Each uses a physiologic parameter, which can be measured, and continuous information is provided to the patient who learns to alter these parameters using relaxation techniques. Patients must have a high level of motivation, as these techniques take a lot of practice to master.

3. E. Positive reinforcement of the undesired behavior is occurring. Most likely this is due to the increased attention from the mother that this behavior evokes. You recommend that she try ignoring this behavior if possible to cause extinction and also to reinforce the desired behavior.

4. B. Modeling is used in social skills training and assertiveness training, in which a live model demonstrates appropriate behaviors during role-playing exercises. Observational learning is enhanced by models that have high status, social power, competence, and some common characteristics with the observer. Aversive therapy uses classical conditioning to link a discomfort (e.g., electric shock) with an undesired behavior. Aversive therapy may be temporarily effective. Token economies are examples of operant conditioning and are used to modify behaviors in ward settings, particularly with psychiatric patients. Flooding is used to treat phobias by keeping patients in the feared (but harmless) situation until their anxiety and fear decrease. Systematic desensitization is used to treat phobias and other irrational anxieties. It begins with imagining a graded hierarchy of anxiety-provoking stimuli while practicing relaxation techniques. An example would be the patient who is fearful of flying but who imagines buying an airline ticket, packing his or her bag, going to the airport, and so on.

CASE 7-5

1. E. Suppression along with sublimation, altruism, anticipation (planning for future internal discomfort or adverse outcomes), asceticism (removing basic pleasurable aspects of experiences),

and humor are the mature defense mechanisms. The others are immature defense mechanisms.

2. D. In phobias, unacceptable internal affects are displaced onto external objects. In hysteria, there is denial, projection, and identification. Obsessional conditions display isolation, reaction formation, and magical undoing. Paranoid conditions are associated with splitting and projection, whereas depression is associated with turning against the self.

3. C. A woman who was physically abused as a child and then starts abusing her children is an example of identification. An example of splitting would be a patient who believes his or her doctor to be wonderful until the doctor is late for an appointment and then decides the doctor is awful. The woman who was sexually abused and then develops multiple personalities provides an example of dissociation. The man who is attracted to his sister-in-law and starts believing that his wife is having an affair is an example of projection. An example of reaction formation would be a man who unconsciously resents his wife and buys her expensive gifts. The man with bowel cancer who decides to worry about it for only 20 minutes a day is an example of suppression. However, denial is an important defense mechanism used by those with serious illness.

4. C. Primary process thinking is associated with the unconscious mind; it involves primitive drives or impulses without logic or a sense of time and is common in young children. Secondary process thinking is logical and is involved with reality; it is associated with the preconscious mind. Transference is the shifting of unconscious emotional attitudes from the patient's past experience of people or objects onto the therapist. These reactions are examined and interpreted in psychoanalysis. Countertransference refers to the therapist's emotional attitude toward the patient and may not be interpreted in the patient's analysis, but it should be closely examined by the therapist. Freud referred to dream work as the process whereby the hidden or latent (unconscious) content of dreams is converted into the reported manifest (actual) content of the dream. He believed that dreams represented wish fulfillment and the gratification of unconscious impulses.

CASE 7-6

1. D. Approximately 30% of people who attempt suicide will have anther attempt, and 10% will succeed. The greatest risk is in the 3 months following an attempt.

2. A. Whites are at higher risk than blacks for suicide. Otherwise, age, being male, chronic medical illness, recent loss of a spouse, and access to a weapon all increase the risk for completed suicide. Women have more attempts (4:1), but men have a higher percentage of completed suicides.

3. A. Fluoxetine is an SSRI and is rarely lethal in overdose. Acetaminophen is associated with hepatic failure; aspirin, with bleeding and metabolic acidosis; imipramine, a tricyclic antidepressant, with QT prolongation and potential heart block or arrhythmia; ibuprofen, with nausea, vomiting, GI bleeding, renal insufficiency, and so on.

4. B. At least 10% of schizophrenics die by suicide, and 25–50% attempt suicide. Risk factors include male gender, youth, substance abuse, high aspirations/lost expectations, multiple relapses, depressed mood, and living alone.

CASE 7-7

1. E. In fact, those who abuse the elderly are often the closest family member, such as a spouse (almost 60%) or child (almost 25%) of the victim. They often have a history of mental or emotional problems, abuse alcohol or illicit substances, are socially isolated, and are in financial difficulty. Characteristics of the victim include physical dependence on others and cognitive impairment, and they tend to deny the abuse for fear of the consequences. It has been reported that up to a third of demented elderly are abused.

2. D. In fact, more premature, low birth-weight infants are abused (approximately 25%) than full-term infants (8%). These children may require more attention from their parents. These children may have mild physical disabilities and may be hyperactive or described as "slow." Most children who are physically abused are younger than 5 years of age. Often these children do not report their injuries to others outside the family unit. Persons who abuse family members are likely to have a personal history of abuse or neglect as a child themselves. Figures reported are as high as 80%, but most abused children do not grow up to be abusive parents themselves. Some of these abused parents may abuse their children if under stress.

3. C. The average number of children being born to women in the United States has decreased from 3.6 in 1960 to 2.0 in the early 1990s, and these decreases are seen in both single and married women. About 25% of families are led by a single parent (55% in African American families), and 90% of these single parents are women. Approximately 60% of children in the United States younger than 18 years of age have both parents who work outside of the home. Approximately 25% of couples are childless, due equally to choice and fertility impairments. The actual percentage of children in the population has decreased from 35% in 1960 to 25% more recently. Approximately 40% of new marriages will divorce, half of these within 5 years.

4. B. Studies have reported that up to 40% of women seen in general practice have been victims of domestic violence. The risk is increased for women who are pregnant. Dangers to the unborn child include poor prenatal care (women may avoid going to the doctor to avoid detection of abuse), miscarriage, antepartum hemorrhage, prematurity, low birth weight, and even stillbirth. Studies have shown that physicians fail to identify these women. The violence tends to follow a three-phase cycle, which starts with increasing levels of tension and criticism, possibly with shoving. The second phase includes increasing anger and violence. This phase is followed by a third phase of apologies and promises to change. Usually the violence continues and may become more severe. It is important that the physician express concern and compassion but not be too controlling or directive. More than a third of female murder victims are killed by their partners. It is important not to pressure patients into filing police reports, as they are able to judge their own safety in this regard. These women should be encouraged to develop a safety plan, which may involve having a bag packed with clothing and important papers (ID, passport, etc.). Domestic violence advocates and social workers can help the patient plan for the future. Legal aid and domestic violence programs are available. It is probably better if both partners attend different group therapies.

CASE 7-8

1. A. Competence is a legal determination. Thus, a physician cannot declare her incompetent. The decision about competence is often made using information from a capacity assessment that is done by a physician. Psychiatrists are most often called upon, but any physician can perform a capacity assessment. Patients require capacity to make any medical decision, whether they are "going along with the doctor" or not. Healthcare proxies can be used to intervene only when the patient lacks capacity or cannot speak for himself or herself. In this case, the patient is severely demented, cannot manage her activities of daily living, and has significant aphasia. She lacks capacity to make treatment decisions, and her healthcare proxy can override her "refusal." Finally, unless her cousin's husband has been designated her proxy, he has no legal right to intervene in her healthcare decisions, especially when the patient's wishes have been clearly documented.

2. C. There are four D's of malpractice: Demonstrating negligence or **dereliction,** demonstrating that the physician did have a relationship and therefore a **duty** to the patient, demonstrating that **damages** occurred (that the patient was injured in some way), and that the damages were caused **directly** by the negligence. Malpractice is a tort, or civil wrong, not a criminal matter. It is unnecessary to prove malicious intent or to show that the physician was paid or that the hospital was vigilant in its hiring practices.

3. C. A Christian Scientist, who does not believe in medical or surgical intervention, may refuse medication or surgery for himself or herself. Although parents are allowed to make medical decisions for their minor children (younger than age 18), they cannot refuse lifesaving treatment (e.g., an emergency appendectomy). Adult Jehovah's Witnesses who are cognitively intact may refuse blood transfusion, even if doing so means death. Patients with early-stage Alzheimer disease often retain capacity, especially for less complex decisions. They may not be able to manipulate large quantities of complex information but may well be able to consent to a biopsy, to appoint a healthcare proxy, and even to make a living will. Having a motor deficit (hemiplegia) does not imply anything about capacity.

4. B. A 35-year-old patient with widely metastatic ovarian cancer who declines further treatment probably has capacity. The 5-year survival for stage IV ovarian cancer is less than 5%, and with no response to chemotherapy the decision to halt treatment would not be inappropriate. The other patients all have psychiatric symptoms that are interfering with their ability to make these decisions. The anorexic is denying the severity of her illness and cannot control her weight, the person with depression inappropriately feels that life is hopeless and there is no reason to remove a skin cancer, the schizophrenic has incorporated the treatment into his delusions, and the man with moderate dementia needs significant homecare but believes that he can manage his postoperative course on his own. In addition, he may be unable to fully understand other risks of that procedure.

CASE 7-9

1. B. Long-term effects of anorexia include cardiac and renal impairments, renal calculi, osteoporosis, impaired fertility, increase rates of perinatal mortality, and dental problems. More than 10%

of those with anorexia will die. Some will recover completely, but others will follow a more chronic course of relapse and remission.

2. B. The associated physical features of bulimia may be divided into two types.

> **(a) Signs and symptoms:** Vomiting leads to callused hands (also called Russell sign), dental erosions, and enlarged parotid glands. Menstrual abnormalities, even amenorrhea, may occur. More severe complications include cardiac/skeletal myopathy from the regular use of ipecac, torn esophagus, and gastric rupture from vomiting. Cardiac arrhythmias may also occur. Those with the nonpurging type have fewer medical complications. Weights may be near normal in most individuals with the disorder.
> **(b) Investigations/labs:** Purging may lead to hyponatremia, hypochloremia, and hypokalemia. Vomiters may develop a metabolic alkalosis, and those who abuse laxatives may develop a metabolic acidosis.

Lanugo hair is associated with anorexia and starvation. Alopecia is not characteristic of bulimia.

3. C. In the intergenerational-experiential school of family therapy, the dysfunctional behavioral problems are viewed as arising from a family developmental fixation. The view of the behavioral-psychoeducational school is that current environmental events shape, maintain, and control interpersonal behaviors. The structural-strategic approach is based on general systems theory as outlined in the text. Some therapists focus on correcting the structure of the family; others focus on the organization and processing of the family.

4. C. Yalom described several curative factors found in groups, including instillation of hope, universality, catharsis, insight, group cohesiveness, altruism, modeling of behavior, development of socializing techniques, and corrective formation of a family group. Group think happens when there are cohesive group members within a group with a strong leader. This can lead to decisions being made without consideration of other intragroup wishes or external opinion. Triangulation is a communication style of a leader-led group. Scapegoating is described in the discussion. None of these are curative factors in a group. Humor is a mature defense mechanism.

CASE 7-10

1. B. Laparoscopic duodenal switch is not an available option to patients with BMIs of less than 40. However, with a BMI of 29 and concurrent obesity-related medical conditions, she is eligible for pharmacologic therapy if she desires. Of course, all patients can benefit from a low-fat, high-fiber diet regimen with moderate exercise. Rigorous exercise can lead to higher rates of injury.

2. C. It is important to assess the degree to which obesity affects the family in order to properly address a child's obesity. Childhood obesity is most commonly affected by eating and exercise habits of the family. No treatment that isolates the child as the sole target of therapy will ever be effective in reducing his or her weight. Therefore, family counseling is often employed and has been shown to be an effective means of treating childhood obesity. Although a child's family may have a strong propensity for obesity, investigating inherited leptin deficiency may not be

appropriate, as this is a very rare cause of obesity, and serum leptin tests are very expensive and only available through special labs. In addition, such investigations rarely lead to changes in management. Lastly, medication and surgery have not been approved for use in children.

3. B. There are many possible causes of dyspnea in an obese person. These include upper airway obstruction, decreased lung volumes from chest wall compression and increased intra-abdominal pressure, and CHF. Given LC's history and physical, he is probably experiencing CHF, a condition associated with obesity. Although this is the most likely cause, other possible causes must be investigated, such as sleep apnea, restrictive lung disease, and CAD. These can be evaluated with the use of a sleep study, a pulmonary function test, and a stress test (probably pharmacologic testing instead of treadmill testing, given his chronic knee pain). He is probably not having an acute MI, given his EKG and negative troponin tests.

4. C. Sympathomimetic drugs are contraindicated in those individuals who have hypertension or cardiac disease, as they may worsen both conditions. However, diet and exercise are always appropriate therapies for obesity. He is also eligible for treatment with orlistat, given his BMI. Finally, with proper medical clearance, he may also be eligible for surgical treatment.

PART VIII: NEUROSCIENCE, PSYCHIATRY, PSYCHOPHARMACOLOGY, AND PSYCHOPATHOLOGY

CASE 8-1

1. B. SSRIs are reported to have fewer side effects and to be safer than either tricyclics or MAOI agents. They do not act as α-adrenergic receptors and hence do not cause orthostatic hypotension. They also do not act as sodium channel inhibitors and therefore do not cause cardiac toxicity. As a group, the SSRIs may cause nervousness, agitation, insomnia, nausea, and headaches. Sexual dysfunction is a common adverse effect of all SSRIs and may cause delayed orgasm or anorgasmia in females and delayed ejaculation in males. Strategies suggested to help with this sexual dysfunction include drug holidays, decreasing the dosage, using agents with shorter half-lives, and the addition of agents such as buspirone, bupropion, yohimbine, or cyproheptadine. Nausea can be minimized by taking the agent with food; insomnia, by taking it in the morning. Sertraline, paroxetine, and fluoxetine are highly protein bound. Therefore, care should be taken in patients who take either digitoxin or warfarin and their levels should be closely monitored. SSRIs should not be combined with MAOI agents to avoid serotoninergic syndrome. SSRIs also inhibit the cytochrome P450 isoenzyme system.

2. D. Although antidepressants are generally used to treat depression, they have a variety of other uses, including the treatment of anxiety (imipramine and SSRIs), bulimia (fluoxetine), enuresis (imipramine), obsessive-compulsive disorder (clomipramine, fluoxetine, and fluvoxamine), narcolepsy (MAOIs and imipramine), panic disorder (imipramine and SSRIs), and pain management (amitriptyline). SNRIs have not been shown to be useful in the treatment of bulimia. Antidepressants may also be used in the treatment of encopresis and attention deficit disorder in children. Trichotillomania is compulsive hair pulling and has been reported to respond to clomipramine.

3. C. Tricyclics have several common side effects related to their mechanism of action. Anticholinergic effects may cause dry mouth, blurred vision, urinary retention, and constipation. These agents should be avoided in those with acute angle glaucoma and prostatic hypertrophy. Antihistaminergic effects may cause sedation, and effects at adrenergic receptors may lead to orthostatic hypotension. Tricyclics are concentrated in conduction tissue and may be fatal in overdose. Priapism is a persistent painful erection that is a surgical emergency. It may be caused rarely by trazodone, which can also cause agranulocytosis. Recent reports have been made of acute liver failure with the newer agent Serzone.

4. E. MAOIs may interact with other CNS active agents, such as other sedatives. Opiates, anesthetics, stimulants, and TCAs can cause serotoninergic syndrome with SSRIs. MAOIs also bind irreversibly to the MAO enzyme. It may take 2 weeks for new enzymes to be formed. MAOIs also cause a reduction on platelet MAO activity, and this can be used to monitor therapeutic efficacy. Tyramine is contained in a variety of foods, such as aged cheeses, beer, wines, meat, yeast extracts, chicken liver, pickled herring, and broad bean pods. MAOIs may block the degradation of tyramine and cause a release of catecholamines, leading to a hypertensive crisis. (Symptoms may include head and neck pain, palpitations, and hyperpraxia, and may lead to convulsions, coma, and death.) Other side effects of MAOIs include anticholinergic side effects, postural hypotension, paresthesia in the limbs, ankle edema, tremor, myoclonus, nausea, and insomnia or precipitation of mania. Atypical features of depression or dysthymia include mood reactivity; significant weight gain or increase in appetite; increased sleeping; heavy, leaden feelings in the limbs; and a long-standing sensitivity to personal rejection.

CASE 8-2

1. C. The risk factors reported in bipolar disorder include age (average age of onset is 30 years), marital status (higher prevalence of bipolar disorder among separated or divorced than among singles), a positive family history of mood disorders, stressful life events, and poor social support. Gender distribution is equal in this disorder, and although there is a strong association between bipolar disorder and substance abuse, it has not been shown to be a risk factor.

2. D. Family members of patients with bipolar disorder have a higher incidence of other psychiatric disorders than do members of the general population. Particularly of note are the increases in both schizoaffective disorder and depression, which has led some researchers to believe that these conditions are in the same spectrum of disorders. None of the other conditions have been shown to be significantly associated with bipolar disorder.

3. E. There have been preliminary reports linking chromosome 18 and bipolar disorder with positive lod scores in an analysis of 22 pedigrees, but this remains controversial. Monozygotic twins have identical genetic genomes, but dizygotic twins share only 50% of their genomes. If monozygotic twins have a higher concordance rate for a disorder than do dizygotic twins, then genetic factors are implicated in the development of the disorder. If monozygotic and dizygotic twins have similar concordance rates for a disorder, then environmental factors may play an important role in the development of the disorder. Some psychiatric conditions, such as Alzheimer disease, appear to have a small number of cases explained by autosomal dominant transmission. Otherwise, most

psychiatric disorders are thought to have polygenic modes of transmission. The diseases shown to be associated with trinucleotide repeat expansions include Huntington disease, fragile X syndrome, myotonic dystrophy, spinal and bulbar muscle atrophy, and dentatorubral-pallidoluysian atrophy, but family pedigrees in both bipolar disorder and schizophrenia are being investigated for a trinucleotide repeat expansion. In these families there was evidence of anticipation, with increased severity of disease phenotype and earlier onsets of illness in subsequent generations. Early linkage studies in bipolar disorder have not been well replicated (e.g., linkage to 11p15 in an Old Amish pedigree).

4. C. Several medical conditions can cause manic symptoms, but if the mood disturbance is thought to have been directly caused by a medical illness, then it should be diagnosed as a mood disorder due to a general medical condition. The following illnesses may present with manic symptoms: Cushing syndrome, hyperthyroidism, multiple sclerosis, and brain tumors. This may also be referred to as secondary mania and may be induced by a variety of other conditions (hemodialysis, surgery, infection [e.g., HIV], neoplasms, and epilepsy) and agents (steroids, isoniazid, levodopa). Patients with this condition tend to be older and usually do not have a family history of bipolar disorder.

CASE 8-3

1. A. Given GZ's pervasive fear of humiliating herself in social situations, her likely diagnosis is social phobia. The probable course of social phobia is chronic and long-standing. People often suffer for years before seeking help.

2. B. The treatment of generalized social phobia is usually an antidepressant, usually an SSRI, and cognitive behavioral therapy. Propranolol is only useful in the limited form of social phobia (e.g., in those with performance anxiety). Long-standing use of high-dose benzodiazepines is not the treatment of choice for any disorder, although clinically one may encounter patients on those regimens. Buspirone may be effective in generalized anxiety disorder.

3. D. Lorazepam is a benzodiazepine. Benzodiazepines bind to the $GABA_A$ receptor, allosterically modifying it so that with GABA binding there is an increase in Cl^- ions. Benzodiazepines cannot open the chloride channel without the presence of GABA. Lorazepam is only glucuronidated and does not have active metabolites.

4. D. Withdrawal seizures. Benzodiazepines are associated with ataxia, drowsiness, tolerance, physical dependence, risk of withdrawal seizures, dizziness, and amnesia. Headaches, constipation, and weight fluctuations are not prominent side effects of these medications.

CASE 8-4

1. D. Exposure and response prevention constitute the basic underlying principle behind behavioral therapy, which has been shown to be beneficial in clinical trials for the treatment of OCD. As this is a psychiatric disorder and not just excessive worry about a real-life problem (he is spending more than 8 hours washing per day), rationalizing with him or educating him is unlikely to affect his behavior or symptoms.

2. A. Serotonin has been most consistently implicated in OCD. This is mainly gleaned from the differential treatment response between serotonergic medications and medications affecting other transmitter systems.

3. E. Using behavioral therapy. Strategies in treating OCD include maximizing the dose of serotonergic medications (SSRIs or clomipramine), augmenting with antipsychotic medications, and using behavioral therapy in addition to pharmacologic management. Although lithium augmentation of antidepressants may have a role in treating refractory depression, and lithium is effective in treating bipolar disorder, there is no literature that suggests it is beneficial in OCD. Stimulants (e.g., methylphenidate) may be used to augment antidepressants in the treatment of major depression. Clozapine is used primarily for treating refractory schizophrenia.

4. B. Occasionally, even with adequate pharmacotherapy and/or behavioral therapy, patients may still experience intractable incapacitating symptoms. In these cases neurosurgery has been used. Obviously, the symptoms must be very severe, and the patient must have proven resistant to multiple psychological and somatic therapies over the course of many years. The success rate is about 50–70%. In general, the surgical procedures used—anterior capsulotomy, cingulotomy, and limbic leukotomy—aim to interrupt the connection between the cortex and the basal ganglia and related structures. Frontal lobotomy is a procedure that was common in the 1940s, with approximately 18,000 lobotomies performed in the United States. It was a fairly nonspecific procedure that caused a great deal of morbidity. Occipital lobe ablation would cause cortical blindness and is not used as a psychiatric treatment. Neither desipramine (a tricyclic antidepressant causing primarily norepinephrine reuptake inhibition) nor acetylcholinesterase inhibitors are efficacious in this disorder.

CASE 8-5

1. C. The symptoms described are consistent with an anticholinergic agent. The only medication on the list that has significant anticholinergic activity is diphenhydramine. Physical symptoms from anticholinergic medications result from postganglionic parasympathetic blockade (antimuscarinic action). They include dilated, poorly reactive pupils; warm, dry skin; facial flushing; dry mouth; tachycardia; GI slowing with constipation; and urinary retention.

2. B. The symptoms of ataxia, ophthalmoplegia (lateral gaze paralysis), and confusion are the classic triad seen in Wernicke encephalopathy. The cause is low thiamine, and it is usually seen in alcoholics. The emergent treatment is IV thiamine, before anything else, especially glucose.

3. E. The symptoms and time frame are classic for alcohol withdrawal delirium, which usually begins 24–72 hours after the last drink. Although individuals may be confused or delirious after general anesthesia, alcohol withdrawal does not classically cause mania. Antibiotics can also cause delirium but are unlikely to cause the autonomic hyperarousal seen in this patient. Cocaine intoxication is associated with hypertension and tachycardia but is unlikely to cause visual hallucinations or significant confusion. Binge cocaine use may be associated with paranoia.

4. B. This gentleman was delirious on admission. Given that 1 month after the event he is no longer delirious but still has cognitive problems (short-term memory, orientation to time,

remembering the name of the street), he probably has an underlying dementia; thus, (A) is incorrect. (B) is the correct answer, describing someone with mild dementia (difficulty with memory and executive functioning) who had a superimposed delirium. (C) is incorrect, as it describes someone who is much more impaired at baseline (probably moderate to severe dementia) and does not explain the delirium or the improvement in symptoms. (D) is incorrect because he does not have the symptoms of dementia pugilistica (which include masked faces, tremor, bradykinesia), and (E) is incorrect because he has no neurologic signs of a large MCA stroke (which would be associated with contralateral hemiparesis).

CASE 8-6

1. C. Vitamin B12 deficiencies, syphilis (the causative agent being *T. pallidum*), hypothyroidism, and various things that can be identified on MRI (strokes, tumors, subdural hematomas, etc.) can all cause the clinical syndrome of dementia. Vitamin C deficiency is not associated with late-life dementia; it causes scurvy, which is characterized by weakness, anemia, mucocutaneous hemorrhage, spongy gums, and brawny induration of the leg muscles. Vitamin K controls the formation of coagulation factors II, VII, IX, and X in the liver. Although there is the possibility that a total body CT scan would reveal a cause of dementia (e.g., a primary malignancy), it is an inappropriately broad test. Ceruloplasmin is tested for Wilson disease. Wilson disease is a progressive and uniformly fatal disorder of copper metabolism that affects one person in 30,000. Unless treated with lifelong uninterrupted treatment with chelating agents, it is always fatal, generally before age 30 years. This woman is too old to have new-onset symptoms. It is an autosomal recessive disorder caused by mutation in gene chromosome 13. In about 40–50% of patients, the disease first affects the CNS and can cause tremors, dystonia, dysarthria, dysphagia, chorea, drooling, and lack of coordination; grossly inappropriate behavior; sudden deterioration of schoolwork; or, rarely, psychosis indistinguishable from schizophrenia or manic-depressive illness.

2. C. The ApoE ε4 allele has been found in 50% of patients with AD. The rare ε2 allele is probably protective against AD. Although mutations on chromosomes 1, 14, and 21 have been associated with AD, they are rare and are more frequently seen in patients with early-onset disease with strong family histories. Trinucleotide CAG repeats on chromosome 4 are seen in Huntington chorea.

3. E. The findings are associated with AD and include tangles (intracellular paired helical filaments of hyperphosphorylated tau protein), plaque (extracellular aggregations of β-amyloid that form the core and are surrounded by many things, including microglia, reactive astrocytes, and dystrophic neuritis), atrophy, ventricular enlargement, and decreased choline acetyltransferase. Alpha-synuclein is the main component of Lewy bodies. When found diffusely in the cortex, they are associated with Lewy body dementia. When they are found in the substantia nigra, they are associated with Parkinson disease. Astrogliosis, neuronal loss, and spongiform change are seen in spongiform encephalitis, such as Kuru or Creutzfeldt-Jakob. Ischemic periventricular leukoencephalopathy is seen in Binswanger disease.

4. A. In general, the frontal lobes are markedly involved in personality, emotions, and executive functioning. They are also inhibitory in terms of controlling behavior. The classic example of a person with a frontal lobe syndrome is Phineas Gage, a foreman of a railway construction gang who, in an accidental explosion, had a tamping iron blown through his head. Before the accident he was capable and efficient. Afterward, he was impatient, profane, and unable to make a plan and execute it. Temporal lesions may cause the inability to encode new memories (e.g., with bilateral hippocampal lesions), whereas occipital lesions are known to cause visual defects and, in severe cases, cortical blindness. Parietal lobe lesions may be associated with anosognosia not recognizing a part of one's body as one's own. Brainstem lesions may be associated with ipsilateral cranial nerve involvement with contralateral weakness or sensory deficit.

CASE 8-7

1. C. DP is perfectionistic, obsessed with order and detail; he also sounds emotionally rigid and inflexible. He sees this as completely ego syntonic (part of himself). This cluster of symptoms is most consistent with OCD. In OCD there needs to be intrusive obsessions, compulsions that often feel excessive or ego dystonic, and the compulsions usually exist to try to counteract the obsessive thoughts. There is no evidence that this man has any of those symptoms. Although people with avoidant personality disorder or schizoid personality disorder may avoid social interactions or want to work at home, they do so for different reasons. Avoidant persons feel inadequate and are hypersensitive to criticism. Schizoid persons are just disinterested in social relationships and are affectively flat and socially withdrawn. Antisocial personality refers not to people who avoid social contact but to those who have a disregard for the rights of others; are exploitative and aggressive, impulsive, and remorseless; and often are involved in illegal behavior.

2. B. GR meets criteria for schizotypal personality disorder, with her ideas of reference, odd beliefs, magical thinking, paranoia, and lack of close social relationships. Correlates of CNS dysfunction seen in schizophrenia have been observed in schizotypal PD, including performance on tests of visual and auditory attention and smooth pursuit eye movement. People with this disorder see their eccentricities as being ego syntonic (i.e., compatible with their sense of self), not ego dystonic. The prevalence of schizotypal PD is increased in the families of schizophrenics, and there is an increased risk of schizophrenia in families of people with schizotypal PD. Although there is an increased risk of schizophrenia, in schizotypal PD only approximately 10–15% will go on to develop schizophrenia. This disorder may be seen slightly more often in men than women, although the M:F ratio may be 1:1.

3. E. ZC displays a pervasive pattern of grandiosity, need for admiration, and lack of empathy, which is consistent with narcissistic PD. People with narcissistic PD are often quite vulnerable to threats to their self-esteem, and they may react defensively with rage, disdain, or indifference but are actually struggling with feelings of shock and humiliation. His feelings of insecurity may be masked by arrogance. He probably has difficulty in sustaining long-term intimate relationships and in accepting feedback. Narcissistic PD is seen in males more often than in females. Histrionic PD is characterized by needing to be the center of attention, being inappropriately seductive, having rapidly shifting shallow emotions, using appearance to draw attention, having an impressionistic style of speech, displaying excessive theatricality, being suggestible, and considering relationships to be more intimate than they are. It is diagnosed most often in women.

4. B. This patient has antisocial PD. He has a long-standing pervasive disregard for and violation of rights of others; he lies, engages in illegal behavior, and is impulsive, aggressive, and remorseless. Antisocial PD is seen in 3% of men, 1% of women, and 20–50% of forensic/prison populations. It is associated with childhood abuse and neglect but is not associated with particular abnormalities on an EEG.

CASE 8-8

1. C. Thioridazine is a low-potency medication associated with sedation and orthostatic hypotension. Haloperidol is a high-potency medication. Typical antipsychotics have their effect through blockade (antagonism) of the D2 receptor. Akathisia refers to an internal sense of restlessness. Parkinsonian symptoms are referred to as *extrapyramidal symptoms*.

2. B. Clozapine is associated with a number of significant side effects, including lowered seizure threshold and agranulocytosis. Perphenazine is a typical mid-potency antipsychotic. Atypical agents usually do have some effect on dopamine receptors, although they may be more potent antagonists at dopamine receptor subtypes (such as D4) rather than the D2 receptors targeted by the typical antipsychotics, or at the 5-HT$_{2A}$ receptor. Antipsychotics do not have their primary action at cholinergic (either nicotinic or muscarinic) receptors.

3. A. In general, all antipsychotic medications, except probably clozapine, can cause the serious side effect of TD. The typical antipsychotics (e.g., chlorpromazine, haloperidol) have been the most studied. The atypical agents may have a lower frequency of TD. TD is an often permanent movement disorder caused by the long-term use of antipsychotic drugs. It is characterized by repetitive, involuntary, purposeless movements, including grimacing, tongue protrusion, lip smacking, rapid eye blinking, and movements of the arms, legs, and trunk. Decreasing the dose of a medication may make the movements more pronounced. Treatment is mainly to switch to an atypical agent and attempt to decrease the medication dose. Akathisia is defined as a subjective sense of restlessness, an inability to sit still. The term *extrapyramidal symptoms* refers to a number of medication side effects that are thought to be associated with antipsychotic blockade of the D2 receptors in the basal ganglia. In general, they include parkinsonian symptoms, acute dystonias, and akathisia. Clozapine causes fewer of these symptoms.

4. C. NMS is a rare, severe complication of antipsychotic treatment consisting of muscular rigidity, dystonia, obtundation, hyperpyrexia, diaphoresis, tachycardia, hypertension, and increased WBC count, CPK, and LFTs. The mortality is approximately 20%. It can be seen at any time in antipsychotic treatment and is usually treated supportively in an intensive care setting. It has a frequency of 0.02–2.4%. Treatment includes rapid external cooling, IV benzodiazepines to decrease muscle rigidity, and discontinuation of the antipsychotic. If antipsychotic medication is necessary, one of a different class can be introduced after 1 or 2 weeks. Malignant hyperthermia is typically a fulminant life-threatening syndrome that occurs when a person with a susceptibility trait is exposed to triggering factors, which include most inhalational anesthetics and succinylcholine. Classic malignant hyperthermia is characterized by hypermetabolism, muscle rigidity, muscle injury, increased sympathetic nervous system activity, and extreme hyperthermia. Death can result from cardiac arrest, brain damage, internal hemorrhaging, or failure of other body systems. It is unlikely that this man has an infectious meningitis.

CASE 8-9

1. A. This presentation is consistent with withdrawal tremors and seizures, which occur within 48 hours after the last drink. Delirium tremens is unlikely, as this condition usually occurs after 48 hours and usually is accompanied by severe autonomic instability and vital sign fluctuations. TN did not report visual hallucinations and therefore is not experiencing hallucinosis. Wernicke encephalopathy is an alcohol-induced organic brain symptom characterized by the classic triad of ataxia, ophthalmoplegia, and altered mental status. Korsakoff syndrome is a persistent amnesia with confabulation (*mnemonic: K is for konfabulation*). Both Wernicke and Korsakoff syndromes are caused by thiamine deficiency. These syndromes are usually present in the stable alcoholic patient. Given TN's apparently normal mental status, these conditions are unlikely etiologies for his presentation.

2. D. Given the recent appearance of black stool and her normal MCV, it is likely that her anemia is caused by an acute event such as a Mallory-Weiss tear in her mucosa at the gastroesophageal junction caused by severe retching from excessive alcohol intake. Such a mucosal tear would produce moderate upper GI hemorrhage that appears as melena (black stool). Chronic etiologies include iron, folate, and vitamin B12 deficiencies as well as anemia of chronic disease. Since her MCV is normal, it is unlikely that she has an iron deficiency anemia or anemia of chronic disease, which produce microcytic anemias. Folate or vitamin B12 deficiency would produce a macrocytic anemia. Lastly, although retching can rupture gastric varices, this would present with more profuse bleeding with frank hematochezia (bright red blood from the rectum), as well as a more fulminant clinical course.

3. B. Ingestion of large amounts of alcohol during college hazing rituals has been associated with CNS depression severe enough to completely depress respiratory drive and result in death. Such severe intoxication must be treated with respiratory support until the patient can metabolize the alcohol. Heroin intoxication is less likely in this case, given the lack of stigmata like pinpoint pupils and track marks, although he can be given naloxone empirically. Benzodiazepine overdose is also possible but less likely. His vital signs and physical exam are inconsistent with a cocaine overdose. Lastly, his glucose level does not suggest an insulin overdose.

4. E. Vitamin K deficiency is associated with coagulopathy due to inability to produce sufficient coagulation factors. Such coagulopathy can predispose an individual to hemorrhagic strokes. Thiamine deficiency can produce altered mental status along with paresthesias. Long-term organic brain syndromes such as Korsakoff syndrome can cause amnestic symptoms with confabulation. Chronic liver disease can predispose someone to hypoglycemic events, which can manifest as syncope. Lastly, chronic liver insufficiency can produce high levels of serum ammonia, which can produce a hepatic encephalopathy and decreased sensorium.

CASE 8-10

1. E. This clinical scenario emphasizes the difficulty in diagnosing the varied clinical manifestations an opiate-dependent person can present with. Given his fever, murmur, and track marks, bacterial endocarditis is possible, with valve vegetations producing a tricuspid stenosis murmur. This is an important consideration in an injection drug user. Acute gastroenteritis is also possible with his 1 day of diarrhea and tender abdomen at the periumbilical region. Viral upper respiratory infections can also produce rhinorrhea, cough due to postnasal drip, *and* concurrent diarrhea. Heroin withdrawal is also possible, given all the symptoms mentioned earlier. This emphasizes the tricky nature of detecting a withdrawal episode in an opiate-dependent person without proper history taking and cooperative disclosure from the patient.

2. D. Although it may seem tempting to give morphine to someone screaming in agony, the appropriate step in this situation is to carefully assess the patient, review her records, and contact her primary care physician to aid in the appropriate management of her pain. Careful attention to any new findings in the history and physical exam can help rule out any serious pathologies, such as spinal tumors or spinal cord impingement. Reviewing records is important to avoid excessive laboratory tests, imaging, and administration of narcotic pain medication. In the ER, the most appropriate medications for pain are nonopioid analgesics, which decrease pain from true inflammatory causes (remember the arachidonic acid pathway and the inhibition of cyclo-oxygenase by ibuprofen and acetaminophen). Ultimately, a single primary care physician should be responsible for prescribing such medication, as it will avoid overprescription and increasing opiate tolerance and dependence. Increased dependence only worsens the pain syndrome when opiate treatment becomes insufficient. Thus, it is inappropriate to administer IV morphine immediately without careful assessment, as it may do a disservice to the patient in the long run.

3. A. Necrotizing fasciitis is a rapidly spreading and rapidly fatal staphylococcal skin infection that can be a complication of injection drug use. Unfortunately, it has a very nonspecific clinical picture. The skin infection may be of any size or morphology, and the only clues that might lead one to suspect necrotizing fasciitis are tenderness out of proportion to exam, fever, other abnormal vital signs, and a general appearance of distress. This man otherwise has a cellulitis and a possible abscess, which are important but less concerning than the diagnosis of necrotizing fasciitis. These infections are usually not life-threatening and can be treated with incision and drainage (for abscesses) and antibiotics. Given his recent heroin injection, he is unlikely to be having withdrawal symptoms. Lastly, given the absence of a murmur, he is unlikely to have bacterial endocarditis, although it is important to keep on your differential in any injection drug user with a fever.

4. E. It is important to remember that a person who appears to be a typical heroin user can have other causes of decreased level of consciousness. Benzodiazepines are also available on the streets and can produce a very similar clinical picture. Unlike heroin, this will respond to flumazenil, not naloxone. Given his lack of response to glucose, hypoglycemia is unlikely to be the cause of his decreased sensorium. Other metabolic abnormalities, such as hyponatremia, can cause altered level of consciousness but mostly present as seizure. Alcohol intoxication is another possible cause of his clinical picture, but given the lack of stigmata and negative breathalyzer exam, it is highly unlikely.

CASE 8-11

1. A. PCP intoxication. This case of acute drug intoxication is a stereotypical presentation of intoxication with a stimulant. It is difficult to pinpoint the drug used from the physical presentation alone, and it is thus important to try to elicit this information so that one can anticipate the duration of action and the therapeutic needs of the patient. However, most cases of acute stimulant intoxication are managed in the same way, with stabilization of vital signs, monitoring, and other supportive measures. The stigmata of vertical nystagmus and moist oral mucosa or hypersalivation lead one to suspect intoxication with PCP. Proper measures to secure the safety of the patient as well as the staff are necessary to counter the hypervigilance and threat of violence that may be induced by this drug.

2. E. All the preceding cases can result in the above presentation. The first three cases of withdrawal emphasize the fact that all three drugs act on the GABA$_A$ receptor, and therapy with lorazepam, a GABA$_A$ receptor agonist, will suppress withdrawal symptoms. Methamphetamine overdose may also present in such a manner, emphasizing the dichotomous nature of physical dependence. Withdrawal generally produces symptoms that are opposite to the effects produced by the drug. Thus, sedative withdrawal can also look like stimulant intoxication. Lastly, just because a person has no stigmata of alcoholism does not mean he is not experiencing alcohol withdrawal.

3. D. Given her unique presentation of severe coma with an intact respiratory drive, she is likely presenting with an acute GHB overdose. This is a relatively new drug and has been used by sexual offenders as a sedative and amnestic for would-be victims. It is in liquid form and can be slipped into a drink. Moderate doses produce agitation, hallucinations, miosis, drowsiness, vomiting, and dizziness. Higher doses can produce seizures and coma. Such symptoms usually resolve within 8 hours of ingestion. Benzodiazepine, barbiturate, and alcoholic overdose can produce severe coma but always with accompanying respiratory depression. Lastly, ketamine is a stimulant and would rarely present in this manner.

4. B. The classic drug of abuse that is associated with chest pain is cocaine, which produces an unstable angina (Prinzmetal angina) thought to be due to acute coronary vasospasm. Any sympathomimetic drug can produce chest pain, which can be exacerbated by the tachycardia and hypertension associated with such intoxication. Although asthma can produce chest pressure, her clinical picture is inconsistent with asthma. Given her age, she is unlikely to have hypertension and associated CAD (although it still should be asked). The hypertension and tachycardia she has now are most likely due to some sort of sympathetic stimulation, most likely due to intoxication with a sympathomimetic. Although family history of early MI is a cardiac risk factor and should be inquired about, she is unlikely to have atherosclerosis associated with familial types of MI, given her age. Lastly, while exogenous estrogen use is theoretically associated with hypercoagulability, intravascular thrombosis, and increased cardiac risk, current low-dose oral contraceptives with combination estrogen and progesterone are not associated with increased cardiac risk. Therefore, this is less concerning than a possible history of drug use.

CASE 8-12

1. D. It is rare to have a disorder of written expression without another learning disorder, and the specific prevalence of this disorder is unknown. Approximately 60–80% of those diagnosed with reading disorder are males, and about 4% of schoolchildren

have this disorder. It has been estimated that approximately 1% of schoolchildren have mathematics disorder. Learning disorders are often found in association with medical disorders, such as FAS or lead poisoning.

2. E. Down syndrome may also be called mongolism and has several characteristic features, which include epicanthic folds; cataracts; strabismus; small, round head with high cheekbones; small nose and ears; high arched palate; protruding tongue; short neck and limbs; single palmar creases; ulnar loops; and hypotonic muscles. Umbilical hernias are common, as is deafness. Associated medical complications include congenital heart defects in 40% (ASDs, VSDs, TOF, and PDA); congenital cataracts; nystagmus; GI abnormalities such as duodenal atresia, pyloric stenosis, and imperforate anus; Hirschsprung disease; hypothyroidism; leukemia; epilepsy; and the neuropathologic changes of Alzheimer disease in their 30s, with onset of dementia in their 40s. In 95% of cases it is caused by trisomy 21(22) but can be caused by a translocation in 5% of cases. Prognathism (the jaw and facial skeleton jutting forward), a large, long head, floppy ears, hypertelorism (increased distance between two orbits), blue eyes, single palmar creases, hyperextendable joints, and macro-orchidism (postpuberty) are associated with fragile X syndrome in males. It is the most common inherited cause of mental retardation and is a triple repeat expansion. It occurs in 1 in 1200 males and in 1 in 2400 females. The fragile site is at Q27-28 on the X chromosome.

3. B. The life expectancy of individuals with mental retardation is directly related to their level of intellectual functioning and the etiology of their impairments. Those with mild mental retardation have increased mortality rates twice that of the general population. However, this rate increases drastically with the increases in mental impairment. Prevalence rates of psychiatric disorders among those with mental retardation range from 30 to 70%. Disorders seen may include the full spectrum of psychiatric disorders, particularly mood disorders, autism, and schizophrenia. Impulsive aggressive behaviors may be common. Those more severely impaired individuals may not present with symptoms like hallucinations and delusions. Self-injurious behavior may occur. Most individuals with mild mental retardation function quite well in the community, either with their families or in a group care setting.

4. C. Rett syndrome has only been reported in females and is thought to be fatal in males. The onset is after a period of normal postnatal development around the age of 5 months. Head growth slows down, causing microcephaly. Previously acquired purposeful movements are lost, and these girls develop characteristic stereotypic hand-wringing or hand-washing movements. They lose social engagement early in the illness but may make some progress as an adolescent. Coordination of the limbs and gait, impaired receptive and expressive language, and severe psychomotor retardation develop. These girls tend to suffer from moderate to severe mental retardation.

PART IX: EPIDEMIOLOGY, BIOSTATISTICS, AND HEALTH POLICY

CASE 9-1

1. D. Given the set of numbers {1,2,4,6,7,8,9}, the sum of these numbers is 37 and there are seven values, so the mean is $37/7 = 5$ $2/7$, or 5.28. The median, which is the center of an odd number of values, is the number 6, with 1, 2, and 4 below and 7, 8, and 9 above.

2. D. Given the set of numbers {1,1,1,1,2,3,5,5,6,6,7,7,9,9}, there are 14 numbers, and their sum is 63. Thus the mean is 4.5; clearly, the median is 5; and the mode is 1. Thus, the answer is (D), which is a mode of 1 and a mean of 4.5.

3. E. What a 95% CI tells you is that if you repeated the same experiment that you did to get your summary statistic (e.g., the mean or proportion), an infinite number of times, 95% of the time you would get a value that falls within the 95% CI. It does not tell you that the true value you are seeking is going to fall within your CI, particularly because your experiment may be faulty or biased; thus, the true value may be missed by the CI. Even with a perfectly performed experiment, the CI is not used to tell you about the true value; it gives just the results of that particular experiment.

4. B. The question asks, "In what type of distribution is the mean greater than the median?" The mean will equal the median in normal and uniform distributions. In a symmetric bimodal distribution this will also be true. In a skewed-to-the-left distribution, the median will be greater than the mean, whereas in a skewed-to-the-right distribution, the mean will be greater than the median.

CASE 9-2

1. B. A type II error is made when you do not reject the null hypothesis when it should be rejected. This is a false-negative study result. The ability to avoid a type II error is statistical power, in this case 0.96. Thus, the probability that a type II error was made is $1 - 0.96 = 0.04$.

2. D. In this study design, you are attempting to determine whether there is a difference in any of these groups of patients with respect to the risk for type 2 diabetes. The test that is needed must be able to compare proportions between multiple groups. The only one that can do that is the chi-square test. The student t test is to compare two means; the z test is to compare the proportions of two groups. A power analysis is performed to measure the power of a particular study to reject the null hypothesis. A Bonferroni correction is performed when making more than one comparison, using, for example, a student t test. Using a cutoff of the test that allows a 5% chance of type I error goes awry when you make many comparisons of outcomes in

the same study. For example, if you compared 100 different means, on average you would expect five of them to meet the $p = .05$ requirement. Thus, a Bonferroni or, more commonly, the student-Newman-Keuls test can be used to adjust the cutoff when making multiple comparisons.

3. A. From the Thumbnail in this case, you can see that a type I error is that of a false-positive test as described by answer choice (A). Answer choice (D) describes a false-negative result, which is that of a type II error. Answer choices (B) and (C) are true-positive and true-negative results, respectively.

4. E. Type I error is that of having a false-positive result. So type I error equals the number of false-positive results over the total number of patients with true results that are negative or not diseased. Type II error is the false-negative mistake. Thus, type II error equals the number of false negatives over the total number of patients with disease, or with true results that are positive (Table A-2).

CASE 9-3

1. E. For the disease described there is actually only the benefit of knowledge of disease to be gained from diagnosis. Thus, the goal for a screening program would be to have as few false-positive test results as possible. This would happen with the greatest specificity. Although it is often difficult to measure the tradeoff between sensitivity and specificity, in this particular case it is likely that increasing the specificity to 99% is worth quite a drop in sensitivity.

2. A. We only know three of the four boxes in the 2 × 2 table. We know that there are six false positives. Thus, the remaining four positive tests must be true positives. Since there are exactly 10 people with disease, there must be six false negatives. Using this information we can calculate the sensitivity, but not the specificity. Sensitivity is $a/(a + c) = 4/10 = 0.4$, or 40%.

3. E. In the diabetes screening test we only know three of the four boxes in the 2 × 2 table as well. Ninety of the 100 positive screens have diabetes, so they must be true positives. The remaining 10 must be false positives. Since there are 100 people with diabetes, there must be 10 false negatives as well. So we can calculate PPV but not NPV. The PPV is equal to $90/100 = 0.9$.

TABLE A-2

Study Results	True Results	
	Positive	Negative
Positive	True positive—85	False positive—50 Type I error = 50/1000 = 0.05
Negative	False negative—15 Type II error = 15/100 = 0.15	True negative—950

4. C. Remember that

$$LR(+) = \frac{\text{Prob(pos test given disease)}}{\text{Prob(pos test given no disease)}} = \frac{a/(a+c)}{b/(b+d)}$$

$$= \frac{\text{sensitivity}}{1 - \text{specificity}}$$

So to determine the positive likelihood ratio [LR(+)], one must calculate the sensitivity and specificity first. In this screening test, 90 of the 100 diabetics were identified, giving a 0.9 (or 90%) sensitivity. The specificity is all of the true negatives over the nondiabetics; that would be 890 divided by 900 = 0.9889 (or 98.89%). Thus, the likelihood ratio is 0.9/0.0111 = 81.081.

CASE 9-4

1. C. Despite wanting to form a supportive relationship with this patient, allay her fears, and answer her questions, as a physician it is important to be able to prioritize seriously ill patients above less ill patients. In this scenario, the patient with possible appendicitis is top priority, despite patient number 1 having been in the ED the longest. Thus, when radiology pages you regarding this patient, you should answer this page as soon as possible to determine whether this patient needs surgery. However, there are better ways to excuse yourself from your third patient. If you tell her, "I will be right back" and then do not come back for a long time, she is likely to become annoyed. However, if you acknowledge her concerns by consulting plastic surgery and explain quickly that you have another sick patient who requires your care, she is likely to understand and to feel that her waiting is justified. Telling her, "no one will notice this scar" does not acknowledge her concerns about scarring and is inappropriately paternalistic.

2. B. In this setting of an emergent procedure needing to be performed, rapid, efficient action is the most important thing. While in most cases it is best to document events as they occur, a physician

in this case should act first and worry about documentation second. Further, there is never an indication to change prior documentation or adjust timing on notes to make it seem as if they were being written prior to when they actually were written. It is useful to communicate the plan of action to the nurse, who is likely to document at some point what that plan was. However, you cannot rely on other practitioners to do your documentation, as everyone may have a different viewpoint on how events occurred. The best way to document an event of this sort is to deal with the emergency, perform the cesarean section, and move the patient to recovery. Once there, discuss the timing of events with nursing and anesthesia and write a note that reflects your best understanding of what occurred.

3. D. It is unclear why this patient has changed physicians. He may have already undergone an extensive work-up for his chronic back pain that you do not need to repeat. If this was a first visit for this symptom, ibuprofen and an x-ray would be a reasonable way to begin management. However, for this patient, who has likely already used ibuprofen and had x-rays, it is unlikely to contribute to his care. It is also folly to assume that a patient has had the appropriate work-up thus far, as he may have switched providers a number of times and not had good continuity of care. Thus, the most important thing to do is to acknowledge his prior care and attempt to assemble a plan of care with his prior practitioner that is acknowledged as workable by you and the patient.

4. D. Answer (A) is the only one that has malpractice. However, because this action did not result in any harm, it is unlikely to lead to a lawsuit. Answers (B), (C), and (E) all involve the physician communicating in an ongoing way with the patient and her family. Although answer (D) results in excellent care, because the physician does not follow up with the patient during her acute event she may feel abandoned. Furthermore, by waiting to follow up with the patient after discharge, if she ends up in a nursing home, goes to a rehabilitation facility, or dies, the physician will not have the opportunity to see the patient at all.

INDEX

Note: Page numbers referencing figures are italicized and followed by an "f". Page numbers referencing tables are italicized and followed by a "t".

A

A. fumigatus (*Aspergillus fumigatus*), 61–63
α-1,4-glycosidic linkage, 184
α-1,6 bond, 184
abdominal disease, 15
Abiotrophia, 9
ABPA (allergic bronchopulmonary aspergillosis), 62
abscesses, staphylococcal, 2
absorption, 98, 101
abuse, 271–272
acamprosate, 311
ACAT (acyl-CoA:cholesterol acyltransferase), 198
accelerated rejection, *80t*
accutane, 243–244
ACE-Is (angiotensin-converting enzyme inhibitors), 112–113
acetylcholinesterase inhibitors (AChEIs), 300
acetyl-CoA carboxylase, 189
acetyl-CoA molecule, 182
α-chain genes, 76
AChEIs (acetylcholinesterase inhibitors), 300
acid-fast stain, 30
acquisition phase, 262
acting out, 266
Actinomyces, 15
actinomycetoma, 14
active TB infection, 31
activity, beta-blockers, *106t*
acute flaccid paralysis, 50
acute giardiasis, 22
acute HIV, 47–49
acute rejection, *80t*
acute rheumatic fever, 6
acyclovir (ACV), *44f*, 167–168
acyl-CoA:cholesterol acyltransferase (ACAT), 198
AD (Alzheimer Disease), 300
AD (autosomal dominant) inheritance, 216–217
ADC (AIDS dementia complex), 300
A-delta fibers, 119
adenoviruses, 22, 59
ADPKD (autosomal dominant polycystic kidney disease), 227
adulterants, 314
affinity, 83
α-glycerol phosphate shuttle, 187
agnosia, 299
α-hemolytic streptococci, *6f*, 8–10
AIDS dementia complex (ADC), 300
alanine, 182
alcohol dependence, 318
alcoholism, 310–313
alkylating agents, 173–174
allergic bronchopulmonary aspergillosis (ABPA), 62
Alphaviridae, *51t*
altered mental status, 317–320
alternative pathway, complement system, 87
altruism, 266
Alzheimer Disease (AD), 300
American College of Obstetricians and Gynecologists, 334
amifostine, 173
amiloride, 110
amino acid nitrogen, 205

aminoglycosides, 12, 161–162
aminopenicillins, 149–150
aminotransferases, 205
ammonia levels, 205
amniocentesis, 331
amoxicillin, 6
amphetamines, 317, 319
amphotericin B (ampho B), 62, 64–66, 69, 169–170
ampicillin, 19
amyloid plaques, 300
anaphylaxis, 149
anergic, 84
aneuploidy, 230
Angelman syndrome, 234–235
angina pectoris, 103
angiotensin receptor blockers (ARBs), 114–115
angiotensin-converting enzyme inhibitors (ACE-Is), 112–113
animal contacts, fevers spread by, *72t*
animal phobias, 290
anorexia nervosa, 276–277
anthracyclines, 171–172
antianaerobic agents, 165–166
antibiotic treatment
    C. difficile colitis, 17
    clostridial infections, 18
    complications of, 17
    gram-positive rods, 15
    N. meningitides, 19–20
    pneumonia, 37
    Pseudomonas aeruginosa, 26
    S. viridans, 9
    staphylococcus aureus, 3–4
    streptococcal pharyngitis, 6
antibiotic-associated colitis, 165
antibodies, 83–84
antibody-mediated immunity, 84–85
anticipation, 216–217
anticoagulant agents, 116–118
anticonvulsants, 122–124
antidepressants
    adverse effects of, 128
    anxiety disorders and, 291
    main classes of, *285t*
    psychopharmacology, 259
antifungals, 62, 66, 169–170
antigen presentation, 84
antigen-dependent somatic mutation, 83
antigen-independent rearrangement, 83
antigen-presenting cells, 76
anti-HIV antibody, 47
antimetabolites, 175–176
antimicrobial peptides, 87
antipsychotics, 129, 259, 307–308
antistaphylococcal penicillins, 149–150
antiviral treatment
    cytomegalovirus, 45–46
    hepatitis B, 55
    herpes simplex virus, 43, *44f*
    herpes viruses, 167–168
    influenza, 58

Index

anxiety disorders
    agents used for, 125–126
    behavioral techniques, 263
    overview, 290–292
anxious personality disorder, 303–304
aortic arches, 249–250
aphasia, 299
apo C-II (apolipoprotein C-II), 198
ApoE ε4 gene, 302
ApoE gene, 302
apolipoprotein C-II (apo C-II), 198
apraxia, 299
AR (autosomal recessive) diseases, 185, 219–220
arboviruses, 50, 51t
ARBs (angiotensin receptor blockers), 114–115
Arcanobacterium haemolyticum, 5
arginase, 205
argininosuccinate lyase, 205
argininosuccinate synthetase, 205
arthropod-borne viruses, 50
ascites, 175
ascorbic acid (vitamin C), 211
ASDs (atrial septal defects), 230
aseptic meningitis, 43
aspergillomas, 62
Aspergillus fumigatus (*A. fumigatus*), 61–63
Aspergillus pneumonia, 62
asterixis, 205
asthma, agents for, 140–142
asymmetric distributions, 326f
Ataxia telangiectasia, 94t
atenolol, 106
atherosclerosis, 199
atherosclerotic plaques, 103
ATP synthase, 187
atrial septal defects (ASDs), 230
atrioventricular (AV) node, 108
atypical antipsychotics, 308
atypical pneumonia, 37
autoimmune diseases, 48t, 83–86
autosomal dominant (AD) inheritance, 216–217
autosomal dominant polycystic kidney disease (ADPKD), 227
autosomal recessive (AR) diseases, 185, 219–220
AV (atrioventricular) node, 108
aversive conditioning, 262
avidin, 211
avidity, 83
azalide azithromycin, 154
azithromycin, 154
azoles, 66, 69, 169–170

B

B lymphocytes, 83–84
β₂-agonists, asthma, 140–141
Babinski reflex, 254t
Bacille Calmette-Guérin (BCG) vaccine, 31
Bacillus cereus, 22
bacitracin, 5–6
bacterial etiologies
    of diarrhea, 22
    of pharyngitis, 5
bacterial meningitis, 19, 151
bacterial organisms
    diagnostic tests, 48t
    sensitivity and specificity, 331t
Bacteroides species, 165
barbiturates, 292, 317, 318
basal metabolic rate (BMR), 279
β-carotene, 211

B-cell defects, 93t
B-cell isotype switching, 77
B-cell receptor (BCR) complex, 84
BCG (Bacille Calmette-Guérin) vaccine, 31
β-chain genes, 76
BCR (B-cell receptor) complex, 84
behavioral therapy, 265, 294
behavioral tolerance, 310
behavioral-psychoeducational therapy, 277
bejel, 41t
bell-and-pad technique, 262
benazepril, 112t
benzathine penicillin, 40
benzodiazepines (BZDs), 126t, 260, 292, 311, 317
benztropine, 307
bepridil, 108, 109t
beriberi, 209
Bernoulli distribution, 327
beta-blockers
    hyperthyroidism, 131
    overview, 105–107
    social phobias, 291
β-hemolytic streptococci, 5–7
bilaminar germ disc, 243
bile acids
    overview, 198–200
    sequestrants, 139
bimodal distribution, 326f, 327
Binswanger disease, 299–300
bioavailability, 98, 101
bioenergetics, 182, 205–206
biotin, 211
bipolar disorders, 287–289
β-lactam antibiotics, 37
β-lactamase inhibitors, 3
Blastomyces dermatitidis, 69
blood–injection–injury phobias, 290
bloody diarrhea, 24
B-lymphocyte immunodeficiencies, 94
BMR (basal metabolic rate), 279
boils, 34
bone lesions, 227
borderline personality disorder (BPD), 303
Borrelia, 41t
β-oxidation, fatty acid, 189–190
BPD (borderline personality disorder), 303
branchial arch anomalies, 249–250
breast cancer, 143
bronchopulmonary infections, 35
bulimia, 276–277
Bunyaviridae, 51t
bupropion, 127
buspirone, 126t, 292
BZDs (benzodiazepines), 126t, 260, 292, 311, 317

C

C. albicans (*Candida albicans*), 66–67
C fibers, 119
C. neoformans (*Cryptococcus neoformans*), 64–65
C1r/C1s components, 88f
C3a component, 89f
C3b component, 88f
C3bBb component, 88f
C4a component, 88f
C4b/C2b components, 88f
C5 component, 89f
C5a component, 89f
C5b component, 89f
C6 component, 89f

Index